Injury & Trauma Sou_____

Learning Disabilities Sourcebook, 3rd Edition

Leukemia Sourcebook

Liver Disorders Sourcebook

Medical Tests Sourcebook, 4th Edition

Men's Health Concerns Sourcebook, 3rd Edition

Mental Health Disorders Sourcebook, 4th Edition

Mental Retardation Sourcebook

Movement Disorders Sourcebook, 2nd Edition

Multiple Sclerosis Sourcebook

Muscular Dystrophy Sourcebook

Obesity Sourcebook

Osteoporosis Sourcebook

Pain Sourcebook, 3rd Edition

Pediatric Cancer Sourcebook

Physical & Mental Issues in Aging Sourcebook

Podiatry Sourcebook, 2nd Edition

Pregnancy & Birth Sourcebook, 3rd Edition

Prostate & Urological Disorders Sourcebook

Prostate Cancer Sourcebook

Rehabilitation Sourcebook

Respiratory Disorders Sourcebook, 2nd Edition

Sexually Transmitted Diseases Sourcebook, 4th Edition

Sleep Disorders Sourcebook, 3rd Edition

Smoking Concerns Sourcebook

Sports Injuries Sourcebook, 4th Edition

Stress-Related Disorders Sourcebook, 2nd Edition

Stroke Sourcebook, 2nd Edition

Surgery Sourcebook, 2nd Edition

Thyroid Disorders Sourcebook

Transplantation Sourcebook

Traveler's Health Sourcebook

Urinary Tract & Kidney Diseases & Disorders Sourcebook, 2nd Edition

Vegetarian Sourcebook

Women's Health Concerns Sourcebook, 3rd Edition

Workplace Health & Safety Sourcebook

Worldwide Health Sourcebook

Teen Health Series

Abuse & Violence Information for Teens

Accident & Safety Information for Teens

Alcohol Information for Teens, 2nd Edition

Allergy Information for Teens

Asthma Information for Teens, 2nd Edition

Body Information for Teens

Cancer Information for Teens, 2nd Edition

Complementary & Alternative Medicine Information for Teens

Diabetes Information for Teens, 2nd Edition

Diet Information for Teens, 3rd Edition

Drug Information for Teens, 3rd Edition

Eating Disorders Information for Teens, 2nd Edition

Fitness Information for Teens, 2nd Edition

Learning Disabilities Information for Teens

Mental Health Information for Teens, 3rd Edition

Pregnancy Information for Teens, 2nd Edition

Sexual Health Information for Teens, 3rd Edition

Skin Health Information for Teens, 2nd Edition

Sleep Information for Teens

Sports Injuries Information for Teens, 2nd Edition

Stress Information for Teens

Suicide Information for Teens, 2nd Edition

Tobacco Information for Teens, 2nd Edition

Cancer

SOURCEBOOK

Sixth Edition

Health Reference Series

Sixth Edition

Cancer
SOURCEBOOK

*Basic Consumer Health Information about Major
Forms and Stages of Cancer, Featuring Facts about
Head and Neck Cancers, Lung Cancers, Gastrointestinal
Cancers, Genitourinary Cancers, Lymphomas, Blood
Cell Cancers, Endocrine Cancers, Skin Cancers,
Bone Cancers, Metastatic Cancers, and More*

*Along with Facts about Cancer Treatments, Cancer
Risks and Prevention, a Glossary of Related Terms,
Statistical Data, and a Directory of Resources
for Additional Information*

Edited by
Karen Bellenir

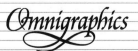

P.O. Box 31-1640, Detroit, MI 48231

Bibliographic Note
Because this page cannot legibly accommodate all the copyright notices, the Bibliographic Note portion of the Preface constitutes an extension of the copyright notice.

Edited by Karen Bellenir

Health Reference Series

Karen Bellenir, *Managing Editor*
David A. Cooke, MD, FACP, *Medical Consultant*
Elizabeth Collins, *Research and Permissions Coordinator*
Cherry Edwards, *Permissions Assistant*
EdIndex, Services for Publishers, *Indexers*

* * *

Omnigraphics, Inc.
Matthew P. Barbour, *Senior Vice President*
Kevin M. Hayes, *Operations Manager*

* * *

Peter E. Ruffner, *Publisher*

Copyright © 2011 Omnigraphics, Inc.
ISBN 978-0-7808-1145-4

Library of Congress Cataloging-in-Publication Data

Cancer sourcebook : basic consumer health information about major forms and stages of cancer, featuring facts about head and neck cancers, lung cancers, gastrointestinal cancers, genitourinary cancers, lymphomas, blood cell cancers, endocrine cancers, skin cancers, bone cancers, metastatic cancers, and more; along with facts about cancer treatments, cancer risks and prevention ... / edited by Karen Bellenir. -- 6th ed.
    p. cm. -- (Health Reference series)
  Includes bibliographical references and index.
  Summary: "Provides basic consumer health information about risks, prevention, and treatment of major forms of cancer. Includes index, glossary of related terms, and other resources"-- Provided by publisher.
  ISBN 978-0-7808-1145-4 (hardcover : alk. paper) 1. Cancer--Popular works. 2. Cancer--Handbooks, manuals, etc. I. Bellenir, Karen.
  RC263.C294 2011
  616.99'4--dc22
                                                        2011003804

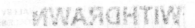

Table of Contents

Visit www.healthreferenceseries.com to view *A Contents Guide to the Health Reference Series*, a listing of more than 15,000 topics and the volumes in which they are covered.

Part II: Common Types of Cancer

Cancers Affecting the Brain and Central Nervous System

Cancers Affecting the Endocrine System

Cancers Affecting the Eyes, Mouth, and Neck

Cancers that Affect the Lungs

Cancers Affecting the Digestive Tract

Cancers Affecting the Urinary Tract

Part IV: Recurrent and Advanced Cancer

Part V: Cancer Research

Part VI: Additional Help and Information

Preface

About This Book

Every year, nearly 1.5 million Americans receive a diagnosis of cancer. Cancer is not a single disease, however. It is many different diseases that all share one common characteristic: Some of the body's cells do not die when they should. Instead they continue to grow and divide. Through this process, cancer cells can damage the body's tissues and organs, leading to a broad array of symptoms and even death. The cellular changes that lead to the development of cancer are sometimes inherited but they may also result from environmental or lifestyle factors. Although the survival rates for many types of cancer have improved in recent years and innovative treatment protocols are being developed, cancer remains the second leading cause of death in the United States.

Cancer Sourcebook, Sixth Edition provides updated information about common types of cancer affecting the head, neck, central nervous system, endocrine system, lungs, digestive and urinary tracts, blood cells, immune system, skin, bones, and other body systems. It explains how people can reduce their risk of cancer by adopting a healthy lifestyle, addressing issues related to cancer risk, and taking advantage of screening exams. Various treatment choices—including surgery, chemotherapy, radiation therapy, bone marrow transplantation, and biological therapies—are discussed, and facts are provided about cancer clinical trials and other ongoing research. The book concludes with a glossary of related terms, a directory of national cancer organizations, and suggestions for finding community-based resources.

Readers seeking additional information about specific cancers, a wide variety of cancer-related topics, or disease management issues, may wish to consult the following additional volumes within Omnigraphics' *Health Reference Series*:

- *Breast Cancer Sourcebook, 3rd Edition* offers facts about breast health and breast cancer, including information about risk factors, prevention efforts, screening and diagnostic methods, treatment options, and post-treatment follow-up care.

- *Cancer Sourcebook for Women, 4th Edition* provides additional details about gynecologic cancers and other cancers of special concern to women. It also describes benign conditions of the female reproductive system, cancer screening and prevention programs, and women's issues in cancer treatment and survivorship.

- *Cancer Survivorship Sourcebook* addresses such issues as the physical, educational, emotional, social, and financial needs of cancer patients beginning with diagnosis and continuing through treatment and beyond. It also includes facts about clinical trials and offers suggestions for dealing with the side effects of cancer treatments.

- *Disease Management Sourcebook* looks at how patients and their loved ones can cope with chronic and serious illnesses. It talks about navigating the health care system, communicating with health care providers, assessing health care quality, and making informed health care decisions.

- *Leukemia Sourcebook* details the symptoms, diagnosis, and treatments of adult and childhood forms of acute and chronic leukemia.

- *Pediatric Cancer Sourcebook* provides facts about the types of cancer most commonly found in infants, children, and adolescents. It also includes suggestions and coping strategies for parents and other caregivers.

- *Prostate Cancer Sourcebook* discusses the detection, diagnosis, and treatment of prostate cancer and non-malignant prostate conditions.

How to Use This Book

This book is divided into parts and chapters. Parts focus on broad areas of interest. Chapters are devoted to single topics within a part, and sections explore aspects of some topics in greater detail.

Part I: Cancer Risk Factors and Cancer Prevention discusses hereditary, lifestyle, and environmental factors that can sometimes set the stage for the growth of cancer. It explains which factors can be prevented and which factors are unavoidable. Statistical information about cancer prevalence, mortality, and survival is also provided, along with facts about specific population groups that suffer disproportionately from cancer.

Part II: Common Types of Cancer includes a head-to-toe list of the most frequently occurring types of cancer. Individual chapters describe the development, identification, and treatment of cancers that affect the various components of the body, including the brain and central nervous system, endocrine system, respiratory system, blood and immune system, digestive and urinary tracts, and reproductive organs, as well as the bones and skin.

Part III: Cancer-Related Tests and Treatments describes the screening methods used to find cancers at their earliest stages and the procedures most commonly used in cancer diagnosis and treatment. These include medical imaging tests, surgical procedures, chemotherapy, radiation therapy, and bone marrow transplantation. The part concludes with a chapter that discusses complementary and alternative medicine (CAM) practices used in cancer care.

Part IV: Recurrent and Advanced Cancer explains the factors that cause cancer to spread to distant parts of the body and to come back again after a time of remission. A chapter on end-of-life care describes some of the decisions cancer patients and their families may face and offers suggestions regarding ways to make wishes known.

Part V: Cancer Research discusses cancer treatment trials and other studies of new medications. Emerging therapies for cancer treatment and prevention, including vaccines, gene therapy, and proton therapy, are also described.

Part VI: Additional Help and Information includes a glossary of terms, a directory of national cancer organizations, and suggestions for finding local resources. A chapter offering cautionary guidance about cancer-related health fraud, especially on the internet, is also provided.

Bibliographic Note

This volume contains documents and excerpts from publications issued by the following U.S. government agencies: Agency for Healthcare

Research and Quality; National Cancer Institute; National Institute of Diabetes and Digestive and Kidney Diseases; U.S. Environmental Protection Agency; and the U.S. Food and Drug Administration.

In addition, this volume contains copyrighted documents from the following organizations: American Institute for Cancer Research; American Society of Clinical Oncology; Canadian Cancer Society; Cancer Project; Cancer Research UK; National Association for Proton Therapy; Nemours Foundation; and the Vanderbilt-Ingram Cancer Center.

Full citation information is provided on the first page of each chapter or section. Every effort has been made to secure all necessary rights to reprint the copyrighted material. If any omissions have been made, please contact Omnigraphics to make corrections for future editions.

Acknowledgements

In addition to the organizations listed above, special thanks are due to research and permissions coordinator, Liz Collins, permissions assistant, Cherry Edwards; editorial assistant, Zachary Klimecki; and prepress service provider, WhimsyInk.

About the Health Reference Series

The *Health Reference Series* is designed to provide basic medical information for patients, families, caregivers, and the general public. Each volume takes a particular topic and provides comprehensive coverage. This is especially important for people who may be dealing with a newly diagnosed disease or a chronic disorder in themselves or in a family member. People looking for preventive guidance, information about disease warning signs, medical statistics, and risk factors for health problems will also find answers to their questions in the *Health Reference Series*. The *Series*, however, is not intended to serve as a tool for diagnosing illness, in prescribing treatments, or as a substitute for the physician/patient relationship. All people concerned about medical symptoms or the possibility of disease are encouraged to seek professional care from an appropriate health care provider.

A Note about Spelling and Style

Health Reference Series editors use *Stedman's Medical Dictionary* as an authority for questions related to the spelling of medical terms and the *Chicago Manual of Style* for questions related to grammatical structures, punctuation, and other editorial concerns. Consistent adherence is not always possible, however, because the individual volumes within the *Series* include many documents from a wide variety of different producers and copyright holders, and the editor's primary goal is to present material from each source as accurately as is possible following the terms specified by each document's producer. This sometimes means that information in different chapters or sections may follow other guidelines and alternate spelling authorities. For example, occasionally a copyright holder may require that eponymous terms be shown in possessive forms (Crohn's disease vs. Crohn disease) or that British spelling norms be retained (leukaemia vs. leukemia).

Locating Information within the Health Reference Series

The *Health Reference Series* contains a wealth of information about a wide variety of medical topics. Ensuring easy access to all the fact sheets, research reports, in-depth discussions, and other material contained within the individual books of the *Series* remains one of our highest priorities. As the *Series* continues to grow in size and scope, however, locating the precise information needed by a reader may become more challenging.

A Contents Guide to the Health Reference Series was developed to direct readers to the specific volumes that address their concerns. It presents an extensive list of diseases, treatments, and other topics of general interest compiled from the Tables of Contents and major index headings. To access *A Contents Guide to the Health Reference Series*, visit www.healthreferenceseries.com.

Medical Consultant

Medical consultation services are provided to the *Health Reference Series* editors by David A. Cooke, MD, FACP. Dr. Cooke is a graduate of Brandeis University, and he received his M.D. degree from the University of Michigan. He completed residency training at the University of Wisconsin Hospital and Clinics. He is board-certified in Internal Medicine. Dr. Cooke currently works as part of the University of Michigan Health System and practices in Ann Arbor, MI. In his free time, he enjoys writing, science fiction, and spending time with his family.

Our Advisory Board

We would like to thank the following board members for providing guidance to the development of this *Series*:

- Dr. Lynda Baker, Associate Professor of Library and Information Science, Wayne State University, Detroit, MI

- Nancy Bulgarelli, William Beaumont Hospital Library, Royal Oak, MI

- Karen Imarisio, Bloomfield Township Public Library, Bloomfield Township, MI

- Karen Morgan, Mardigian Library, University of Michigan-Dearborn, Dearborn, MI

- Rosemary Orlando, St. Clair Shores Public Library, St. Clair Shores, MI

Health Reference Series Update Policy

The inaugural book in the *Health Reference Series* was the first edition of *Cancer Sourcebook* published in 1989. Since then, the *Series* has been enthusiastically received by librarians and in the medical community. In order to maintain the standard of providing high-quality health information for the layperson the editorial staff at Omnigraphics felt it was necessary to implement a policy of updating volumes when warranted.

Medical researchers have been making tremendous strides, and it is the purpose of the *Health Reference Series* to stay current with the most recent advances. Each decision to update a volume is made on an individual basis. Some of the considerations include how much new information is available and the feedback we receive from people who use the books. If there is a topic you would like to see added to the update list, or an area of medical concern you feel has not been adequately addressed, please write to:

Editor
Health Reference Series
Omnigraphics, Inc.
P.O. Box 31-1640
Detroit, MI 48231
E-mail: editorial@omnigraphics.com

Part One

Cancer Risk Factors and Cancer Prevention

Chapter 1

Questions and Answers about Cancer

Cancer is the second leading cause of death in the United States. However, improvements in cancer detection, diagnosis, and treatment have increased the survival rate for many types of cancer.

What is cancer?

Cancer is a group of many related diseases that begin in cells, the body's basic building blocks. To understand cancer, it is helpful to know what happens when normal cells become cancerous.

The body is made up of many types of cells. Normally, cells grow and divide to produce more cells as they are needed to keep the body healthy. Sometimes, this orderly process goes wrong. New cells form when the body does not need them, and old cells do not die when they should. The extra cells form a mass of tissue called a growth or tumor. Not all tumors are cancerous; tumors can be benign or malignant.

Benign tumors are not cancer: They can often be removed and, in most cases, they do not come back. Cells in benign tumors do not spread to other parts of the body. Most important, benign tumors are rarely a threat to life.

Malignant tumors are cancer: Cells in malignant tumors are abnormal and divide without control or order. Cancer cells invade and

---

From "Cancer: Questions and Answers," National Cancer Institute (www .cancer.gov), June 6, 2005. Reviewed by David A. Cooke, MD, FACP, September 2010.

destroy the tissue around them. Cancer cells can also break away from a malignant tumor and enter the bloodstream or lymphatic system.

Blood vessels include a network of arteries, capillaries, and veins through which the blood circulates in the body. The lymphatic system carries lymph and white blood cells through lymphatic vessels (thin tubes) to all the tissues of the body. By moving through the bloodstream or lymphatic system, cancer can spread from the primary (original) cancer site to form new tumors in other organs. The spread of cancer is called metastasis.

What causes cancer?

Scientists have learned that cancer is caused by changes in genes that normally control the growth and death of cells. Certain lifestyle and environmental factors can change some normal genes into genes that allow the growth of cancer. Many gene changes that lead to cancer are the result of tobacco use, diet, exposure to ultraviolet (UV) radiation from the sun, or exposure to carcinogens (cancer-causing substances) in the workplace or in the environment. Some gene alterations are inherited (from one or both parents). However, having an inherited gene alteration does not always mean that the person will develop cancer; it only means that the chance of getting cancer is increased. Scientists continue to examine the factors that may increase or decrease a person's chance of developing cancer.

Although being infected with certain viruses, such as the human papillomavirus (HPV), hepatitis B and C (HepB and HepC), and human immunodeficiency virus (HIV), increases the risk of some types of cancer, cancer itself is not contagious. A person cannot catch cancer from someone who has this disease. Scientists also know that an injury or bruise does not cause cancer.

Can cancer be prevented?

Although there is no guaranteed way to prevent cancer, people can reduce their risk (chance) of developing cancer by following these guidelines:

- Not using tobacco products
- Choosing foods with less fat and eating more vegetables, fruits, and whole grains
- Exercising regularly and maintaining a lean weight
- Avoiding the harmful rays of the sun, using sunscreen, and wearing clothing that protects the skin

- Talking with a doctor about the possible benefits of drugs proven to reduce the risk of certain cancers

Although many risk factors can be avoided, some, such as inherited conditions, are unavoidable. Still, it is helpful to be aware of them. It is also important to keep in mind that not everyone with a particular risk factor for cancer actually gets the disease; in fact, most do not. People who have an increased likelihood of developing cancer can help protect themselves by avoiding risk factors whenever possible and by getting regular checkups so that, if cancer develops, it is likely to be found and treated early. Treatment is often more effective when cancer is detected early. Screening exams, such as sigmoidoscopy or the fecal occult blood test, mammography, and the Pap test, can detect precancerous conditions (which can be treated before they turn into cancer) and early-stage cancer.

The National Cancer Institute (NCI) is conducting many cancer prevention studies to explore ways to reduce the risk of developing cancer. These studies are evaluating dietary supplements, chemopreventive agents, nutrition, personal behaviors, and other factors that may prevent cancer.

What are some of the common signs and symptoms of cancer?

Cancer can cause a variety of symptoms. Possible signs of cancer include the following:

- New thickening or lump in the breast or any other part of the body
- New mole or an obvious change in the appearance of an existing wart or mole
- A sore that does not heal
- Nagging cough or hoarseness
- Changes in bowel or bladder habits
- Persistent indigestion or difficulty swallowing
- Unexplained changes in weight
- Unusual bleeding or discharge

When these or other symptoms occur, they are not always caused by cancer. They can be caused by infections, benign tumors, or other problems. It is important to see a doctor about any of these symptoms or about other physical changes. Only a doctor can make a diagnosis. A person with these or other symptoms should not wait to feel pain because early cancer usually does not cause pain.

If symptoms occur, the doctor may perform a physical examination, order blood work and other tests, and/or recommend a biopsy. In most cases, a biopsy is the only way to know for certain whether cancer is present. During a biopsy, the doctor removes a sample of tissue from the abnormal area. A pathologist studies the tissue under a microscope to identify cancer cells.

How is cancer treated?

Cancer treatment can include surgery, radiation therapy, chemotherapy, hormone therapy, and biological therapy. The doctor may use one method or a combination of methods, depending on the type and location of the cancer, whether the disease has spread, the patient's age and general health, and other factors. Because treatment for cancer can also damage healthy cells and tissues, it often causes side effects. Some patients may worry that the side effects of treatment are worse than the disease. However, patients and doctors generally discuss the treatment options, weighing the likely benefits of killing cancer cells and the risks of possible side effects. Doctors can suggest ways to reduce or eliminate problems that may occur during and after treatment.

Surgery is an operation to remove cancer. The side effects of surgery depend on many factors, including the size and location of the tumor, the type of operation, and the patient's general health. Patients have some pain after surgery, but this pain can be controlled with medicine. It is also common for patients to feel tired or weak for a while after surgery.

Patients may worry that having a biopsy or other type of surgery for cancer will spread the disease. This is a very rare occurrence because surgeons take special precautions to prevent cancer from spreading during surgery. Also, exposing cancer to air during surgery does not cause the disease to spread.

Radiation therapy (also called radiotherapy) uses high-energy rays to kill cancer cells in a targeted area. Radiation can be given externally by a machine that aims radiation at the tumor area. It can also be given internally; needles, seeds, wires, or catheters containing a radioactive substance are placed directly in or near the tumor. Radiation treatments are painless. The side effects are usually temporary, and most can be treated or controlled. Patients are likely to feel very tired, especially in the later weeks of treatment. Radiation therapy may also cause a decrease in the number of white blood cells, which help protect the body against infection. With external radiation, it is also common to have temporary hair loss in the treated area and for the skin to become red, dry, tender, and itchy.

There is no risk of radiation exposure from coming in contact with a patient undergoing external radiation therapy. External radiation does not cause the body to become radioactive. With internal radiation (also called implant radiation), a patient may need to stay in the hospital, away from other people, while the radiation level is highest. Implants may be permanent or temporary. The amount of radiation in a permanent implant goes down to a safe level before the person leaves the hospital. With a temporary implant, there is no radioactivity left in the body after the implant is removed.

Chemotherapy is the use of drugs that kill cancer cells throughout the body. Healthy cells can also be harmed, especially those that divide quickly. The doctor may use one drug or a combination of drugs. The side effects of chemotherapy depend mainly on the drug(s) and the dose(s) the patient receives. Hair loss is a common side effect of chemotherapy; however, not all anticancer drugs cause loss of hair. Anticancer drugs may also cause temporary fatigue, poor appetite, nausea and vomiting, diarrhea, and mouth and lip sores. Drugs that prevent or reduce nausea and vomiting can help with some of these side effects. Normal cells usually recover when chemotherapy is over, so most side effects gradually go away after treatment ends.

Hormone therapy is used to treat certain cancers that depend on hormones for their growth. It works by keeping cancer cells from getting or using the hormones they need to grow. This treatment may include the use of drugs that stop the production of certain hormones or that change the way hormones work. Another type of hormone therapy is surgery to remove organs that make hormones. For example, the ovaries may be removed to treat breast cancer, or the testicles may be removed to treat prostate cancer.

Hormone therapy can cause a number of side effects. Patients may feel tired, or have fluid retention, weight gain, hot flashes, nausea and vomiting, changes in appetite, and, in some cases, blood clots. Hormone therapy may also cause bone loss in premenopausal women. Depending on the type of hormone therapy used, these side effects may be temporary, long lasting, or permanent.

Biological therapy uses the body's immune system, directly or indirectly, to fight disease and to lessen some of the side effects of cancer treatment. Monoclonal antibodies, interferon, interleukin-2, and colony-stimulating factors are some types of biological therapy.

The side effects caused by biological therapy vary with the specific treatment. In general, these treatments tend to cause flu-like symptoms, such as chills, fever, muscle aches, weakness, loss of appetite, nausea, vomiting, and diarrhea. Patients also may bleed or bruise easily, get a skin rash, or have swelling. These problems can be severe, but they go away after the treatment stops.

Are clinical trials (research studies) available? Where can people get more information about clinical trials?

Yes. Clinical trials are an important treatment option for many cancer patients. To develop new, more effective treatments, and better ways to use current treatments, the NCI is sponsoring clinical trials in many hospitals and cancer centers around the country. Clinical trials are a critical step in the development of new methods of treatment. Before any new treatment can be recommended for general use, doctors conduct clinical trials to find out whether the treatment is safe for patients and effective against the disease.

People interested in taking part in a clinical trial should talk with their doctor.

Does cancer always cause pain?

Having cancer does not always mean having pain. Whether a patient has pain may depend on the type of cancer, the extent of the disease, and the patient's tolerance for pain. Most pain occurs when the cancer grows and presses against bones, organs, or nerves. Pain may also be a side effect of treatment. However, pain can generally be relieved or reduced with prescription medicines or over-the-counter drugs recommended by the doctor. Other ways to reduce pain, such as relaxation exercises, may also be useful. Pain should not be accepted as an unavoidable part of having cancer. It is important for patients to talk about pain so steps can be taken to help relieve it. The fear of addiction or "losing control" should not stop patients from taking pain medication. Patients who take medications for cancer pain, as prescribed by their doctor, rarely become addicted to them. In addition, changing the dose or type of medication can usually help if the patient has troublesome side effects.

Chapter 2

Cancer Statistics

Chapter Contents

Section 2.1

Understanding Statistics on Incidence, Prevalence, and Mortality

Key Messages

- Statistics are used to help doctors understand who is at risk for cancer.

- Several types of statistics are used to determine cancer risk for large groups of people: incidence, prevalence, and mortality.

- Understanding your risk of cancer can help you receive appropriate screening tests and make lifestyle choices to reduce cancer risk.

Many people may want to know their individual risk of being diagnosed with cancer. Statistics are used to determine the risk of cancer for groups of people and can be helpful to estimate your risk of cancer based on individual aspects that are similar to the groups at risk. However, statistics cannot tell you if you will develop cancer. Read below to learn more about the types of statistics used to estimate cancer risk.

Estimating How Many People Will Be Diagnosed with Cancer during the Year

Incidence is used to determine an estimate of the number of the people diagnosed with cancer in a given population (for example, all men in the United States) over a specific period of time (typically one year). Expected incidence of cancer cases for the current year is calculated by using the number of cancer cases that occurred each year over a range of years and fitting those numbers to a statistical model, which predicts the number of new cases that are expected for the current year. The range may be used differently in different statistical reports and for different types of statistics.

- **Example:** In the American Cancer Society's publication, *Cancer Facts & Figures 2010*, cancer incidence for 2010 was calculated by using the number of cancer cases from 1995 to 2006.

Incidence is frequently given as an incidence rate that states the number of people estimated to be diagnosed with cancer per 100,000 people.

- **Example:** The 2010 incidence rate for prostate cancer in the United States is about 156, which means that almost 156 out of every 100,000 men in the United States are expected to be diagnosed with prostate cancer in 2010.

Incidence is often stated as an age-adjusted incidence rate. The number of people who fall into different age groups varies (for example, there are many more 30 to 40 year olds than 80 to 90 year olds). This is referred to as age distribution. Incidence rates can be adjusted to account for these age distribution differences so that populations can be compared.

- **Example:** Florida has a large number of older adults, while most people who live in Alaska, by comparison, are young. Because the incidence of breast cancer increases with age, the annual absolute incidence rate of invasive breast cancer is much higher in Florida than in Alaska. However, when adjusted for age, the annual age-adjusted incidence rate (cases per 100,000 women) for Alaska was higher than that of Florida from 2002–2006: 114.1 in Florida compared with 126.4 in Alaska.

Incidence statistics can be given for large populations, such as all people in the United States, or for more specific population groups, such as only women ages 20 to 24. Large population statistics are usually estimates based on information collected from a smaller sample of the whole population. When these statistics describe particular population groups, they are usually referred to as "specific."

- **Example:** The age-specific incidence rate for breast cancer in 20-year-olds to 24-year-olds is 1.6 (per 100,000 women).

Incidence statistics may also be given for several cancers combined, for specific types of cancer, for specific stages of a type of cancer, or for specific cancer risk factors (anything that increases a person's chance of developing a type of cancer).

11

Calculating How Many People Have or Have Had Cancer

Prevalence is used to describe the number of people in a specific population that have a certain type of cancer at a specific point in time. While incidence describes the estimated number of new cases of a cancer, prevalence can describe all cases, including newly diagnosed and people who are being treated or who have been treated for cancer in the past. Prevalence can be expressed in terms of an absolute number or as a percentage.

- **Example:** The estimated prevalence of ovarian cancer in the United States in 2007 was 177,162. This means that 177,162 of the women in the United States were living with or had a history of ovarian cancer.

Prevalence rates express the number of cases of cancer per 100,000 people.

- **Example:** The estimated prevalence rate for ovarian cancer in the United States in 2007 was 59. This means, in 2007, almost 59 out of every 100,000 women were living with or had a history of ovarian cancer.

Like incidence, prevalence can also be used for large populations, specific population groups, several cancers combined, specific types of cancer, specific stages of a type of cancer, or cancer risk factors.

- **Example:** Genetic mutations in either one of two specific genes, BRCA1 and BRCA2, are associated with increased breast cancer risk. It is estimated that the prevalence of mutations of one of these two genes is less than 1%. This means that less than 1% of women have a mutated BRCA1 or BRCA2 gene. However, the prevalence of a BRCA gene mutation among women with breast cancer is approximately 5% to 10%. This means that out of all women who have breast cancer, 5% to 10% have a BRCA gene mutation. The increased prevalence of BRCA gene mutations among women with breast cancer means that a woman with a BRCA gene mutation has an increased risk of breast cancer.

Calculating How Many People Die from Cancer

In cancer statistics, mortality is used to describe the number of deaths from cancer during a specific time period. The cancer mortality rate describes the number of deaths from cancer per 100,000 people during a specific time period, usually one year. Mortality rates can be calculated for specific types of cancer and for specific subsets of the population (such as children under 12, smokers, or women with the BRCA1 gene mutation). As with incidence rates, mortality rates can also be given as age-adjusted mortality rates.

Mortality rates can change dramatically with advances in treatment, screening, and prevention.

- **Example:** The age-adjusted mortality rate for Hodgkin lymphoma in the United States in the early 1960s was greater than 1.55 (1.55 deaths per 100,000 people). Following the introduction of combination chemotherapy in the late 1960s, the rate dropped to less than 0.5 by the 1990s.

Estimating a Person's Risk of Cancer to Recommend Screening

By looking at the incidence and prevalence statistics for different types of cancer in various groups of people, researchers can estimate which groups of people may have an increased risk of developing certain types of cancer. Statistics tell us that older women are at higher risk for breast cancer than younger women, black men are at higher risk for prostate cancer than white men, and people who drink alcohol often are at higher risk for liver cancer than people who don't drink alcohol.

Risk information from incidence and prevalence statistics is combined with mortality statistics to provide some of the basis for cancer screening recommendations.

- **Example:** Prevalence and incidence statistics show that colorectal cancer is among the most common cancers in the United States. Age-specific prevalence and incidence rates also show that colorectal cancer is most common in people over age 50. The mortality rates for colorectal cancer show that treatment is much more successful when cancer is found early than if the cancer has spread. Therefore, combining these pieces of information, doctors recommend that routine screening for colorectal cancer begin at age 50 to increase the likelihood of prevention or early detection.

Other risk factors, such as family history, presence of other illnesses, and various lifestyle factors, are also taken into account when making screening recommendations specific to an individual.

Points to Remember

- Statistics are estimates that describe trends in large numbers of people. Statistics cannot be used to predict what will actually happen to a single person.

- Incidence, prevalence, and mortality statistics for different cancer stages, age groups, or time periods can vary dramatically. People are encouraged to ask their doctor for the most appropriate statistics based on their individual medical condition.

- As with any medical information, talk with your doctor for clarification if cancer-related statistics seem unclear.

Section 2.2

The Role Statistics Play in Predicting a Patient's Prognosis

"Understanding Prognosis and Cancer Statistics: Questions and Answers," National Cancer Institute (www.cancer.gov), March 7, 2008.

What is a prognosis?

People facing cancer are naturally concerned about what the future holds. A prognosis gives an idea of the likely course and outcome of a disease—that is, the chance that a patient will recover or have a recurrence (return of the cancer).

What factors affect a patient's prognosis?

Many factors affect a person's prognosis. Some of the most important are the type and location of the cancer, the stage of the disease (the extent to which the cancer has metastasized, or spread), and its grade (how abnormal the cancer cells look and how quickly the cancer is likely to grow and spread). In addition, for hematologic cancers (cancers of the blood or bone marrow) such as leukemias and lymphomas, the presence of chromosomal abnormalities and abnormalities in the patient's complete blood count (CBC) can affect a person's prognosis. Other factors that may also affect the prognosis include the person's age, general health, and response to treatment.

How do statistics contribute to predicting a patient's prognosis?

When doctors discuss a person's prognosis, they carefully consider all factors that could affect that person's disease and treatment and then try to predict what might happen. The doctor bases the prognosis on information researchers have collected over many years about hundreds or even thousands of people with cancer.

When possible, the doctor uses statistics based on groups of people whose situations are most similar to that of an individual patient. Several types of statistics might be used to discuss prognosis. Some commonly used statistics are described below:

- Survival rate indicates the percentage of people with a certain type and stage of cancer who survive for a specific period of time after their diagnosis. For example, 55 out of 100 people with a certain type of cancer will live for at least five years, and the other 45 people will not. Survival statistics may further categorize the people who die by cause of death because some will die from un-related causes. For example, of the 45 people mentioned above, 35 may die from their cancer and 10 may die from other causes.

- The five-year survival rate indicates the percentage of people who are alive five years after their cancer diagnosis, whether they have few or no signs or symptoms of cancer, are free of disease, or are having treatment. Five-year survival rates are used as a standard way of discussing prognosis as well as a way to compare the value of one treatment with another. It does not mean that a patient can expect to live for only five years after treatment or that there are no cures for cancer.

- Disease-free or recurrence-free survival rates represent how long one survives free of the disease, rather than until death.

Because survival rates are based on large groups of people, they cannot be used to predict what will happen to a particular patient. No two patients are exactly alike, and treatment and responses to treatment vary greatly.

The doctor may speak of a favorable prognosis if the cancer is likely to respond well to treatment. The prognosis may be unfavorable if the cancer is likely to be difficult to control. It is important to keep in mind, however, that a prognosis is only a prediction. Again, doctors cannot be absolutely certain about the outcome for a particular patient.

Is it helpful to know the prognosis?

Cancer patients and their loved ones face many unknowns. Understanding cancer and what to expect can help patients and their loved ones plan treatment, think about lifestyle changes, and make decisions about their quality of life and finances. Many people with cancer want to know their prognosis. They find it easier to cope when they know the statistics. They may ask their doctor or search for statistics such as survival rates on their own. Other people find statistical information confusing and frightening, and they think it is too impersonal to be of use to them.

The doctor who is most familiar with a patient's situation is in the best position to discuss the prognosis and to explain what the statistics may mean for that person. At the same time, it is important to understand that even the doctor cannot tell exactly what to expect. In fact, a person's prognosis may change if the cancer progresses or if treatment is successful.

Seeking information about the prognosis is a personal decision. It is up to each patient to decide how much information he or she wants and how to deal with it.

What is the prognosis if a patient decides not to have treatment?

Because everyone's situation is different, this question can be difficult to answer. Prognostic statistics often come from studies comparing new treatments with best available treatments, not with "no treatment." Therefore, it is not always easy for doctors to accurately estimate prognosis for patients who decide not to have treatment. However, as mentioned above, the doctor who is most familiar with a patient's situation is in the best position to discuss prognosis, taking into account individual characteristics of the patient that can affect the overall situation.

There are many reasons patients decide not to have treatment. One reason may be concern about side effects related to treatment. Patients should discuss this concern with their doctor and cancer nurse. Many medications are available to prevent or control the side effects caused by cancer therapies. Another reason patients might decide not to have treatment is that their type of cancer does not have a good prognosis even when treated. In these cases, patients may want to explore clinical trials (research studies). A clinical trial may offer access to new drugs that may be more promising than the standard treatments available.

Section 2.3

Incidence, Mortality, and Survival Rates for Common Cancers

Statistics in this section were excerpted from "SEER Stat Fact Sheets" and are based on Surveillance Epidemiology and End Results (SEER) incidence and National Center for Health Statistics (NCHS) mortality statistics. Most can be found within this document: Horner MJ, Ries LAG, Krapcho M, Neyman N, Aminou R, Howlader N, Altekruse SF, Feuer EJ, Huang L, Mariotto A, Miller BA, Lewis DR, Eisner MP, Stinchcomb DG, Edwards BK (eds). *SEER Cancer Statistics Review, 1975-2006*, National Cancer Institute. Bethesda, MD, http://seer.cancer.gov/csr/1975_2006/, based on November 2008 SEER data submission, posted to the SEER web site, 2009.

Cancer, Totals for All Sites

It is estimated that 1,479,350 men and women (766,130 men and 713,220 women) will be diagnosed with cancer and 562,340 men and women will die of cancer of all sites in 2009.

Surveillance Epidemiology and End Results (SEER) Incidence: From 2002–2006, the median age at diagnosis for cancer of all sites was 66 years of age. Approximately 1.1% were diagnosed under age 20; 2.7% between 20 and 34; 5.8% between 35 and 44; 13.9% between 45 and 54; 21.8% between 55 and 64; 24.9% between 65 and 74; 22.2% between 75 and 84; and 7.6% 85 or more years of age.

U.S. Mortality: From 2002–2006, the median age at death for cancer of all sites was 73 years of age. Approximately 0.4% died under age 20; 0.8% between 20 and 34; 2.7% between 35 and 44; 9.0% between 45 and 54; 17.5% between 55 and 64; 25.2% between 65 and 74; 29.9% between 75 and 84; and 14.6% 85 or more years of age.

Table 2.1. Incidence Rates by Race

Race/Ethnicity	Male	Female
All Races	541.8 per 100,000 men	408.5 per 100,000 women
White	544.3 per 100,000 men	420.5 per 100,000 women
Black	633.7 per 100,000 men	398.9 per 100,000 women
Asian/Pacific Islander	349.1 per 100,000 men	287.5 per 100,000 women
American Indian/ Alaska Native	331.0 per 100,000 men	302.2 per 100,000 women
Hispanic	409.7 per 100,000 men	312.5 per 100,000 women

For additional details regarding these statistics, visit http://seer.cancer.gov/statfacts/html/all.html.

Table 2.2. Death Rates by Race

Race/Ethnicity	Male	Female
All Races	229.9 per 100,000 men	157.8 per 100,000 women
White	226.7 per 100,000 men	157.3 per 100,000 women
Black	304.2 per 100,000 men	183.7 per 100,000 women
Asian/Pacific Islander	135.4 per 100,000 men	95.1 per 100,000 women
American Indian/ Alaska Native	183.3 per 100,000 men	140.1 per 100,000 women
Hispanic	154.7 per 100,000 men	103.9 per 100,000 women

For additional details regarding these statistics, visit http://seer.cancer.gov/statfacts/html/all.html.

Survival: Survival examines how long after diagnosis people live. Cancer survival is measured in a number of different ways depending on the intended purpose. The survival rates presented here are based on the relative survival rate, which measures the survival of the cancer patients in comparison to the general population to estimate the effect of cancer. The overall five-year relative survival rate for 1999–2005 from 17 SEER geographic areas was 66.1%. Five-year relative survival rates by race and sex were: 67.0% for white men; 66.9% for white women; 60.6% for black men; 55.2% for black women.

Lifetime Risk: Based on rates from 2004–2006, 40.58% of men and women born today will be diagnosed with cancer at some time during their lifetime. These statistics are called the lifetime risk (the probability of developing cancer in the course of one's lifespan). Sometimes it is more useful to look at the probability of developing cancer between two age groups. For example, 20.45% of men will develop cancer between their 50th and 70th birthdays compared to 15.33% for women.

Prevalence: On January 1, 2006, in the United States there were approximately 11,384,892 men and women alive who had a history of cancer—5,168,889 men and 6,216,003 women. This includes any person alive on January 1, 2006 who had been diagnosed with cancer at any point prior to January 1, 2006 and includes persons with active disease and those who are cured of their disease. Prevalence can also be expressed as a percentage, and it can also be calculated for a specific amount of time prior to January 1, 2006 such as diagnosed within five years of January 1, 2006.

Anal Cancer

It is estimated that 5,290 men and women (2,100 men and 3,190 women) will be diagnosed with, and 710 men and women will die of, cancer of the anus, anal canal, and anorectum in 2009.

SEER incidence: From 2002–2006, the median age at diagnosis for cancer of the anus, anal canal, and anorectum was 61 years of age. Approximately 0.0% were diagnosed under age 20; 1.2% between 20 and 34; 10.5% between 35 and 44; 23.6% between 45 and 54; 23.0% between 55 and 64; 19.0% between 65 and 74; 16.2% between 75 and 84; and 6.4% 85 or more years of age.

U.S. mortality: From 2002–2006, the median age at death for cancer of the anus, anal canal, and anorectum was 65 years of age. Approximately 0.0% died under age 20; 1.0% between 20 and 34; 7.5% between 35 and 44; 18.5% between 45 and 54; 22.1% between 55 and 64; 19.3% between 65 and 74; 20.7% between 75 and 84; and 10.9% 85 or more years of age.

Survival: The overall five-year relative survival rate for 1999–2005 from 17 SEER geographic areas was 66.3%. Five-year relative survival rates by race and sex were: 61.8% for white men; 70.3% for white women; 53.7% for black men; 65.7% for black women.

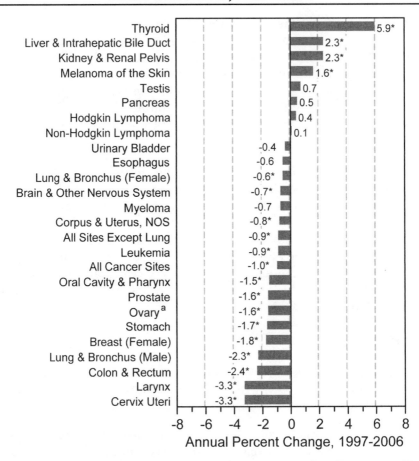

Figure 2.1. *Trends in Seer incidence Rates (Source: SEER 13 areas (San Francisco, Connecticut, Detroit, Hawaii, Iowa, New Mexico, Seattle, Utah, Atlanta, San Jose-Monterey, Los Angeles, Alaska Native Registry and Rural Georgia) and US Mortality Files, National Center for Health Statistics, Centers for Disease Control and Prevention.*

For sex-specific cancer sites, the population was limited to the population of the appropriate sex. Underlying rates are per 100,000 and age-adjusted to the 2000 US Std Population (19 age groups - Census P25-1103). *The Annual Percent Change is significantly different from zero (p<.05). ªOvary excludes borderline cases or histologies 8442, 8451, 8462, 8472, and 8473.)

Bone Cancer

It is estimated that 2,570 men and women (1,430 men and 1,140 women) will be diagnosed with and 1,470 men and women will die of cancer of the bones and joints in 2009.

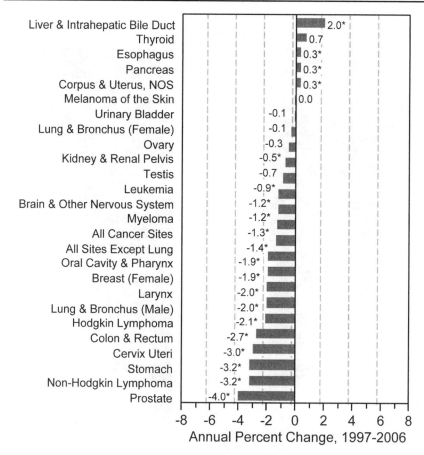

Figure 2.2. *Trends in U.S. Cancer Death Rates (Source: SEER 13 areas (San Francisco, Connecticut, Detroit, Hawaii, Iowa, New Mexico, Seattle, Utah, Atlanta, San Jose-Monterey, Los Angeles, Alaska Native Registry and Rural Georgia) and US Mortality Files, National Center for Health Statistics, Centers for Disease Control and Prevention.*

For sex-specific cancer sites, the population was limited to the population of the appropriate sex. Underlying rates are per 100,000 and age-adjusted to the 2000 US Std Population (19 age groups - Census P25-1103). *The Annual Percent Change is significantly different from zero (p<.05).)

SEER incidence: From 2002–2006, the median age at diagnosis for cancer of the bones and joints was 39 years of age. Approximately 29.4% were diagnosed under age 20; 16.1% between 20 and 34; 10.7% between 35 and 44; 12.8% between 45 and 54; 10.3% between 55 and 64; 8.8% between 65 and 74; 8.2% between 75 and 84; and 3.8% 85 or more years of age.

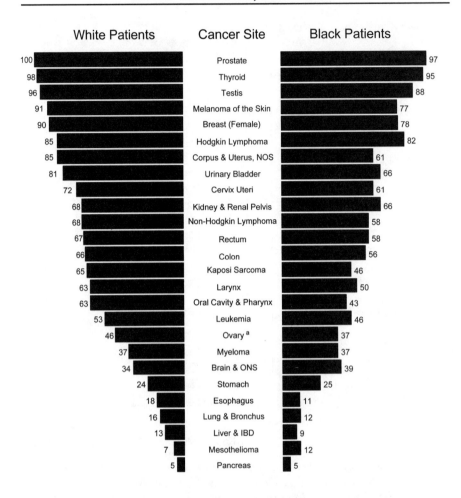

White Patients	Cancer Site	Black Patients
100	Prostate	97
98	Thyroid	95
96	Testis	88
91	Melanoma of the Skin	77
90	Breast (Female)	78
85	Hodgkin Lymphoma	82
85	Corpus & Uterus, NOS	61
81	Urinary Bladder	66
72	Cervix Uteri	61
68	Kidney & Renal Pelvis	66
68	Non-Hodgkin Lymphoma	58
67	Rectum	58
66	Colon	56
65	Kaposi Sarcoma	46
63	Larynx	50
63	Oral Cavity & Pharynx	43
53	Leukemia	46
46	Ovary [a]	37
37	Myeloma	37
34	Brain & ONS	39
24	Stomach	25
18	Esophagus	11
16	Lung & Bronchus	12
13	Liver & IBD	9
7	Mesothelioma	12
5	Pancreas	5

Figure 2.3. *5-Year Relative Survival Rates SEER Program, 1999–2006, Both Sexes, by Race (Source: SEER 17 areas (San Francisco, Connecticut, Detroit, Hawaii, Iowa, New Mexico, Seattle, Utah, Atlanta, San Jose-Monterey, Los Angeles, Alaska Native Registry, Rural Georgia, California excluding SF/SJM/LA, Kentucky, Louisiana, and New Jersey) and US Mortality Files, National Center for Health Statistics, Centers for Disease Control and Prevention. [a]Rates are per 100,000 and age-adjusted to the 2000 US Std Population (19 age groups - Census P25-1103). [b]Rates for American Indian/Alaska Native are based on the CHSDA (Contract Health Service Delivery Area) counties. Hispanic is not mutually exclusive from whites, blacks, Asian/Pacific Islanders, and American Indians/ Alaska Natives. Incidence data for Hispanics are based on NHIA and exclude cases from the Alaska Native Registry and Kentucky. Mortality data for Hispanics exclude cases from Minnesota, New Hampshire, and North Dakota.*

U.S. mortality: From 2002–2006, the median age at death for cancer of the bones and joints was 58 years of age. Approximately 14.5% died under age 20; 14.4% between 20 and 34; 7.0% between 35 and 44; 9.9% between 45 and 54; 11.9% between 55 and 64; 13.7% between 65 and 74; 17.9% between 75 and 84; and 10.8% 85 or more years of age.

Survival: The overall five-year relative survival rate for 1999–2005 from 17 SEER geographic areas was 68.4%. Five-year relative survival rates by race and sex were: 64.4% for white men; 72.9% for white women; 65.2% for black men; 67.3% for black women.

Brain and Other Nervous System Cancer

It is estimated that 22,070 men and women (12,010 men and 10,060 women) will be diagnosed with and 12,920 men and women will die of cancer of the brain and other nervous system in 2009.

SEER incidence: From 2002–2006, the median age at diagnosis for cancer of the brain and other nervous system was 56 years of age. Approximately 13.2% were diagnosed under age 20; 9.3% between 20 and 34; 10.1% between 35 and 44; 15.0% between 45 and 54; 17.6% between 55 and 64; 16.4% between 65 and 74; 14.2% between 75 and 84; and 4.2% 85 or more years of age.

U.S. mortality: From 2002–2006, the median age at death for cancer of the brain and other nervous system was 64 years of age. Approximately 4.3% died under age 20; 3.8% between 20 and 34; 7.4% between 35 and 44; 15.2% between 45 and 54; 21.3% between 55 and 64; 22.3% between 65 and 74; 19.5% between 75 and 84; and 6.1% 85 or more years of age.

Survival: The overall five-year relative survival rate for 1999–2005 from 17 SEER geographic areas was 34.8%. Five-year relative survival rates by race and sex were: 32.4% for white men; 36.1% for white women; 33.9% for black men; 43.7% for black women.

Breast Cancer

It is estimated that 192,370 women will be diagnosed with and 40,170 women will die of cancer of the breast in 2009.

SEER incidence: From 2002–2006, the median age at diagnosis for cancer of the breast was 61 years of age. Approximately 0.0% were diagnosed under age 20; 1.9% between 20 and 34; 10.5% between 35 and 44; 22.5% between 45 and 54; 23.7% between 55 and 64; 19.6% between 65 and 74; 16.2% between 75 and 84; and 5.5% 85 or more years of age.

U.S. mortality: From 2002–2006, the median age at death for cancer of the breast was 68 years of age. Approximately 0.0% died under age 20; 1.0% between 20 and 34; 6.2% between 35 and 44; 15.1% between 45 and 54; 20.3% between 55 and 64; 19.8% between 65 and 74; 22.8% between 75 and 84; and 14.9% 85 or more years of age.

Survival: The overall five-year relative survival rate for 1999–2005 from 17 SEER geographic areas was 89.1%. Five-year relative survival rates by race were: 90.3% for white women; 77.9% for black women.

Cervical Cancer

It is estimated that 11,270 women will be diagnosed with and 4,070 women will die of cancer of the cervix uteri in 2009.

SEER incidence: From 2002–2006, the median age at diagnosis for cancer of the cervix uteri was 48 years of age. Approximately 0.2% were diagnosed under age 20; 14.9% between 20 and 34; 26.2% between 35 and 44; 23.5% between 45 and 54; 15.8% between 55 and 64; 10.4% between 65 and 74; 6.6% between 75 and 84; and 2.5% 85 or more years of age.

U.S. mortality: From 2002–2006, the median age at death for cancer of the cervix uteri was 57 years of age. Approximately 0.0% died under age 20; 5.3% between 20 and 34; 16.2% between 35 and 44; 23.2% between 45 and 54; 20.1% between 55 and 64; 15.2% between 65 and 74; 13.1% between 75 and 84; and 6.9% 85 or more years of age.

Survival: The overall five-year relative survival rate for 1999–2005 from 17 SEER geographic areas was 70.6%. Five-year relative survival rates by race were: 72.0% for white women; 61.4% for black women.

Colorectal Cancer

It is estimated that 146,970 men and women (75,590 men and 71,380 women) will be diagnosed with and 49,920 men and women will die of cancer of the colon and rectum in 2009.

SEER incidence: From 2002–2006, the median age at diagnosis for cancer of the colon and rectum was 71 years of age. Approximately

0.1% were diagnosed under age 20; 1.1% between 20 and 34; 3.8% between 35 and 44; 12.0% between 45 and 54; 18.7% between 55 and 64; 24.7% between 65 and 74; 27.7% between 75 and 84; and 12.1% 85 or more years of age.

U.S. mortality: From 2002–2006, the median age at death for cancer of the colon and rectum was 75 years of age. Approximately 0.0% died under age 20; 0.6% between 20 and 34; 2.4% between 35 and 44; 8.0% between 45 and 54; 15.2% between 55 and 64; 22.6% between 65 and 74; 30.8% between 75 and 84; and 20.4% 85 or more years of age.

Survival: The overall five-year relative survival rate for 1999–2005 from 17 SEER geographic areas was 65.2%. Five-year relative survival rates by race and sex were: 66.3% for white men; 65.9% for white women; 55.5% for black men; 56.7% for black women.

Corpus and Uterus Cancer

It is estimated that 42,160 women will be diagnosed with and 7,780 women will die of cancer of the corpus and uterus, not otherwise specified (NOS) in 2009.

SEER incidence: From 2002–2006, the median age at diagnosis for cancer of the corpus and uterus, NOS was 62 years of age. Approximately 0.0% were diagnosed under age 20; 1.5% between 20 and 34; 6.4% between 35 and 44; 19.0% between 45 and 54; 29.9% between 55 and 64; 22.4% between 65 and 74; 15.6% between 75 and 84; and 5.1% 85 or more years of age.

U.S. mortality: From 2002–2006, the median age at death for cancer of the corpus and uterus, NOS was 72 years of age. Approximately 0.0% died under age 20; 0.4% between 20 and 34; 2.2% between 35 and 44; 8.0% between 45 and 54; 19.2% between 55 and 64; 26.3% between 65 and 74; 28.2% between 75 and 84; and 15.8% 85 or more years of age.

Survival: The overall five-year relative survival rate for 1999–2005 from 17 SEER geographic areas was 82.9%. Five-year relative survival rates by race were: 84.7% for white women; 61.3% for black women.

Endocrine Cancers (Other than Thyroid)

It is estimated that 2,130 men and women (1,070 men and 1,060 women) will be diagnosed with and 840 men and women will die of cancers of the endocrine system other than thyroid cancer (which is listed separately) in 2009.

SEER incidence: From 2002–2006, the median age at diagnosis for other cancer of the endocrine system was 51 years of age. Approximately 22.7% were diagnosed under age 20; 7.6% between 20 and 34; 10.4% between 35 and 44; 14.7% between 45 and 54; 17.3% between 55 and 64; 14.6% between 65 and 74; 10.1% between 75 and 84; and 2.5% 85 or more years of age.

U.S. mortality: From 2002-2006, the median age at death for other cancer of the endocrine system was 56 years of age. Approximately 21.4% died under age 20; 5.5% between 20 and 34; 7.2% between 35 and 44; 13.6% between 45 and 54; 15.2% between 55 and 64; 16.7% between 65 and 74; 14.6% between 75 and 84; and 5.7% 85 or more years of age.

Survival: The overall five-year relative survival rate for 1999–2005 from 17 SEER geographic areas was 62.4%. Five-year relative survival rates by race and sex were: 62.4% for white men; 60.0% for white women; 62.4% for black men; 67.1% for black women.

Esophageal Cancer

It is estimated that 16,470 men and women (12,940 men and 3,530 women) will be diagnosed with and 14,530 men and women will die of cancer of the esophagus in 2009.

SEER incidence: From 2002–2006, the median age at diagnosis for cancer of the esophagus was 68 years of age. Approximately 0.0% were diagnosed under age 20; 0.4% between 20 and 34; 2.4% between 35 and 44; 12.2% between 45 and 54; 24.0% between 55 and 64; 28.1% between 65 and 74; 24.8% between 75 and 84; and 8.1% 85 or more years of age.

U.S. mortality: From 2002–2006, the median age at death for cancer of the esophagus was 70 years of age. Approximately 0.0% died under age 20; 0.3% between 20 and 34; 2.3% between 35 and 44; 11.0% between 45 and 54; 22.9% between 55 and 64; 27.7% between 65 and 74; 26.4% between 75 and 84; and 9.4% 85 or more years of age.

Survival: The overall five-year relative survival rate for 1999–2005 from 17 SEER geographic areas was 16.8%. Five-year relative survival rates by race and sex were: 17.6% for white men; 17.6% for white women; 9.8% for black men; 13.4% for black women.

Eye Cancer

It is estimated that 2,350 men and women (1,200 men and 1,150 women) will be diagnosed with and 230 men and women will die of cancer of the eye and orbit in 2009.

SEER incidence: From 2002–2006, the median age at diagnosis for cancer of the eye and orbit was 60 years of age. Approximately 13.9% were diagnosed under age 20; 3.6% between 20 and 34; 7.3% between 35 and 44; 14.1% between 45 and 54; 19.6% between 55 and 64; 18.9% between 65 and 74; 17.0% between 75 and 84; and 5.5% 85 or more years of age.

U.S. mortality: From 2002–2006, the median age at death for cancer of the eye and orbit was 69 years of age. Approximately 3.7% died under age 20; 1.5% between 20 and 34; 4.5% between 35 and 44; 11.6% between 45 and 54; 19.4% between 55 and 64; 21.8% between 65 and 74; 24.4% between 75 and 84; and 13.0% 85 or more years of age.

Survival: The overall five-year relative survival rate for 1999–2005 from 17 SEER geographic areas was 83.8%. Five-year relative survival rates by race and sex were: 81.6% for white men; 85.5% for white women; 83.3% for black men; 84.1% for black women.

Kidney Cancer and Cancer of the Renal Pelvis

It is estimated that 57,760 men and women (35,430 men and 22,330 women) will be diagnosed with and 12,980 men and women will die of cancer of the kidney and renal pelvis in 2009.

SEER incidence: From 2002–2006, the median age at diagnosis for cancer of the kidney and renal pelvis was 64 years of age. Approximately 1.3% were diagnosed under age 20; 1.5% between 20 and 34; 6.1% between 35 and 44; 16.4% between 45 and 54; 24.6% between 55 and 64; 24.3% between 65 and 74; 20.0% between 75 and 84; and 5.7% 85 or more years of age.

U.S. mortality: From 2002–2006, the median age at death for cancer of the kidney and renal pelvis was 71 years of age. Approximately 0.5% died under age 20; 0.5% between 20 and 34; 2.4% between 35 and 44; 10.2% between 45 and 54; 20.0% between 55 and 64; 25.4% between 65 and 74; 27.9% between 75 and 84; and 13.2% 85 or more years of age.

Survival: The overall five-year relative survival rate for 1999–2005 from 17 SEER geographic areas was 68.4%. Five-year relative survival rates by race and sex were: 68.1% for white men; 69.1% for white women; 64.7% for black men; 67.4% for black women.

Laryngeal Cancer

It is estimated that 12,290 men and women (9,920 men and 2,370 women) will be diagnosed with and 3,660 men and women will die of cancer of the larynx in 2009.

SEER incidence: From 2002–2006, the median age at diagnosis for cancer of the larynx was 65 years of age. Approximately 0.0% were diagnosed under age 20; 0.5% between 20 and 34; 3.4% between 35 and 44; 15.5% between 45 and 54; 28.7% between 55 and 64; 29.0% between 65 and 74; 18.1% between 75 and 84; and 4.7% 85 or more years of age.

U.S. mortality: From 2002–2006, the median age at death for cancer of the larynx was 69 years of age. Approximately 0.0% died under age 20; 0.1% between 20 and 34; 1.8% between 35 and 44; 11.5% between 45 and 54; 24.9% between 55 and 64; 29.2% between 65 and 74; 24.3% between 75 and 84; and 8.1% 85 or more years of age.

Survival: The overall five-year relative survival rate for 1999–2005 from 17 SEER geographic areas was 61.6%. Five-year relative survival rates by race and sex were: 64.0% for white men; 59.6% for white women; 51.6% for black men; 46.1% for black women.

Leukemia

It is estimated that 44,790 men and women (25,630 men and 19,160 women) will be diagnosed with and 21,870 men and women will die of leukemia in 2009.

SEER incidence: From 2002–2006, the median age at diagnosis for leukemia was 66 years of age. Approximately 11.1% were diagnosed under age 20; 4.7% between 20 and 34; 5.5% between 35 and 44; 10.1% between 45 and 54; 15.0% between 55 and 64; 19.8% between 65 and 74; 23.3% between 75 and 84; and 10.5% 85 or more years of age.

U.S. mortality: From 2002–2006, the median age at death for leukemia was 74 years of age. Approximately 3.0% died under age 20; 3.2% between 20 and 34; 3.4% between 35 and 44; 6.5% between 45 and 54; 12.4% between 55 and 64; 21.9% between 65 and 74; 31.6% between 75 and 84; and 17.9% 85 or more years of age.

Survival: The overall five-year relative survival rate for 1999-2005 from 17 SEER geographic areas was 53.1%. Five-year relative survival rates by race and sex were: 53.8% for white men; 53.0% for white women; 45.5% for black men; 46.1% for black women.

Liver and Intrahepatic Bile Duct Cancer

It is estimated that 22,620 men and women (16,410 men and 6,210 women) will be diagnosed with and 18,160 men and women will die of cancer of the liver and intrahepatic bile duct in 2009.

SEER incidence: From 2002–2006, the median age at diagnosis for cancer of the liver and intrahepatic bile duct was 64 years of age. Approximately 1.1% were diagnosed under age 20; 1.0% between 20 and 34; 3.7% between 35 and 44; 20.3% between 45 and 54; 24.6% between 55 and 64; 23.5% between 65 and 74; 19.8% between 75 and 84; and 5.9% 85 or more years of age.

U.S. mortality: From 2002–2006, the median age at death for cancer of the liver and intrahepatic bile duct was 70 years of age. Approximately 0.3% died under age 20; 0.7% between 20 and 34; 2.5% between 35 and 44; 15.0% between 45 and 54; 20.5% between 55 and 64; 24.1% between 65 and 74; 26.2% between 75 and 84; and 10.7% 85 or more years of age.

Survival: The overall five-year relative survival rate for 1999–2005 from 17 SEER geographic areas was 13.1%. Five-year relative survival rates by race and sex were: 12.4% for white men; 13.6% for white women; 8.3% for black men; 10.0% for black women.

Lung Cancer

It is estimated that 219,440 men and women (116,090 men and 103,350 women) will be diagnosed with and 159,390 men and women will die of cancer of the lung and bronchus in 2009.

SEER incidence: From 2002–2006, the median age at diagnosis for cancer of the lung and bronchus was 71 years of age. Approximately 0.0% were diagnosed under age 20; 0.2% between 20 and 34; 1.8% between 35 and 44; 8.8% between 45 and 54; 21.0% between 55 and 64; 31.4% between 65 and 74; 29.1% between 75 and 84; and 7.7% 85 or more years of age.

U.S. mortality: From 2002–2006, the median age at death for cancer of the lung and bronchus was 72 years of age. Approximately 0.0% died under age 20; 0.1% between 20 and 34; 1.5% between 35 and 44; 7.9% between 45 and 54; 19.6% between 55 and 64; 30.9% between 65 and 74; 30.7% between 75 and 84; and 9.3% 85 or more years of age.

Survival: The overall five-year relative survival rate for 1999–2005 from 17 SEER geographic areas was 15.6%. Five-year relative survival rates by race and sex were: 13.7% for white men; 18.3% for white women; 10.8% for black men; 14.5% for black women.

Lymphoma

It is estimated that 74,490 men and women (40,630 men and 33,860 women) will be diagnosed with and 20,790 men and women will die of lymphoma in 2009.

SEER incidence: From 2002–2006, the median age at diagnosis for lymphoma was 64 years of age. Approximately 3.0% were diagnosed under age 20; 7.5% between 20 and 34; 8.4% between 35 and 44; 13.7% between 45 and 54; 17.8% between 55 and 64; 20.4% between 65 and 74; 21.4% between 75 and 84; and 7.8% 85 or more years of age.

U.S. mortality: From 2002–2006, the median age at death for lymphoma was 75 years of age. Approximately 0.6% died under age 20; 2.3% between 20 and 34; 3.2% between 35 and 44; 7.4% between 45 and 54; 14.0% between 55 and 64; 22.5% between 65 and 74; 33.0% between 75 and 84; and 17.0% 85 or more years of age.

Survival: The overall five-year relative survival rate for 1999–2005 from 17 SEER geographic areas was 69.9%. Five-year relative survival rates by race and sex were: 69.0% for white men; 72.6% for white women; 58.4% for black men; 68.6% for black women.

Myeloma

It is estimated that 20,580 men and women (11,680 men and 8,900 women) will be diagnosed with and 10,580 men and women will die of myeloma in 2009.

SEER incidence: From 2002–2006, the median age at diagnosis for myeloma was 70 years of age. Approximately 0.0% were diagnosed under age 20; 0.5% between 20 and 34; 3.3% between 35 and 44; 11.9% between 45 and 54; 20.7% between 55 and 64; 26.5% between 65 and 74; 27.6% between 75 and 84; and 9.5% 85 or more years of age.

U.S. mortality: From 2002–2006, the median age at death for myeloma was 74 years of age. Approximately 0.0% died under age 20; 0.1% between 20 and 34; 1.3% between 35 and 44; 6.4% between 45 and 54; 15.7% between 55 and 64; 26.8% between 65 and 74; 34.9% between 75 and 84; and 14.9% 85 or more years of age.

Survival: The overall five-year relative survival rate for 1999-2005 from 17 SEER geographic areas was 37.1%. Five-year relative survival rates by race and sex were: 38.6% for white men; 34.9% for white women; 36.0% for black men; 37.2% for black women.

Oral Cancer

It is estimated that 35,720 men and women (25,240 men and 10,480 women) will be diagnosed with and 7,600 men and women will die of cancer of the oral cavity and pharynx in 2009.

SEER incidence: From 2002–2006, the median age at diagnosis for cancer of the oral cavity and pharynx was 62 years of age. Approximately 0.6% were diagnosed under age 20; 2.4% between 20 and 34; 6.8% between 35 and 44; 20.9% between 45 and 54; 26.2% between 55 and 64; 21.3% between 65 and 74; 16.1% between 75 and 84; and 5.8% 85 or more years of age.

U.S. mortality: From 2002–2006, the median age at death for cancer of the oral cavity and pharynx was 68 years of age. Approximately 0.2% died under age 20; 0.8% between 20 and 34; 3.4% between 35 and 44; 14.6% between 45 and 54; 23.6% between 55 and 64; 23.9% between 65 and 74; 22.2% between 75 and 84; and 11.2% 85 or more years of age.

Survival: The overall five-year relative survival rate for 1999–2005 from 17 SEER geographic areas was 61.0%. Five-year relative survival rates by race and sex were: 62.4% for white men; 63.8% for white women; 38.2% for black men; 53.2% for black women.

Ovarian Cancer

It is estimated that 21,550 women will be diagnosed with and 14,600 women will die of cancer of the ovary in 2009.

SEER incidence: From 2002–2006, the median age at diagnosis for cancer of the ovary was 63 years of age. Approximately 1.3% were diagnosed under age 20; 3.5% between 20 and 34; 7.4% between 35 and 44; 18.9% between 45 and 54; 22.3% between 55 and 64; 19.9% between 65 and 74; 19.0% between 75 and 84; and 7.6% 85 or more years of age.

U.S. mortality: From 2002–2006, the median age at death for cancer of the ovary was 71 years of age. Approximately 0.1% died under age 20; 0.7% between 20 and 34; 3.0% between 35 and 44; 11.3% between 45 and 54; 19.7% between 55 and 64; 24.4% between 65 and 74; 28.1% between 75 and 84; and 12.7% 85 or more years of age.

Survival: The overall five-year relative survival rate for 1999-2005 from 17 SEER geographic areas was 45.9%. Five-year relative survival rates by race were: 45.8% for white women; 37.4% for black women.

Pancreatic Cancer

It is estimated that 42,470 men and women (21,050 men and 21,420 women) will be diagnosed with and 35,240 men and women will die of cancer of the pancreas in 2009.

SEER incidence: From 2002–2006, the median age at diagnosis for cancer of the pancreas was 72 years of age. Approximately 0.0% were diagnosed under age 20; 0.4% between 20 and 34; 2.4% between 35 and 44; 9.6% between 45 and 54; 19.2% between 55 and 64; 26.1% between 65 and 74; 29.4% between 75 and 84; and 12.8% 85 or more years of age.

U.S. Mortality: From 2002–2006, the median age at death for cancer of the pancreas was 73 years of age. Approximately 0.0% died under age 20; 0.2% between 20 and 34; 1.7% between 35 and 44; 8.2% between 45 and 54; 17.9% between 55 and 64; 25.9% between 65 and 74; 31.1% between 75 and 84; and 14.9% 85 or more years of age.

Survival: The overall five-year relative survival rate for 1999–2005 from 17 SEER geographic areas was 5.5%. Five-year relative survival rates by race and sex were: 5.5% for white men; 5.5% for white women; 4.5% for black men; 6.2% for black women.

Prostate Cancer

It is estimated that 192,280 men will be diagnosed with and 27,360 men will die of cancer of the prostate in 2009.

SEER incidence: From 2002–2006, the median age at diagnosis for cancer of the prostate was 68 years of age. Approximately 0.0% were diagnosed under age 20; 0.0% between 20 and 34; 0.6% between 35 and 44; 8.7% between 45 and 54; 29.0% between 55 and 64; 35.6% between 65 and 74; 21.4% between 75 and 84; and 4.7% 85 or more years of age.

U.S. mortality: From 2002–2006, the median age at death for cancer of the prostate was 80 years of age. Approximately 0.0% died under age 20; 0.0% between 20 and 34; 0.1% between 35 and 44; 1.4% between 45 and 54; 7.2% between 55 and 64; 20.1% between 65 and 74; 40.9% between 75 and 84; and 30.3% 85 or more years of age.

Survival: The overall five-year relative survival rate for 1999–2005 from 17 SEER geographic areas was 99.7%. Five-year relative survival rates by race were: 99.9% for white men; 96.5% for black men.

Skin Cancer

The statistics in this section exclude basal cell and squamous cell carcinoma. It is estimated that 74,610 men and women (42,920 men and 31,690 women) will be diagnosed with and 11,590 men and women will die of cancer of the skin in 2009.

SEER incidence: From 2002-2006, the median age at diagnosis for cancer of the skin was 60 years of age. Approximately 0.9% were diagnosed under age 20; 7.7% between 20 and 34; 12.0% between 35 and 44; 18.3% between 45 and 54; 19.4% between 55 and 64; 17.8% between 65 and 74; 17.6% between 75 and 84; and 6.3% 85 or more years of age.

U.S. mortality: From 2002-2006, the median age at death for cancer of the skin was 70 years of age. Approximately 0.1% died under age 20; 2.3% between 20 and 34; 5.7% between 35 and 44; 13.0% between 45 and 54; 18.3% between 55 and 64; 20.7% between 65 and 74; 25.1% between 75 and 84; and 14.8% 85 or more years of age.

Survival: The overall five-year relative survival rate for 1999–2005 from 17 SEER geographic areas was 91.1%. Five-year relative survival rates by race and sex were: 88.6% for white men; 93.7% for white women; 86.2% for black men; 91.1% for black women.

Small Intestine Cancer

It is estimated that 6,230 men and women (3,240 men and 2,990 women) will be diagnosed with and 1,110 men and women will die of cancer of the small intestine in 2009.

SEER incidence: From 2002–2006, the median age at diagnosis for cancer of the small intestine was 67 years of age. Approximately 0.2% were diagnosed under age 20; 1.8% between 20 and 34; 6.0% between 35 and 44; 14.9% between 45 and 54; 21.9% between 55 and 64; 24.8% between 65 and 74; 22.2% between 75 and 84; and 8.1% 85 or more years of age.

U.S. mortality: From 2002–2006, the median age at death for cancer of the small intestine was 71 years of age. Approximately 0.0% died under age 20; 0.9% between 20 and 34; 4.1% between 35 and 44; 10.5% between 45 and 54; 18.3% between 55 and 64; 24.1% between 65 and 74; 28.9% between 75 and 84; and 13.3% 85 or more years of age.

Survival: The overall five-year relative survival rate for 1999–2005 from 17 SEER geographic areas was 61.7%. Five-year relative survival rates by race and sex were: 63.7% for white men; 63.8% for white women; 50.3% for black men; 55.3% for black women.

Soft Tissue Cancer

It is estimated that 10,660 men and women (5,780 men and 4,880 women) will be diagnosed with and 3,820 men and women will die of cancer of the soft tissue including heart in 2009.

SEER incidence: From 2002–2006, the median age at diagnosis for cancer of the soft tissue including heart was 57 years of age. Approximately 9.9% were diagnosed under age 20; 9.8% between 20 and 34; 11.2% between 35 and 44; 14.9% between 45 and 54; 15.7% between 55 and 64; 15.5% between 65 and 74; 16.3% between 75 and 84; and 6.7% 85 or more years of age.

U.S. mortality: From 2002–2006, the median age at death for cancer of the soft tissue including heart was 65 years of age. Approximately 4.1% died under age 20; 6.5% between 20 and 34; 7.3% between 35 and 44; 13.5% between 45 and 54; 17.5% between 55 and 64; 19.2% between 65 and 74; 21.7% between 75 and 84; and 10.2% 85 or more years of age.

Survival: The overall five-year relative survival rate for 1999–2005 from 17 SEER geographic areas was 67.2%. Five-year relative survival rates by race and sex were: 67.5% for white men; 68.2% for white women; 61.4% for black men; 60.5% for black women.

Stomach Cancer

It is estimated that 21,130 men and women (12,820 men and 8,310 women) will be diagnosed with and 10,620 men and women will die of cancer of the stomach in 2009.

SEER incidence: From 2002–2006, the median age at diagnosis for cancer of the stomach was 71 years of age. Approximately 0.1% were diagnosed under age 20; 1.5% between 20 and 34; 4.8% between 35 and 44; 11.6% between 45 and 54; 17.7% between 55 and 64; 24.6% between 65 and 74; 27.7% between 75 and 84; and 12.0% 85 or more years of age.

U.S. mortality: From 2002–2006, the median age at death for cancer of the stomach was 73 years of age. Approximately 0.0% died under age 20; 1.2% between 20 and 34; 3.9% between 35 and 44; 9.7% between 45 and 54; 15.7% between 55 and 64; 22.8% between 65 and 74; 29.5% between 75 and 84; and 17.2% 85 or more years of age.

Survival: The overall five-year relative survival rate for 1999–2005 from 17 SEER geographic areas was 25.7%. Five-year relative survival rates by race and sex were: 22.5% for white men; 26.7% for white women; 22.6% for black men; 28.4% for black women.

Testicular Cancer

It is estimated that 8,400 men will be diagnosed with and 380 men will die of cancer of the testis in 2009.

SEER incidence: From 2002–2006, the median age at diagnosis for cancer of the testis was 34 years of age. Approximately 5.5% were diagnosed under age 20; 46.6% between 20 and 34; 28.9% between 35 and 44; 13.5% between 45 and 54; 3.5% between 55 and 64; 1.1% between 65 and 74; 0.6% between 75 and 84; and 0.2% 85 or more years of age.

U.S. mortality: From 2002–2006, the median age at death for cancer of the testis was 40 years of age. Approximately 2.9% died under age 20; 32.0% between 20 and 34; 25.4% between 35 and 44; 18.4% between 45 and 54; 8.9% between 55 and 64; 5.2% between 65 and 74; 4.3% between 75 and 84; and 2.8% 85 or more years of age.

Survival: The overall five-year relative survival rate for 1999–2005 from 17 SEER geographic areas was 95.3%. Five-year relative survival rates by race were: 95.6% for white men; 88.4% for black men.

Thyroid Cancer

It is estimated that 37,200 men and women (10,000 men and 27,200 women) will be diagnosed with and 1,630 men and women will die of cancer of the thyroid in 2009.

SEER incidence: From 2002–2006, the median age at diagnosis for cancer of the thyroid was 48 years of age. Approximately 1.8% were diagnosed under age 20; 16.9% between 20 and 34; 22.0% between 35 and 44; 23.8% between 45 and 54; 16.9% between 55 and 64; 11.1% between 65 and 74; 6.2% between 75 and 84; and 1.4% 85 or more years of age.

U.S. mortality: From 2002–2006, the median age at death for cancer of the thyroid was 73 years of age. Approximately 0.1% died under age 20; 0.9% between 20 and 34; 2.6% between 35 and 44; 8.5% between 45 and 54; 17.0% between 55 and 64; 24.0% between 65 and 74; 30.3% between 75 and 84; and 16.6% 85 or more years of age.

Survival: The overall five-year relative survival rate for 1999–2005 from 17 SEER geographic areas was 97.3%. Five-year relative survival rates by race and sex were: 94.8% for white men; 98.2% for white women; 91.4% for black men; 95.5% for black women.

Urinary Bladder Cancer

It is estimated that 70,980 men and women (52,810 men and 18,170 women) will be diagnosed with and 14,330 men and women will die of cancer of the urinary bladder in 2009.

SEER incidence: From 2002–2006, the median age at diagnosis for cancer of the urinary bladder was 73 years of age. Approximately 0.1% were diagnosed under age 20; 0.5% between 20 and 34; 2.0% between 35 and 44; 7.5% between 45 and 54; 17.8% between 55 and 64; 27.5% between 65 and 74; 32.1% between 75 and 84; and 12.5% 85 or more years of age.

U.S. mortality: From 2002–2006, the median age at death for cancer of the urinary bladder was 78 years of age. Approximately 0.0% died under age 20; 0.1% between 20 and 34; 0.9% between 35 and 44; 4.0% between 45 and 54; 11.1% between 55 and 64; 21.5% between 65 and 74; 36.9% between 75 and 84; and 25.4% 85 or more years of age.

Survival: The overall five-year relative survival rate for 1999–2005 from 17 SEER geographic areas was 80.0%. Five-year relative survival rates by race and sex were: 81.7% for white men; 77.0% for white women; 71.5% for black men; 57.3% for black women.

Vulvar Cancer

It is estimated that 3,580 women will be diagnosed with and 900 women will die of cancer of the vulva in 2009.

SEER incidence: From 2002–2006, the median age at diagnosis for cancer of the vulva was 68 years of age. Approximately 0.2% were diagnosed under age 20; 2.3% between 20 and 34; 8.3% between 35 and 44; 16.1% between 45 and 54; 16.8% between 55 and 64; 17.1% between 65 and 74; 24.7% between 75 and 84; and 14.4% 85 or more years of age.

U.S. mortality: From 2002–2006, the median age at death for cancer of the vulva was 79 years of age. Approximately 0.0% died under age 20; 0.7% between 20 and 34; 2.3% between 35 and 44; 6.5% between 45 and 54; 10.9% between 55 and 64; 17.4% between 65 and 74; 32.7% between 75 and 84; and 29.4% 85 or more years of age.

Survival: The overall five-year relative survival rate for 1999-2005 from 17 SEER geographic areas was 76.1%. Five-year relative survival rates by race were: 76.5% for white women; 70.1% for black women.

Chapter 3

Cancer Health Disparities

How does the National Cancer Institute (NCI) define "cancer health disparities?"

The National Cancer Institute (NCI) defines "cancer health disparities" as adverse differences in cancer incidence (new cases), cancer prevalence (all existing cases), cancer death (mortality), cancer survivorship, and burden of cancer or related health conditions that exist among specific population groups in the United States. These population groups may be characterized by age, disability, education, ethnicity, gender, geographic location, income, or race. People who are poor, lack health insurance, and are medically underserved (have limited or no access to effective health care)—regardless of ethnic and racial background—often bear a greater burden of disease than the general population.

A close look at cancer incidence and death statistics reveals that certain groups in this country suffer disproportionately from cancer and its associated effects, including premature death. For example, African Americans/Blacks, Asian Americans, Hispanic/Latinos, American Indians, Alaska Natives, and underserved Whites are more likely than the general population to have higher incidence and death statistics for certain types of cancer.

From "Cancer Health Disparities," National Cancer Institute (www.cancer.gov), March 11, 2008.

What factors contribute to cancer health disparities?

Complex and interrelated factors contribute to the observed disparities in cancer incidence and death among racial, ethnic, and underserved groups. The most obvious factors are associated with a lack of
health care coverage and low socioeconomic status (SES).

SES is most often based on a person's income, education level, occupation, and other factors, such as social status in the community
and where he or she lives. Studies have found that SES, more than
race or ethnicity, predicts the likelihood of an individual's or a group's
access to education, certain occupations, health insurance, and living
conditions—including conditions where exposure to environmental
toxins is most common—all of which are associated with the risk of
developing and surviving cancer. SES, in particular, appears to play a
major role in influencing the prevalence of behavioral risk factors for
cancer (for example, tobacco smoking, physical inactivity, obesity, and
excessive alcohol intake, and health status), as well as in following
cancer screening recommendations.

Research also shows that individuals from medically underserved
populations are more likely to be diagnosed with late-stage diseases
that might have been treated more effectively or cured if diagnosed
earlier. Financial, physical, and cultural beliefs are also barriers that
prevent individuals or groups from obtaining effective health care.

How does NCI gather data on cancer incidence and death for various population groups in the United States?

The Surveillance, Epidemiology, and End Results (SEER) Program
is NCI's authoritative source for information about cancer incidence
and survival. SEER collects cancer incidence and survival data from
cancer registries that cover approximately 26% of the U.S. population.
Over several decades, SEER has worked diligently to better represent
racial, ethnic, and socioeconomic diversity and currently covers 23%
of African Americans/Blacks, 40% of Hispanic/Latinos, 42% of American Indians and Alaska Natives, 53% of Asian Americans, and 70%
of Hawaiian/Pacific Islanders living in the United States. In addition,
SEER statistics reflect the U.S. population in regard to poverty and
education, with both urban and rural groups represented. The *Methods for Measuring Cancer Disparities: A Review Using Data Relevant
to Healthy People 2010 Cancer-Related Objectives* report (http://seer
.cancer.gov/publications/disparities/) describes how data are collected
to measure cancer health disparities.

The incidence and death statistics presented in this chapter are from Tables I-23 through I-28 of the *SEER Cancer Statistics Review, 1975–2004*. These statistics are most often reported as the numbers of new cases of invasive cancer and cancer deaths per year per 100,000 persons in the U.S. population. When the statistics focus on cancer incidence and death in a single gender—for example, on female breast cancer or male prostate cancer—the numbers are per 100,000 persons of that gender. In addition, the SEER statistics are age-adjusted to the 2000 U.S. standard population. Age-adjustment is done because different population groups may not be comparable with respect to age. Age-adjustment allows cancer incidence and death statistics (expressed below as cancer incidence and death "rates") for these population groups to be compared.

What are the overall cancer incidence and death rates for different populations living in the United States?

Although cancer deaths have declined for both Whites and African Americans/Blacks living in the United States, African Americans/Blacks continue to suffer the greatest burden for each of the most common types of cancer. For all cancers combined, the death rate is 25% higher for African Americans/Blacks than for Whites. Incidence and death rates for all cancers among U.S. racial/ethnic groups are shown in Table 3.1.

Table 3.1. Overall Cancer Incidence and Death Rates, All Sites

Racial/Ethnic Group	Incidence	Death
All	470.1	192.7
African American/Black	504.1	238.8
Asian/Pacific Islander	314.9	115.5
Hispanic/Latino	356.0	129.1
American Indian/Alaska Native	297.6	160.4
White	477.5	190.7

Statistics are for 2000–2004, age-adjusted to the 2000 U.S. standard million population, and represent the number of new cases of invasive cancer and deaths per year per 100,000 men and women.

How do breast cancer incidence and death rates differ for women from different racial or ethnic groups?

In the United States, White women have the highest incidence rate for breast cancer, although African American/Black women are most likely to die from the disease. Breast cancer incidence and death rates are lower for women from other racial and ethnic groups than for White and African American/Black women. Incidence and death rates for female breast cancer are shown in Table 3.2.

Table 3.2. Female Breast Cancer Incidence and Death Rates

Racial/Ethnic Group	Incidence	Death
All	127.8	25.5
African American/Black	118.3	33.8
Asian/Pacific Islander	89.0	12.6
Hispanic/Latino	89.3	16.1
American Indian/Alaska Native	69.8	16.1
White	132.5	25.0

Statistics are for 2000–2004, age-adjusted to the 2000 U.S. standard million population, and represent the number of new cases of invasive cancer and deaths per year per 100,000 women.

What factors might contribute to the higher breast cancer death rate observed in African American/Black women?

Lack of medical coverage, barriers to early detection and screening, and unequal access to improvements in cancer treatment may contribute to observed differences in survival between African American/Black and White women. In addition, recent NCI-supported research indicates that aggressive breast tumors are more common in younger African American/Black and Hispanic/Latino women living in low SES areas. This more aggressive form of breast cancer is less responsive to standard cancer treatments and is associated with poorer survival.

How do cervical cancer incidence and death rates differ for women from different racial or ethnic groups?

Compared to White women in the general population, African American/Black women are more likely to be diagnosed with cervical cancer. Hispanic/Latino women, however, have the highest cervical cancer incidence rate. Interestingly, White women living in Appalachia suffer a disproportionately higher risk for developing cervical cancer than other White women. The highest death rate from cervical cancer is among African American/Black women. Incidence and death rates for cervical cancer are shown in Table 3.3.

Table 3.3. Cervical Cancer Incidence and Death Rates

Racial/Ethnic Group	Incidence	Death
All	8.7	2.6
African American/Black	11.4	4.9
Asian/Pacific Islander	8.0	2.4
Hispanic/Latino	13.8	3.3
American Indian/Alaska Native	6.6	4.0
White	8.5	2.3

Statistics are for 2000–2004, age-adjusted to the 2000 U.S. standard million population, and represent the number of new cases of invasive cancer and deaths per year per 100,000 women.

What factors might contribute to the greater burden of cervical cancer among Hispanic/Latino and African American/Black women?

The disproportionate burden of cervical cancer in Hispanic/Latino and African American/Black women is primarily due to a lack of screening. In an effort to understand this disparity in cervical cancer screening, NCI conducted a study of regions within the United States where cervical cancer incidence rates are high. They found that cervical cancer rates reflected a larger problem of unequal access to health care. The *Excess Cervical Cancer Mortality: A Marker for Low Access to Health Care in Poor Communities* report (http://crchd.cancer.gov/ attachments/excess-cervcanmort.pdf) supports reaching these medically underserved groups through culturally sensitive trained care providers; increasing the number of female health providers, particularly those of the same race or ethnicity; and removing cultural and economic barriers to break down resistance to screening for cervical and other cancers.

41

Persistent infection with certain strains of the human papillomavirus (HPV) is the major cause of most cases of cervical cancer. An HPV vaccine is now available that targets two strains of the virus that are associated with development of cervical cancer and account for approximately 70% of all cases of cervical cancer worldwide. This vaccine prevents infection by two HPV strains and has the potential to reduce cervical cancer-related health disparities both in the United States and around the world.

How do prostate cancer incidence and death rates differ for men from different racial or ethnic groups?

African American/Black men have the highest incidence rate for prostate cancer in the United States and are more than twice as likely as White men to die of the disease. The lowest death rates for prostate cancer are found in Asian/Pacific Islander men. Incidence and death rates for prostate cancer are shown in Table 3.4.

Table 3.4. Prostate Cancer Incidence and Death Rates

Racial/Ethnic Group	Incidence	Death
All	168.0	27.9
African American/Black	255.5	62.3
Asian/Pacific Islander	96.5	11.3
Hispanic/Latino	140.8	21.2
American Indian/Alaska Native	68.2	21.5
White	161.4	25.6

Statistics are for 2000–2004, age-adjusted to the 2000 U.S. standard million population, and represent the number of new cases of invasive cancer and deaths per year per 100,000 men.

What factors might contribute to the disproportionate burden of prostate cancer among African American/Black men?

The higher incidence of prostate cancer in African American/Black men compared with men from other racial/ethnic groups prompted the hypothesis that genetic factors might account, in part, for the observed differences. Recent findings from NCI's Cancer Genetic Markers of Susceptibility (CGEMS) program (http://cgems.cancer.gov/) and other investigations support this hypothesis. Researchers have identified changes—called variants—in human DNA that are associated with the risk of developing prostate cancer. Different combinations of these variants have been found in men from different racial/ethnic backgrounds, and each combination is associated with higher or lower risk for prostate cancer. Nearly all of the variants associated with an increased risk of developing prostate cancer were found most often in African American/Black men, and certain combinations of these variants were associated with a five-fold increased risk of prostate cancer in men of this racial/ethnic group.

In addition, research has shown that low SES, lack of health insurance coverage, unequal access to health care services, and absence of ties to a primary care physician are barriers to screening for prostate cancer and the timely diagnosis of this disease, making African American/Black men less likely to receive regular physical examinations and screening for prostate cancer.

Do incidence and death rates differ for colorectal or lung cancer among various racial and ethnic groups?

African American/Black men and women have the highest incidence and death rates for both colorectal and lung cancers, while Hispanic/Latinos have the lowest rates. Colorectal and lung cancer incidence and death rates are shown in Table 3.5.

Table 3.5. Colorectal and Lung Cancer Incidence and Death Rates

Racial/Ethnic Group	Colorectal		Lung and Bronchus	
	Incidence	Death	Incidence	Death
All	51.6	19.4	64.5	54.7
African American/Black	62.1	26.7	76.6	62.0
Asian/Pacific Islander	41.6	12.3	39.4	26.9
Hispanic/Latino	39.3	13.6	33.3	23.6
American Indian/Alaska Native	40.8	17.0	44.0	39.9
White	51.2	18.9	65.7	55.0

Statistics are for 2000–2004, age-adjusted to the 2000 U.S. standard million population, and represent the number of new cases of invasive cancer and deaths per year per 100,000 men and women.

Which cancers are diagnosed most often in Asian/Pacific Islander populations?

Asian Americans and Pacific Islanders have the highest incidence rates for both liver and stomach cancer and are twice as likely to die from these cancers as Whites. Incidence and death rates for stomach, liver, and bile duct cancers are shown in Table 3.6.

Table 3.6. Liver and Stomach Cancer

Racial/Ethnic Group	Liver and Bile Duct		Stomach	
	Incidence	Death	Incidence	Death
All	6.2	4.9	8.1	4.2
African American/Black	7.6	6.5	12.5	8.2
Asian/Pacific Islander	13.9	10.6	14.3	8.0
Hispanic/Latino	9.7	7.6	12.3	6.8
American Indian/Alaska Native	9.7	8.4	11.5	7.2
White	5.2	4.5	7.1	3.7

Statistics are for 2000–2004, age-adjusted to the 2000 U.S. standard million population, and represent the number of new cases of invasive cancer and deaths per year per 100,000 men and women.

Why is stomach cancer more commonly diagnosed in Asian/Pacific Islander populations?

Asian/Pacific Islanders, similar to Hispanic/Latinos, have lower incidence rates than Whites for most common cancers. However, they suffer more often from cancers that are related to infections. One risk factor for stomach cancer is infection with a bacterium called *Helicobacter pylori*, or *H. pylori*. Although additional study is needed, infection with *H. pylori* may explain, in part, why Asian/Pacific Islander populations have higher rates for this type of cancer.

Which cancer is more commonly diagnosed in American Indian and Alaska Native populations?

American Indians and Alaska Natives have higher incidence and death rates for kidney cancer than other racial/ethnic groups. However, these rates should be viewed with caution because the data currently available for American Indian/Alaska Native populations are not representative. An analysis of cancer incidence and mortality data within Native American populations is the focus of the *Annual Report to the Nation on the Status of Cancer 197–2004, Featuring Cancer in American Indians and Alaska Natives* (http://www.interscience.wiley .com/cancer/report2007), a yearly publication that summarizes the latest cancer statistics. Incidence and death rates for kidney and renal pelvis cancers are shown in Table 3.7.

Table 3.7. Kidney Cancer Incidence and Death Rates (Kidney and Renal Pelvis)

Racial/Ethnic Group	Incidence	Death
All	12.8	4.2
African American/Black	14.3	4.1
Asian/Pacific Islander	6.3	1.7
Hispanic/Latino	12.4	3.6
American Indian/Alaska Native	14.7	6.5
White	13.3	4.3

Statistics are for 2000–2004, age-adjusted to the 2000 U.S. standard million population, and represent the number of new cases of invasive cancer and deaths per year per 100,000 men and women.

How is NCI working in a coordinated way to reduce cancer health disparities?

NCI has a longstanding history of pursuing research aimed at understanding and addressing cancer health disparities. As many as 20 years ago, NCI established the Special Populations Studies Branch to study groups of people within the United States who suffer a greater burden of cancer. NCI's commitment to underserved populations continued to grow and mature over the years, and, in 2001, the institute established the Center to Reduce Cancer Health Disparities (CRCHD) to serve as the cornerstone of NCI's efforts to reduce the unequal burden of cancer in our nation.

Today, CRCHD is working to strengthen and integrate NCI's studies in basic, clinical, translational, and community-based research that offer opportunities to advance our understanding of cancer-related health disparities and ways to effectively address them. CRCHD manages specific programs and grants aimed at examining the diverse aspects of cancer-related disparities. These programs are addressing the cultural barriers and biases that racial and ethnic minorities encounter in obtaining appropriate and timely treatment, as well as financial and physical restraints that prevent underserved populations from obtaining quality health care. CRCHD is also leading NCI's efforts to train students and investigators from diverse populations to pursue research in cancer, as well as research examining factors that contribute to cancer health disparities.

CRCHD also cosponsors an annual Cancer Health Disparities Summit. During this three-day meeting, NCI-funded researchers from training, education, and outreach programs gather to discuss both disparities issues that are present in their communities and possible solutions for these issues.

What are some of NCI's programs and projects aimed at addressing cancer health disparities and increasing access to quality cancer care for medically underserved communities?

NCI and its divisions support diverse research programs that address the behavioral, biological, treatment, prevention, and economic issues that all contribute to cancer health disparities. The programs listed below highlight NCI's commitment to addressing the needs of the medically underserved.

NCI Community Cancer Centers Program (NCCCP)
http://ncccp.cancer.gov/index.htm

In 2007, NCI launched the pilot phase of the NCCCP, an initiative that aims to bring the latest advances in cancer care to patients in their own communities. Over the next three years, 16 community hospitals and health care systems will work with NCI to identify the best strategies for delivering state-of-the-art cancer care to the greatest number of Americans in the communities in which they live. The program seeks to bring more Americans into a system of high-quality cancer care, increase participation in clinical trials, reduce cancer health care disparities, and improve information sharing among community cancer centers. The NCCCP will focus on underserved communities and groups that are disproportionately affected by cancer.

The Centers for Population Health and Health Disparities (CPHHD)
http://cancercontrol.cancer.gov/populationhealthcenters

Initiated in 2003, the CPHHD supports a transdisciplinary approach to overcoming health disparities. The eight centers of the CPHHD initiative are supported by a collaboration of NCI and other National Institutes of Health institutes and offices. NCI supports five of the eight centers that address cancer health disparities through innovative research to understand the complex interaction of the social and physical environment, in combination with behavioral and biological factors that determine health and disease in diverse populations.

The Community Networks Program (CNP)
http://crchd.cancer.gov/cnp/background.html

The CNP aims to reduce cancer health disparities through community-based education, training, and research among racial and ethnic minorities and medically underserved populations. The overall goal of this program is to significantly improve access to—and use of—beneficial cancer interventions and treatments in communities experiencing cancer health disparities.

Minority-Based Community Clinical Oncology Program (MB-CCOP)
http://prevention.cancer.gov/programs-resources/programs/ccop

Initiated in 1990, the MB-CCOP provides underserved cancer patients with access to state-of-the-art cancer treatment and prevention in their own communities. In addition, as part of NCI's effort to reduce cancer health disparities in minority populations, the program encourages physicians who are practicing in these communities to become involved in NCI-approved clinical trials. Over the past decade, more than 5,500 minority patients have enrolled in both treatment and prevention clinical trials sponsored by NCI through the MB-CCOP network.

The Cancer Disparities Research Partnership (CDRP) Program
http://www3.cancer.gov/rrp/CDRP/index.html

The CDRP is a unique research program that supports the planning, development, and conduct of radiation oncology clinical trials in institutions that care for a disproportionate number of medically underserved, low-income, ethnic and minority populations that have not been traditionally involved in NCI-sponsored research. The CDRP works to establish partnerships between large comprehensive centers and smaller community centers so that the smaller centers can build and sustain an effective radiation oncology clinical trial program.

Patient Navigation Program (PNP)
http://crchd.cancer.gov/pnp/background.html

The PNP was developed to help guide cancer patients from underserved populations through the complex journey of seeking treatment and overcoming language, financial, and cultural barriers that often undermine their care. The PNP places patients in contact with trained, culturally sensitive health care workers, or "navigators," from local communities. Navigators help minority cancer patients obtain accurate information about their diagnosis and treatment procedures, assist in gaining access to hospitals and clinics, provide guidance on financial assistance, and help with tracking their medical records and obtaining prescriptions.

Southern Community Cohort Study
http://epi.grants.cancer.gov/ResPort/Southern.html

This NCI-funded study will follow about 100,000 residents from six southeastern states—two-thirds of whom are African American/Black—to determine what roles diet, lifestyle, occupation, and environmental factors play in the development of common types of cancer, such as prostate, lung, breast, and colon cancers.

Cancer Information Service (CIS)
http://www.cancer.gov/cancertopics/factsheet/Information/CIS

NCI established the CIS in 1975 to educate people about cancer prevention, risk factors, early detection, symptoms, diagnosis, treatment, and research. The three components of this program—the Partnership Program, Information Service, and Research Program—work together to reach many audiences, particularly those who are adversely affected by health disparities. Through a network of 15 regional offices across the country, the CIS serves the United States and its territories. Each regional center collaborates with partners in their communities to disseminate cancer control information and develop education programs to improve the health of minority and medically underserved populations. Currently, there are over 600 partners from nonprofit, private, and other government organizations at the national, regional, and state levels that are working with the CIS Partnership Program. Through the Information Service, CIS information specialists provide the latest, most-accurate information about cancer by telephone (800-4-CANCER), instant messaging, and e-mail through NCI's Web site. The CIS Research Program participates in cancer control and health communications research that supports NCI's priorities and programs. To date, the CIS has collaborated on more than 50 studies that have helped researchers learn better ways to communicate with people about healthy lifestyles, health risks, and how to prevent, diagnose, and treat cancer.

NCI Spanish-language Web Site
http://www.cancer.gov/espanol

NCI launched its Spanish-language website in April 2007 to address the language and cultural barriers that many Hispanic/Latinos face when seeking cancer-related information. NCI's Spanish website is not simply a translation of information available on the English-language website; the content is tailored to meet the needs and concerns of the Hispanic community. The Spanish website is a complement to existing Spanish-language resources from NCI, such as those available through the Cancer Information Service (CIS) and the NCI Publications Locator (http://www.cancer.gov/Publications). NCI established the CIS in 1975 to educate people about cancer prevention, risk factors, early detection, symptoms, diagnosis, treatment, and research. CIS information specialists provide the latest, most-accurate information about cancer by telephone (800-4-CANCER), instant messaging, and e-mail.

Continuing Umbrella of Research Experiences (CURE) and Minority Institutions / Cancer Center Partnership (MI/CCP) Programs
http://minorityopportunities.nci.nih.gov/mTraining/index.html
http://minorityopportunities.nci.nih.gov/institutions/miccp.html

NCI supports training programs for students and investigators from diverse populations. The CURE program provides long-term funding to qualified minority students interested in pursuing scientific and cancer-related careers. The MI/CCP program provides funding to support NCI Cancer Centers and other institutions in recruiting minorities to pursue cancer research.

The Network for Cancer Control Research Among American Indian / Alaska Native Populations (AI/AN)
http://crchd.cancer.gov/spn/aian-spcn-pilot.html

The network is an NCI program that fosters collaborations between American Indian/Alaska Native researchers and other researchers and educators. The program's goals are to facilitate the exchange of cancer control information among researchers and to encourage American Indian researchers and medical students to become involved in their community health care programs. The network established the Native Cancer Information Resource Center (Native C.I.R.C.L.E.) in 1998, which serves as a clearinghouse for cancer educational materials that are specific to American Indian and Alaska Native communities.

NCI's Atlas of Cancer Mortality in the United States, 1950–94
http://www3.cancer.gov/atlasplus/new.html

NCI's *Atlas of Cancer Mortality in the United States, 1950–94* is a book of maps, text, tables, and figures showing the geographic patterns of cancer death rates throughout the United States from 1951–1994 for more than 40 types of cancer. Included are maps of cancer mortality specific to African Americans/Blacks. These maps can be used to pinpoint areas of high cancer mortality in the United States and provide avenues to focus future cancer health disparities research.

Tobacco Research Network on Disparities (TReND) Program
http://dccps.nci.nih.gov/tcrb/trend/index.html

To address the high rates of lung cancer in minority populations, NCI, in collaboration with the American Legacy Foundation, initiated the TReND program. This program supports collaborations among researchers to develop new solutions that address tobacco use in underserved communities and to better understand tobacco-related health disparities.

Chapter 4

Lifestyle Issues and Cancer Risk

Chapter Contents

Section 4.1

Tobacco Use and Cancer Risk

From "Tobacco, Smoking and Cancer: The Evidence," © 2009 Cancer Research UK (www.cancerresearchuk.org). Reprinted with permission. Complete text including references is available at http://info.cancerresearchuk.org/healthy living/smokingandtobacco/howdoweknow. Accessed July 2010.

Smoking is the single biggest cause of cancer in the world.

Experts agree that smoking is the single biggest cause of cancer in the world. Smoking causes over a quarter of cancer deaths in developed countries. Around half of current smokers will be killed by their habit if they continue to smoke. And 25–40% of smokers will die in middle age.

Smoking causes even more deaths from other respiratory diseases and heart conditions than from cancer. If current trends continue, scientists estimate that tobacco will kill about one billion people in the twenty-first century.

Smoking greatly increases the risk of lung cancer.

Studies from Europe, Japan, and North America have shown that 9 in 10 lung cancers are caused by smoking. In 2002, lung cancer killed around 33,600 people—about one person every 15 minutes.

Tobacco smoke was first shown to cause lung cancer in 1950. This study found that people who smoked 15–24 cigarettes a day had 26 times the lung cancer risk of non-smokers. And people who smoked less than 15 cigarettes a day still had 8 times the lung cancer risk of non-smokers.

After these first results came out, United Kingdom (UK) scientists began a large study of smoking in British doctors, which Cancer Research UK has helped to fund. This British Doctors' Study has provided much of our current knowledge about the dangers of smoking.

The people with the highest lung cancer risks are those who:

- smoke the most cigarettes per day,
- smoke over long periods of time, and
- start smoking young.

We cannot exactly calculate a person's lung cancer risk based on how many cigarettes they smoke or the number years they have been a smoker. But studies have shown that lung cancer risk is greatest among those who smoke the most cigarettes over the longest period of time.

The length of time spent smoking seems to be the more important of these two factors. The British Doctors' Study found that people who had smoked for 45 years had 100 times the lung cancer risk of people who had smoked for 15 years, regardless of whether they smoked heavily or moderately. And smoking one packet a day for 40 years is about 8 times more dangerous than smoking two packets a day for 20 years.

Even light or irregular smoking can increase the risk of cancer. One study found that even people who smoked 1–4 cigarettes a day had much greater risks of dying from lung cancer or heart disease, while another found that even people who smoke just 2 cigarettes a day are more likely to develop cancers of the mouth and oesophagus (food pipe). And the European Prospective Investigation into Cancer and Nutrition (EPIC) study found that occasional smokers who have never smoked daily, still have higher risks of most cancers, and double the risk of bladder cancer.

Starting smoking at an early age increases the risk of cancer even more. One study found that young smokers are especially vulnerable to DNA damage caused by chemicals in cigarette smoke. And when they quit, they have higher levels of DNA damage than people who started smoking later in life.

Smoking is a major cause of several types of cancer.

Smoking also increases your risk of cancers of the bladder, cervix, kidney, larynx (voice box), pharynx (upper throat), nose, mouth, esophagus (food pipe), pancreas, stomach, liver, and some types of leukemia. And smokers are seven times more likely to die of these cancer than non-smokers.

There is some evidence that smoking could also cause other cancers including bowel cancer and Hodgkin's lymphoma.

Smoking is the most important preventable cause of bladder cancer and causes two in three cases in men and one in three cases in women. It increases the risk of this disease by 3–5 times.

Smoking doubles the risk of kidney cancer, and causes one in four cases in men, and one in ten cases in women.

Smoking is the number one cause of mouth and esophageal cancers, and together with alcohol, causes about nine in ten cases of these cancers. By the age of 75, a non-smoker has a 1 in 125 chance of developing these cancers, but a smoker's odds are 1 in 16.

Smoking is the only established preventable cause of pancreatic cancer, one of the most dangerous types of cancer in the UK. It causes over a quarter of pancreatic cancer cases.

Smoking is the most important preventable cause of stomach cancer and causes about one in five cases.

There is some evidence to suggest that smoking may increase the risk of breast cancer, bowel cancer, and lymphomas but more research will be needed to say for sure.

Stopping smoking can reduce your risk.

A large number of studies have shown that stopping smoking can greatly reduce the risk of smoking-related cancers. And the earlier you stop, the better. The last results from the Doctors' Study show that stopping smoking at 50 halved the excess risk of cancer overall, while stopping at 30 avoided almost all of it.

However, it's never too late to quit. One study found that even people who quit in their sixties can experience health benefits and gain valuable years of life.

The effects of stopping vary depending on the cancer. For example, ten years after stopping, a person's risk of lung cancer falls to about half that of a smoker. And the increased oral and laryngeal cancer risks practically disappear within ten years of stopping. But the risks of bladder cancer are still higher than normal 20 years after stopping.

Cutting down the number of cigarettes you smoke slightly reduces your risk of lung cancer, but you'll only experience the full health benefits if you stop altogether. One study found that even smokers who halved the number of cigarettes they smoked had similar risks of dying from heart disease and only slightly lower risks of dying from cancer.

Tobacco smoke contains many dangerous chemicals.

Scientists have identified about 4,000 different chemicals in tobacco smoke. According to the International Agency for Research into Cancer and the European Network for Smoking Prevention, at least 80 of these chemicals could cause cancer. Many of the other thousands of chemicals are toxic and harmful to your health, including carbon monoxide, hydrogen cyanide and ammonia.

One study compared the amounts of cancer-causing chemicals in tobacco smoke with their ability to cause cancer. It concluded that the chemicals in smoke most likely to increase our risk of cancer include 1,3-butadiene, arsenic, benzene and cadmium.

Cigarettes contain at least 599 different additives including chocolate, vanilla, sugar, liquorice, herbs, and spices. These are not toxic but they make cigarettes taste nicer and ensure that smokers want to continue smoking.

Tobacco smoke contains significant amounts of dangerous chemicals.

Carbon monoxide is the fourth most common chemical in tobacco smoke and can make up 3–5% of its volume. Many of the other toxins are present in lower amounts, but some can still cause major damage at low concentrations.

Even single poisons can lead to substantial cancer risks. For example, benzene is a known cause of leukemia. One study estimated that the benzene in cigarettes is responsible for between 10–50% of the leukemia deaths caused by smoking.

Some studies have suggested that radioactive polonium-210 could account for much of the lung cancer risk caused by smoking. Polonium-210 becomes concentrated in hotspots in smokers' airways, subjecting them to very high doses of high-energy alpha-radiation. One study estimated that smoking 1.5 packs a day leads to as much radiation exposure as having 300 chest X-rays a year.

Chemicals in tobacco smoke can build up to harmful amounts.

Many tobacco poisons disable the cleaning systems that our bodies use to remove toxins. Cadmium overwhelms cleaner enzymes that mop up toxins and convert them into more harmless forms. And many gases such as hydrogen cyanide and ammonia kill cilia, tiny hairs in our airways that help to clear away toxins.

So over time, tobacco poisons can build up to high levels in our blood, substantially increasing our risks of cancer and other diseases. By comparing the levels of toxins in smokers and non-smokers, some studies have found that smokers can have:

- twice as much cadmium in their blood;
- four times as much polonium-210 in their lungs;
- ten times as much benzene in their breath;
- ten times as much arsenic in their blood.

For most of us, much of our exposure to cancer-causing chemicals like benzene, formaldehyde, cadmium, and nitrosamines comes from breathing in tobacco smoke. For example, one study found that smoking households have four times as much benzene in the air as non-smoking households.

The chemicals in smoke are more dangerous in combination than individually.

The cocktail of chemicals in tobacco smoke is even more dangerous as a mix.

Chemicals such as nitrosamines, benzo(a)pyrene, benzene, acrolein, cadmium, and polonium-210 can damage DNA. Studies have shown that benzo[a]pyrene damages a gene called p53 that normally protects our cells from cancer.

One study found that chromium makes polycyclic aromatic hydrocarbons (PAHs) stick more strongly to DNA increasing the chances of serious DNA damage. Others have found that chemicals like arsenic, cadmium, and nickel stop our cells from repairing DNA damage. This worsens the effects of chemicals like benzo(a)pyrene and makes it even more likely that damaged cells will eventually turn cancerous.

The poisons in cigarettes can affect almost every organ in the body.

The many toxins in tobacco smoke can harm many different parts of your body.

Many tobacco poisons can damage your heart and its blood vessels. By comparing the amounts and strengths of different chemicals, one study found that hydrogen cyanide and arsenic alone can cause major damage to our bodies' blood network.

Acrolein, acetaldehyde, and formaldehyde are most likely to cause diseases in our lungs and airways. Gases like hydrogen sulfide and pyridine can also irritate our airways, radioactive polonium-210 deposits damage surrounding cells, and nitrogen oxide constricts the airways, making breathing more difficult.

A protein called hemoglobin carries oxygen round our bloodstream. But carbon monoxide and nitrogen oxide stick more strongly to hemoglobin than oxygen, and reduce the levels of oxygen in our blood. This starves our organs of this vital gas.

Toluene can interfere with the development of brain cells. It also disrupts the insulating sheath that surrounds nerve cells, making them less efficient at carrying signals.

Nicotine is a very addictive drug.

The Royal College of Physicians compared nicotine to other supposedly "harder" drugs such as heroin and cocaine. They looked at many things including how these drugs cause addiction, how difficult it is to stop using them, and how many deaths they caused. The panel concluded that nicotine causes addiction in much the same way as heroin or cocaine and is just as addictive, if not more so, than these "harder" drugs.

Smokers associate smoking with feeling good because nicotine makes the brain release dopamine—a chemical linked to feelings of pleasure. Smokers can also make mental links between abstract things like the taste of cigarettes or the feeling of smoking. These behaviors can become just as addictive as the nicotine itself.

Smokers are still exposed to dangerous chemicals if they smoke filtered or 'low-tar' cigarettes.

Filters do not block out the many toxic gases in smoke, such as hydrogen cyanide, ammonia, and carbon monoxide. They also do nothing to reduce levels of sidestream smoke from the burning end of the cigarette.

Some of the most dangerous chemicals in tobacco smoke, like hydrogen cyanide, are present as gases, and do not count as part of tar. This means that cigarettes with less tar are not necessarily any less dangerous.

Besides, researchers have found that people who smoked low-tar brands smoked harder and more frequently to satisfy their nicotine cravings. For example, in one study, low-tar smokers inhaled 40% more smoke per cigarette and ended up with similar nicotine levels as smokers who use normal brands.

And some smokers block filters with fingers or saliva. One Canadian study showed that over half of discarded cigarette butts showed blocked filters.

According to one study, low-tar smokers ended up inhaling about 80% more smoke, and had similar levels of cancer-causing chemicals in their blood. They can also inhale over twice as much tar and nicotine as smokers of normal brands.

Alcohol and other substances worsen the effect of smoking.

Tobacco, as well as alcohol, can cause mouth, esophageal, and liver cancers. Scientists have also found that together, their effects are much worse. And while alcohol does not cause stomach cancer, it can worsen the risk of this disease in smokers.

One study found that together, smoking and drinking increased liver cancer risk by ten times. And a Spanish team found that people who smoke and drink heavily could increase their risk of esophageal cancer by up to 50 times. This problem is made even worse because heavy drinkers and smokers often have poor diets.

Smoking also interacts with many other cancer risk factors and worsens their effects. For example the lung cancer risk due to exposure to high levels of radon gas is 25 times higher in smokers than in non-smokers.

Second-hand smoking also causes cancer and kills thousands of people every year.

Several studies have shown that breathing in other people's smoke causes cancer in non-smokers. Second-hand smoke contains several cancer causing chemicals. Many of these chemicals are present in higher concentrations than in the smoke inhaled by the smoker themselves.

One study analyzed 55 studies from around the world found that non-smoking spouses of people who smoke at home have 27% higher risks of lung cancer. And a review of 22 studies found that people exposed to second-hand smoke in the workplace have 24% higher risks of lung cancer. Those who were exposed to the highest levels of second-hand smoke at work had twice the risks of lung cancer.

One study estimates that passive smoking may kill over 11,000 people every year in the UK from cancer, heart disease, strokes, and other diseases.

Second-hand smoking also causes other health problems in non-smokers including asthma and heart disease. One study showed that even 30 minutes of exposure to second-hand smoke can reduce blood flow in a non-smoker's heart.

Children are especially at risk from second-hand smoking.

Children are particularly at risk because they breathe faster than adults and have underdeveloped immune systems. A study by the Royal College of Physicians showed that about 17,000 children in the UK are admitted to hospital every year because of illnesses caused by second-hand smoke.

A large study of over 300,000 people found that children who were frequently exposed to cigarette smoke at home had a higher risks of lung cancer as adults. Another study found that children in households where both parents smoke have a 72% higher risk of respiratory diseases. And the EPIC study found that exposing children to second-hand smoke increases the risk of bladder cancer later on in life by a third.

Childhood exposure to second-hand smoke had also been linked to a wide range of other conditions including asthma, sudden infant death syndrome (or cot death), childhood meningitis, and mental disabilities.

Smoking while pregnant can harm your baby.

Smoking during pregnancy hinders the blood flow to the placenta, which reduces the amount of nutrients that reach the baby. Because of this, women who smoke while pregnant have lighter babies than those who don't smoke. And low birth weight can lead to higher risks of diseases and death in infancy and early childhood.

There is also evidence that women exposed to second-hand smoke during pregnancy also have lighter babies.

Smoking during pregnancy has also been linked to other pregnancy complications including miscarriage, stillbirth, ectopic pregnancy, and cot death. It may also have consequences for the physical and mental development of the child.

Smokeless tobacco can also cause cancer.

Smokeless tobacco, also known as chewing tobacco or snuff, is popular in South Asian communities in the UK. Many studies have shown that smokeless tobacco can cause oral cancer and may cause pancreatic cancer. One study found that people who used smokeless tobacco had almost 50 times higher oral cancer risks than those who didn't.

The most dangerous chemicals in smokeless tobacco are called tobacco-specific nitrosamines (TSNAs). One review found that people who use smokeless tobacco expose themselves to up to a thousand times more TSNAs than non-smokers, and up to 50 times more than smokers.

Smokeless tobacco is also as addictive as cigarettes. Some studies found that the amount of nicotine absorbed from smokeless tobacco is three to four times greater than that deliver by a cigarette. The nicotine is also absorbed more slowly and stays in the bloodstream for a longer time.

A Swedish type of smokeless tobacco called *snus* is often promoted as "safe," but studies have found that even this can increase the risk of esophageal, stomach, and pancreatic cancers.

Section 4.2

Facts about Alcohol Use and Cancer Risk

Excerpted from "Alcohol, The Forgotten Cancer Risk," by Karen
Collins, MS, RD, CDN. © 2008 American Institute for Cancer Research
(www.aicr.org). Reprinted with permission.

Are alcoholic drinks linked to cancer?

There is strong evidence that alcoholic beverages increase risk of
developing cancers of the mouth, pharynx, larynx, and esophagus,
both pre- and post-menopausal breast cancer, and colorectal cancer in
men. Drinking alcoholic beverages probably increases risk of colorectal
cancer in women and liver cancer in both men and women. Your risk
of lung cancer rises dramatically if you drink alcohol and smoke.

How does drinking alcoholic beverages increase my cancer risk?

Some tissues in the body, such as the mouth and esophagus, are
directly exposed to alcohol. This can cause cell damage that sparks the
cancer process. Years of drinking can lead to liver damage that may
eventually turn to liver cancer. Experts cannot yet clearly explain how
drinking alcohol leads to breast cancer, but the association between
alcohol and the disease is apparent in study after study.

Should I avoid alcohol completely to lower my cancer risk?

Even small amounts of alcohol increase your risk for certain cancers,
so the American Institute for Cancer Research (AICR) does not recommend alcohol consumption. However, moderate alcohol consumption—no
more than one drink per day for women and two for men—may protect
against coronary heart disease and type 2 diabetes. If you choose to
drink, keep to these limits. Heavier drinking raises the risk of cancer,
heart disease, high blood pressure, stroke, osteoporosis, malnutrition,
inflammation of the pancreas, damage to the brain, liver cirrhosis, accidents, violence, and suicide. Alcohol causes birth defects too. If you are
pregnant or may become pregnant, do not drink any alcohol.

There are other ways to lower your risk of heart disease, and most of them also lower your risk for cancer. In addition to eating a mostly plant-based diet, AICR advises getting at least 30 minutes of physical activity daily and maintaining a healthy weight.

Table 4.1. One Drink Equals

1   bottle or can (12 fluid ounces) of regular beer, approximately 140–180 calories (Note: light beer has about 70–125 calories per 12 ounces; and non-alcoholic beer has fewer calories than light beer—check the label.)

1.5 fluid ounces of 80-proof liquor such as bourbon and vodka, approximately 100 calories

1   fluid ounce of 100-proof liquor such as bourbon and vodka, approximately 80 calories

5   fluid ounces of wine, approximately 100–140 calories

1   bottle (12 fluid ounces) of alcoholic lemonade or other carbonated drink, ranging from 220 to more than 300 calories

Research on cancer risk suggests that the type of drink does not matter, but the amount does. Remember the limits: no more than two drinks daily for men and no more than one daily for women.

Why is moderate drinking different for men and women?

Women metabolize alcohol more slowly than men, so alcohol stays in a woman's bloodstream longer. Also, men tend to have more muscle than women; alcohol can be diluted into water held in muscle tissue, but not into fat tissue.

A woman's risk for breast cancer—the most frequently diagnosed cancer in women—increases with greater alcohol consumption. Women at high risk for breast cancer should consider not drinking.

Women metabolize alcohol differently than men, so liver disease and other alcohol-related health problems develop faster in women than in men who drink the same amount.

Cutting Down on Alcohol

Any reduction in alcohol consumption will lower your risk for developing cancer. Here are a few tips to help you cut back or lessen the effect of drinking.

- At home, stock your refrigerator with plenty of thirst-quenching alternatives like flavored waters and seltzers.

- During the cocktail hour, sip on non-alcoholic drinks like sparkling water with a twist of lime. For something more filling and with a little zip, try tomato or vegetable juice with lemon and a drop or two of hot sauce. Sparkling apple cider or club soda mixed with cranberry juice are both refreshing and quite suitable for a celebration.

- Sip slowly and avoid pressure from others to drink faster.

- Avoid salty snacks that increase your thirst unless you plan to quench it with water.

- Keep track of how much you're drinking by refilling your own glass and avoiding topping off your drinks.

- Look for a low alcohol or non-alcoholic beer. Some wine shops and grocery stores sell non-alcoholic wines too.

- When entertaining, place a large glass filled with water by each plate for your guests to satisfy their thirst with something non-caloric and non-alcoholic.

- At parties, serve a non-alcoholic punch, and dilute wine by mixing it with club soda and/or juice.

- When dining out, be aware that waiters and bartenders often serve larger-than-standard drinks.

Remember what responsible drinking means: Never drink and drive. Minors and pregnant women should not drink alcohol at all.

Section 4.3

Questions and Answers about Obesity and Cancer Risk

Excerpted from "Obesity and Cancer: Questions and Answers,"
National Cancer Institute (www.cancer.gov), March 16, 2004. Revised
by David A. Cooke, MD, FACP, September 2010.

What is obesity?

People who are obese have an abnormally high and unhealthy proportion of body fat. To measure obesity, researchers commonly use a formula based on weight and height known as the body mass index (BMI). BMI is the ratio of weight (in kilograms) to height (in meters) squared. BMI provides a more accurate measure of obesity or being overweight than does weight alone.

Guidelines established by the National Institutes of Health (NIH) place adults age 20 and older into one of four categories based on their BMI (1):

- <18.5 underweight

- 18.5 to 24.9 healthy

- 25.0 to 29.9 overweight

- >30.0 obese

Table 4.2 can be used to determine BMI category. (Find the height, and move across the chart to the appropriate weight.)

Compared with people in the healthy weight category, those who are overweight or obese are at greater risk for many diseases, including diabetes, high blood pressure, cardiovascular diseases, stroke, and certain cancers. Obesity lowers life expectancy.

What have scientists learned about the relationship between obesity and cancer?

In 2001, experts concluded that cancers of the colon, breast (postmenopausal), endometrium (the lining of the uterus), kidney, and esophagus

63

are associated with obesity. Subsequent research has confirmed substantial links between obesity and cancers of the liver, gallbladder, stomach, ovaries, and pancreas. Risk of prostate cancer, Hodgkin disease, and non-Hodgkin lymphoma have also been linked to obesity.

Obesity and physical inactivity may account for 25 to 30% of several major cancers—colon, breast (postmenopausal), endometrial, kidney, and cancer of the esophagus.

Preventing weight gain can reduce the risk of many cancers. Experts recommend that people establish habits of healthy eating and physical activity early in life to prevent overweight and obesity. Those who are already overweight or obese are advised to avoid additional weight gain, and to lose weight through a low-calorie diet and exercise. Even a weight loss of only 5 to 10% of total weight can provide health benefits.

How many people get cancer by being overweight or obese? How many die?

In 2002, about 41,000 new cases of cancer in the United States were estimated to be due to obesity. This means that about 3.2% of all new cancers are linked to obesity.

A recent report estimated that, in the United States, 14% of deaths from cancer in men and 20% of deaths in women were due to overweight and obesity.

Does obesity increase the risk of breast cancer?

The effect of obesity on breast cancer risk depends on a woman's menopausal status. Before menopause, obese women have a lower risk of developing breast cancer than do women of a healthy weight. However, after menopause, obese women have 1.5 times the risk of women of a healthy weight.

Obese women are also at increased risk of dying from breast cancer after menopause compared with lean women. Scientists estimate that about 11,000 to 18,000 deaths per year from breast cancer in U.S. women over age 50 might be avoided if women could maintain a BMI under 25 throughout their adult lives.

Obesity seems to increase the risk of breast cancer only among postmenopausal women who do not use menopausal hormones. Among women who use menopausal hormones, there is no significant difference in breast cancer risk between obese women and women of a healthy weight.

Both the increased risk of developing breast cancer and dying from it after menopause are believed to be due to increased levels of estrogen

Table 4.2. Body Mass Index (Source: From "Diagnosis of Diabetes," National Diabetes Information Clearinghouse (www.diabetes.niddk.nih.gov), October 2008).

	Normal						Overweight					Obese										Extreme Obesity														
BMI	19	20	21	22	23	24	25	26	27	28	29	30	31	32	33	34	35	36	37	38	39	40	41	42	43	44	45	46	47	48	49	50	51	52	53	54
Height (inches)												Body Weight (pounds)																								
58	91	96	100	105	110	115	119	124	129	134	138	143	148	153	158	162	167	172	177	181	186	191	196	201	205	210	215	220	224	229	234	239	244	248	253	258
59	94	99	104	109	114	119	124	128	133	138	143	148	153	158	163	168	173	178	183	188	193	198	203	208	212	217	222	227	232	237	242	247	252	257	262	267
60	97	102	107	112	118	123	128	133	138	143	148	153	158	163	168	174	179	184	189	194	199	204	209	215	220	225	230	235	240	245	250	255	261	266	271	276
61	100	106	111	116	122	127	132	137	143	148	153	158	164	169	174	180	185	190	195	201	206	211	217	222	227	232	238	243	248	254	259	264	269	275	280	285
62	104	109	115	120	126	131	136	142	147	153	158	164	169	175	180	186	191	196	202	207	213	218	224	229	235	240	246	251	256	262	267	273	278	284	289	295
63	107	113	118	124	130	135	141	146	152	158	163	169	175	180	186	191	197	203	208	214	220	225	231	237	242	248	254	259	265	270	278	282	287	293	299	304
64	110	116	122	128	134	140	145	151	157	163	169	174	180	186	192	197	204	209	215	221	227	232	238	244	250	256	262	267	273	279	285	291	296	302	308	314
65	114	120	126	132	138	144	150	156	162	168	174	180	186	192	198	204	210	216	222	228	234	240	246	252	258	264	270	276	282	288	294	300	306	312	318	324
66	118	124	130	136	142	148	155	161	167	173	179	186	192	198	204	210	216	223	229	235	241	247	253	260	266	272	278	284	291	297	303	309	315	322	328	334
67	121	127	134	140	146	153	159	166	172	178	185	191	198	204	211	217	223	230	236	242	249	255	261	268	274	280	287	293	299	306	312	319	325	331	338	344
68	125	131	138	144	151	158	164	171	177	184	190	197	203	210	216	223	230	236	243	249	256	262	269	276	282	289	295	302	308	315	322	328	335	341	348	354
69	128	135	142	149	155	162	169	176	182	189	196	203	209	216	223	230	236	243	250	257	263	270	277	284	291	297	304	311	318	324	331	338	345	351	358	365
70	132	139	146	153	160	167	174	181	188	195	202	209	216	222	229	236	243	250	257	264	271	278	285	292	299	306	313	320	327	334	341	348	355	362	369	376
71	136	143	150	157	165	172	179	186	193	200	208	215	222	229	236	243	250	257	265	272	279	286	293	301	308	315	322	329	338	343	351	358	365	372	379	386
72	140	147	154	162	169	177	184	191	199	206	213	221	228	235	242	250	258	265	272	279	287	294	302	309	316	324	331	338	346	353	361	368	375	383	390	397
73	144	151	159	166	174	182	189	197	204	212	219	227	235	242	250	257	265	272	280	288	295	302	310	318	325	333	340	348	355	363	371	378	386	393	401	408
74	148	155	163	171	179	186	194	202	210	218	225	233	241	249	256	264	272	280	287	295	303	311	319	326	334	342	350	358	365	373	381	389	396	404	412	420
75	152	160	168	176	184	192	200	208	216	224	232	240	248	256	264	272	279	287	295	303	311	319	327	335	343	351	359	367	375	383	391	399	407	415	423	431
76	156	164	172	180	189	197	205	213	221	230	238	246	254	263	271	279	287	295	304	312	320	328	336	344	353	361	369	377	385	394	402	410	418	426	435	443

Source: Adapted from *Clinical Guidelines on the Identification, Evaluation, and Treatment of Overweight and Obesity in Adults: The Evidence Report.*

in obese women. Before menopause, the ovaries are the primary source of estrogen. However, estrogen is also produced in fat tissue and, after menopause, when the ovaries stop producing hormones, fat tissue becomes the most important estrogen source. Estrogen levels in postmenopausal women are 50 to 100% higher among heavy versus lean women. Estrogen-sensitive tissues are therefore exposed to more estrogen stimulation in heavy women, leading to a more rapid growth of estrogen-responsive breast tumors.

Another factor related to the higher breast cancer death rates in obese women is that breast cancer is more likely to be detected at a later stage in obese women than in lean women. This is because the detection of a breast tumor is more difficult in obese versus lean women.

Weight gain during adulthood has been found to be the most consistent and strongest predictor of breast cancer risk in studies in which it has been examined. The distribution of body fat may also affect breast cancer risk. Women with a large amount of abdominal fat have a greater breast cancer risk than those whose fat is distributed over the hips, buttocks, and lower extremities. Results from studies on the effect of abdominal fat are much less consistent than studies on weight gain or BMI.

Does obesity increase the risk of cancer of the uterus?

Obesity has been consistently associated with uterine (endometrial) cancer. Obese women have two to four times greater risk of developing the disease than do women of a healthy weight, regardless of menopausal status. Increased risk has also been demonstrated among overweight women. Obesity has been estimated to account for about 40% of endometrial cancer cases in affluent societies.

It is unclear why obesity is a risk factor for endometrial cancer; however, it has been suggested that lifetime exposure to hormones and high levels of estrogen and insulin in obese women may be contributing factors.

Does obesity increase the risk of colon cancer?

Colon cancer occurs more frequently in people who are obese than in those of a healthy weight. An increased risk of colon cancer has been consistently reported for men with high BMIs. The relationship between BMI and risk in women, however, has been found to be weaker or absent.

Unlike for breast and endometrial cancer, estrogen appears to be protective for colon cancer for women overall. However, obesity and estrogen status also interact in influencing colon cancer risk. Women with a high BMI who are either premenopausal or postmenopausal and taking estrogens have an increased risk of colon cancer similar to that found for men with a high BMI. In contrast, women with a high BMI who are postmenopausal and not taking estrogens do not have an increased risk of colon cancer.

A number of mechanisms have been proposed for the adverse effect of obesity on colon cancer risk. One of the major hypotheses is that high levels of insulin or insulin-related growth factors in obese people may promote tumor development.

Does obesity increase the risk of kidney cancer?

Studies have consistently found a link between a type of kidney cancer (renal cell carcinoma) and obesity in women, with some studies finding risk among obese women to be two to four times the risk of women of a healthy weight.

Results of studies including men have been more variable, ranging from an association similar to that seen in women, to a weak association, to no association at all. A meta-analysis (where several studies are combined into a single report), which found an equal association of risk among men and women, estimated the kidney cancer risk to be 36% higher for an overweight person and 84% higher for an obese person compared to those with a healthy weight.

The mechanisms by which obesity may increase renal cell cancer risk are not well understood. An increased exposure to sex steroids, estrogen and androgen, is one possible mechanism.

Does obesity increase the risk of cancer of the esophagus or stomach?

Overweight and obese individuals are two times more likely than healthy weight people to develop a type of esophageal cancer called esophageal adenocarcinoma. A smaller increase in risk has been found for gastric cardia cancer, a type of stomach cancer that begins in the area of the stomach next to the esophagus. Most studies have not observed increases in risk with obesity in another type of esophageal cancer, squamous cell cancer. An increased risk of esophageal adenocarcinoma has also been associated with weight gain, smoking, and being younger than age 59.

The mechanisms by which obesity increases risk of adenocarcinoma of the esophagus and gastric cardia are not well understood. One of the leading mechanisms proposed has been that increases in gastric reflux due to obesity may increase risk. However, in the few studies that have examined this issue, risk associated with BMI was similar for those with and without gastric reflux.

Does obesity increase the risk of prostate cancer?

Of the more than 35 studies on prostate cancer risk, most conclude that there is no association with obesity. Some report that obese men are at higher risk than men of healthy weight, particularly for more aggressive tumors. One study found an increased risk among men with high waist-to-hip ratios, suggesting that abdominal fat may be a more appropriate measure of body size in relation to prostate cancer. Studies examining BMI and prostate cancer mortality have had conflicting results.

Despite the lack of association between obesity and prostate cancer incidence, a number of studies have examined potential biological factors that are related to obesity, such as insulin-related growth factors, leptin, and other hormones. Results of these studies are inconsistent, but generally, risk has been linked to men with higher levels of leptin, insulin, and IGF-1 (insulin-like growth factor-1).

Is there any evidence that obesity is linked to cancer of the gallbladder, ovaries, or pancreas?

An increased risk of gallbladder cancer has been found to be associated with obesity, particularly among women. This may be due to the higher frequency of gallstones in obese individuals, as gallstones are considered a strong risk factor for gallbladder cancer. However, there is not enough evidence to draw firm conclusions.

It is unclear whether obesity affects ovarian cancer risk. Some studies report an increased risk among obese women, whereas others have found no association. A recent report found an increased risk in women who were overweight or obese in adolescence or young adulthood; no increased risk was found in older obese women.

Studies evaluating the relationship between obesity and pancreatic cancer have been inconsistent, but have increasingly supported a relationship. One recent study found that obesity increases the risk of pancreatic cancer only among those who are not physically active. A recent meta-analysis reported that obese people may have a 19% higher risk of pancreatic cancer than those with a healthy BMI. The results, however, were not conclusive. A large Swedish study published in 2005 found significantly increased cancer risk associated with obesity and large waist circumference.

Does losing weight lower the risk of cancer?

There is insufficient evidence that intentional weight loss will affect cancer risk for any cancer. A very limited number of observational studies have examined the effect of weight loss, and a few found some decreased risk for breast cancer among women who have lost weight. However, most of these studies have not been able to evaluate whether the weight loss was intentional or related to other health problems.

Does regular physical activity lower the risk of cancer?

There have been no controlled clinical trials on the effect of regular physical activity on the risk of developing cancer. However, observational studies have examined the possible association between physical activity and a lower risk of developing colon or breast cancer:

- **Colon cancer:** In 2002, a major review of observational trials found that physical activity reduced colon cancer risk by 50%. This risk reduction occurred even with moderate levels of physical activity. For example, one study showed that even moderate exercise, such as brisk walking for three to four hours per week, can lower colon cancer risk. A limited number of studies have examined the effect of physical activity on colon cancer risk for both lean and obese people. Most of these studies have found a protective effect of physical activity across all levels of BMI.

- **Breast cancer:** The pattern of the association between physical activity and breast cancer risk is somewhat different. Most studies on breast cancer have focused on postmenopausal women. A recent study from the Women's Health Initiative found that physical activity among postmenopausal women at a level of walking about 30 minutes per day was associated with a 20% reduction in breast cancer risk. However, this reduction in risk was greatest among women who were of normal weight. For these women, physical activity was associated with a 37% decrease in risk. The protective effect of physical activity was not found among overweight or obese women.

What biological mechanisms are thought to be involved in explaining the link between obesity and cancer?

The biological mechanism that explains how obesity increases cancer risk may be different for different cancers. The exact mechanisms are not known for any of the cancers. However, possible mechanisms include alterations in sex hormones (for example, estrogen, progesterone, and androgens), and insulin and IGF-1 in obese people that may account for their increased risk for cancers of the breast, endometrium, and colon. Sex-hormone binding globulin, the major carrier protein for certain sex hormones in the plasma, may also be involved in the altered risk for these cancers in obese people.

Section 4.4

The Roles of Exercise and Stress Management in Reducing Cancer Risk

Excerpted from "Cancer Facts: The Roles of Exercise and Stress Management," © The Cancer Project, a program of Physicians Committee for Responsible Medicine, 2010. Used by permission. For the complete text of this document, including references, visit www.cancerproject.org/diet_cancer/facts/exercise.php.

Healthy foods, physical activity, and reducing stress are increasingly recognized as vital ingredients of cancer prevention and survival. While genetics play a role in predisposing some people to cancer, other factors play a much greater role. In fact, much of what appears to "run in the family" results from shared exposure to environmental factors, such as cancer-promoting chemicals or dietary patterns. Many factors, including diet, physical activity, viral and bacterial infections, radiation, and exposure to carcinogens all influence one's risk of developing cancer.

In the past two decades, a wealth of research has revealed that emotional factors and a lack of exercise can alter the body's resistance to cancer. Changing exercise patterns and emotional states could therefore play a powerful role in preventing or surviving the disease—a role no less important than making appropriate dietary changes.

Immunity against Cancer

Cancer begins with a major change in a normal, living cell. The transformation from a normal cell to a cancer cell is triggered by damage to the DNA, for example, by radiation or a carcinogenic chemical. The cells generally undergo cellular division more rapidly than the cells from which they originate. When a cancer cell divides, it forms two new cancer cells. The process continues until a mass of cells is created, called a tumor. The dangerous nature of cancer stems from the abnormal cells' ability to invade other tissues and travel through the blood and lymphatic vessels to other areas of the body, a process called metastasis.

Each of us is constantly exposed to carcinogens in our food, air, and water, resulting in the production of cancer cells within the body. Ordinarily, however, our immune system recognizes and destroys these cells before they have a chance to multiply. (The same thing happens to the vast majority of viruses and bacteria entering our bodies.) Given this fact, simply having abnormal cells develop is not the only factor in determining the course of cancer. The primary threat of cancer may result instead from the body's inability to eliminate the abnormal cells.

The immune system provides the body with a way to seek out and destroy cancer cells. Among the main anti-cancer components of this system are specialized white blood cells, known as T-lymphocytes or T-cells, which travel throughout the body to detect unusual cells. Some lymphocytes can produce various anticancer chemicals, such as tumor necrosis factor, interleukin, and interferon. These are the body's equivalent of chemotherapy, except they don't harm healthy cells as chemotherapy does.

The body's most immediate and powerful protection against cancer, however, results from the action of natural killer cells (NK cells), a specialized form of lymphocyte. NK cells descend directly on a microscopic tumor and begin devouring and disintegrating the tissue. As a consequence, many tumors never make it beyond the early stages.

Stress and Immunity

Stress affects us physically and psychologically. In the case of a perceived threat, the body undergoes a build-up of internal tension characterized by increased heart rate, blood pressure, and muscular tension, to prepare for swift and powerful action. In primitive times, these bodily changes probably helped us adapt to dangerous situations, such as sudden storms or attacks. In many cases, however, these aspects of the stress response are inappropriate in the context of modern society. You don't need tight muscles and a rapid heart rate, for example, in trying to resolve a business dispute or a conflict at home.

Under stressful circumstances, the brain signals the adrenal glands to produce corticosteroids, hormones which weaken the immune response. Corticosteroids exert such a powerful immune-suppressive effect that synthetic steroids (for example, cortisone) are widely used as drugs to suppress immunity in allergic conditions and the rejection of transplanted organs. Cancerous processes are accelerated in the presence of large amounts of corticosteroids as well as other stress-related hormones.

Among the stress-related emotional factors now thought to play a role in reducing cancer resistance are depression, grief, repressed anger, hopelessness, helplessness, and a high degree of passivity or social conformity. Certain cancers have also been associated with distressing life events. For example, the risk of developing breast cancer is significantly higher if the woman has experienced the loss of a spouse or close friend. A recent review notes that, in fact, major stressful life events can contribute to cancer morbidity.

No scientific evidence has yet found that stress and emotions can directly cause cancer. The most plausible link is an indirect effect via the immune system. When immunity is weakened by stress, particularly in the presence of biological stressors such as a fatty diet or environmental pollution, then cancer can thrive and grow.

Exercise against Cancer

The evidence that exercise may play an effective role against cancer is accumulating fast. Regular exercise has been associated with a decrease in the risk of colorectal, breast, and lung cancers. In a large-scale study of 17,148 Harvard alumni, men who burned as few as 500 calories a week in exercise—the equivalent of about an hour's worth of brisk walking or less than 10 minutes of walking a day—had death rates 15 to 20% lower than men who were almost completely sedentary. Men who burned 2,000 calories a week (about four hours of brisk walking per week) had about 35% lower cancer mortality. The researchers concluded that the more exercise you get (up to a point), the lower your risk of premature death from cancer or heart disease. The Harvard study found that the risk of colon cancer, the second leading cause of cancer-related death in the U.S., was dramatically reduced by exercise.

Prostate cancer is the most common cancer affecting men today. In the Harvard study, alumni who expended greater than 4,000 calories per week (equivalent to about eight hours of brisk walking) were at a reduced risk of developing prostate cancer compared to their inactive counterparts.

For women, a history of moderate, recreational exercise is associated with a reduced risk of breast, uterine, cervical, and ovarian cancers, although not all studies have shown this effect. Findings from a 1993 study suggest that women engaged in moderate or high levels of physical activity may have a reduced risk of endometrial cancer; women engaged in the lowest level of physical activity had four times greater risk of cancer.

There are many mechanisms by which exercise and physical activity contribute to decreased cancer risk. It has been postulated that individuals who regularly engage in physical activity also practice healthful eating habits including eating less meat and other fatty foods, abstaining from tobacco use, and moderating alcohol consumption, in addition to helping control energy balance through caloric intake and expenditure. In addition, exercise and physical activity have a number of positive physiological effects on the body.

Two explanations for the reduction in cancer among those who exercise are: (1) an increase in gastrointestinal transit speed, which results in lower amounts of carcinogens in food being absorbed or exposed to the intestinal wall; and (2) a decrease in the level of circulating estrogen levels, which in turn reduces the risk of certain cancers, particularly breast cancer and cancers of the female reproductive system.

Exercise may also have a direct effect on the immune system. David Nieman and coworkers at Loma Linda University in California found that brisk walking (45 minutes, five times a week, for 15 weeks) boosts the body's resistance to disease by boosting NK cell activity. This was reflected in the fact that, compared to a non-walking, sedentary group, people in the walking group contracted the same number of colds and flus, but the number of days they suffered cold and flu symptoms was cut in half.

Managing Stress

Reducing stress helps cut your risk of heart problems, strengthens your immune system, and reduces anxiety. If you are relaxed, you are more likely to stick to a healthful lifestyle and less likely to depend on sedatives of daily martinis that many people use to deal with stress.

First, get plenty of sleep. You know the amount of sleep you need to feel well. And if you can spare the time, a short nap before dinner is a great stress reducer. At work, take a break every now and then to move around, take a deep breath, stretch, and have a big yawn.

Here are three simple exercises that melt away stress. These techniques work by turning off external stimuli and relaxing your muscles. When your body is relaxed, your mind tends to let go of tension, too. Twice a day, try any one of these for several minutes. They also help if you are having trouble falling asleep.

For each exercise, sit in a comfortable chair or lie on your back in a quiet room. Unplug the phone and use a "Do Not Disturb" sign. If you should happen to doze off, don't worry. That is a sign that your body wants more rest.

Relaxation Breathing

For about 30 seconds, simply relax with your eyes closed, thinking about nothing at all. Then start to pay attention to your breathing. Let your breathing slow down naturally, like a person sleeping. Feel the cool air come in through your nose with each inhalation, and feel your breath leave as you exhale. Imagine that tension is leaving your body with each exhalation.

Now imagine that, as you breathe in, the air comes into your nostrils and caresses your face like a gentle breeze. As you breathe out, the exhalation carries away the tension from your face. As you breathe slowly in and out, tension gradually leaves your body and you become more and more relaxed.

Now imagine that, as you breathe in, the gentle air enters your nose and spreads relaxation up over the top of your head. As you exhale, imagine the tension leaving this area and passing out of your body. Then imagine the next breath carrying relaxation over your face, your scalp, and both sides of your head. As you exhale, let the tension flow out easily.

If other thoughts come to mind, simply return to paying attention to your breathing. Your breathing is slow and easy, with no effort at all. Let your body relax.

Now let your breath carry relaxation to your neck. As you exhale, tension passes out of your neck and out of your body with the exhaled air. Then feel a breath carry relaxation to your shoulders. As you exhale, tension leaves your shoulders and passes out of your body.

Now, one breath at a time, focus your attention on each part of your body from the top down: your upper arms, forearms, hands, chest, stomach, hips, thighs, knees, calves, ankles, and feet. Imagine each breath of air carrying relaxation into each part of your body. As you breathe out, tension passes out through your nostrils.

This relaxing exercise will take several minutes, and you can do it at whatever pace is comfortable for you. When you have finished, allow yourself to sit quietly for two minutes or more.

Muscle Relaxation Sequence

As in the previous exercise, focus on one body part at a time from the head down. This time, tighten and release the muscles in each body part, one at a time. This allows the muscles to achieve a deep state of relaxation.

Start by sitting quietly for about 30 seconds. Allow your breathing to slow down naturally. Now gently raise your eyebrows for a second, and then relax. You may briefly feel tension in the front and back of your head, followed by relaxation. Breathe slowly in and out. Now gently tighten the muscles of your face into a slight grimace for about one second, then let them totally relax. Take a normal breath in and out, and feel your face relaxing. Then gently clench your jaw and release it. This tightens and then relaxes the muscles of the cheeks and above the ears.

Tighten the muscles of your neck and release them. After a moment, raise your shoulders and drop them. Let each body part relax in sequence. Take your time, and allow your body to completely relax after each tightening. Tighten and release the muscles of your upper arm and then your forearm. Ball your hand into a fist for a moment and then release it. Feel the tension leave each body part. Continue slow and relaxed breathing.

Then briefly tighten and release, in succession, the muscles of your chest, your abdomen, your thighs, calves, and feet. When you are finished, notice whether tension remains in any part of your body. If it does, imagine that body part gradually releasing tension as you breathe slowly in and out.

Enjoy the feeling of relaxation for a few minutes before getting up.

Listening to Breathing

This exercise can be used anywhere, whether you are on a stage waiting to give a speech or tossing and turning in a hotel bed unable to wind down from the stresses of the day. It uses imaginary sounds with no meaning to focus your attention away from the events of the day.

Sit quietly or lie on your back. Listen to your breathing, and let your breathing slow down. Imagine that as you breathe in, the inhalation makes a sound like the word so. As you exhale, imagine that your breathing sounds like the word hum. You need not make these sounds; just imagine them as you inhale and exhale.

Let your breathing slow down a little more, and slowly imagine the word so with each inhalation. Slowly and silently say hum to yourself as you slowly exhale. Repeat this for several minutes. If you find your mind drifting to something else, gently come back to listening to your breathing. You can also use this technique for just a few seconds, if you like, as a quick stress reducer.

Section 4.5

Sun Exposure and Cancer Risk

"Sun Safety," August 2010, reprinted with permission from www.kids health.org. Copyright © 2007 The Nemours Foundation. This information was provided by KidsHealth, one of the largest resources online for medically reviewed health information written for parents, kids, and teens. For more articles like this one, visit www.KidsHealth.org, or www .TeensHealth.org.

We all need some sun exposure; it's our primary source of vitamin D, which helps us absorb calcium for stronger, healthier bones. But it doesn't take much time in the sun for most people to get the vitamin D they need, and repeated unprotected exposure to the sun's ultraviolet rays can cause skin damage, eye damage, immune system suppression, and skin cancer. Even people in their twenties can develop skin cancer.

Most kids rack up between 50% and 80% of their lifetime sun exposure before age 18, so it's important that parents teach their children how to enjoy fun in the sun safely. With the right precautions, you can greatly reduce your child's chance of developing skin cancer.

Facts about Sun Exposure

The sun radiates light to the earth, and part of that light consists of invisible ultraviolet (UV) rays. When these rays reach the skin, they cause tanning, burning, and other skin damage.

Sunlight contains three types of ultraviolet rays: UVA, UVB, and UVC.

1. UVA rays cause skin aging and wrinkling and contribute to skin cancer, such as melanoma. Because UVA rays pass effortlessly through the ozone layer (the protective layer of atmosphere, or shield, surrounding the earth), they make up the majority of our sun exposure. Beware of tanning beds because they use UVA rays as well as UVB rays. A UVA tan does not help protect the skin from further sun damage; it merely produces color and a false sense of protection from the sun.

2. UVB rays are also dangerous, causing sunburns, cataracts (clouding of the eye lens), and effects on the immune system. They also contribute to skin cancer. Melanoma, the most dangerous form of skin cancer, is thought to be associated with severe UVB sunburns that occur before the age of 20. Most UVB rays are absorbed by the ozone layer, but enough of these rays pass through to cause serious damage.

3. UVC rays are the most dangerous, but fortunately, these rays are blocked by the ozone layer and don't reach the earth.

What's important is to protect your family from exposure to UVA and UVB, the rays that cause skin damage.

Melanin: The Body's First Line of Defense

UV rays react with a chemical called melanin that's found in skin. Melanin is the first defense against the sun because it absorbs dangerous UV rays before they do serious skin damage. Melanin is found in different concentrations and colors, resulting in different skin colors. The lighter someone's natural skin color, the less melanin it has to absorb UV rays and protect itself. The darker a person's natural skin color, the more melanin it has to protect itself. (But both dark- and light-skinned kids need protection from UV rays because any tanning or burning causes skin damage.)

Also, anyone with a fair complexion—lighter skin and eye color—is more likely to have freckles because there's less melanin in the skin. Although freckles are harmless, being outside in the sun may help cause them or make them darker.

As the melanin increases in response to sun exposure, the skin tans. But even that "healthy" tan may be a sign of sun damage. The risk of damage increases with the amount and intensity of exposure. Those who are chronically exposed to the sun, such as farmers, boaters, and sunbathers, are at much greater risk. A sunburn develops when the amount of UV exposure is greater than what can be protected against by the skin's melanin.

Unprotected sun exposure is even more dangerous for kids with:

*   moles on their skin (or whose parents have a tendency to develop moles);

*   very fair skin and hair;

*   a family history of skin cancer, including melanoma.

You should be especially careful about sun protection if your child has one or more of these high-risk characteristics.

Also, not all sunlight is "equal" in UV concentration. The intensity of the sun's rays depends upon the time of year, as well as the altitude and latitude of your location. UV rays are strongest during summer. Remember that the timing of this season varies by location; if you travel to a foreign country during its summer season, you'll need to pack the strongest sun protection you can find.

Extra protection is also required near the equator, where the sun is strongest, and at high altitudes, where the air and cloud cover are thinner, allowing more damaging UV rays to get through the atmosphere. Even during winter months, if your family goes skiing in the mountains, be sure to apply plenty of sunscreen; UV rays reflect off both snow and water, increasing the probability of sunburn.

With the right precautions, kids can safely play in the sun. Here are the most effective strategies:

Avoid the Strongest Rays of the Day

First, seek shade when the sun is at its highest overhead and therefore strongest (usually 10 a.m. until 4 p.m. in the northern hemisphere). If kids must be in the sun between these hours, be sure to apply and reapply protective sunscreen—even if they're just playing in the backyard. Most sun damage occurs as a result of incidental exposure during day-to-day activities, not at the beach.

Even on cloudy, cool, or overcast days, UV rays travel through the clouds and reflect off sand, water, and even concrete. Clouds and pollution don't filter out UV rays, and they can give a false sense of protection. This "invisible sun" can cause unexpected sunburn and skin damage. Often, kids are unaware that they're developing a sunburn on cooler or windy days because the temperature or breeze keeps skin feeling cool on the surface.

Make sure your kids don't use tanning beds at any time, even to "prepare" for a trip to a warm climate. Both UVA and UVA/UVB tanning beds produce sunburn. And there is an increase in the risk of melanoma in people who have used tanning beds before the age of 35.

Cover Up

One of the best ways to protect your family from the sun is to cover up and shield skin from UV rays. Ensure that clothes will screen out harmful UV rays by placing your hand inside the garments and making sure you can't see it through them.

Because infants have thinner skin and underdeveloped melanin, their skin burns more easily than that of older kids. But sunscreen should not be applied to babies under six months of age, so they absolutely must be kept out of the sun whenever possible. If your infant must be in the sun, dress him or her in clothing that covers the body, including hats with wide brims to shadow the face. Use an umbrella to create shade.

Even older kids need to escape the sun. For all-day outdoor affairs, bring along a wide umbrella or a pop-up tent to play in. If it's not too hot outside and won't make kids even more uncomfortable, have them wear light long-sleeved shirts and/or long pants. Before heading to the beach or park, call ahead to find out if certain areas offer rentals of umbrellas, tents, and other sun-protective gear.

Use Sunscreen Consistently

Lots of good sunscreens are available for kids, including formulations for sensitive skin, brands with fun scents like watermelon, long-lasting waterproof and sweat-proof versions, and easy-application varieties in spray bottles.

What matters most in a sunscreen is the degree of protection from UV rays it provides. When faced with the overwhelming sea of sunscreen choices at drugstores, concentrate on the SPF (sun protection factor) numbers on the labels.

For kids age six months and older, select an SPF of 30 or higher to prevent both sunburn and tanning. Choose a sunscreen that states on the label that it protects against both UVA and UVB rays (referred to as "broad-spectrum" sunscreen). In general, sunscreens provide better protections against UVB rays than UVA rays, making signs of skin aging a risk even with consistent use of sunscreen. To avoid possible skin allergy, don't use sunscreens with PABA; if your child has sensitive skin, look for a product with the active ingredient titanium dioxide (a chemical-free block).

To get a tanned appearance, teens might try self-tanning lotions. These offer an alternative to ultraviolet exposure, but only minimal (or no) protection from UV light.

For sunscreen to do its job, it must be applied correctly. Be sure to:

- Apply sunscreen whenever kids will be in the sun.

- Apply sunscreen about 15 to 30 minutes before kids go outside so that a good layer of protection can form. Don't forget about lips, hands, ears, feet, shoulders, and behind the neck. Lift up bathing suit straps and apply sunscreen underneath them (in case the straps shift as a child moves).

- Don't try to stretch out a bottle of sunscreen; apply it generously.

- Reapply sunscreen often, approximately every two to three hours, as recommended by the American Academy of Dermatology. Reapply after a child has been sweating or swimming.

- Apply a waterproof sunscreen if kids will be around water or swimming. Water reflects and intensifies the sun's rays, so kids need protection that lasts. Waterproof sunscreens may last up to 80 minutes in the water, and some are also sweat- and rub-proof. But regardless of the waterproof label, be sure to reapply sunscreen when kids come out of the water.

Keep in mind that every child needs extra sun protection. The American Academy of Dermatology recommends that all kids—regardless of their skin tone—wear sunscreen with an SPF of 30 or higher. Although dark skin has more protective melanin and tans more easily than it burns, remember that tanning is also a sign of sun damage. Dark-skinned kids also can develop painful sunburns.

Use Protective Eyewear for Kids

Sun exposure damages the eyes as well as the skin. Even one day in the sun can result in a burned cornea (the outermost, clear membrane layer of the eye). Cumulative exposure can lead to cataracts (clouding of the eye lens, which leads to blurred vision) later in life. The best way to protect eyes is to wear sunglasses.

Not all sunglasses provide the same level of ultraviolet protection; darkened plastic or glass lenses without special UV filters just trick the eyes into a false sense of safety. Purchase sunglasses with labels ensuring that they provide 100% UV protection.

But not all kids enjoy wearing sunglasses, especially the first few times. To encourage them to wear them, let kids select a style they like—many manufacturers make fun, multicolored frames or ones embossed with cartoon characters. And don't forget that kids want to be like grown-ups. If you wear sunglasses regularly, your kids may be willing to follow your example. Providing sunglasses early in childhood will encourage the habit of wearing them in the future.

Double-Check Medications

Some medications increase the skin's sensitivity to UV rays. As a result, even kids with skin that tends not to burn easily can develop a severe sunburn in just minutes when taking certain medications. Fair-skinned kids, of course, are even more vulnerable.

Ask your doctor or pharmacist if any prescription (especially antibiotics and acne medications) and over-the-counter medications your child is taking can increase sun sensitivity. If so, always take extra sun precautions. The best protection is simply covering up or staying indoors; even sunscreen can't always protect skin from sun sensitivity caused by medications.

If Your Child Gets a Sunburn

A sunburn can sneak up on kids, especially after a long day at the beach or park. Often, they seem fine during the day but then gradually develop an "after-burn" later that evening that can be painful and hot and even make them feel sick.

When kids get sunburned, they usually experience pain and a sensation of heat—symptoms that tend to become more severe several hours after sun exposure. Some also develop chills. Because the sun has dried their skin, it can become itchy and tight. Sunburned skin begins to peel about a week after the sunburn. Encourage your child not to scratch or peel off loose skin because skin underneath the sunburn is vulnerable to infection.

If your child does get a sunburn, these tips may help:

- Have your child take a cool (not cold) bath, or gently apply cool, wet compresses to the skin to help alleviate pain and heat.

- To ease discomfort, apply pure aloe vera gel (available in most pharmacies) to any sunburned areas.

- Give your child an anti-inflammatory medication like ibuprofen or use acetaminophen to lessen the pain and itching. (Do not, however, give aspirin to children or teens.) Over-the-counter diphenhydramine may also help reduce itching and swelling.

- Apply topical moisturizing cream to rehydrate the skin and treat itching. For the more seriously sunburned areas, apply a thin layer of 1% hydrocortisone cream to help with pain. (Do not use petroleum-based products, because they prevent excess heat and sweat from escaping. Also, avoid first-aid products that contain benzocaine, which may cause skin irritation or allergy.)

If the sunburn is severe and blisters develop, call your doctor. Until you can see your doctor, tell your child not to scratch, pop, or squeeze the blisters, which can become easily infected and can result in scarring. Keep your child in the shade until the sunburn is healed. Any additional sun exposure will only increase the severity of the burn and increase pain.

Be Sun Safe Yourself

Don't forget: Being a good role model by wearing sunscreen and limiting your time in the sun not only reduces your risk of sun damage, but teaches your kids good sun sense.

Section 4.6

Indoor Tanning and Cancer Risk

"Indoor Tanning," June 2009, reprinted with permission from www.kids health.org. Copyright © 2009 The Nemours Foundation. This information was provided by KidsHealth, one of the largest resources online for medically reviewed health information written for parents, kids, and teens. For more articles like this one, visit www.KidsHealth.org, or www.TeensHealth.org.

You know that basking in the sun is bad for you—sun worshippers have prematurely aging skin, wrinkles, and maybe even skin cancer to look forward to. But you're no fan of the Morticia Addams look either.

Tempted to try a tanning salon? Maybe you've heard that sunbeds only use "safe" UVA light, avoiding the UVB light that causes burning. But unfortunately it's not that simple. UVA rays can cause just as much—if not more—damage than UVB rays because they penetrate the skin more deeply. In fact, doctors say that the use of tanning salons is one reason they're treating more young patients for skin cancer.

Indoor Tanning vs. Sunlight

The sun's rays contain two types of ultraviolet radiation that affect your skin: UVA and UVB. UVB radiation burns the upper layers of skin (the epidermis), causing sunburns. UVA radiation penetrates to the lower layers of the epidermis, where it triggers cells called melanocytes (pronounced: mel-an-oh-sites) to produce melanin. Melanin is the brown pigment that causes tanning.

Both UVA and UVB rays contribute to skin aging. Both types also can cause potentially cancerous changes in your cells' DNA. And, according to a recent study, radiation from just 10 indoor-tanning sessions in two weeks can suppress a person's cancer-fighting immune system.

Although tanning beds use UVA light, the concentration of UVA rays from a tanning bed is greater than that from the sun. And despite manufacturer claims, some tanning lamps do also emit UVB light. So if you try indoor tanning, you'll absorb far more rays in the long run, significantly age your skin, and put yourself at even greater risk for skin cancer.

What Tanning Salons Don't Tell You

A 2002 study published in the *Journal of the National Cancer Institute* found that users of tanning beds and lamps had substantially increased risks of basal and squamous cell carcinoma, the two most common types of skin cancer.

And don't expect tanning salon employees to warn you about the perils of using their facilities. Despite federal guidelines on how much exposure people should have to tanning equipment, most of the tanning parlors in a 2005 survey said customers could come in as often as they wanted. And more than a third of the tanning salons denied that indoor tanning can cause skin cancer or prematurely age the skin.

How can they get away with statements that aren't true? Tanning salons are a $2 billion industry in the United States and they want your business. Additionally, not all states regulate tanning equipment, and the federal government is still working out guidelines. So there are no structures in place to govern how salons are operated—including how well they maintain their equipment.

Minimizing Your Risk

People who have tanned in the past already have skin damage—even if they can't see it yet—and need to be very cautious about additional UV exposure. Like everyone else, they should wear sunscreen or sun-protective clothing (or both) while outdoors, and a dermatologist should check their skin periodically for suspicious moles or other lesions.

But you don't have to go without that sun-bronzed look. The new generation of self-tanners and spray-on tans offer easy, realistic results at a reasonable price. Just be sure to use a daily sunblock with an SPF of at least 15 when you go outdoors since fake tanners don't protect you against sunburn.

Chapter 5

Hereditary Cancer Risks

Hereditary Cancer

Cancer is a common disease with complex causes, many of which are not completely understood. Recent advances in cancer genetics have led to the identification of genes that, when altered, create a significantly increased risk for certain cancers. Although most cancers are not due to single, inherited gene alterations, for many common cancers as many as 5–10% are due to hereditary cancer syndromes.

Some of the features seen in families with hereditary cancer syndromes may include:

- clustering of certain types of cancers in a family;

- cancer occurring at younger ages than expected;

- cancer in several close relatives;

- cancer in more than one generation;

- more than one type of cancer in the same individual

- families that include diagnoses of rare cancers.

Hereditary Breast and Ovarian Cancer

Background

Breast cancer is the most common type of cancer among women in the United States, with more than 200,000 new cases diagnosed each year. In fact, about one in eight women will develop breast cancer sometime during her lifetime.

Ovarian cancer is less common, with over 23,000 diagnoses each year in the United States. Around one in 55 women will develop ovarian cancer during her lifetime.

Breast and/or Ovarian Cancer in Families

Some kinds of cancer, including breast and ovarian, can run in families. Although most cases are not hereditary, about 5–10% of breast and ovarian cancer cases may be hereditary, associated with an inheritance of a single genetic alteration.

Breast and Ovarian Cancer Genes

Mutations in two genes, discovered in the 1990s, are involved in the majority of families with early onset breast and/or ovarian cancer. These genes are called BRCA1 and BRCA2. ("BR" stands for breast and "CA" stands for cancer. The numbers "1" and "2" represent the order in which they were found.)

Hereditary Breast and Ovarian Cancer Risks

Everyone has BRCA1 and BRCA2 genes, but in some individuals there is an alteration, or change, in one of these genes. For women who have inherited an alteration in either BRCA1 or BRCA2 the risk of developing breast cancer by the age of 70 is approximately 50–85%. (This compares to a risk of 7% by age 70 for women in the general population.) The lifetime ovarian cancer risk for women with a BRCA1 or BRCA2 alteration ranges between 10–45% (compared to a 1-2% risk by age 70 for women in the general population).

Am I at an Increased Risk for Carrying an Alteration in BRCA1 or BRCA2?

- Have you had a diagnosis of breast cancer before age 40?

- Have you had bilateral breast cancer or have you had breast cancer and ovarian cancer?

- Have you been diagnosed with breast cancer or ovarian cancer?

- Do you have several close relatives who have had breast cancer (especially before age 50) and/or ovarian cancer?

- Do you have any male relatives who have had breast cancer?

- Does your family have Ashkenazi Jewish ancestry and have you and/or a close relative been diagnosed with breast cancer and/or ovarian cancer?

- Do you have a blood relative who has had a positive genetic test for an inherited alteration in one of the genes associated with hereditary breast/ovarian cancer syndrome, BRCA1 or BRCA2?

If you answered "YES" to any of these questions, you may be at an increased risk for carrying an alteration in one of the genes associated with hereditary breast/ovarian cancer syndrome.

Hereditary Colon Cancer

Background

Cancer of the colon or rectum, colorectal cancer, is the third most common type of cancer in the United States, with nearly 150,000 diagnoses every year. About one in 18 individuals in this country will develop colorectal cancer sometime during his or her lifetime.

Colon Cancer in Families

Most cases of colorectal cancer are not hereditary. However, an estimated 5% of colon cancer cases are due to inherited alterations in single cancer susceptibility genes. An alteration of this type can be passed from generation to generation and increase the risk of developing colon and other cancers.

The most common hereditary colorectal cancer syndromes are called hereditary non-polyposis colorectal cancer (HNPCC) and familial adenomatous polyposis (FAP). There are other rare genetic conditions, as well, which can increase the risk of colorectal cancer.

Hereditary Non-Polyposis Colorectal Cancer (HNPCC) or Lynch syndrome

Hereditary non-polyposis colorectal cancer, also known as Lynch syndrome, is a hereditary condition characterized by an increased risk of colorectal, uterine, and other cancers, which can develop at earlier ages than one would expect in the general population. In addition to colon and uterine cancer, individuals with HNPCC are at an increased risk for cancer of the ovary, stomach, urinary tract, small bowel, and bile duct. HNPCC accounts for approximately 2%–4% of all colon cancers.

Familial Adenomatous Polyposis (FAP)

Familial adenomatous polyposis is an inherited condition characterized by the development of hundreds to thousands of polyps in the colon and rectum at a young age, usually in the teens to 20s. A subtype of FAP (called attenuated FAP) is characterized by fewer polyps and later age of onset. The major risk of FAP is development of colorectal cancer if not recognized and managed appropriately. Other features sometimes seen in FAP include polyps in the small intestine and stomach, soft-tissue tumors of the skin, jawbone growths, and brain tumors. FAP accounts for approximately 1% of all colon cancers.

Am I at Increased Risk for Carrying a Colon Cancer Susceptibility Gene?

- Have you or any family members been diagnosed with colon or rectal cancer or polyps at an early age (before age 50)?

- Do you have a close relative who has been diagnosed with colon cancer more than once (separate cancers, diagnosed at the same or different time) or colon cancer and another cancer such as uterine or ovarian.

- Does anyone in the family have a history of multiple colon polyps?

- Do you have a blood relative who has been found to carry an alteration in a colon cancer susceptibility gene?

If you answered "YES" to any of these questions, you may be at increased risk for carrying an alteration in a colon cancer susceptibility gene. Familial cancer risk counseling can help you to understand your cancer risks and the management options available to you.

Rare Hereditary Cancer

Cancer can run in families because of shared environmental exposures, simply by chance; or possibly a combination of shared exposures and inherited susceptibility. However, in some families cancer is due to inheritance of an altered or mutated gene with increased risks of cancers associated with an hereditary cancer syndrome. There are several hereditary cancer syndromes that may often go unrecognized because they are not common. Several of these syndromes are described below. Our understanding of these syndromes is advancing rapidly. If your personal or family history is of concern to you or if your history sounds consistent with any of the syndromes described below, then cancer risk counseling and risk assessment may be helpful in clarifying your family cancer risks and in helping to plan appropriate cancer prevention strategies.

Multiple Endocrine Neoplasia Syndromes (MEN)

Multiple endocrine neoplasia (MEN) is an inherited disorder that leads to the growth of tumors in specific endocrine glands. There are two main types of MEN: MEN 1 and MEN 2. Families with MEN 1 are at an increased risk for developing parathyroid tumors, pancreatic tumors and/or pituitary tumors. MEN 2 is further subdivided to three subtypes: MEN 2A, FMTC (familial medullary thyroid cancer), and MEN 2B. Families with MEN 2 are at an increased risk to develop medullary thyroid cancers, and depending on the subtype of MEN 2, some families may also be at an increased risk to develop pheochromocytoma (tumors of the adrenal gland), parathyroid tumors, and/or mucosal neuromas on the lips and tongue.

The diagnosis and classification of MEN depends on your family and medical history, a clinical examination and genetic testing. If you have a personal and/or family history of medullary thyroid carcinoma, parathyroid tumors, pituitary tumors or other endocrine tumors, seeking cancer risk assessment and counsel may be a valuable service for you and your family.

Li-Fraumeni Syndrome

Li-Fraumeni syndrome is a rare inherited cancer syndrome. Families with Li-Fraumeni have an increased risk for osteosarcomas (bone tumors), soft-tissue sarcomas, pre-menopausal breast cancer, brain tumors, adrenal cortical tumors, and acute leukemias. Family members with Li-Fraumeni syndrome are specifically at an increased risk for some childhood cancers and multiple cancers originating in different tissues.

If you have had early onset cancer, such as breast cancer, brain tumor, acute leukemia, soft tissue sarcomas, bone sarcomas, or adrenal cortical carcinoma, or if you have several family members with early onset cancer, or individuals in your family with more than one cancer diagnosis, such as sarcoma and breast cancer, then cancer risk assessment may be valuable in providing information and a plan of surveillance for you or your family.

Von Hippel-Lindau Syndrome

Von Hippel-Lindau (VHL) disease is an inherited condition characterized by abnormal growth of blood vessels in certain parts of the body. People with VHL are at risk to develop growths in their blood capillaries called angiomas or hemangioblastomas. These growths may develop in the retinas, certain areas of the brain, the spinal cord, the adrenal glands and other parts of the body. Lesions in the retina may cause retinal detachment and eventual blindness. Angiomas in the brain or spinal cord may press on nerve or brain tissue and cause symptoms such as headaches, problems with balance in walking, or weakness of arms and legs. People with VHL can also develop cysts and tumors in the kidney, pancreas, liver, or adrenal glands or in some cases renal cell carcinoma.

If you have had angiomas, and/or hemangioblastomas, or if you have several family members with angiomas, and/or hemangioblastomas, you may benefit from an evaluation and cancer risk counseling.

Familial Malignant Melanoma Syndrome

The incidence of melanoma is approximately one in 70 in the Caucasian population; approximately 5 to 10% of cutaneous malignant melanoma is thought to be hereditary (familial malignant melanoma syndrome). These families are characterized by multiple family members with early age of onset malignant melanoma. These families are also at an increased risk for pancreatic cancer. Approximately 20–40% of families with familial malignant melanoma syndrome have an alteration (mutation) in a gene called CDKN4A (p16).

If you have two or more relatives on the same side of the family affected with malignant melanoma (especially at an early age), or if you and/or a close relative have a history of multiple primary melanoma, or if you have a family history of both malignant melanoma and pancreatic cancer you may benefit from cancer risk assessment and counseling.

Is Genetic Testing Right for Me?

Genetic testing for alterations in some cancer susceptibility genes is now available. The decision to undergo genetic testing is a very personal one and there are many issues to consider before making this decision. Cancer risk assessment and counseling is an important step before making the decision to pursue genetic testing. If you are concerned about your risk of cancer, cancer risk counseling can help you better understand your risks and the options available to you and your family.

Chapter 6

Infectious Diseases and Cancer Risk

Chapter Contents

Section 6.1

Human Papillomaviruses and Cancer: Questions and Answers

Excerpted from "Human Papillomaviruses and Cancer: Questions and Answers," National Cancer Institute (www.cancer.gov), February 14, 2008.

What are human papillomaviruses, and how are they transmitted?

Human papillomaviruses (HPVs) are a group of more than 100 related viruses. They are called papillomaviruses because certain types may cause warts, or papillomas, which are benign (noncancerous) tumors. The HPVs that cause the common warts which grow on hands and feet are different from those that cause growths in the throat or genital area. Some types of HPV are associated with certain types of cancer. These are called high-risk, oncogenic, or carcinogenic HPVs.

Genital HPV infections are very common and are sexually transmitted. Of the more than 100 types of HPV, more than 30 types can be passed from one person to another through sexual contact. Although HPVs are usually transmitted sexually, doctors cannot say for certain when infection occurred. Most HPV infections occur without any symptoms and go away without any treatment over the course of a few years. However, HPV infection sometimes persists for many years, with or without causing cell abnormalities. This can increase a woman's risk of developing cervical cancer.

What are genital warts?

Some types of HPV may cause warts to appear on or around the genitals or anus. Genital warts (technically known as condylomata acuminata) are most commonly associated with two HPV types, HPV-6 and HPV-11. Warts may appear within several weeks after sexual contact with a person who is infected with HPV, or they may take months or years to appear, or they may never appear. HPVs may also cause flat, abnormal growths in the genital area and on the cervix (the lower part of the uterus that extends into the vagina). However, HPV infections of the cervix usually do not cause any symptoms.

What is the association between HPV infection and cancer?

Persistent HPV infections are now recognized as the major cause of cervical cancer. In 2007, it was estimated that 11,000 women in the United States would be diagnosed with this type of cancer and nearly 4,000 would die from it. Cervical cancer strikes nearly half a million women each year worldwide, claiming a quarter of a million lives. Studies also suggest that HPVs may play a role in some cancers of the anus, vulva, vagina, and penile cancer (cancer of the penis).

Studies have also found that oral HPV infection is a strong risk factor for oropharyngeal cancer (cancer that forms in tissues of the oropharynx, which is the middle part of the throat and includes the soft palate, the base of the tongue, and the tonsils). Researchers found that an oral HPV infection and past HPV exposure increase the risk of oropharyngeal squamous cell cancer, regardless of tobacco and alcohol use, two other important risk factors for this disease. However, combining HPV exposure and heavy tobacco and alcohol use did not have an additive effect.

Are there specific types of HPV that are associated with cancer?

Some types of HPV are referred to as "low-risk" viruses because they rarely cause lesions that develop into cancer. HPV types that are more likely to lead to the development of cancer are referred to as "high-risk." Both high-risk and low-risk types of HPV can cause the growth of abnormal cells, but only the high-risk types of HPV lead to cancer. Sexually transmitted, high-risk HPVs include types 16, 18, 31, 33, 35, 39, 45, 51, 52, 56, 58, 59, 66, 68, and 73. These high-risk types of HPV cause growths on the cervix that are usually flat and nearly invisible, as compared with the external warts caused by low-risk types HPV-6 and HPV-11. HPV types 16 and 18 together cause about 70% of cervical cancers. It is important to note, however, that the great majority of high-risk HPV infections go away on their own and do not cause cancer.

What are the risk factors for HPV infection and cervical cancer?

Having many sexual partners is a risk factor for HPV infection. Although most HPV infections go away on their own without causing any type of abnormality, infection with high-risk HPV types increases the chance that mild abnormalities will develop and progress to more severe abnormalities or cervical cancer. However, even among the women who do develop abnormal cell changes with high-risk types of HPV, only a small percentage would develop cervical cancer if the abnormal cells were not removed. As a general rule, the more severe the abnormal cell change, the greater the risk of cancer. Studies suggest that whether a woman develops cervical cancer depends on a variety of factors acting together with high-risk HPVs. The factors that may increase the risk of cervical cancer in women with HPV infection include smoking and having many children.

Can HPV infection be prevented?

The surest way to eliminate risk for genital HPV infection is to refrain from any genital contact with another individual.

For those who choose to be sexually active, a long-term, mutually monogamous relationship with an uninfected partner is the strategy most likely to prevent genital HPV infection. However, it is difficult to determine whether a partner who has been sexually active in the past is currently infected.

HPV infection can occur in both male and female genital areas that are covered or protected by a latex condom, as well as in areas that are not covered. Although the degree of protection provided by condoms in preventing HPV infection is unknown, condom use has been associated with a lower rate of cervical cancer.

In 2006, the U.S. Food and Drug Administration (FDA) approved Gardasil®, a vaccine that is highly effective in preventing infection with types 16 and 18, two "high-risk" HPVs that cause most (70%) cervical cancers, and types 6 and 11, which cause most (90%) genital warts. [Note: FDA approved Cervarix, a second vaccine for the prevention of HPV types 16 and 18, in October 2009.]

How are HPV infections detected?

Testing samples of cervical cells is an effective way to identify high-risk types of HPV that may be present. The FDA has approved an HPV test as a follow-up for women who have an ambiguous Pap test (a screening test to detect cervical cell changes) and, for women over the age of 30, for general cervical cancer screening. This HPV test can identify at least 13 of the high-risk types of HPV associated with the development of cervical cancer. This test, which looks for viral DNA, is performed by collecting cells from the cervix and then sending them to a laboratory for analysis. The test can detect high-risk types of HPV even before there are any conclusive visible changes to the cervical cells. There are currently no approved tests to detect HPV infection in men.

What tests are used to screen for and diagnose precancerous cervical conditions?

A Pap test is the standard way to check for any cervical cell changes. A Pap test is usually done as part of a gynecologic exam. The U.S. Preventive Services Task Force guidelines recommend that women have a Pap test at least once every three years, beginning about three years after they begin to have sexual intercourse, but no later than age 21.

Because the HPV test can detect high-risk types of HPV in cervical cells, the FDA approved this test as a useful addition to the Pap test to help health care providers decide which women with atypical squamous cells of undetermined significance (ASCUS) need further testing, such as colposcopy and biopsy of any abnormal areas. (Colposcopy is a procedure in which a lighted magnifying instrument called a colposcope is used to examine the vagina and cervix. Biopsy is the removal of a small piece of tissue for diagnosis.) In addition, the HPV test can be a helpful addition to the Pap test for general screening of women age 30 and over.

What are the treatment options for HPV infection?

Although there is currently no medical cure for human papillomavirus infection, the lesions and warts these viruses cause can be treated. Methods commonly used to treat lesions include cryosurgery (freezing that destroys tissue), LEEP (loop electrosurgical excision procedure, the removal of tissue using a hot wire loop), and conventional surgery. Similar treatments may be used for external genital warts. In addition, some drugs may be used to treat external genital warts.

Section 6.2

HIV Infection and Cancer Risk

Excerpted from "HIV Infection and Cancer Risk,"
National Cancer Institute (www.cancer.gov), January 29, 2010.

Do people infected with human immunodeficiency virus (HIV) have an increased risk of cancer?

Yes. People infected with HIV have a substantially higher risk of some types of cancer than uninfected people of the same age. Three of these cancers are known as "acquired immunodeficiency syndrome (AIDS)-defining cancers" or "AIDS-defining malignancies": Kaposi sarcoma, non-Hodgkin lymphoma, and cervical cancer. A diagnosis of any one of these cancers marks the point at which HIV infection has progressed to AIDS.

People infected with HIV are about 800 times more likely than uninfected people to be diagnosed with Kaposi sarcoma, at least seven times more likely to be diagnosed with non-Hodgkin lymphoma, and, among women, at least three times more likely to be diagnosed with cervical cancer.

In addition, people infected with HIV are also at higher risk of several other types of cancer. These "non-AIDS-defining cancers" include anal cancer, Hodgkin lymphoma, liver cancer, and lung cancer.

People infected with HIV are at least nine times more likely to be diagnosed with anal cancer than uninfected people, at least ten times more likely to be diagnosed with Hodgkin lymphoma, and three to four times as likely to be diagnosed with liver and lung cancers.

People infected with HIV do not have increased risks of breast, colorectal, prostate, or many other common types of cancer. Screening for these cancers in HIV-infected people should follow current guidelines.

Why do people infected with HIV have a higher risk of cancer?

Infection with HIV weakens the immune system and reduces the body's ability to destroy cancer cells and fight infections that may lead to cancer.

Many people infected with HIV are also infected with other viruses that increase the risk of certain cancers. The following are the most important of these cancer-causing viruses:

- Human herpesvirus 8 (HHV8), also known as Kaposi sarcoma-associated herpesvirus (KSHV), is the cause of Kaposi sarcoma.

- Epstein Barr virus (EBV) causes some subtypes of non-Hodgkin and Hodgkin lymphoma.

- Human papillomavirus (HPV) causes cervical cancer and some types of anal, penile, vaginal, vulvar, and head and neck cancer.

- Hepatitis B virus (HBV) and hepatitis C virus (HCV) both can cause liver cancer.

Infection with most of these viruses is more common among people infected with HIV than among uninfected people.

In addition, the prevalence of some traditional risk factors for cancer, especially smoking (a known cause of lung cancer) and heavy alcohol use (which can increase the risk of liver cancer), is higher among people infected with HIV.

Has the introduction of antiretroviral therapy changed the cancer risk of people infected with HIV?

The introduction of highly active antiretroviral therapy (HAART) in the mid-1990s greatly reduced the incidence of Kaposi sarcoma and non-Hodgkin lymphoma among people infected with HIV. HAART lowers the amount of HIV circulating in the blood, thereby allowing partial restoration of immune system function. Although lower than before, the risk of these two cancers is still much higher among people infected with HIV than among people in the general population. This persistently high risk may be due, at least in part, to the fact that immune system function remains substantially impaired in people treated with HAART. In addition, over time, HIV can develop resistance to the drugs used in HAART, and many people infected with HIV have had difficulty in accessing medical care or taking their medication as prescribed.

Although the introduction of HAART has led to reductions in the incidence of Kaposi sarcoma and non-Hodgkin lymphoma among HIV-infected individuals, it has not reduced the incidence of cervical cancer, which has essentially remained unchanged. Moreover, the incidence of several non-AIDS-defining cancers, particularly Hodgkin lymphoma and anal cancer, may have been increasing among HIV-infected individuals since the introduction of HAART. The influence of HAART on the risk of these other cancer types is not well understood.

What can people infected with HIV do to reduce their risk of cancer or to find cancer early?

Taking HAART as indicated based on current HIV treatment guidelines lowers the risk of the major AIDS-defining cancers and increases overall survival.

The risk of lung cancer can be reduced by quitting smoking. Because HIV-infected people have a higher risk of lung cancer, it is especially important that they do not smoke. Help with quitting smoking is available through the National Cancer Institute's (NCI) smoking quitline at 877-44U-QUIT (877-448-7848). NCI is a part of the National Institutes of Health (NIH).

The higher incidence of liver cancer among HIV-infected people appears to be related to more frequent co-infection with hepatitis virus (particularly HCV) and alcohol abuse/dependence than among uninfected people. Therefore, HIV-infected individuals should know their hepatitis status. If blood tests show that they have previously been infected with HBV or HCV, they should consider reducing their alcohol consumption. In addition, if they currently have viral hepatitis, they should discuss with their health care provider whether HBV- or HCV-suppressing therapy is an option for them. Some drugs may be used for both HBV-suppressing therapy and HAART.

Because HIV-infected women have a higher risk of cervical cancer, it is important that they be screened regularly for this disease. Studies have suggested that Pap test abnormalities are more common among HIV-infected women and that HPV DNA tests may not be as effective as Pap tests in screening these women for cervical cancer.

Some researchers recommend anal Pap smear screening to detect and treat early lesions before they progress to anal cancer. This type of screening may be most beneficial for men who have had sexual intercourse with other men. HIV-infected patients should discuss such screening with their medical providers.

Section 6.3

Kaposi Sarcoma-Associated Herpesvirus

"Kaposi Sarcoma-Associated Herpesvirus," © 2009 Cancer Research UK (www
.cancerresearchuk.org). Reprinted with permission. Complete text including
references is available at http://info.cancerresearchuk.org/cancerstats/causes/
infectiousagents/kaposisarcoma/index.htm. Accessed January 2010.

This section contains information on Kaposi sarcoma-associated
herpesvirus (KSHV) including Kaposi sarcoma, primary effusion lymphoma, and multicentric Castleman disease.

Kaposi sarcoma-associated herpesvirus (KSHV, also known as
HHV8) is more closely related to Epstein-Barr virus (EBV) than it is
to other human herpesviruses, but it has its own unique complement
of latent cycle genes.

Like EBV, it preferentially infects and establishes latency in B
lymphocytes, but its effects in B cell growth are more subtle. The virus
also infects, and can replicate in, certain types of endothelial cells.
Quite unusually for a human herpesvirus, KSHV prevalence varies
widely in different human populations. More than 50% people in many
African countries carry KSHV, but this falls to 10% or less in Eastern
European/Mediterranean countries and < 1% in Northern Europe. The
circumstances under which KSHV infection leads to cancer strongly
indicate that a fine balance exists between this potentially dangerous
virus and the host's immune defences.

Kaposi Sarcoma

Classic Kaposi sarcoma (KS) was first described as a slow-growing
endothelial cell tumour seen in elderly men of Mediterranean or Eastern European descent; subsequently a slightly more aggressive form of
the disease (so called 'endemic' KS) was recognized at higher rates in
African populations. With the onset of the AIDS epidemic the worldwide incidence of this cancer has increased dramatically in the past 25
years, and a much more aggressive form of KS is now the commonest
tumor among HIV-infected people in Africa. KS also became common
among a subset of HIV patients in the West, but the incidence is now

falling with the introduction of effective anti-HIV drug therapy. KS is also appearing among the small proportion of transplant recipients who happen to be infected with KSHV; this clearly shows that the KSHV-host balance is delicately poised and any reduction in host immune competence leaves the individual at high risk of malignancy. All cases of KS worldwide, whether classic, endemic, or HIV-associated, are positive for the KSHV genome and express a subset of KSHV proteins in the tumor cells.

Primary Effusion Lymphoma

Primary effusion lymphoma (PEL) is a unique B cell malignancy which is seen very rarely and only in immunosuppressed patients, either KSHV-infected AIDS-patients or in KSHV-infected transplant recipients receiving high doses of immunosuppression. It is consistently KSHV genome-positive and its development is thought to require a combination of virus infection and as yet poorly characterized cellular genetic changes. In many cases, the EBV genome is also present in the tumor cells but the significance of this is not understood.

Multicentric Castleman Disease

Multicentric Castleman disease (MCD) is a B cell lymphoproliferative lesion which can be quite variable in appearance and about which little is known. It is found at low incidence in immunocompetent people, where about half of cases have the KSHV genome in tumor cells. MCD incidence is again higher in AIDS patients and all such tumors are KSHV-genome positive.

Section 6.4

Hepatitis Viruses and Cancer Risk

This section contains information on hepatitis viruses, including hepatitis B and hepatitis C.

Chronic infection with hepatitis B and C causes 75–80% of liver cancers diagnosed worldwide. High prevalence areas are also those with the highest incidence rates for liver cancer. Other causes of the disease include liver damaging agents, such as alcohol, which become more important in countries such as where hepatitis virus infection is less prevalent.

Hepatitis B Virus

Hepatitis B virus (HBV), an agent that specifically infects and replicates in liver cells, is highly prevalent in many areas of the world, especially in South East Asia and sub-Saharan Africa. This not only explains the high rates of hepatitis (inflammation of the liver) in these populations but is very likely to be responsible for their increased incidence of primary liver cancer. Thus chronic HBV carriers have a 20–100-fold higher risk of liver cancer than uninfected individuals. Tumors tend to arise after 30 years or more of chronic HBV infection and the great majority show evidence of clonally integrated HBV DNA sequences in the tumor cells.

Such evidence strongly suggests a causative role for HBV in liver carcinogenesis, but the precise mechanism through which HBV acts is still not understood. In most cases the HBV genome is not integrated near cellular oncogenes and although some HBV proteins have interesting effects on cell growth in the laboratory, the virus does not consistently express those viral proteins when it is present in tumor cells. A more likely scenario is that many virus-infected liver cells are destroyed as a result of immunological attack rather than by virus

101

replication per se. Such damage stimulates the remaining cells to grow and divide, thereby increasing the risk of genetic accidents. In addition, subsequent infection of regenerating cells can lead to chance integration of viral DNA into their genome, further promoting cell genomic instability.

Together these effects would enhance the chances of a HBV-infected liver cell accumulating the series of genetic changes necessary for its malignant conversion. Other co-factors may act independently of HBV; evidence suggests that one such co-factor might be the presence in the diet of certain carcinogenic chemicals arising from the use of poorly preserved foodstuffs.

Hepatitis C Virus

In contrast to HBV, which may act through a combination of direct and indirect mechanisms, the infection of the liver with hepatitis C virus (HCV), is thought to increase the risk of liver cancer by purely indirect means. Worldwide, 0.5 to 2% of the population have current or past infection with hepatitis C. Despite the similarity in name, HCV is quite different from HBV; it is an RNA virus and never converts its genome into a DNA copy, and so there is no risk of integrating viral sequences accidentally into the cell genome. However, like HBV, it damages liver cells and causes continual re-growth; this alone is enough to increase the risk of genetic accidents leading to liver cancer. There is also an increased risk of non-Hodgkin lymphoma (NHL) among people infected with hepatitis C; the mechanism underlying this association is still not understood.

Section 6.5

Human T-Lymphotropic Virus Type 1 (HTLV1) and Cancer Risk

"HTLV1 Retrovirus," © 2009 Cancer Research UK (www.cancerresearchuk .org). Reprinted with permission. Complete text including references is available at http://info.cancerresearchuk.org/cancerstats/causes/infectiousagents/ htlvretrovirus.htm. Accessed January 2010.

Human T lymphotropic virus type 1 (HTLV1) was the first human retrovirus to be discovered and is endemic in certain areas (especially SW Japan, the Caribbean, and parts of Africa and South America) where up to 10% or more of the population may be infected.

The virus naturally infects CD4+ T lymphocytes and can be transmitted between close contacts through blood transfer or from mother to infant through cells in breast milk. In most cases the infection is harmless. However, as many as one in 20 infected individuals eventually develop a type of adult T cell leukemia in which every tumor cell carries a clonally integrated HTLV1 provirus.

HTLV1 differs from the standard "chronically oncogenic" and "acutely oncogenic" retroviruses in its mechanism of action; it appears to drive cell growth through expression of a particular viral protein, Tax, in latently-infected cells.

Tax can transactivate expression of a number of key cellular genes that enhance cell growth. The best examples are the genes encoding interleukin 2 (a T cell growth factor) and the interleukin 2 receptor (a molecule that allows cells to respond to the growth factor). As a consequence, the infected cells not only make their own growth signals, but also respond to them.

HTLV1 induces a rather weak growth transformation of T cells in the laboratory but, in the body, is probably never sufficiently strong to induce T cell leukemia on its own. However, a virally infected cell in which growth controls have even partly broken down, is more susceptible to further genetic accidents. During persistent infection a gradual build-up of HTLV1-positive T cells which have accumulated additional genetic changes may occur. Eventually this can lead to selection and outgrowth of a fully malignant, HTLV1-positive clone. At this stage malignant cell growth can occur in the absence of tax gene expression.

Section 6.6

Epstein-Barr Virus and Cancer Risk

This section contains information on Epstein-Barr virus including
post-transplant lymphoma, Burkitt lymphoma, Hodgkin lymphoma,
and nasopharyngeal carcinoma.

Epstein-Barr virus is a herpesvirus that is widespread in all human
populations. Infection usually occurs in childhood but if delayed until
adolescence can result in infectious mononucleosis (glandular fever).
EBV is distantly related to other herpesviruses like herpes simplex (the
cause of cold sores) or varicella-zoster (the cause of chicken pox). Like
them, EBV can replicate fully in epithelial cells, in this case in pharyngeal cells lining the inner mucosal surfaces of the mouth and nose.

Unlike other herpesviruses, Epstein-Barr virus has a unique set
of growth activating genes which it uses to establish a latent growth-
transforming infection of its main target cell, the B lymphocyte. The
growth of latently-infected B cells is normally controlled by the host
immune response, particularly the T cell response, and so the great
majority of people are able to carry this potentially dangerous virus
all their life without any ill effect. In certain circumstances, however,
long-term virus carriage can result in the appearance a number of
EBV-positive tumors.

Post-Transplant Lymphoma

Patients receiving T cell-suppressive drugs to prevent rejection of
a transplanted organ have reduced immune control over various persistent virus infections, including EBV. Strongly immunosuppressed
patients are at high risk of developing post-transplant lymphoma
(PTL), a tumor caused by EBV-transformed B cells growing out in the
absence of T cell control. A similar tumor is seen in late-stage AIDS
patients whose T cell control has been destroyed by HIV infection.

Burkitt Lymphoma

EBV is also strongly linked to a second B cell tumour, endemic Burkitt lymphoma (BL), the commonest cancer of childhood in many parts of equatorial Africa and in New Guinea.

Every tumor is EBV genome-positive and continues to express at least one virus latent protein. In addition, every tumor has acquired a chromosomal translocation leading to uncontrolled expression of the cellular oncogene, c-myc. EBV infection and the c-myc translocation appear to be independent changes that together drive the B cell to full malignancy. Chronic malarial infection is another key co-factor in tumor development and this explains the unusual geographic distribution of the disease. The malarial parasite is thought to act as a chronic immune stimulus to B cells, increasing the number of cells in active growth and therefore at risk of accidental c-myc translocation. BL is a rare childhood tumor in the Western world. Over the last 25 years, however, BL has appeared unexpectedly in HIV infected adults as an early symptom of AIDS, with HIV seeming to mimic some of the chronic immune stimulation seen from malaria in Africa. In contrast to endemic BL, only a minority of childhood and AIDS-associated BL are EBV positive.

Hodgkin Lymphoma

Hodgkin lymphoma (HL) is a third tumor of B cell origin that is linked to EBV. The disease occurs in all human populations at a roughly similar frequency. Some 40% of HL cases in Western countries are EBV genome-positive, and the association with EBV is even higher in many other parts of the world. Cellular genetic changes, as yet poorly understood, are crucial to HL development. In those tumors where EBV is present, the continued expression of a number of key viral latent proteins strongly suggests that the virus is contributing actively to tumor growth.

Nasopharyngeal Carcinoma

Nasopharyngeal carcinoma (NPC) is a cancer of the epithelial cells lining the nasal cavity. It is seen worldwide but is most common throughout South East Asia, especially in southern China. All cases of NPC worldwide are EBV-associated and express viral latent proteins in every cell, strongly suggesting that the virus is key to tumor development. The difference in NPC incidence in different human populations cannot be explained by the prevalence of EBV infection, since most people worldwide carry the virus. Instead it is thought to reflect the essential role of two other co-factors in NPC development, firstly some genetic susceptibility among southern Chinese, South East Asian, and Inuit people and secondly the influence of chemical carcinogens in the local diet.

Section 6.7

Helicobacter Pylori
and Cancer Risk

From "*H. pylori* and Cancer: Fact Sheet," National Cancer Institute (www.cancer.gov), October 17, 2006.

What is Helicobacter pylori?

Helicobacter pylori, or *H. pylori*, is a spiral-shaped bacterium that is able to grow in the human stomach. Normally, the acidic stomach environment prevents the survival of viruses, bacteria, and other microorganisms. However, *H. pylori* has evolved to be uniquely suited to thrive in the harsh stomach environment. *H. pylori* bacteria secrete urease, a special enzyme that converts urea to ammonia. Ammonia reduces the acidity of the stomach, making it a more hospitable home for *H. pylori*.

The ability to survive in the stomach provides *H. pylori* with a useful hiding place. White blood cells that would normally recognize and attack invading bacteria are unable to cross from blood vessels into the stomach lining. Instead, the ineffective white blood cells continue to respond to the site of infection, where they die and release nutrients that feed *H. pylori*.

H. pylori has co-existed with humans for thousands of years. However, because scientists believed the stomach was a sterile organ, this bacterium was not discovered until the 1980s. Some other gut bacteria actually aid their human hosts in the absorption of nutrients and defense against other, more dangerous, microbes. Because *H. pylori* is relatively newly discovered, the complex interactions between this microbe and humans, including its risks and benefits, are still being discovered.

How was the association between H. pylori and disease established?

In the 1980s, scientists began to notice the presence of curved bacteria, which later became known as *H. pylori*, in tissue samples taken from patients with ulcers of the stomach and upper small intestine. Believing that no bacteria could survive the harsh stomach environment, most scientists thought these mysterious bacteria were either due to contamination of tissue samples or just another harmless species of bacteria like many found in the gut. However, Australian researchers Barry J. Marshall, M.D., and J. Robin Warren, M.D., were convinced that the bacteria were actually the cause of ulcers. Marshall, frustrated with the lack of a good animal model of infection, infected himself with the curved bacteria. He became ill, developed inflammation of the stomach, and was able to culture the bacteria from his own ulcers, thereby proving the microbe to be the cause of stomach ulcers. For their discovery of *H. pylori* and its role in gastric ulcer formation, Marshall and Warren were awarded the 2005 Nobel Prize in Medicine.

What is the prevalence of infection with H. pylori?

Human infection with *H. pylori* is common; the Centers for Disease Control and Prevention estimate that approximately two-thirds of the world's population harbors the bacterium, with infection rates much higher in developing nations than in Europe and North America.

H. pylori is thought to be spread either through contaminated food and water or through direct mouth-to-mouth contact. In most populations, the bacterium is first acquired during childhood. Children living in crowded conditions and with a lower socioeconomic status are more likely to become infected.

It has been estimated that between 2% to 20% of people infected with *H. pylori* will develop ulcers. Some evidence also links *H. pylori* infection to gastric cancer, gastric mucosa-associated lymphoid tissue (MALT) lymphoma, and perhaps pancreatic cancer and cardiovascular disease. However, the majority of people infected with *H. pylori* will not become ill from the bacteria.

What is peptic ulcer disease?

Peptic ulcers are holes in the lining of the stomach or upper small intestine (duodenum) that extend deep into the muscular layers of these organs. An ulcer forms when surface cells become inflamed, die, and are shed. The damage can be caused by mechanical abrasion, infection, or inflammation, which results from an overreaction of immune cells.

Peptic ulcer disease (PUD) is responsible for over three million visits to the doctor per year in the United States. Stomach pain similar to heartburn or indigestion is the most prevalent symptom of a stomach ulcer. Other symptoms may include loss of appetite, weight loss, vomiting, blood in the stool, or anemia.

Before the 1980s, due to its high acid content, scientists believed the stomach was sterile, and mistakenly attributed PUD to stress and spicy foods. Now, research has shown that bacterial toxins released by *H. pylori* and the inflammation that results from infection can damage the stomach lining and cause peptic ulcers. Although statistics vary depending on geographical region, *H. pylori* is responsible for the large majority of peptic ulcers.

What is gastric cancer?

Gastric cancer, or cancer of the stomach, was once considered a single entity. Now, epidemiologists divide this cancer into two main classes: gastric cardia cancer (which is cancer of the top inch of the stomach, where it meets the esophagus) and non-cardia gastric cancer (cancer in all other areas of the stomach). This classification was adopted because these two types of stomach cancer have different risk factors and different patterns of occurrence. For example, *H. pylori* has been established as a strong risk factor for non-cardia gastric cancer, whereas its association with gastric cardia cancer is controversial.

In 2006, there will be an estimated 22,280 new cases of gastric cancer and approximately 11,430 deaths due to the disease in the U.S. Gastric cancer is the second most common cause of cancer-related deaths in the world, killing approximately 700,000 people in 2002. Gastric cancer is more common in developing countries than in the U.S.

Overall gastric cancer incidence rates are decreasing. However, this decline is mainly in non-cardia gastric cancer rates. In contrast, gastric cardia cancer rates are increasing, particularly in Western countries, such as the U.S. and many parts of Europe. Gastric cardia cancer, which was once very uncommon, now constitutes nearly half of all stomach cancers in white males in the U.S.

Infection with *H. pylori* is the most important risk factor for gastric cancer. Other risk factors include chronic gastritis (inflammation of the stomach); older age; being male; a diet high in salted, smoked, or poorly preserved foods and low in fruits and vegetables; certain types of anemia; smoking cigarettes; and a family history of stomach cancers.

What is pancreatic cancer?

Pancreatic cancer is cancer of the pancreas, a six-inch gland shaped like a thin pear. The pancreas is found behind the stomach and in front of the spine. It produces juices that help digest food as well as hormones, such as insulin, which help control blood sugar levels. The digestive juices are produced by exocrine pancreas cells and the hormones are produced by endocrine pancreas cells. About 95% of pancreatic cancers begin in exocrine cells.

It is estimated that 32,180 new cases of pancreatic cancer will be diagnosed in the United States in 2006. Only 20% of patients survive one year after diagnosis; an estimated 31,800 people will die from the disease in 2006, making it the fifth leading cause of cancer deaths in the United States.

Very little is known about what causes pancreatic cancer or how to prevent it. Long-term diabetes, obesity, and certain inherited genetic conditions are considered risk factors. In addition, smokers are twice as likely as nonsmokers to be diagnosed with pancreatic cancer.

What is gastric MALT lymphoma?

Cancer affecting the mucosa-associated lymphoid tissue (MALT) in the stomach, or gastric MALT lymphoma, is a rare type of non-Hodgkin lymphoma characterized by B lymphocytes, a type of immune cell, that slowly multiply in the stomach lining. The lining of the stomach normally lacks lymphoid (immune system) tissue, but this tissue nearly always appears in response to colonization of the lining by *H. pylori* bacteria. MALT lymphomas account for approximately 4% of all cases of lymphoma.

Is there evidence that shows that H. pylori *infection increases the risk of gastric cancer?*

Many studies have demonstrated a link between *H. pylori* infection and gastric cancers. In 1994, the International Agency for Research on Cancer (IARC) classified *H. pylori* as a carcinogen, or cancer-causing agent, despite conflicting results at the time.

Since then, colonization of the stomach with *H. pylori* has been increasingly accepted as an important risk factor for gastric cancers. However, this association varies by region of the stomach. In 2001, a combined analysis of 12 *H. pylori* and gastric cancer studies estimated that the risk of non-cardia gastric cancer was nearly six times higher for *H. pylori*-infected people than for uninfected people. Data show that infection with *H. pylori* plays an important role in the development of non-cardia gastric cancer, but its association with gastric cardia cancer is less clear.

What evidence shows that H. pylori *infection increases the risk of pancreatic cancer?*

Observational findings show that many people who had surgery to treat peptic ulcers developed pancreatic cancer up to 20 years later. In addition, one study found that out of 92 pancreatic cancer patients, 65% tested positive for *H. pylori*, while only 45% of non-cancer control participants tested positive. Although the study group was small and patients were not tested for *H. pylori* until after they were diagnosed with cancer, this study concluded that a positive association exists between *H. pylori* and pancreatic cancer.

What evidence shows that H. pylori *infection increases the risk of MALT lymphoma?*

Nearly all patients with gastric MALT lymphoma are infected with *H. pylori*, and the risk of developing this tumor is over six times higher in infected people than in uninfected people. Furthermore, up to 80% of patients with gastric MALT lymphoma achieve complete remission of their tumors after treatment with *H. pylori*-eradicating antibiotic therapy.

The exact incidence of gastric MALT lymphoma in *H. pylori*-infected persons is unknown, but these tumors occur in less than 1% of infected individuals.

What is the Alpha-Tocopherol, Beta-Carotene (ATBC) Cancer Prevention Study?

From 1985 to 1993, the Alpha-Tocopherol, Beta-Carotene (ATBC) Cancer Prevention Study in Finland studied a group of 29,133 male smokers between the ages of 50 and 69 years to determine whether daily supplementation with alpha-tocopherol, beta-carotene, or both, would reduce the number of lung or other cancers. After the original trial period ended, researchers continued to follow the participants.

What is the link between H. pylori *and gastric cancer, according to the ATBC follow-up study?*

Through April 1999, the Finnish Cancer Registry diagnosed 234 participants of the ATBC study with gastric cancer. Each of these participants was randomly matched by age with a cancer-free control participant. *H. pylori* infection status was determined from blood samples initially obtained from each study participant at the time of enrollment in the study. Comparing cancer subjects with non-cancer controls, the ATBC gastric cancer follow-up study concluded that infection with *H. pylori* was a strong risk factor for non-cardia gastric cancer and increased risk for the disease nearly eight-fold. In contrast, the study found that presence of the bacteria decreased the risk of cardia gastric cancer by about two-thirds.

There is little debate that *H. pylori* increases risk of non-cardia gastric cancer. However, the inverse association between *H. pylori* and gastric cardia cancer is relatively new. Only one study other than the ATBC has demonstrated statistically significant data to support the association of *H. pylori* and decreased risk of gastric cardia cancer, while others have reported conflicting results. Time trends of gastric cancer rates support the ATBC study results. In recent years, the number of *H. pylori* infections in developed countries has decreased, most likely due to changes in diet, refrigeration, better hygiene, and increased antibiotic use. The decline in *H. pylori* infection in developed countries has coincided with a decline in rates of non-cardia gastric cancer, but a rise in rates of gastric cardia cancer and certain types of esophageal cancer.

The ATBC Study has the advantage of examining blood samples collected years before cancer diagnosis. *H. pylori* bacteria prefer to grow on normal stomach cells rather than pre-cancerous cells, meaning that the development of advanced gastric cancer may result in lower numbers of the bacteria present in the stomach. By determining *H. pylori* status only after diagnosis of cancer, some previous studies may have underestimated the infection rate in participants with gastric cancer.

What is the link between H. pylori *and pancreatic cancer, according to the ATBC follow-up study?*

Similar to the ATBC follow-up study for gastric cancer, a pancreatic cancer follow-up study identified all cases of pancreatic cancer diagnosed through December 1995.

This follow-up study compared the levels of antibodies to *H. pylori* from blood samples taken at the start of the study (before the cancer was diagnosed). Researchers examined a group of 121 men who developed pancreatic cancer and compared them to a subgroup of 226 men who did not develop cancer but were similar in age and other characteristics. ATBC study participants infected with *H. pylori* were approximately twice as likely to develop pancreatic cancer as those without the bacteria.

How can **H. pylori** *infection decrease the risk of some cancers while increasing the risk of others?*

H. pylori infection is associated with a reduced risk of gastric cardia cancer. It is not clear why this bacterium could be inversely related to risk of cardia gastric cancer. One hypothesis is that the *H. pylori* urease enzyme reduces acid production in the stomach during colonization, thereby decreasing acid reflux into the esophagus, a major risk for cancers affecting regions of the upper stomach and esophagus.

What role do antibiotics play in gastric cancer rates?

The results of the ATBC gastric cancer study and others suggest that caution might be needed in wide-spread *H. pylori* eradication programs. The possibility of an inverse relationship between the bacterium and cardia gastric cancer is supported by correlating the decrease in *H. pylori* infection rates in Western countries during the past century, the result of improved hygiene and widespread antibiotic use, to lower rates of non-cardia cancer and higher rates of cardia cancer in these same regions.

What is CagA-positive **H. pylori** *and how does it affect risk of cancer?*

H. pylori bacteria use a needle-like appendage to inject CagA, a toxin produced by cytotoxin-associated gene A, into the junctions where two stomach lining cells meet. Not all strains of *H. pylori* carry the CagA gene; those that do are classified as CagA-positive. This toxin alters the structure of stomach cells and allows the bacteria to attach themselves more easily. Long-term exposure to CagA causes chronic inflammation.

Scientists may not be able to definitively attribute CagA alone to increased development of cancer because CagA-positive and CagA-negative strains also have other genetic differences. While results are conflicting, recent research suggests that infection with CagA-positive strains of *H. pylori* further increases the risk of gastric cancer above the risk associated with CagA-negative strains. Laboratory studies show that CagA-induced cellular changes can lead to accumulation of genetic mutations involved in the development of malignancies. This link is supported by a combined analysis of 16 studies that found a two-fold increase in the risk of non-cardia gastric cancer associated with CagA-positive *H. pylori* as compared to CagA-negative *H. pylori*.

The ATBC study determined *H. pylori* infection status at the time of study enrollment between 1985 and 1988 by the presence of antibodies directed against either the whole bacteria or the CagA toxin. The gastric cancer follow-up study reported that CagA-positive *H. pylori* strains had a stronger association with risk of non-cardia gastric cancer, as compared with Cag-A negative strains, although this difference was not statistically significant. In the ATBC pancreatic cancer study, infection with CagA-positive *H. pylori* strains were associated with an approximately two-fold increase in risk for the disease over people in the study who were not infected.

Chapter 7

Hormonal Therapies and Cancer Risk

Chapter Contents

Section 7.1

Oral Contraceptives and Cancer Risk

Excerpted from "Oral Contraceptives and Cancer Risk: Questions and Answers," National Cancer Institute (www.cancer.gov), May 2006.

Oral contraceptives (OCs) first became available to American women in the early 1960s. The convenience, effectiveness, and reversibility of action of birth control pills (popularly known as "the pill") have made them the most popular form of birth control in the United States. However, concerns have been raised about the role that the hormones in OCs might play in a number of cancers, and how hormone-based OCs contribute to their development. Sufficient time has elapsed since the introduction of OCs to allow investigators to study large numbers of women who took birth control pills for many years.

This section addresses only what is known about OC use and the risk of developing cancer. It does not deal with other serious side effects of OC use, such as the increased risk of cardiovascular disease for certain groups of women. Recently, alternative methods of delivering hormones for contraception have been developed, including a topical patch, vaginal ring, and intrauterine delivery system, but these products are too new to have been tested in clinical trials (research studies) for long-term safety and other effects.

What types of oral contraceptives are available in the United States? Why do researchers believe that oral contraceptives may influence cancer risk?

Currently, two types of OCs are available in the United States. The most commonly prescribed OC contains two man-made versions of natural female hormones (estrogen and progesterone) that are similar to the hormones the ovaries normally produce. This type of pill is often called a "combined oral contraceptive." The second type of OC available in the United States is called the minipill. It contains only a type of progesterone.

Estrogen stimulates the growth and development of the uterus at puberty, causes the endometrium (the inner lining of the uterus) to thicken during the first half of the menstrual cycle, and influences breast tissue throughout life, but particularly from puberty to menopause.

Progesterone, which is produced during the last half of the menstrual cycle, prepares the endometrium to receive the egg. If the egg is fertilized, progesterone secretion continues, preventing release of additional eggs from the ovaries. For this reason, progesterone is called the "pregnancy-supporting" hormone, and scientists believe that it has valuable contraceptive effects. The man-made progesterone used in OCs is called progestogen or progestin.

Because medical research suggests that some cancers depend on naturally occurring sex hormones for their development and growth, scientists have been investigating a possible link between OC use and cancer risk. Researchers have focused a great deal of attention on OC users over the past 40 years. This scrutiny has produced a wealth of data on OC use and the development of certain cancers, although results of these studies have not always been consistent. The risk of endometrial and ovarian cancers is reduced with the use of OCs, while the risk of breast and cervical cancers is increased.

How do oral contraceptives affect breast cancer risk?

A woman's risk of developing breast cancer depends on several factors, some of which are related to her natural hormones. Hormonal factors that increase the risk of breast cancer include conditions that may allow high levels of hormones to persist for long periods of time, such as beginning menstruation at an early age (before age 12), experiencing menopause at a late age (after age 55), having a first child after age 30, and not having children at all.

A 1996 analysis of worldwide epidemiologic data conducted by the Collaborative Group on Hormonal Factors in Breast Cancer found that women who were current or recent users of birth control pills had a slightly elevated risk of developing breast cancer. The risk was highest for women who started using OCs as teenagers. However, 10 or more years after women stopped using OCs, their risk of developing breast cancer returned to the same level as if they had never used birth control pills, regardless of family history of breast cancer, reproductive history, geographic area of residence, ethnic background, differences in study design, dose and type of hormone, or duration of use. In addition, breast cancers diagnosed in women after 10 or more years of not using OCs were less advanced than breast cancers diagnosed in women who had never used OCs. To conduct this analysis, the researchers examined the results of 54 studies. The analysis involved 53,297 women with breast cancer and 100,239 women without breast cancer. More than 200 researchers participated in this combined analysis of their original studies, which represented about 90% of the epidemiological studies throughout the world that had investigated the possible relationship between OCs and breast cancer.

The findings of the Women's Contraceptive and Reproductive Experiences (Women's CARE) study were in contrast to those described above. The Women's CARE study examined the use of OCs as a risk factor for breast cancer in women ages 35 to 64. Researchers interviewed 4,575 women who were diagnosed with breast cancer between 1994 and 1998, and 4,682 women who did not have breast cancer. Investigators collected detailed information about the participants' use of OCs, reproductive history, health, and family history. The results, which were published in 2002, indicated that current or former use of OCs did not significantly increase the risk of breast cancer. The findings were similar for white and black women. Factors such as longer periods of use, higher doses of estrogen, initiation of OC use before age 20, and OC use by women with a family history of breast cancer were not associated with an increased risk of the disease.

In a National Cancer Institute (NCI)-sponsored study published in 2003, researchers examined risk factors for breast cancer among women ages 20 to 34 compared with women ages 35 to 54. Women diagnosed with breast cancer were asked whether they had used OCs for more than six months before diagnosis and, if so, whether the most recent use had been within five years, five to 10 years, or more than 10 years. The results indicated that the risk was highest for women who used OCs within five years prior to diagnosis, particularly in the younger group.

How do oral contraceptives affect ovarian and endometrial cancer risk?

Studies have consistently shown that using OCs reduces the risk of ovarian cancer. In a 1992 analysis of 20 studies of OC use and ovarian cancer, researchers from Harvard Medical School found that the risk of ovarian cancer decreased with increasing duration of OC use. Results showed a 10 to 12% decrease in risk after one year of use, and approximately a 50% decrease after five years of use.

Researchers have studied how the amount or type of hormones in OCs affects ovarian cancer risk reduction. One of the studies used in the Harvard analysis, the Cancer and Steroid Hormone Study (CASH), found that the reduction in ovarian cancer risk was the same regardless of the type or amount of estrogen or progestin in the pill. A more recent analysis of data from the CASH study, however, indicated that OC formulations with high levels of progestin reduced ovarian cancer risk more than preparations with low progestin levels. In another recent study, the Steroid Hormones and Reproductions (SHARE) study, researchers investigated new, lower-dose progestins that have varying androgenic properties (testosterone-like effects). They found no difference in ovarian cancer risk between androgenic and nonandrogenic pills.

OC use in women at increased risk of ovarian cancer due to BRCA1 and BRCA2 genetic mutations has been studied. One study showed a reduction in risk, but a more recent study showed no effect.

The use of OCs has been shown to significantly reduce the risk of endometrial cancer. This protective effect increases with the length of time OCs are used, and continues for many years after a woman stops using OCs.

How do oral contraceptives affect cervical cancer risk?

Evidence shows that long-term use of OCs (five or more years) may be associated with an increased risk of cancer of the cervix (the narrow, lower portion of the uterus). Although OC use may increase the risk of cervical cancer, human papillomavirus (HPV) is recognized as the major cause of this disease. Approximately 14 types of HPV have been identified as having the potential to cause cancer, and HPVs have been found in 99% of cervical cancer biopsy specimens worldwide.

A 2003 analysis by the International Agency for Research on Cancer (IARC) found an increased risk of cervical cancer with longer use of OCs. Researchers analyzed data from 28 studies that included 12,531 women with cervical cancer. The data suggested that the risk of cervical cancer may decrease after OC use stops. In another IARC report, data from eight studies were combined to assess the effect of OC use on cervical cancer risk in HPV-positive women. Researchers found a fourfold increase in risk among women who had used OCs for longer than five years. Risk was also increased among women who began using OCs before age 20 and women who had used OCs within the past five years. The IARC is planning a study to reanalyze all data related to OC use and cervical cancer risk.

How do oral contraceptives affect liver cancer risk?

Several studies have found that OCs increase the risk of liver cancer in populations usually considered low risk, such as white women in the United States and Europe who do not have liver disease. In these studies, women who used OCs for longer periods of time were found to be at increased risk for liver cancer. However, OCs did not increase the risk of liver cancer in Asian and African women, who are considered high risk for this disease. Researchers believe this is because other risk factors, such as hepatitis infection, outweigh the effect of OCs.

What screening tests are available for the cancers described?

Studies have found that regular breast cancer screening with mammograms reduces the number of deaths from breast cancer for women ages 40 to 69. Women who are at increased risk for breast cancer should seek medical advice about when to begin having mammograms and how often to be screened. A high-quality mammogram, with a clinical breast exam (an exam done by a professional health care provider), is the most effective way to detect breast cancer early.

Abnormal changes in the cervix can often be detected by a Pap test and treated before cancer develops. Women who have begun to have sexual intercourse or are age 21 should check with their doctor about having a Pap test. Researchers are working on developing screening tests for ovarian and endometrial cancer.

Women who are concerned about their risk for cancer are encouraged to talk with their health care provider.

Section 7.2

Menopausal Hormone Replacement Therapy Use and Cancer

Excerpted from "Menopausal Hormone Replacement Use and Cancer," National Cancer Institute (www.cancer.gov), January 2007.

What is menopause?

Menopause is the time in a woman's life when menstruation (having a period) ends. It is part of a biological process that begins, for most women, in their mid-thirties. During this time, the ovaries gradually produce lower levels of natural sex hormones—estrogen and progesterone. Estrogen promotes the normal development of a woman's breasts and uterus, controls the cycle of ovulation (when an ovary releases an egg into a fallopian tube), and affects many aspects of a woman's physical and emotional health. Progesterone controls menstruation and prepares the lining of the uterus to receive the fertilized egg.

"Natural menopause" occurs when a woman has her last menstrual period, or stops menstruating, and is considered complete when menstruation has stopped for one year. This usually occurs between ages 45 and 55, with variations in timing from woman to woman. Women who undergo surgery to remove both ovaries (an operation called bilateral oophorectomy) experience "surgical menopause," an immediate end to menstruation caused by lack of hormones produced by the ovaries.

By the time a woman has reached natural menopause, estrogen output has decreased significantly. Even though low levels of this hormone are produced by other organs after menopause, these levels are only about one-tenth of the level found in premenopausal women. Progesterone is nearly absent in menopausal women.

What are menopausal hormones and why are they used?

Doctors may recommend menopausal hormones to counter some of the problems often associated with the onset of menopause (hot flashes, night sweats, sleeplessness, and vaginal dryness) or to prevent some long-term conditions that are more common in postmenopausal

121

women, such as osteoporosis (a condition characterized by a decrease in bone mass and density, causing bones to become fragile). Menopausal hormone use (sometimes referred to as hormone replacement therapy or postmenopausal hormone use) usually involves treatment with either estrogen alone or estrogen in combination with progesterone or progestin, a synthetic hormone with effects similar to those of progesterone. Among women who are prescribed menopausal hormones, women who have undergone a hysterectomy (surgery to remove the uterus and, sometimes, the cervix) are generally given estrogen alone. Women who have not undergone this surgery are given estrogen plus progestin, which is known to have a lower risk of causing endometrial cancer (cancer of the lining of the uterus).

How does medical research determine the benefits and risks of taking menopausal hormones?

Researchers commonly conduct two very different, yet important types of studies with people to examine the benefits and risks of hormone use: clinical trials and observational studies. In clinical trials, the participants are given either hormones or placebos (look-alike pills that do not contain any drug) to determine the effect of the hormones on various conditions and diseases. In observational studies, the investigators do not try to affect the outcome; they compare the health status of women taking hormones to that of women not taking hormones.

What has medical research found out about the risks and benefits of hormone use after menopause?

The most comprehensive evidence about the risks and benefits of taking hormones after menopause to prevent disease comes from the Women's Health Initiative (WHI) Hormone Program, which was sponsored by the National Heart, Lung, and Blood Institute (NHLBI) and the National Cancer Institute (NCI), parts of the National Institutes of Health (NIH). This research program examined the effects of menopausal hormones on women's health. The WHI Hormone Program involved two studies—the use of estrogen plus progestin for women with a uterus (the Estrogen-plus-Progestin Study), and the use of estrogen alone for women without a uterus (the Estrogen-Alone Study). In both hormone therapy studies, women were randomly assigned to receive either the hormone medication being studied or the placebo.

The WHI Estrogen-plus-Progestin Study was stopped in July 2002, when investigators reported that the overall risks of estrogen plus progestin, specifically Prempro™, outweighed the benefits. The researchers found that use of this estrogen-plus-progestin pill increased the risk of breast cancer, heart disease, stroke, blood clots, and urinary incontinence. However, the risk of colorectal cancer and hip fractures was lower among women using estrogen plus progestin than among those taking the placebo. In addition, the WHI Memory Study showed that estrogen plus progestin doubled the risk for developing dementia (a decline in mental ability in which the patient can no longer function independently on a day-to-day basis) in postmenopausal women age 65 and older. The risk increased for all types of dementia, including Alzheimer's disease.

The WHI Estrogen-Alone Study, which involved Premarin™, was stopped in February 2004, when the researchers concluded that estrogen alone increased the risk of stroke and blood clots. In contrast with the WHI Estrogen-plus-Progestin Study, the risk of breast cancer was decreased in women using estrogen alone compared with those taking the placebo. Use of estrogen alone did not increase or decrease the risk of colorectal cancer. Similar to the results seen in the Estrogen-plus-Progestin Study, women using estrogen alone had an increased risk of urinary incontinence and a decreased risk of hip fractures.

Another large epidemiologic study, the Million Women Study, enrolled 1.3 million women in the United Kingdom. This study evaluated health outcomes in women using and not using menopausal hormones. Several analyses have been published to date, and many more are expected in the future.

How does menopausal hormone use affect breast cancer risk and survival?

The WHI Estrogen-plus-Progestin Study concluded that estrogen plus progestin increases the risk of invasive breast cancer. After five years of follow-up, women taking these hormones had a 24% increase in breast cancer risk compared with women taking the placebo. The increase amounted to an additional 8 cases of breast cancer for every 10,000 women taking estrogen plus progestin for one year compared with 10,000 women taking the placebo.

A detailed analysis of data from the WHI Estrogen-plus-Progestin Study showed that, among women taking estrogen plus progestin, the breast cancers were slightly larger and diagnosed at more advanced stages compared with breast cancers in women taking the placebo. Among women taking estrogen plus progestin, 25.4% of the cancers had spread outside the breast to nearby organs or lymph nodes compared with 16.0% among nonusers. Women taking estrogen plus progestin also had more abnormal mammograms (breast x-rays that require additional evaluation) than the women taking the placebo.

The WHI Estrogen-Alone Study concluded that taking estrogen did not increase the risk of breast cancer in women with a prior hysterectomy, at least for the seven years of follow-up in the study. Further analysis of data from the study indicated a 20% decrease in risk of breast cancer in women taking estrogen alone, although this decrease was seen mainly in the occurrence of early-stage breast cancer and ductal breast cancer (a specific type that begins in the lining of the milk ducts in the breast). The observed reduction amounted to six fewer cases of breast cancer for every 10,000 women taking estrogen for one year compared with 10,000 nonusers, but this lower incidence was not statistically significant; that is, the lower incidence could have arisen by chance rather than being related to estrogen-alone use. The Estrogen-Alone Study also showed a substantial increase in the frequency of abnormal mammograms.

A comprehensive review of data from 51 epidemiological (population) studies published in the 1980s and 1990s found a statistically significant increase in breast cancer risk among current or recent users of any hormone replacement therapy compared with the risk among nonusers. Most women in the analysis (88%) had used estrogen alone, and data for estrogen-plus-progestin users was not analyzed separately. Analysis of the pooled data also showed that the risk of breast cancer increased with increasing duration of hormone use, and this effect was more prominent in women with low body weight or a low body mass index. However, breast cancers in hormone users were less likely to have spread to other parts of the body compared with the breast cancers in nonusers. The increase in breast cancer risk largely, if not completely, disappeared about five years after cessation of hormone use.

As part of the Million Women Study, researchers examined six types of breast cancer among users and nonusers of menopausal hormones. The results showed that the effects of hormone use varied among breast cancer types. Overall, breast cancer risk was significantly increased among current users, although the risk was lower among women with higher body mass index.

What are the effects of hormone use on the risk of endometrial cancer?

Studies have shown that long-term exposure of the uterus to estrogen alone increases a woman's risk of endometrial cancer. The risk associated with estrogen plus progestin appears to be much less, but some data suggest that the risk is still increased compared with the risk for nonusers. The long-term effects of estrogen plus progestin on endometrial cancer risk remain uncertain.

The WHI Estrogen-plus-Progestin Study showed that endometrial cancer rates for women taking estrogen plus progestin daily were the same as or possibly less than those for women taking the placebo pill. Uterine bleeding, however, was a common side effect, leading to more frequent biopsies and ultrasounds for women taking estrogen plus progestin compared with those taking a placebo.

The Million Women Study confirmed a lower risk of endometrial cancer in women taking estrogen plus progestin in comparison with those taking estrogen only or tibolone, a synthetic steroid that is not available in the United States.

How does menopausal hormone use affect the risk of ovarian cancer?

Several observational studies have found that the use of estrogen alone is associated with a slightly increased risk of ovarian cancer for women who used this hormone for 10 or more years. One observational study that followed 44,241 menopausal women for approximately 20 years concluded that women who used estrogen alone for 10 or more years were twice as likely to develop ovarian cancer compared with women who did not use menopausal hormones. Another large observational study also found an association between estrogen use and death due to ovarian cancer. In this study, the increased risk appeared to be limited to women who used estrogen for 10 or more years.

The results from the Million Women Study showed that women currently using menopausal hormones had an increased risk of developing ovarian cancer and a 20% likelihood of dying from the disease compared with nonusers. However, the increased risk disappeared after hormone use stopped.

Data from the WHI Estrogen-plus-Progestin Study indicate that there may be an increased risk of ovarian cancer with use of estrogen plus progestin. After 5.6 years of follow-up, a 58% increased risk of ovarian cancer was reported in women using estrogen plus progestin compared with nonusers, but the increased risk was not statistically significant. One observational study suggested that regimens of estrogen plus progestin do not increase the risk of ovarian cancer if progestin is used for more than 15 days per month, but this study was too small to draw firm conclusions. More research is needed to clarify the relationship between menopausal hormone use, particularly for estrogen plus progestin, and the risk of ovarian cancer.

How does menopausal hormone use affect the risk of colorectal cancer?

After five years of follow-up of women taking estrogen plus progestin, the WHI Estrogen-plus-Progestin Study reported a 37% reduction in colorectal cancer cases compared with women taking the placebo. On average, the researchers found that if a group of 10,000 women takes estrogen plus progestin for a year, six fewer cases of colon cancer will occur than in a group of nonusers. These findings are consistent with observational studies, which have suggested that the use of postmenopausal hormones may reduce the risk of colorectal cancer. The WHI Estrogen-Alone Study concluded that estrogen alone had no significant effect on colorectal cancer risk.

Should women with a history of cancer take menopausal hormones?

One of the roles of naturally occurring estrogen is to promote the normal growth of cells in the breast and uterus. For this reason, it is generally believed that menopausal estrogen use by women who have already been diagnosed with breast cancer may promote further tumor growth. Studies of hormone use to treat menopausal symptoms in breast cancer survivors have produced conflicting results.

In one trial, 434 breast cancer survivors receiving either estrogen alone or estrogen plus progestin were followed for two years before the study was stopped because researchers concluded that even short-term use of hormone replacement therapy posed an unacceptable risk of breast cancer recurrence. Among these study participants, 26 women in the group receiving hormone replacement therapy had another occurrence of breast cancer compared with seven women in the group receiving no hormone replacement therapy. In another study, which included 378 women who were followed for four years, 11 women receiving hormone replacement therapy had another occurrence of breast cancer compared with 13 women receiving no hormone replacement therapy, so the risk of breast cancer recurrence was not increased. A review of 15 studies comprising a total of 1,416 breast cancer survivors and 1,998 women without a history of breast cancer found no increase in risk of cancer recurrence with hormone replacement therapy use.

There is limited research on the risks associated with menopausal hormone use by women who have had other cancers, particularly gynecological cancers. One review of the published research found that no firm conclusion could be drawn about the safety of hormone use in women with a history of cancer. However, survivors of gastric and bladder cancer and meningioma may be at higher risk of a recurrence. Survivors of gynecological cancers may be at higher risk because these cancers tend to be more hormone-dependent, but more studies are needed.

Does the way in which hormones are administered make a difference?

Most of the data on the long-term health effects of hormones come from studies in which hormones (estrogen alone or estrogen plus progestin) are administered orally in the form of pills. Hormones in the form of transdermal patches or gels are also used to treat menopause-related symptoms. Estrogen-containing vaginal creams and rings can be used specifically for vaginal dryness. Progesterone is also available as a pill or gel. The amount of estrogen that enters the bloodstream from estrogen-containing vaginal creams and rings depends on the types of hormones and the dose. Generally, vaginal administration of hormones results in lower levels of circulating hormones compared with an equivalent oral dose. Because the vaginal epithelium (thin layer of tissue that covers the vagina) responds to very small doses of estrogen, low-dose estrogen-containing creams or gels can be used.

What should women do if they are concerned about taking menopausal hormones?

Although menopausal hormones have short-term benefits such as relief from hot flashes and vaginal dryness, several health concerns are associated with their use. Women should discuss with their health care provider whether to take menopausal hormones and what alternatives may be appropriate for them. The U.S. Food and Drug Administration (FDA) currently advises women to use menopausal hormones for the shortest time and at the lowest dose possible to control symptoms. The FDA publication Menopause and hormones provides additional information about the risks and benefits of hormone use for menopausal symptoms. This resource is available at http://www.fda.gov/For Consumers/ByAudience/ForWomen/ucm118624.htm on the internet.

What are the alternatives for women who choose not to take menopausal hormones?

To decrease the risk of chronic disease, women can adopt a healthy lifestyle by exercising regularly, eating a healthy diet, limiting the consumption of alcohol, and not starting to smoke or, for smokers, trying to quit. Eating foods rich in calcium and vitamin D or taking dietary supplements containing these nutrients can help prevent osteoporosis. Results from the WHI showed that taking calcium and vitamin D supplements provided some benefit in preserving bone mass and preventing hip fractures, particularly in women age 60 and older. Although generally well tolerated, these supplements were associated with an increased risk of kidney stones. Other drugs, such as alendronate (Fosamax®), raloxifene (Evista®), and risedronate (Actonel®), have been shown to prevent bone loss. In addition, parathyroid hormone (Forteo®) is approved by the FDA for osteoporosis treatment.

Short-term menopause-related problems may go away on their own and frequently require no therapy at all. Local therapy for specific symptoms, such as vaginal dryness and urinary bladder conditions, is available. Some women seek relief from menopausal symptoms with nonprescription complementary and alternative therapies containing estrogen-like compounds. Some sources of these estrogen-like compounds include soy-based products, whole grain cereal, oilseeds (primarily flaxseed), legumes, and the botanical black cohosh. The benefits and risks of most of these agents have not been proven, however.

One NIH-funded study, the Herbal Alternatives (HALT) for Menopause Study, involved 351 women, some of whom were postmenopausal while others were approaching menopause. All of these women experienced hot flashes and night sweats and were given herbal supplements, menopausal hormones, or no therapy. Women in the herbal supplement groups received black cohosh alone, a multibotanical supplement (including black cohosh), or the multibotanical supplement plus counseling to increase their intake of dietary soy. Women in the herbal supplement groups had no significant reduction in the number of hot flashes and night sweats compared with women who received no therapy. The women who received menopausal hormones had significantly fewer menopausal symptoms compared with the women who received no therapy.

Women should talk with their doctor about the option best for them.

What research still needs to be done?

Unresolved questions include whether different forms of the hormones, lower doses, different hormones, or different methods of administration are safer or more effective; whether risks and/ or benefits persist after women stop taking hormones; whether women might be able to take hormones safely for a short period of time; and whether certain subgroups of women, including women with a history of cancer, might be at higher or lower risk than the general population.

The WHI continues to evaluate the longer-term effects of calcium and vitamin D supplements on preserving bone mass, preventing hip fractures, and reducing colon cancer risk, and continues long-term follow-up of women in the hormone trials.

The NIH continues to sponsor research to evaluate the effects of estrogen-like compounds on menopausal symptoms and long-term health after menopause. Several NCI-sponsored studies are evaluating the effectiveness of nonhormonal treatments, such as the botanical St. John's wort and the antidepressant drug citalopram hydrobromide, in reducing hot flashes in women with a history of breast cancer.

Section 7.3

Risk of Ovarian Cancer from Hormone Therapy Confirmed

Excerpted from "Risk of Ovarian Cancer from Hormone Therapy Confirmed," National Cancer Institute (www.cancer.gov), August 2009.

Women who have taken hormone therapy are at a higher risk of developing ovarian cancer than women who have not, according to a nationwide study involving nearly 910,000 women in Denmark. The findings, which confirm and extend the results of previous studies, suggest that the risk of ovarian cancer should be a factor when women consider using hormone therapy to treat postmenopausal symptoms. The study is reported in the July 15, 2009 issue of the *Journal of the American Medical Association*.

Lina Steinrud Mørch of Copenhagen University and her colleagues used detailed information from national registries to detect an increased risk of ovarian cancer among former and current hormone users, compared with non-users. A woman's risk did not seem to depend on the type of hormones, the duration of use, or the mode of administration. The findings translate into about one extra ovarian cancer per approximately 8,300 women taking hormone therapy each year.

Since the Women's Health Initiative reported in 2002 that combination hormone therapy (estrogen plus progestin) was associated with an increased risk of breast cancer, several studies have linked estrogen-alone therapy to the risk of ovarian cancer. There have also been hints of an increased risk from combination therapy, and these are now confirmed.

"Here we see that combination therapy had essentially the same amount of increased risk as estrogen-alone therapy," said Dr. Garnet Anderson, an ovarian cancer researcher at the Fred Hutchinson Cancer Research Center. The results, she added, are not likely to alter the current guidelines on hormone therapy, which urge women to use the smallest possible dose for the shortest time period.

Hormone therapy may have caused approximately 140 extra cases of ovarian cancer in Denmark during the study period, or 5% of the ovarian cancers. "Even though this share seems low, ovarian cancer remains highly fatal, so accordingly this risk warrants consideration when deciding whether to use hormone therapy," the authors concluded.

Section 7.4

Diethylstilbestrol (DES) and Cancer Risk

Excerpted From "DES: Questions and Answers,"
National Cancer Institute (www.cancer.gov), November 2006.

What is DES?

DES (diethylstilbestrol) is a synthetic form of estrogen, a female hormone. It was prescribed between 1938 and 1971 to help women with certain complications of pregnancy. Use of DES declined following studies in the 1950s that showed it was not effective in preventing pregnancy complications. When given during the first five months of a pregnancy, DES can interfere with the development of the reproductive system in a fetus. For this reason, although DES and other estrogens may be prescribed for some medical problems, they are no longer used during pregnancy.

What health problems might DES-exposed daughters have?

In 1971, DES was linked to clear cell adenocarcinoma in a small number of daughters of women who had used DES during pregnancy. This uncommon cancer of the vagina or cervix is usually diagnosed between age 15 and 25 in DES-exposed daughters. Some cases have been reported in women in their thirties and forties. The risk to women older than age 40 is still unknown, because the women first exposed to DES in utero are just reaching their fifties, and information about their risk has not been gathered. The overall risk of an exposed daughter to develop this type of cancer is estimated to be approximately one in 1,000 (0.1%). Although clear cell adenocarcinoma is extremely rare, it is important that DES-exposed daughters be aware of the risk and have regular physical examinations.

Scientists found a link between DES exposure before birth and an increased risk of developing abnormal cells in the tissue of the cervix and vagina. Physicians use a number of terms to describe these abnormal cells, including dysplasia, cervical intraepithelial neoplasia, and squamous intraepithelial lesions. These abnormal cells resemble cancer cells in appearance; however, they do not invade nearby healthy tissue

131

as cancer cells do. Although these conditions are not cancer, they may develop into cancer if left untreated. DES-exposed daughters should have a yearly Pap test and pelvic exam to check for abnormal cells. DES-exposed daughters may also have structural changes in the vagina, uterus, or cervix, as well as irregular menstruation and an increased risk of miscarriage, ectopic (tubal) pregnancy, infertility, and premature births.

Evidence from a recent study suggests that daughters of women who took DES during pregnancy may have a slightly increased risk of breast cancer after age 40. The risk of breast cancer for DES-exposed women over age 40 was 1.9 times the risk of breast cancer for unexposed women of the same ages. The increased risk association was present for all breast cancer risk factors examined, and did not differ by tumor receptor status, tumor size, or lymph node involvement.

Although this evidence suggests that prenatal DES exposure increases the risk of breast cancer, breast cancer is still a relatively rare event among DES-exposed women. For every 1,000 DES-exposed women aged 45 to 49, 4 new cases of breast cancer per year would be expected, compared with 2 new cases per year in every 1,000 unexposed women.

While the greater risk above age 40 is statistically significant, that is, is more than would be expected to happen by chance alone, it is still based on relatively small numbers. The actual risk could be quite a bit lower or higher. Therefore, additional research is needed to be sure that the increased risk was caused by DES.

What health problems might DES-exposed sons have?

There is some evidence that DES-exposed sons may have testicular abnormalities, such as undescended testicles or abnormally small testicles. The risk for testicular or prostate cancer is unclear; studies of the association between DES exposure in utero and testicular cancer have produced mixed results. In addition, investigations of abnormalities of the urogenital system among DES-exposed sons have not produced clear answers.

What health problems might DES-exposed mothers have?

Women who used DES may have a slightly increased risk of breast cancer. Current research indicates that the risk of breast cancer in DES-exposed mothers is approximately 30% higher than the risk for women who have not been exposed to this drug. This risk has been stable over time, and does not seem to increase as the mothers become older. Additional research is needed to clarify this issue and whether DES-exposed mothers are at higher risk for any other types of cancer.

How can people find out if they took DES during pregnancy or were exposed to DES in utero?

It has been estimated that five to 10 million people were exposed to DES during pregnancy. Many of these people are not aware that they were exposed. A woman who was pregnant between 1938 and 1971 and had problems or a history of problems during pregnancy may have been given DES or a similar drug. Women who think they used a hormone such as DES during pregnancy, or people who think that their mother used DES during pregnancy, can contact the attending physician or the hospital where the delivery took place to request a review of the medical records. If any pills were taken during pregnancy, obstetrical records should be checked to determine the name of the drug. Mothers and children have a right to this information.

However, finding medical records after a long period of time can be difficult. If the doctor has retired or died, another doctor may have taken over the practice as well as the records. The county medical society or health department may know where the records have been stored. Some pharmacies keep records for a long time and can be contacted regarding prescription dispensing information. Military medical records are kept for 25 years. In many cases, however, it may be impossible to determine whether DES was used.

What should DES-exposed daughters do?

It is important for women who believe they may have been exposed to DES before birth to be aware of the possible health effects of DES and inform their doctor of their exposure. It is important that the physician be familiar with possible problems associated with DES exposure, because some problems, such as clear cell adenocarcinoma, are likely to be found only when the doctor is looking for them. A thorough examination may include the following:

- **Pelvic examination:** A doctor performs a physical examination of the reproductive organs. An examination of the rectum also should be done.

- **Palpation:** As part of a pelvic examination, the doctor feels the vagina, uterus, cervix, and ovaries for any lumps. Often palpation provides the only evidence that an abnormal growth is present.

- **Pap test:** A routine cervical Pap test is not adequate for DES-exposed daughters. The cervical Pap test must be supplemented with a special Pap test of the vagina called a "four-quadrant" Pap test, in which cell samples are taken from all sides of the upper vagina.

133

- **Iodine staining of the cervix and vagina:** An iodine solution is used to temporarily stain the linings of the cervix and vagina to detect adenosis (a noncancerous but abnormal growth of glandular tissue) or other abnormal tissue.

- **Colposcopy:** In colposcopy, a magnifying instrument is used to view the vagina and cervix. Some doctors do not perform colposcopy routinely. However, if the Pap test result is not normal, it is very important to check for abnormal tissue.

- **Biopsy:** Small samples of any tissue that appears abnormal on colposcopy are removed and examined under a microscope to see whether cancer cells are present.

- **Breast examinations:** Researchers are continuing to study whether DES-exposed daughters have a higher risk of breast cancer than unexposed daughters; therefore, DES-exposed daughters should continue to rigorously follow the routine breast cancer screening recommendations for their age group.

What should DES-exposed mothers do?

A woman who took DES while pregnant (or suspects she may have taken it) should inform her doctor. She should try to learn the dosage, when the medication was started, and how it was used. She also should inform her children who were exposed before birth so that this information can be included in their medical records. DES-exposed mothers should have regular breast cancer screenings and yearly medical checkups that include a pelvic examination and a Pap test.

What should DES-exposed sons do?

DES-exposed sons should inform their physician of their exposure and be examined periodically. While the level of risk of developing testicular cancer is unclear among DES-exposed sons, males with undescended testicles or unusually small testicles have an increased risk of developing testicular cancer, whether or not they were exposed to DES.

Is it safe for DES-exposed daughters to use oral contraceptives or hormone replacement therapy?

Each woman should discuss this important question with her doctor. Although studies have not shown that the use of birth control pills or hormone replacement therapy are unsafe for DES-exposed daughters, some doctors believe these women should avoid these medications because they contain estrogen. Structural changes in the vagina or cervix should cause no problems with the use of other forms of contraception, such as diaphragms or spermicides.

Do DES-exposed daughters have unusual problems with fertility and pregnancy?

Multiple studies have found an increased risk of premature births, miscarriage, and ectopic pregnancy associated with DES exposure. In an analysis of data published in 2000, researchers found that DES daughters were three times more likely to have had premature births and four times more likely to have had a miscarriage or ectopic pregnancy than unexposed daughters. Full-term infants were delivered in the first pregnancies of 64.1% of exposed women compared with 84.5% of unexposed women.

Early studies investigating a possible link between DES exposure and infertility produced conflicting results. However, a study published in 2001 that compared DES-exposed and unexposed daughters found that DES-exposed daughters have a higher risk of infertility than unexposed women, and the increased risk of infertility is mainly due to uterine or tubal problems.

What is the focus of current research on DES exposure?

Researchers continue to study DES-exposed daughters as they move into the menopausal years. The cancer risks for exposed daughters and sons are also being studied to determine if they differ from the unexposed population. In addition, researchers are studying possible health effects on the grandchildren of mothers who were exposed to DES during pregnancy (also called third-generation daughters or DES granddaughters).

Two published studies have examined DES granddaughters for possible abnormalities. A 1995 study found that the age menstruation began was not affected by the mother's exposure to DES. In a 2002 study, researchers compared DES granddaughters' pelvic exams to the results of their mothers' first pelvic exams. None of the granddaughters' pelvic exams showed changes usually associated with DES exposure. The researchers concluded that third-generation effects of in utero DES exposure are unlikely.

A recent and larger study using questionnaires to daughters of mothers who were exposed in utero to DES (granddaughters), however, shows a slight effect on menstrual periods—later attainment of menstrual regularization and more irregular periods—in the exposed granddaughters compared with the unexposed granddaughters. Also, there was a suggestion that infertility was greater among the exposed, and the exposed tended to have fewer births. Because a number of these associations are based on small numbers of events, researchers will continue to study these women to further clarify these findings.

Researchers are also following up on the observation that exposure to DES may lead to an increased risk of breast cancer. A 2006 analysis found that DES exposure in utero was associated with a slightly increased risk of breast cancer. The experience of the women thus far suggests that increased risk might be restricted to women age 40 or older. Further follow-up is needed to confirm this and to characterize risk as the women age.

A study published in 2003 found little support for the hypothesis that in utero exposure to DES influences the psychosexual characteristics (the likelihood of ever having been married, age at first intercourse, number of sexual partners, and having had a same-sex sexual partner in adulthood) of adult men and women.

Chapter 8

Radiation and Cancer Risk

Chapter Contents

Section 8.1

The Difference between Ionizing and Non-Ionizing Radiation

Excerpted from, "Ionizing and Non-Ionizing Radiation,"
Environmental Protection Agency (www.epa.gov),
October 2009.

Radiation having a wide range of energies form the electromagnetic spectrum, which is illustrated in Figure 8.1. The spectrum has two major divisions:

- non-ionizing radiation
- ionizing radiation

Radiation that has enough energy to move atoms in a molecule around or cause them to vibrate, but not enough to remove electrons, is referred to as "non-ionizing radiation." Examples of this kind of radiation are sound waves, visible light, and microwaves.

Radiation that falls within the ionizing radiation" range has enough energy to remove tightly bound electrons from atoms, thus creating ions. This is the type of radiation that people usually think of as 'radiation.' We take advantage of its properties to generate electric power, to kill cancer cells, and in many manufacturing processes.

The energy of the radiation shown on the spectrum in Figure 8.1 increases from left to right as the frequency rises.

Nonionizing Radiation

We take advantage of the properties of non-ionizing radiation for common tasks:

- Microwave radiation—telecommunications and heating food
- Infrared radiation—infrared lamps to keep food warm in restaurants
- Radio waves—broadcasting

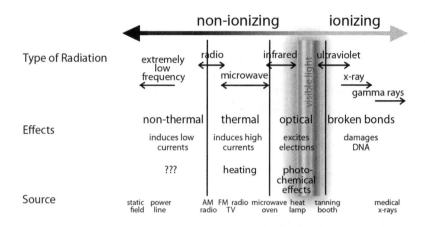

Figure 8.1. *Types of Radiation in the Electromagnetic Spectrum*

Non-ionizing radiation ranges from extremely low frequency radiation, shown on the far left through the audible, microwave, and visible portions of the spectrum into the ultraviolet range.

Extremely low-frequency radiation has very long wave lengths (on the order of a million meters or more) and frequencies in the range of 100 Hertz or cycles per second or less. Radio frequencies have wave lengths of between 1 and 100 meters and frequencies in the range of 1 million to 100 million Hertz. Microwaves that we use to heat food have wavelengths that are about 1 hundredth of a meter long and have frequencies of about 2.5 billion Hertz.

Ionizing Radiation

Higher frequency ultraviolet radiation begins to have enough energy to break chemical bonds. X-ray and gamma ray radiation, which are at the upper end of magnetic radiation have very high frequency—in the range of 100 billion billion Hertz—and very short wavelengths—1 million millionth of a meter. Radiation in this range has extremely high energy. It has enough energy to strip off electrons or, in the case of very high-energy radiation, break up the nucleus of atoms.

Ionization is the process in which a charged portion of a molecule (usually an electron) is given enough energy to break away from the atom. This process results in the formation of two charged particles or ions: the molecule with a net positive charge, and the free electron with a negative charge.

Each ionization releases approximately 33 electron volts (eV) of energy. Material surrounding the atom absorbs the energy. Compared to other types of radiation that may be absorbed, ionizing radiation deposits a large amount of energy into a small area. In fact, the 33 eV from one ionization is more than enough energy to disrupt the chemical bond between two carbon atoms. All ionizing radiation is capable, directly or indirectly, of removing electrons from most molecules.

There are three main kinds of ionizing radiation:

- Alpha particles, which include two protons and two neutrons

- Beta particles, which are essentially electrons

- Gamma rays and x-rays, which are pure energy (photons)

Section 8.2

How Radiation Affects Cancer Risk

Excerpted from, "Health Effects," Environmental Protection
Agency (www.epa.gov), February 2010.

How does radiation cause health effects?

Radioactive materials that decay spontaneously produce ionizing
radiation, which has sufficient energy to strip away electrons from atoms
(creating two charged ions) or to break some chemical bonds. Any living
tissue in the human body can be damaged by ionizing radiation in a
unique manner. The body attempts to repair the damage, but sometimes
the damage is of a nature that cannot be repaired or it is too severe or
widespread to be repaired. Also mistakes made in the natural repair
process can lead to cancerous cells. The most common forms of ionizing
radiation are alpha and beta particles, or gamma and X-rays.

What kinds of health effects does exposure to radiation cause?

In general, the amount and duration of radiation exposure affects
the severity or type of health effect. There are two broad categories of
health effects: stochastic and non-stochastic.

Stochastic health effects: Stochastic effects are associated with
long-term, low-level (chronic) exposure to radiation. ("Stochastic" refers to the likelihood that something will happen.) Increased levels
of exposure make these health effects more likely to occur, but do not
influence the type or severity of the effect.

Cancer is considered by most people the primary health effect from
radiation exposure. Simply put, cancer is the uncontrolled growth of
cells. Ordinarily, natural processes control the rate at which cells grow
and replace themselves. They also control the body's processes for repairing or replacing damaged tissue. Damage occurring at the cellular
or molecular level, can disrupt the control processes, permitting the

141

uncontrolled growth of cells—cancer. This is why ionizing radiation's ability to break chemical bonds in atoms and molecules makes it such a potent carcinogen.

Other stochastic effects also occur. Radiation can cause changes in DNA, the "blueprints" that ensure cell repair and replacement produces a perfect copy of the original cell. Changes in DNA are called mutations.

Sometimes the body fails to repair these mutations or even creates mutations during repair. The mutations can be teratogenic or genetic. Teratogenic mutations are caused by exposure of the fetus in the uterus and affect only the individual who was exposed. Genetic mutations are passed on to offspring.

Non-stochastic health effects: Non-stochastic effects appear in cases of exposure to high levels of radiation, and become more severe as the exposure increases. Short-term, high-level exposure is referred to as 'acute' exposure.

Many non-cancerous health effects of radiation are non-stochastic. Unlike cancer, health effects from 'acute' exposure to radiation usually appear quickly. Acute health effects include burns and radiation sickness. Radiation sickness is also called 'radiation poisoning.' It can cause premature aging or even death. If the dose is fatal, death usually occurs within two months. The symptoms of radiation sickness include: nausea, weakness, hair loss, skin burns or diminished organ function.

Medical patients receiving radiation treatments often experience acute effects, because they are receiving relatively high "bursts" of radiation during treatment.

Is any amount of radiation safe?

There is no firm basis for setting a "safe" level of exposure above background for stochastic effects. Many sources emit radiation that is well below natural background levels. This makes it extremely difficult to isolate its stochastic effects. In setting limits, EPA makes the conservative (cautious) assumption that any increase in radiation exposure is accompanied by an increased risk of stochastic effects.

Some scientists assert that low levels of radiation are beneficial to health (this idea is known as hormesis).

However, there do appear to be threshold exposures for the various non-stochastic effects. (Please note that the acute affects in the following table are cumulative. For example, a dose that produces damage to bone marrow will have produced changes in blood chemistry and be accompanied by nausea.)

Table 8.1. Health Effects of Radiation Exposure

Exposure (rem)	Health Effect	Time to Onset (without treatment)
5–10	changes in blood chemistry	
50	nausea	hours
55	fatigue	
70	vomiting	
75	hair loss	2–3 weeks
90	diarrhea	
100	hemorrhage	
400	possible death	within 2 months
1,000	destruction of intestinal lining, internal bleeding, and death	1–2 weeks
2,000	damage to central nervous system, loss of consciousness	minutes
	death	hours to days

How do we know radiation causes cancer?

Basically, we have learned through observation. When people first began working with radioactive materials, scientists didn't understand radioactive decay, and reports of illness were scattered.

As the use of radioactive materials and reports of illness became more frequent, scientists began to notice patterns in the illnesses. People working with radioactive materials and x-rays developed particular types of uncommon medical conditions. For example, scientists recognized as early at 1910 that radiation caused skin cancer. Scientists began to keep track of the health effects, and soon set up careful scientific studies of groups of people who had been exposed.

Among the best known long-term studies are those of Japanese atomic bomb blast survivors, other populations exposed to nuclear testing fallout (for example, natives of the Marshall Islands), and uranium miners.

Aren't children more sensitive to radiation than adults?

Yes, because children are growing more rapidly, there are more cells dividing and a greater opportunity for radiation to disrupt the process.

EPA's radiation protection standards take into account the differences in the sensitivity due to age and gender.

Fetuses are also highly sensitive to radiation. The resulting effects depend on which systems are developing at the time of exposure.

How do the effects of radiation type and exposure pathway influence health?

Both the type of radiation to which the person is exposed and the pathway by which they are exposed influence health effects. Different types of radiation vary in their ability to damage different kinds of tissue. Radiation and radiation emitters (radionuclides) can expose the whole body (direct exposure) or expose tissues inside the body when inhaled or ingested.

All kinds of ionizing radiation can cause cancer and other health effects. The main difference in the ability of alpha and beta particles and gamma and x-rays to cause health effects is the amount of energy they can deposit in a given space. Their energy determines how far they can penetrate into tissue. It also determines how much energy they are able to transmit directly or indirectly to tissues and the resulting damage.

Although an alpha particle and a gamma ray may have the same amount of energy, inside the body the alpha particle will deposit all of its energy in a very small volume of tissue. The gamma radiation will spread energy over a much larger volume. This occurs because alpha particles have a mass that carries the energy, while gamma rays do not.

Do chemical properties of radionuclides contribute to radiation health effects?

The chemical properties of a radionuclide can determine where health effects occur. To function properly many organs require certain elements. They cannot distinguish between radioactive and non-radioactive forms of the element and accumulate one as quickly as the other.

Radioactive iodine concentrates in the thyroid. The thyroid needs iodine to function normally, and cannot tell the difference between stable and radioactive isotopes. As a result, radioactive iodine contributes to thyroid cancer more than other types of cancer.

Calcium, strontium-90 and radium-226 have similar chemical properties. The result is that strontium and radium in the body tend to collect in calcium rich areas, such as bones and teeth. They contribute to bone cancer.

What is the cancer risk from radiation? How does it compare to the risk of cancer from other sources?

Each radionuclide represents a somewhat different health risk. However, health physicists currently estimate that overall, if each person in a group of 10,000 people exposed to 1 rem of ionizing radiation, in small doses over a life time, we would expect 5 or 6 more people to die of cancer than would otherwise.

In this group of 10,000 people, we can expect about 2,000 to die of cancer from all non-radiation causes. The accumulated exposure to 1 rem of radiation, would increase that number to about 2005 or 2006.

To give you an idea of the usual rate of exposure, most people receive about 3 tenths of a rem (300 mrem) every year from natural background sources of radiation (mostly radon).

Section 8.3

Radon and Cancer

Excerpted from "Radon and Cancer Risk," National Cancer Institute (www.cancer.gov), July 2004. Reviewed by David A. Cooke, MD, FACP, September 2010.

What is radon?

Radon is a radioactive gas released from the normal decay of uranium in rocks and soil. It is an invisible, odorless, tasteless gas that seeps up through the ground and diffuses into the air. In a few areas, depending on local geology, radon dissolves into ground water and can be released into the air when the water is used. Radon gas usually exists at very low levels outdoors. However, in areas without adequate ventilation, such as underground mines, radon can accumulate to levels that substantially increase the risk of lung cancer.

How is the general population exposed to radon?

Radon is present in nearly all air. Everyone breathes radon in every day, usually at very low levels. However, people who inhale high levels of radon are at an increased risk for developing lung cancer.

Radon can enter homes through cracks in floors, walls, or foundations, and collect indoors. It can also be released from building materials, or from water obtained from wells that contain radon. Radon levels can be higher in homes that are well insulated, tightly sealed, and/or built on uranium-rich soil. Because of their closeness to the ground, basement and first floors typically have the highest radon levels.

How does radon cause cancer?

Radon decays quickly, giving off tiny radioactive particles. When inhaled, these radioactive particles can damage the cells that line the lung. Long-term exposure to radon can lead to lung cancer, the only cancer proven to be associated with inhaling radon.

How many people develop lung cancer because of exposure to radon?

Cigarette smoking is the most common cause of lung cancer. Radon represents a far smaller risk for this disease, but it is the second leading cause of lung cancer in the United States. Scientists estimate that approximately 15,000 to 22,000 lung cancer deaths per year are related to radon.

Although the association between radon exposure and smoking is not well understood, exposure to the combination of radon gas and cigarette smoke creates a greater risk for lung cancer than either factor alone. The majority of radon-related cancer deaths occur among smokers.

How did scientists discover that radon plays a role in the development of lung cancer?

Radon was identified as a health problem when scientists noted that underground uranium miners who were exposed to it died of lung cancer at high rates. Results of miner studies have been confirmed by experimental animal studies, which show higher rates of lung tumors among rodents exposed to high radon levels.

What have scientists learned about the relationship between radon and lung cancer?

Scientists agree that radon causes lung cancer in humans. Recent research has focused on specifying the effect of residential radon on lung cancer risk. In these studies, scientists measure radon levels in the homes of people who have lung cancer and compare them to the levels of radon in the homes of people who have not developed lung cancer.

One of these studies, funded by the National Institute of Environmental Health Sciences, examined residential radon exposure in Iowa among females who had lived in their current home for at least 20 years. This study included 413 females with lung cancer and 614 females without lung cancer. During the study, radon levels were tested in homes, lung cancer tissues were examined, and the scientists collected information about home characteristics and other topics. Results from this study suggested a link between exposure to radon and lung cancer.

Scientists have conducted more studies like this in other regions of the United States and around the world. Many of these studies have demonstrated an association between residential exposure to radon and lung cancer, but this finding has not been observed in all studies. The inconsistencies between studies are due in part to the small size of some studies, the varying levels of radon in many homes, and the difficulty of measuring a person's exposure to radon over time.

Researchers have combined and analyzed data from all radon studies conducted in Canada and the United States. By combining the data from these studies, scientists were able to analyze data from thousands of people. The results of this analysis demonstrated a slightly increased risk of lung cancer associated with exposure to household radon. This increased risk was consistent with the level of risk estimated based on studies of underground miners.

Researchers are also investigating more precise ways to measure a person's exposure to radon over time. In a study published in 2002, scientists examined radon exposure among people in Sweden who had not smoked daily for more than a year. This study included 110 people with lung cancer and 231 people without lung cancer. As with previous studies, the scientists measured radon levels of indoor air. The researchers also used a new technique of analyzing glass to estimate radon exposure over time. Using this technique, the scientists took measurements from glass in an object (for example, a mirror or picture frame) that was at least 15 years old and had been in the person's home throughout that time, even if the person had moved from one home to another. In this study, both of the techniques for measuring radon demonstrated a relationship between long-term exposure to radon and lung cancer, and supported the results of previous studies.

How can people know if they have an elevated level of radon in their homes?

Testing is the only way to know if a person's home has elevated radon levels. Indoor radon levels are affected by the soil composition under and around the house, and the ease with which radon enters the house. Homes that are next door to each other can have different indoor radon levels, making a neighbor's test result a poor predictor of radon risk. In addition, precipitation, barometric pressure, and other influences can cause radon levels to vary from month to month or day to day, which is why both short- and long-term tests are available.

Short-term detectors measure radon levels for two days to 90 days, depending on the device. Long-term tests determine the average concentration for more than 90 days. Because radon levels can vary from day to day and month to month, a long-term test is a better indicator of average radon level. Both tests are relatively easy to use and inexpensive. A state or local radon official can explain the differences between testing devices and recommend the most appropriate test for a person's needs and conditions.

The U.S. Environmental Protection Agency (EPA) recommends taking action to reduce radon in homes that have a radon level at or above 4 picocuries per liter (pCi/L). About one in 15 U.S. homes is estimated to have radon levels at or above this EPA action level. Scientists estimate that lung cancer deaths could be reduced by 2–4%, or about 5,000 deaths, by lowering radon levels in homes exceeding the EPA's action level.

The cost of a radon reduction depends on the size and design of a home and the radon reduction methods that are needed. These costs typically range from $800 to $2,500, with an average cost of $1,200.

Where can people find more information about radon?

The following organizations can provide additional resources that readers may find helpful:

- The EPA website contains news, information, and publications on radon. It is located at http://www.epa.gov/iaq/radon on the internet.

- The National Safety Council (NSC), in partnership with the EPA, operates a Radon Hotline. To reach an automated system for ordering materials and listen to informational recordings, call 800-SOS-RADON (800-767-7236).

- To contact an information specialist, dial 800-55-RADON (800-557-2366) or send an e-mail to airqual@nsc.org.

- More information about radon and its testing can be found on the NSC's website at http://www.nsc.org/issues/radon/ on the internet.

- The Indoor Air Quality Information Clearinghouse (IAQ INFO) is operated by the EPA. To order publications or contact an information specialist, dial 800-438-4318. Alternatively, IAQ INFO can be reached by e-mail at iaqinfo@aol.com, by fax at 703-356-5386, or by mail at Post Office Box 37133, Washington, DC 20013-7133.

- The National Hispanic Indoor Air Quality Helpline is a service of the National Alliance for Hispanic Health, in partnership with the EPA. The Helpline provides bilingual (Spanish/English) information about indoor air pollutants. To speak with an information specialist, call 800-SALUD-12 (800-725-8312).

Section 8.4

Medical X-Rays: Benefits and Risks

Excerpted from "Medical X-Rays," U.S. Food and Drug Administration (www.fda.gov), August 2009.

Description

X-rays refer to radiation, waves or particles that travel through the air like light or radio signals. X-ray energy is high enough that some radiation passes through objects (such as internal organs, body tissues, and clothing) and onto x-ray detectors (such as film or a detector linked to a computer monitor). In general, objects that are more dense (such as bones and calcium deposits) absorb more of the radiation from the x-rays and don't allow as much to pass through them. These objects leave a different image on the detector than less dense objects. Specially trained or experienced physicians can read these images to diagnose medical conditions or injuries.

Procedures

Medical x-rays are used in many types of examinations and procedures. Here are some examples:

- X-ray radiography (to find orthopedic damage, tumors, pneumonias, foreign objects, etc)

- Mammography (to image the internal structures of breasts)

- CT (computed tomography) (to produce cross-sectional images of the body)

- Fluoroscopy (to dynamically visualize the body for example to see where to remove plaque from coronary arteries or where to place stents to keep those arteries open)

- Radiation therapy in cancer treatment

Risks/Benefits

Medical x-rays have increased the ability to detect disease or injury early enough for a medical problem to be managed, treated, or cured. When applied and performed appropriately, these procedures can improve health and may even save a person's life.

X-ray energy also has a small potential to harm living tissue. The most significant risks are a small increase in the possibility that a person exposed to x-rays will develop cancer later in life and cataracts and skin burns only at very high levels of radiation exposure and in only very few procedures.

The risk of developing cancer from radiation exposure is generally small, and it depends on at least three factors—the amount of radiation dose, the age at exposure, and the sex of the person exposed:

- The lifetime risk of cancer increases the larger the dose and the more x-ray exams a patient undergoes.

- The lifetime risk of cancer is larger for a patient who received x-rays at a younger age than for one who receives them at an older age.

- Women are at a somewhat higher lifetime risk than men for developing radiation-associated cancer after receiving the same exposures at the same ages.

Information for Patients

Here are some tips for reducing your radiation risks and contribute to your successful examination or procedure:

- Keep a "medical x-ray history" with the names of your radiological exams or procedures, the dates and places where you had them, and the physicians who referred you for those exams.

- Make your current healthcare providers aware of your medical x-ray history.

- Ask your healthcare provider about whether or not alternatives to x-ray exams would allow the provider to make a good assessment or provide appropriate treatment for your medical situation.

- Provide interpreting physicians and referring physicians with recent x-ray images and radiology reports.

- Inform radiologists or x-ray technologists in advance if you are pregnant or think you may be pregnant.

Section 8.5

Iodine-131 and Cancer Risk

Excerpted from "Get the Facts about Exposure to I-131 Radiation,"
National Cancer Institute (www.cancer.gov), August 2003.
Reviewed by David A. Cooke, MD, FACP, September 2010.

Introduction

During the Cold War in the 1950s and early 1960s, the U.S. government conducted about one hundred nuclear weapons (atomic bomb) tests in the atmosphere at a test site in Nevada. The radioactive substances released by these tests are known as "fallout." They were carried thousands of miles away from the test site by winds. As a result, people living in the United States at the time of the testing were exposed to varying levels of radiation.

Among the numerous radioactive substances released in fallout, there has been a great deal of concern about and study of one radioactive form of iodine--called iodine-131, or I-131. I-131 collects in the thyroid gland. People exposed to I-131, especially during childhood, may have an increased risk of thyroid disease, including thyroid cancer. Thyroid cancer is uncommon and is usually curable. Typically, it is a slow-growing cancer that is highly treatable. About 95 out of 100 people who are diagnosed with thyroid cancer survive the disease for at least five years after diagnosis.

The thyroid controls many body processes, including heart rate, blood pressure, and body temperature, as well as childhood growth and development. It is located in the front of the neck, just above the top of the breastbone and overlying the windpipe.

This section is designed to provide information about I-131 and its possible effects on the thyroid gland. Although the potential of developing thyroid cancer from exposure to I-131 is small, it is important for Americans who grew up during the atomic bomb testing between 1951 and 1963 to be aware of risks.

How Americans Were Exposed to I-131

During the Cold War, the United States developed and tested nuclear weapons in an effort to deter and to be fully prepared for nuclear attacks from other nations. Most of the aboveground U.S. nuclear tests were conducted in Nevada from 1951 to 1963. As a result of these tests, potentially health-harming radioactive materials were released into the atmosphere and produced fallout.

I-131 was among the radioactive materials released by the atomic bomb tests. It was carried thousands of miles away from the test areas on the winds. Because of wind and rainfall patterns, the distribution of fallout varied widely after each test. Therefore, although all areas of the U.S. received fallout from at least one nuclear weapons test, certain areas of North America received more fallout than others.

Scientists estimate that the larger amounts of I-131 fell over some parts of Utah, Colorado, Idaho, Nevada, and Montana. But I-131 traveled to all states, particularly those in the Midwestern, Eastern, and Northeastern United States. Some of the I-131 collected on pastures and on grasses, where it was consumed by cows and goats. When consumed by cows or goats, I-131 collects in the animals' milk. Eating beef from cows exposed to I-131 carried little risk. Much of the health risk associated with I-131 occurred among milk-drinkers—usually children. From what is known about thyroid cancer and radiation, scientists think that people who were children during the period of atomic bomb testing are at higher risk for developing thyroid cancer.

In addition to nuclear testing in Nevada, Americans were exposed to I-131 through:

- Nuclear testing elsewhere in the world (mainly in the 1950s and 1960s)

- Nuclear power plant accidents (such as the Chornobyl accident in 1986, also known as Chernobyl)

- Releases from atomic weapons production plants (such as the Hanford facility in Washington state from 1944 to 1957)

Scientists are working to find out more about ways to measure and address potential I-131 exposure from other sources. Scientists are also working to find out more about other radioactive substances released by fallout and about their possible effects on human health.

The Search for Answers

Congress directed government health agencies to investigate the I-131 problem many years ago, and to make recommendations to Americans who might have related health risks. Gathering information turned out to be very complicated. Record-keeping was incomplete at the time of the bomb testing. Much of the information needed to calculate an individual's dose of I-131 and associated risk is either unreliable or unavailable.

Despite such challenges, government agencies organized expert scientific teams that have devoted many years to learning more about I-131. Reports were published in 1997 and 1999. This information continues the effort to educate the American people about the potential health risks from exposure to I-131 from the Nevada Test Site during the Cold War years.

I-131's Rapid Breakdown

Like all radioactive substances, I-131 releases radiation as it breaks down. It is this radiation that can injure human tissues. But I-131's steady breakdown means that the amount of I-131 present in the environment after a bomb test steadily decreased. Therefore, farm animals that grazed in fields within a few days after a test would have consumed higher levels of I-131 than animals grazing later.

The Milk Connection

People younger than 15 at the time of aboveground testing (between 1951 and 1963) who drank milk, and who lived in the Mountain West, Midwestern, Eastern, and Northeastern United States, probably have a higher thyroid cancer risk from exposure to I-131 in fallout than other people. Their thyroid glands were still developing during the testing period. And they were more likely to have consumed milk contaminated with I-131. The amount of I-131 people absorbed depends on:

- Their age during the testing period (between 1951 and 1963)
- The amount and source of milk they drank in those years
- Where they lived during the testing period

Age and residence during the Cold War years are usually known. But few people can recall the exact amounts or sources of the milk they drank as children. While the amount of milk consumed is important in determining exposure to I-131, it is also important to know the source of the milk. Fresh milk from backyard or farm cows and goats usually contained more I-131 than store-bought milk. This is because processing and shipping milk allowed more time for the I-131 to break down.

About Thyroid Disease

There are two main types of thyroid diseases noncancerous thyroid disease and thyroid cancer.

Noncancerous Thyroid Disease

Some thyroid diseases are caused by changes in the amount of thyroid hormones that enter the body from the thyroid gland. Doctors can screen for these with a simple blood test.

Noncancerous thyroid disease also includes lumps, or nodules, in the thyroid gland that are benign and not cancerous.

Thyroid Cancer

Thyroid cancer occurs when a lump, or nodule, in the thyroid gland is cancerous.

Thyroid and I-131

Exposure to I-131 may increase a person's risk of developing thyroid cancer. It is thought that risk is higher for people who have had multiple exposures and for people exposed at a younger age. Thyroid cancer accounts for less than 2% of all cancers diagnosed in the United States. Typically, it is a slow-growing cancer that is highly treatable and usually curable. About 95 out of 100 people who are diagnosed with thyroid cancer survive the disease for at least five years, and about 92 out of 100 people survive the disease for at least 20 years after diagnosis.

The cause of most cases of thyroid cancer is not known. Exposure to I-131 can increase the risk of thyroid cancer. But even among people who have documented exposures to I-131, few develop this cancer. It is known that children have a higher-than-average risk of developing thyroid cancer many years later if they were exposed to radiation. This knowledge comes from studies of people exposed to x-ray treatments for childhood cancer or noncancerous head and neck conditions, or as a result of direct radiation from the atomic bombings of Hiroshima and Nagasaki.

The thyroid gland in adults, however, appears to be more resistant to the effects of radiation. There appears to be little risk of developing thyroid cancer from exposure to I-131 or other radiation sources as an adult.

There is no single or specific symptom of thyroid cancer. Doctors screen for thyroid cancer by feeling the gland, to check for a lump or nodule. If a doctor feels a nodule, it does not mean cancer is present. Most thyroid nodules found during a medical exam are not cancer.

If thyroid cancer is found, it is treated by removing the thyroid gland. People who undergo surgery will need to take thyroid hormone replacement pills for the rest of their lives. Although this is inconvenient and expensive, cancer survival rates are excellent. In fact, the cause of death among people who once had thyroid cancer is rarely the result of the return or spread of the same cancer.

Living with a serious disease like thyroid cancer isn't easy. A cancer diagnosis can be devastating. Some people find they need help coping with the emotional and practical aspects of their disease. Doctors and other health professionals can help with concerns about treatment and managing side effects. Support groups can help also. The National Cancer Institute's Cancer Information Service can help put you in touch with support groups in your community. Call 800-4-CANCER for more information.

Who's at Risk?

How can people reach a sound decision about their risk of thyroid cancer? When is it time to visit a doctor?

Scientists estimate that about 25% of the radioactive materials released during atomic bomb testing in Nevada reached the ground somewhere in the United States. But information about where the wind carried these materials is not precise. In addition, most adults cannot remember exact details of their milk-drinking habits in childhood.

Still, scientists and doctors think that I-131 exposure is a potential risk factor for thyroid cancer, and that some Americans have a higher risk than others. A "personal risk profile" includes four key points that may influence a person's decision to visit a doctor or other health professional for evaluation:

Age: People who are now 40 years of age or older, particularly those born between 1936 and 1963 and who were children at the time of testing, are at higher risk.

Milk drinking: Childhood milk drinkers, particularly those who drank large quantities of milk or those who drank unprocessed milk from farm or backyard cows and goats, have increased risk.

Childhood residence: The Mountain West, Midwest, East, and Northeast areas of the United States generally were more affected by I-131 fallout from nuclear testing.

Medical signs: A lump or nodule that an individual can see or feel in the area of the thyroid gland requires attention. If you can see or feel a lump or nodule, it is important that you see a doctor.

How Do Doctors Diagnose and Treat Thyroid Cancer?

There are two methods of investigating a thyroid lump or nodule:

- **Ultrasound:** To locate and describe the lump

- **Biopsy:** To determine if the lump is cancerous

Thyroid ultrasound creates pictures by bouncing sound waves off the gland. This technique is painless and quick. But it cannot determine whether a lump is cancerous. The ultrasound device uses sound waves that people cannot hear. A computer uses the echoes to create a picture called a sonogram. From the picture, the doctor can see:

- How many nodules are present

- How big they are

- Whether they are solid or filled with fluid

Confirmation of cancer requires biopsy, usually using fine needle aspiration. Cells removed from a nodule during biopsy are directly examined in the laboratory with a microscope.

Fine needle aspiration biopsy—in which a few cells are withdrawn from a nodule in a thin, hollow needle—is fast and carries minimal risk. Most people with a thyroid nodule who have a biopsy turn out not to have thyroid cancer. But even noncancerous nodules require medical follow-up. If a diagnosis cannot be made from the biopsy, the doctor may operate to remove the nodule. A pathologist then checks the tissue for cancer cells.

If thyroid cancer is found, it is treated by removing the thyroid gland. People who undergo surgery will need to take thyroid hormone replacement pills for the rest of their lives.

Unlike many other far more common and threatening cancers, thyroid cancer is generally cured by surgery, often along with postoperative radioiodine treatment. People who think they may be at risk for thyroid cancer should discuss this concern with their doctor. The doctor may suggest a schedule for checkups.

Key Facts

- I-131 breaks down rapidly in the atmosphere and environment

- Exposure was highest in the first few days after each nuclear test explosion

- Most exposure occurred through drinking fresh milk

- People received little exposure from eating fruits and leafy vegetables as compared to drinking fresh milk because although I-131 was deposited on fruits and leafy vegetables, the I-131 in fallout was deposited only on the surface; people generally wash or peel fruits and leafy vegetables

- Thyroid cancer is uncommon, usually curable, and approximately two to three times more common in women

Reliable information about I-131's impact on human health has been difficult to collect, but scientists think risk for thyroid cancer increases with exposure, but even among people exposed to I-131, few develop this cancer. In addition, people exposed as children have a higher risk than people exposed as adults.

The National Cancer Institute's website (www.cancer.gov) offers additional information about I-131. You can search for the keyword "I-131" to locate their dose estimator or call their Cancer Information Service at 800-4-CANCER. If you are concerned about exposure to I-131 and its possible effect on your thyroid health, your health care professional can help you determine if any specific attention is required.

Section 8.6

Magnetic Field Exposure and Cancer

Excerpted from "Magnetic Field Exposure and Cancer: Questions and Answers," National Cancer Institute (www.cancer.gov), April 2005. Reviewed by David A. Cooke, MD, FACP, September 2010.

What are electric and magnetic fields?

Electricity is the movement of electrons, or current, through a wire. The type of electricity that runs through power lines and in houses is alternating current (AC). AC power produces two types of fields (areas of energy)—an electric field and a magnetic field. An electric field is produced by voltage, which is the pressure used to push the electrons through the wire, much like water being pushed through a pipe. As the voltage increases, the electric field increases in strength. A magnetic field results from the flow of current through wires or electrical devices and increases in strength as the current increases. These two fields together are referred to as electric and magnetic fields, or EMFs.

Both electric and magnetic fields are present around appliances and power lines. However, electric fields are easily shielded or weakened by walls and other objects, whereas magnetic fields can pass through buildings, humans, and most other materials. Since magnetic fields are most likely to penetrate the body, they are the component of EMFs that are usually studied in relation to cancer.

The focus of this chapter is on extremely low-frequency magnetic fields. Examples of devices that emit these fields include power lines and electrical appliances, such as electric shavers, hair dryers, computers, televisions, electric blankets, and heated waterbeds. Most electrical appliances have to be turned on to produce a magnetic field. The strength of a magnetic field decreases rapidly with increased distance from the source.

Is there a link between magnetic field exposure at home and cancer in children?

Numerous epidemiological (population) studies and comprehensive reviews have evaluated magnetic field exposure and risk of cancer in

158

children. Since the two most common cancers in children are leukemia and brain tumors, most of the research has focused on these two types. A study in 1979 pointed to a possible association between living near electric power lines and childhood leukemia. Among more recent studies, findings have been mixed. Some have found an association; others have not. These studies are discussed in the following paragraphs. Currently, researchers conclude that there is limited evidence that magnetic fields from power lines cause childhood leukemia, and that there is inadequate evidence that these magnetic fields cause other cancers in children. Researchers have not found a consistent relationship between magnetic fields from power lines or appliances and childhood brain tumors.

In one large study by the National Cancer Institute (NCI) and the Children's Oncology Group, researchers measured magnetic fields directly in homes. This study found that children living in homes with high magnetic field levels did not have an increased risk of childhood acute lymphoblastic leukemia. The one exception may have been children living in homes that had fields greater than 0.4 microtesla (μT), a very high level that occurs in few residences. Another study conducted by NCI researchers reported that children living close to overhead power lines based on distance measurements were not at greater risk of leukemia.

To estimate more accurately the risks of leukemia in children from magnetic fields resulting from power lines, researchers pooled (combined) data from many studies. In one pooled study that combined nine well-conducted studies from several countries, including a study from the NCI, a twofold excess risk of childhood leukemia was associated with exposure to magnetic fields above 0.4 μT. In another pooled study that combined 15 studies, a similar increased risk was seen above 0.3 μT. It is difficult to determine if this level of risk represents a real increase or if it results from study bias. Such study bias can be related to the selection of study subjects or possibly to other factors that relate to levels of magnetic field exposure. If magnetic fields caused childhood leukemia, certain patterns would have been found such as increasing risk with increasing levels of magnetic field exposure.

Another way that people can be exposed to magnetic fields is from household electrical appliances. Several studies have investigated this relationship. Although magnetic fields near many electrical appliances are higher than near power lines, appliances contribute less to a person's total exposure to magnetic fields. This is because most appliances are used only for short periods of time, and most are not used close to the body, whereas power lines are always emitting magnetic fields.

In a detailed evaluation, investigators from NCI and the Children's Oncology Group examined whether the use of household electrical appliances by the mother while pregnant and later by the child increased the risk of childhood leukemia. Although some appliances were associated with childhood leukemia, researchers did not find any consistent pattern of increasing risk with increasing years of use or how often the appliance was used. A few other studies have reported mostly inconsistencies or no relation between appliances and risk of childhood cancer.

Occupational exposure of mothers to high levels of magnetic fields during pregnancy has been associated with childhood leukemia in a Canadian study. Similar studies need to be done in other populations to see if this is indeed the case.

Is there a link between magnetic field exposure in the home and cancer in adults?

Although several studies have looked into the relationship of leukemia, brain tumors, and breast cancer in adults exposed to magnetic fields in the home, there are only a few large studies with long-term, magnetic field measurements. No consistent association between magnetic fields and leukemia or brain tumors has been established.

The majority of epidemiological studies have shown no relationship between breast cancer in women and magnetic fields from electrical appliances. Recent studies of breast cancer and magnetic fields in the home have included direct and indirect magnetic field measurements. These studies mostly found no association between breast cancer in females and magnetic fields from power lines or electric blankets. A Norwegian study found a risk for exposure to magnetic fields in the home, and a study in African-American women found that use of electric bedding devices may increase breast cancer risk.

Is there a link between magnetic field exposure at work and cancer in adults?

Several studies conducted in the 1980s and early 1990s reported that people who worked in some electrical occupations (such as power station operators and phone line workers) had higher than expected rates of some types of cancer, particularly leukemia, brain tumors, and male breast cancer. Some occupational studies showed very small increases in risk for leukemia and brain cancer, but these results were based on job titles and not actual measurements. More recently conducted studies that have included both job titles and individual exposure measurements have no consistent finding of an increasing risk of leukemia, brain tumors, or female breast cancer with increasing exposure to magnetic fields at work.

What have scientists learned from animal experiments about the relationship between magnetic field exposure and cancer?

Animal studies have not found that magnetic field exposure is associated with increased risk of cancer. The absence of animal data supporting carcinogenicity makes it biologically less likely that magnetic field exposures in humans, at home or at work, are linked to increased cancer risk.

Chapter 9

Environmental Carcinogens

Cancer: Inside and Outside Factors

Cancer is a renegade system of growth inside the human body. The changes that must occur inside for cancer to flourish are genetic changes, but factors outside the body also play a role.

Humans do not exist in contaminant-free surroundings. Over a lifetime, a person's internal genetic makeup persistently interacts with external factors. Factors outside the body such as diet, smoking, alcohol use, hormone levels, or exposures to certain viruses and cancer-linked chemicals (carcinogens) over time may collectively conspire with internal genetic mutations to destabilize normal checks and balances on growth and maturation.

When most people think of the word "environment," they think of forests, oceans, or mountains. In cancer research, however, scientists define the environment as everything outside the body that enters and interacts with it. This interaction is called an exposure. So, environmental exposures can include such factors as sunshine, radiation, hormones, viruses, bacteria, and chemicals in the air, water, food, and workplace, as well as lifestyle choices like cigarette smoking, excessive alcohol consumption (more than two drinks/day), an unhealthful diet, lack of exercise, or sexual behavior that increases one's exposure.

Excerpted from "Understanding Cancer Series: Cancer and the Environment," National Cancer Institute (www.cancer.gov), September 1, 2006.

Researchers have estimated that as many as two in three cases of cancer (67%) are linked to some type of environmental factor, including use—or abuse—of tobacco, alcohol, and food, as well as exposures to radiation, infectious agents, and substances in the air, water, and soil.

We know that some exposures increase the risk of cancer, but we don't know which specific combinations of environmental factors on the outside of the body combine with gene changes on the inside to lead to cancer. We don't know why two persons can have very similar environmental exposures, yet one gets cancer and the other does not. A number of individual factors are involved and there are complex relationships among them.

The individual chance that someone will develop cancer in response to a particular, single environmental exposure depends on how long and how often that person was exposed. It also depends on the person's exposures to certain environmental factors (including diet, hormones), genetic makeup, age, and gender.

Environmental Carcinogens: The "Nasties" Lineup

Every two years, the federal government publishes a report on environmental exposures that have been linked to cancer. The most recent report included more than 220 substances. It helps to understand which of these exposures have the most impact on the general public.

As you consider these factors one at a time, it is important to remember that an individual accumulates a unique set of responses to his or her unique environment over a lifetime. Lengths and strengths of exposures will vary, and the person's genome itself will change.

Tobacco

Cigarette, cigar, and pipe smoking have been linked to more than a dozen types of cancer, including lung, mouth, bladder, colon, and kidney cancers. Chewing tobacco and snuff increase the risk of oral cancer, and second-hand smoke increases the risk of lung cancer.

Smoking is the single most common cause of cancer, and exposure to cancer-causing substances in tobacco products accounts for about 30% of cancer deaths in the United States. To reduce your cancer risk, don't smoke or use tobacco products. Avoid smoke-filled rooms if possible.

Alcohol

Alcohol is another risk factor. Heavy drinkers have an increased risk of cancers of the mouth, throat, liver, voice box, and esophagus.

There is also some evidence for an increased risk of breast cancer. Drinkers who also smoke may have an even higher risk of some oral and throat cancers. Drink in moderation, if at all: no more than one or two drinks per day.

Pesticides

About 20 ingredients in pesticides have been found to cause cancer in animals. Studies of people with high exposure to pesticides—farmers, crop duster pilots, pesticide manufacturers—have shown higher rates of blood and lymphatic system cancers in these people, as well as melanoma and cancers of the lip, stomach, brain, lung, and prostate.

Medications

Some chemotherapy drugs used to treat cancer may increase the risk of second cancers later in life. Drugs that suppress the immune system—used to treat some cancers as well as to prepare patients receiving organ transplants—also are associated with increased risk of cancer, particularly lymphoma.

On the other hand, new estrogen-blocking drugs called aromatase inhibitors can decrease the recurrence of breast cancer.

Any medication carries risks and benefits, so always check with a health professional before starting a new drug.

Hormones

Estrogen and progesterone are naturally occurring hormones. Given to women to treat the symptoms of menopause, they have been linked to increased risk of breast cancer.

Estrogen may also increase the risk of endometrial cancer, but progesterone helps protect against this increased risk. Estrogen and progestin (a synthetic form of progesterone) taken together are associated with increased risks of breast cancer, heart disease, stroke, and blood clots. Women who take oral contraceptives, which contain both estrogen and progesterone, may have increases in early-onset breast cancers and liver cancer, but have substantially reduced risks of endometrial and ovarian cancers.

Synthetic Hormones

The synthetic hormone tamoxifen is used in breast cancer therapies to prevent recurrence of disease or to prevent onset in women at high risk for this cancer, but it may increase the risk of endometrial cancer, strokes, and blood clots.

DES (diethylstilbestrol) is another synthetic hormone that was prescribed to pregnant women in the 1940s, 1950s, and 1960s. DES use was discontinued after scientists discovered that women taking it had an increased risk of breast cancer, and that girls born to women taking DES had an increased risk of rare types of vaginal and cervical cancer. Most physical or structural differences associated with exposure to DES are found in the reproductive tract, including a "hood" or collar on the cervix and a T-shaped uterus.

Solvents

Solvents are used in paint removers, grease removers, paint thinners, and dry cleaning. The solvents benzene, carbon tetrachloride, chloroform, and methylene chloride have been linked to human cancer.

The strongest evidence linking a solvent to cancer involves benzene, which is also found in cigarette smoke and gasoline. It increases the risk of leukemia.

If you must work with solvents, work outside or make sure the area is well ventilated.

Fibers and Dusts

Some fibers and dusts can increase the risk of lung-related cancers.

Asbestos is linked to increased risks of lung cancer and mesothelioma, a rare cancer of the lining of the lung and abdominal cavity. In the past, asbestos was widely used in construction, but its use has been restricted. However, workers employed in construction, electrical work, or carpentry may still be exposed through renovations or asbestos-removal projects.

Other fibers and dusts (including silica dust and wood dust) can increase the risks of cancers of the lung, nasal cavities, and sinuses.

Wear a well-fitting mask if your job exposes you to fine particles, fibers, or dust.

Dioxins

Dioxins are byproducts of paper bleaching, smelting, and waste incineration. They are widespread in the environment because they break down very slowly. They also accumulate in fat cells. Most of our exposure to dioxins comes from eating dairy products, fish, and meat.

Polycyclic Aromatic Hydrocarbons

These compounds (known as PAHs) come from the burning of carbon-based material. They are found in wood smoke, car exhaust, cigarette smoke, and charcoal-grilled foods. Sausages and roasted coffees may also contain PAHs. These compounds have been linked to increased risks of lung, skin, and urinary cancers.

Metals

Some metals—including arsenic, beryllium, cadmium, chromium, lead, and nickel—have been associated with several types of cancer, including lung, kidney, brain, skin, and liver cancers.

Vinyl Chloride

Vinyl chloride is used in the plastics industry and has been associated with lung cancer and with angiosarcomas (blood-vessel tumors) of the liver and brain. Most people are not routinely exposed to vinyl chloride unless they work in plastics manufacturing plants. People who live close to such plants also may be exposed through contaminated air.

Benzidine

Benzidine has been known to be associated with cancer since the 1920s. It is used in the production of dyes for paper, textiles, and leather. Exposure to these dyed products is not hazardous, however.

Aflatoxins

Aflatoxins are produced by certain types of fungi that grow on grains and peanuts. People can also be exposed to aflatoxins by eating meat or dairy products from animals that ate contaminated feed. Exposure to high levels of aflatoxins increases the risk of liver cancer. Peanuts are screened for aflatoxins in most countries, including the United States.

Identifying Cancer-Causing Substances

Americans commonly use more than 100,000 chemicals, and this doesn't take into account mixtures or combinations of chemicals. Plus, some chemicals are altered by the atmosphere, water, or incineration.

Scientists have been working for several decades to identify substances that cause cancer. They have three ways to do this: through human studies, animal studies, and laboratory experiments.

Human Studies

Human studies are the way to decide with the most certainty whether a substance causes cancer.

By following groups of people over time, researchers may be able to see whether certain exposures lead to cancer. They also compare a group of people who have been diagnosed with a type of cancer to another group of people without the disease. Sometimes the group with cancer has patterns of exposures very different from the patterns in the group without cancer.

Many environmental causes of cancer have first been noticed in the workplace, because people in certain occupations have higher exposures to some chemicals than do people in the general population.

Animal Studies

Rodents (mice and rats) are commonly used in studies of environmental causes of cancer. They have a relatively short lifespan (two to three years), and their bodies' responses to known cancer-causing chemicals are similar to a human response. Dietary studies in rodents are more difficult, however, due to differences in the digestive systems of rodents and humans.

In animal studies, the chemical exposures are usually at much higher levels than would be seen with human exposure. If an extremely high level of exposure does not lead to cancer, researchers reason that the chemical most likely does not cause cancer at lower levels either.

Laboratory Studies of Human Cells

Researchers study human cells in the laboratory to see whether certain chemicals might cause changes that could lead to cancer.

These studies are often done to see if animal studies—which take longer and are more complex—are actually needed. If a chemical does not cause cancer in laboratory cells, animal studies usually aren't done.

Risk Assessment

How do scientists decide which exposures are high risk and which are low risk? Risk assessment involves three factors:

1. **Potency:** The potential of a given amount of a substance to cause cancer. Benzene, for example, is quite potent because even small amounts of it can increase cancer risk. Other compounds, such as chloroform, are less potent; they require higher exposures to increase the risk by the same degree.

2. **Type of exposure:** Whether the exposure is one-time (acute) or long-term (chronic), and whether it is unavoidable (in the workplace, for example, or in the air we breathe).

3. **Dose response:** A dose-response trend describes what happens to cancer risk as the level of exposure increases or decreases.

Occupational Cancer Risks

Certain occupations carry an increased cancer risk: these include painters; furniture makers; workers in the iron, steel, coal, and rubber industries; and workers involved in shoe manufacturing and repair.

Always use proper protective equipment when handling chemicals, and clean spills immediately.

Ask at your workplace about Material Safety Data Sheets, which contain information about hazardous substances. The National Institute for Occupational Safety and Health (http://www.cdc.gov/niosh/) can answer many of your questions.

Avoidable Risks

While it is always prudent to be aware of environmental exposures to carcinogens, one must also remember that the major environmental factors linked to cancer deaths can be avoided, because most of them involve behavior choices. More than half of all cancer deaths could be prevented by eliminating the use of tobacco products, moderating the use of alcohol, and making better dietary choices.

Part Two

Common Types of Cancer

Chapter 10

Brain Tumors

This chapter is about tumors that begin in the brain (primary brain tumors). Each year in the United States, more than 35,000 people are told they have a tumor that started in the brain.

This information is only about primary brain tumors. Cancer that spreads to the brain from another part of the body is different from a primary brain tumor. Lung cancer, breast cancer, kidney cancer, melanoma, and other types of cancer commonly spread to the brain. When this happens, the tumors are called metastatic brain tumors. People with metastatic brain tumors have different treatment options. Treatment depends mainly on where the cancer started.

This chapter tells about diagnosis, treatment, and supportive care. Learning about medical care for brain tumors can help you take an active part in making choices about your care.

The Brain

The brain is a soft, spongy mass of tissue. It is protected by the bones of the skull, three thin layers of tissue (meninges), and watery fluid (cerebrospinal fluid) that flows through spaces between the meninges and through spaces (ventricles) within the brain.

The brain directs the things we choose to do (like walking and talking) and the things our body does without thinking (like breathing).

Excerpted from "What You Need to Know about Brain Tumors," National Cancer Institute (www.cancer.gov), NIH Publication No. 09-1558, April 29, 2009.

The brain is also in charge of our senses (sight, hearing, touch, taste, and smell), memory, emotions, and personality.

A network of nerves carries messages back and forth between the brain and the rest of the body. Some nerves go directly from the brain to the eyes, ears, and other parts of the head. Other nerves run through the spinal cord to connect the brain with the other parts of the body. Within the brain and spinal cord, glial cells surround nerve cells and hold them in place.

The three major parts of the brain control different activities:

- **Cerebrum:** The cerebrum uses information from our senses to tell us what is going on around us and tells our body how to respond. It controls reading, thinking, learning, speech, and emotions. The cerebrum is divided into the left and right cerebral hemispheres. The right hemisphere controls the muscles on the left side of the body. The left hemisphere controls the muscles on the right side of the body.

- **Cerebellum:** The cerebellum controls balance for walking and standing, and other complex actions.

- **Brain stem:** The brain stem connects the brain with the spinal cord. It controls breathing, body temperature, blood pressure, and other basic body functions.

Tumor Grades and Types

When most normal cells grow old or get damaged, they die, and new cells take their place. Sometimes, this process goes wrong. New cells form when the body doesn't need them, and old or damaged cells don't die as they should. The buildup of extra cells often forms a mass of tissue called a growth or tumor. Primary brain tumors can be benign or malignant.

Benign brain tumors do not contain cancer cells:

- Usually, benign tumors can be removed, and they seldom grow back.

- Benign brain tumors usually have an obvious border or edge. Cells from benign tumors rarely invade tissues around them. They don't spread to other parts of the body.

- However, benign tumors can press on sensitive areas of the brain and cause serious health problems. Unlike benign tumors in most other parts of the body, benign brain tumors are sometimes life threatening.

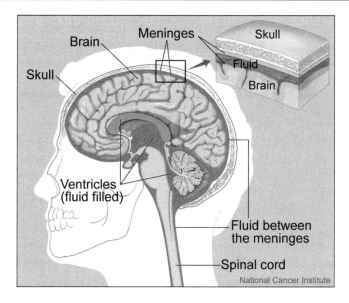

Figure 10.1. *The Brain and Nearby Structures (image by Alan Hoofring, National Cancer Institute).*

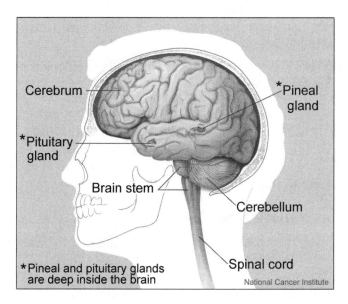

Figure 10.2. *Major Parts of the Brain (image by Alan Hoofring, National Cancer Institute).*

- Benign brain tumors may become malignant.

Malignant brain tumors (also called brain cancer) contain cancer cells:

- Malignant brain tumors are generally more serious and often are a threat to life.
- They are likely to grow rapidly and crowd or invade the nearby healthy brain tissue.
- Cancer cells may break away from malignant brain tumors and spread to other parts of the brain or to the spinal cord. They rarely spread to other parts of the body.

Tumor Grade

Doctors group brain tumors by grade. The grade of a tumor refers to the way the cells look under a microscope.

- **Grade I:** The tissue is benign. The cells look nearly like normal brain cells, and they grow slowly.
- **Grade II:** The tissue is malignant. The cells look less like normal cells than do the cells in a Grade I tumor.
- **Grade III:** The malignant tissue has cells that look very different from normal cells. The abnormal cells are actively growing (anaplastic).
- **Grade IV:** The malignant tissue has cells that look most abnormal and tend to grow quickly.

Cells from low-grade tumors (grades I and II) look more normal and generally grow more slowly than cells from high-grade tumors (grades III and IV). Over time, a low-grade tumor may become a high-grade tumor. However, the change to a high-grade tumor happens more often among adults than children.

Types of Primary Brain Tumors

There are many types of primary brain tumors. Primary brain tumors are named according to the type of cells or the part of the brain in which they begin. For example, most primary brain tumors begin in glial cells. This type of tumor is called a glioma.

Among adults, the following are the most common types of brain tumors:

- **Astrocytoma:** The tumor arises from star-shaped glial cells called astrocytes. It can be any grade. In adults, an astrocytoma most often arises in the cerebrum.

  - **Grade I or II astrocytoma:** It may be called a low-grade glioma.

  - **Grade III astrocytoma:** It's sometimes called a high-grade or an anaplastic astrocytoma.

  - **Grade IV astrocytoma:** It may be called a glioblastoma or malignant astrocytic glioma.

- **Meningioma:** The tumor arises in the meninges. It can be grade I, II, or III. It's usually benign (grade I) and grows slowly.

- **Oligodendroglioma:** The tumor arises from cells that make the fatty substance that covers and protects nerves. It usually occurs in the cerebrum. It's most common in middle-aged adults. It can be grade II or III.

Among children, the most common types are:

- **Medulloblastoma:** The tumor usually arises in the cerebellum. It's sometimes called a primitive neuroectodermal tumor. It is grade IV.

- **Grade I or II astrocytoma:** In children, this low-grade tumor occurs anywhere in the brain. The most common astrocytoma among children is juvenile pilocytic astrocytoma. It's grade I.

- **Ependymoma:** The tumor arises from cells that line the ventricles or the central canal of the spinal cord. It's most commonly found in children and young adults. It can be grade I, II, or III.

- **Brain stem glioma:** The tumor occurs in the lowest part of the brain. It can be a low-grade or high-grade tumor. The most common type is diffuse intrinsic pontine glioma.

Risk Factors

When you're told that you have a brain tumor, it's natural to wonder what may have caused your disease. But no one knows the exact causes of brain tumors. Doctors seldom know why one person develops a brain tumor and another doesn't.

Researchers are studying whether people with certain risk factors are more likely than others to develop a brain tumor. A risk factor is something that may increase the chance of getting a disease. Studies have found the following risk factors for brain tumors:

- **Ionizing radiation:** Ionizing radiation from high dose x-rays (such as radiation therapy from a large machine aimed at the head) and other sources can cause cell damage that leads to a tumor. People exposed to ionizing radiation may have an increased risk of a brain tumor, such as meningioma or glioma.

- **Family history:** It is rare for brain tumors to run in a family. Only a very small number of families have several members with brain tumors.

Researchers are studying whether using cell phones, having had a head injury, or having been exposed to certain chemicals at work or to magnetic fields are important risk factors. Studies have not shown consistent links between these possible risk factors and brain tumors, but additional research is needed.

Symptoms

The symptoms of a brain tumor depend on tumor size, type, and location. Symptoms may be caused when a tumor presses on a nerve or harms a part of the brain. Also, they may be caused when a tumor blocks the fluid that flows through and around the brain, or when the brain swells because of the buildup of fluid. These are the most common symptoms of brain tumors:

- Headaches (usually worse in the morning)
- Nausea and vomiting
- Changes in speech, vision, or hearing
- Problems balancing or walking
- Changes in mood, personality, or ability to concentrate
- Problems with memory
- Muscle jerking or twitching (seizures or convulsions)
- Numbness or tingling in the arms or legs

Most often, these symptoms are not due to a brain tumor. Another health problem could cause them. If you have any of these symptoms, you should tell your doctor so that problems can be diagnosed and treated.

Diagnosis

If you have symptoms that suggest a brain tumor, your doctor will give you a physical exam and ask about your personal and family health history. You may have one or more of the following tests:

Neurologic exam: Your doctor checks your vision, hearing, alertness, muscle strength, coordination, and reflexes. Your doctor also examines your eyes to look for swelling caused by a tumor pressing on the nerve that connects the eye and the brain.

MRI: Magnetic resonnance imaging. A large machine with a strong magnet linked to a computer is used to make detailed pictures of areas inside your head. Sometimes a special dye (contrast material) is injected into a blood vessel in your arm or hand to help show differences in the tissues of the brain. The pictures can show abnormal areas, such as a tumor.

CT scan: Computed tomography. An x-ray machine linked to a computer takes a series of detailed pictures of your head. You may receive contrast material by injection into a blood vessel in your arm or hand. The contrast material makes abnormal areas easier to see.

Other Common Tests

Your doctor may ask for other tests:

Angiogram: Dye injected into the bloodstream makes blood vessels in the brain show up on an x-ray. If a tumor is present, the x-ray may show the tumor or blood vessels that are feeding into the tumor.

Spinal tap: Your doctor may remove a sample of cerebrospinal fluid (the fluid that fills the spaces in and around the brain and spinal cord). This procedure is performed with local anesthesia. The doctor uses a long, thin needle to remove fluid from the lower part of the spinal column. A spinal tap takes about 30 minutes. You must lie flat for several hours afterward to keep from getting a headache. A laboratory checks the fluid for cancer cells or other signs of problems.

Biopsy: The removal of tissue to look for tumor cells is called a biopsy. A pathologist looks at the cells under a microscope to check for abnormal cells. A biopsy can show cancer, tissue changes that may lead to cancer, and other conditions. A biopsy is the only sure way to diagnose a brain tumor, learn what grade it is, and plan treatment.

Surgeons can obtain tissue to look for tumor cells in two ways:

- **Biopsy at the same time as treatment:** The surgeon takes a tissue sample when you have surgery to remove part or all of the tumor.

- **Stereotactic biopsy:** You may get local or general anesthesia and wear a rigid head frame for this procedure. The surgeon makes a small incision in the scalp and drills a small hole (a burr hole) into the skull. CT or MRI is used to guide the needle through the burr hole to the location of the tumor. The surgeon withdraws a sample of tissue with the needle. A needle biopsy may be used when a tumor is deep inside the brain or in a part of the brain that can't be operated on.

However, if the tumor is in the brain stem or certain other areas, the surgeon may not be able to remove tissue from the tumor without harming normal brain tissue. In this case, the doctor uses MRI, CT, or other imaging tests to learn as much as possible about the brain tumor.

A person who needs a biopsy may want to ask the doctor the following questions:

- Why do I need a biopsy? How will the biopsy results affect my treatment plan?

- What kind of biopsy will I have?

- How long will it take? Will I be awake? Will it hurt?

- What are the chances of infection or bleeding after the biopsy? Are there any other risks?

- How soon will I know the results?

- If I do have a brain tumor, who will talk with me about treatment? When?

Treatment

People with brain tumors have several treatment options. The options are surgery, radiation therapy, and chemotherapy. Many people get a combination of treatments. The choice of treatment depends mainly on the type and grade of brain tumor, its location in the brain, its size, and your age and general health. For some types of brain cancer, the doctor also needs to know whether cancer cells were found in the cerebrospinal fluid.

Your doctor can describe your treatment choices, the expected results, and the possible side effects. Because cancer therapy often damages healthy cells and tissues, side effects are common. Before treatment starts, ask your health care team about possible side effects and how treatment may change your normal activities. You and your health care team can work together to develop a treatment plan that meets your medical and personal needs.

You may want to talk with your doctor about taking part in a clinical trial, a research study of new treatment methods.

Your doctor may refer you to a specialist, or you may ask for a referral. Specialists who treat brain tumors include neurologists, neurosurgeons, neuro-oncologists, medical oncologists, radiation oncologists, and neuroradiologists.

Your health care team may also include an oncology nurse, a registered dietitian, a mental health counselor, a social worker, a physical therapist, an occupational therapist, a speech therapist, and a physical medicine specialist. Also, children may need tutors to help with schoolwork.

You may want to ask your doctor these questions before you begin treatment:

- What type of brain tumor do I have?
- Is it benign or malignant?
- What is the grade of the tumor?
- What are my treatment choices? Which do you recommend for me? Why?
- What are the expected benefits of each kind of treatment?
- What can I do to prepare for treatment?
- Will I need to stay in the hospital? If so, for how long?
- What are the risks and possible side effects of each treatment? How can side effects be managed?
- What is the treatment likely to cost? Will my insurance cover it?
- How will treatment affect my normal activities? What is the chance that I will have to learn how to walk, speak, read, or write after treatment?
- Would a research study (clinical trial) be appropriate for me?
- Can you recommend other doctors who could give me a second opinion about my treatment options?
- How often should I have checkups?

Second Opinion

Before starting treatment, you might want a second opinion about your diagnosis and treatment plan. Some people worry that the doctor will be offended if they ask for a second opinion. Usually the opposite is true. Most doctors welcome a second opinion. And many health insurance companies will pay for a second opinion if you or your doctor requests it. Some companies require a second opinion.

If you get a second opinion, the doctor may agree with your first doctor's diagnosis and treatment plan. Or the second doctor may suggest another approach. Either way, you'll have more information and perhaps a greater sense of control. You can feel more confident about the decisions you make, knowing that you've looked at your options.

It may take some time and effort to gather your medical records and see another doctor. In many cases, it's not a problem to take several weeks to get a second opinion. The delay in starting treatment usually won't make treatment less effective. To make sure, you should discuss this delay with your doctor. Some people with a brain tumor need treatment right away.

There are many ways to find a doctor for a second opinion. You can ask your doctor, a local or state medical society, a nearby hospital, or a medical school for names of specialists. Also, you can request a consultation with specialists at the National Institutes of Health Clinical Center in Bethesda, Maryland.

Nutrition

It's important for you to take care of yourself by eating well. You need the right amount of calories to maintain a good weight. You also need enough protein to keep up your strength. Eating well may help you feel better and have more energy.

Sometimes, especially during or soon after treatment, you may not feel like eating. You may be uncomfortable or tired. You may find that foods don't taste as good as they used to. In addition, the side effects of treatment (such as poor appetite, nausea, vomiting, or mouth blisters) can make it hard to eat well. Your doctor, a registered dietitian, or another health care provider can suggest ways to deal with these problems.

Supportive Care

A brain tumor and its treatment can lead to other health problems. You may receive supportive care to prevent or control these problems. You can have supportive care before, during, and after cancer treatment.

It can improve your comfort and quality of life during treatment. Your health care team can help you with the following problems:

- **Swelling of the brain:** Many people with brain tumors need steroids to help relieve swelling of the brain.

- **Seizures:** Brain tumors can cause seizures (convulsions). Certain drugs can help prevent or control seizures.

- **Fluid buildup in the skull:** If fluid builds up in the skull, the surgeon may place a shunt to drain the fluid.

- **Sadness and other feelings:** It's normal to feel sad, anxious, or confused after a diagnosis of a serious illness. Some people find it helpful to talk about their feelings.

Many people with brain tumors receive supportive care along with treatments intended to slow the progress of the disease. Some decide not to have antitumor treatment and receive only supportive care to manage their symptoms.

Rehabilitation

Rehabilitation can be a very important part of the treatment plan. The goals of rehabilitation depend on your needs and how the tumor has affected your ability to carry out daily activities.

Some people may never regain all the abilities they had before the brain tumor and its treatment. But your health care team makes every effort to help you return to normal activities as soon as possible. Several types of therapists can help:

- **Physical therapists:** Brain tumors and their treatment may cause paralysis. They may also cause weakness and problems with balance. Physical therapists help people regain strength and balance.

- **Speech therapists:** Speech therapists help people who have trouble speaking, expressing thoughts, or swallowing.

- **Occupational therapists:** Occupational therapists help people learn to manage activities of daily living, such as eating, using the toilet, bathing, and dressing.

- **Physical medicine specialists:** Medical doctors with special training help people with brain tumors stay as active as possible. They can help people recover lost abilities and return to daily activities.

Children with brain tumors may have special needs. Sometimes children have tutors in the hospital or at home. Children who have problems learning or remembering what they learn may need tutors or special classes when they return to school.

Follow-Up Care

You'll need regular checkups after treatment for a brain tumor. For example, for certain types of brain tumors, checkups may be every three months. Checkups help ensure that any changes in your health are noted and treated if needed. If you have any health problems between checkups, you should contact your doctor.

Your doctor will check for return of the tumor. Also, checkups help detect health problems that can result from cancer treatment. Checkups may include careful physical and neurologic exams, as well as MRI or CT scans. If you have a shunt, your doctor checks to see that it's working well.

Chapter 11

Childhood Brain and Spinal Cord Tumors

General Information about Childhood Brain and Spinal Cord Tumors

A childhood brain or spinal cord tumor is a disease in which abnormal cells form in the tissues of the brain or spinal cord. There are many types of childhood brain and spinal cord tumors. The tumors are formed by the abnormal growth of cells and may begin in different areas of the brain or spinal cord. Tumors may be benign (noncancerous) or malignant (cancerous).

Together, the brain and spinal cord make up the central nervous system (CNS).

The Brain

The brain controls major body functions. It has three major parts:

- The cerebrum is the largest part of the brain. It is at the top of the head. The cerebrum controls thinking, learning, problem solving, emotions, speech, reading, writing, and voluntary movement.

- The cerebellum, which is in the lower back of the brain (near the middle of the back of the head), controls movement, balance, and posture.

Excerpted from PDQ® Cancer Information Summary. National Cancer Institute; Bethesda, MD. "Childhood Brain and Spinal Cord Tumors Treatment Overview (PDQ) - Patient Version." Updated 10/2009. Available at: http://cancer.gov. Accessed January 20, 2010.

185

- The brain stem connects the brain to the spinal cord. It is in the lowest part of the brain (just above the back of the neck). The brain stem controls breathing, heart rate, and the nerves and muscles used in seeing, hearing, walking, talking, and eating.

The Spinal Cord

The spinal cord connects the brain with nerves in most parts of the body. It is a column of nerve tissue that runs from the brain stem down the center of the back. It is covered by three thin layers of tissue called membranes. These membranes are surrounded by the vertebrae (back bones). Spinal cord nerves carry messages between the brain and the rest of the body, such as a signal from the brain to cause muscles to move or from the skin to the brain about the sense of touch.

Brain and Spinal Cord Tumors in Children

Although cancer is rare in children, brain and spinal cord tumors are the third most common type of childhood cancer, after leukemia and lymphoma. Brain tumors can occur in both children and adults. Treatment for children is usually different than treatment for adults.

This chapter describes the treatment of primary brain and spinal cord tumors (tumors that begin in the brain and spinal cord). Treatment of metastatic brain and spinal cord tumors, which are tumors formed by cancer cells that begin in other parts of the body and spread to the brain or spinal cord, is not covered in this summary.

There are different types of childhood brain and spinal cord tumors. Childhood brain and spinal cord tumors are named based on the type of cell they formed in and where the tumor first formed in the CNS.

Types of Childhood Brain and Spinal Cord Tumors

Astrocytomas: Childhood astrocytomas are tumors that form in cells called astrocytes. They can be low-grade or high-grade tumors. The grade of the tumor describes how abnormal the cancer cells look under a microscope and how quickly the tumor is likely to grow and spread. High-grade astrocytomas are fast-growing, malignant tumors. Low-grade astrocytomas are slow-growing tumors that are less likely to be malignant.

Atypical teratoid/rhabdoid tumor: Childhood atypical teratoid/rhabdoid tumors are fast-growing tumors that often form in the cerebellum. They may also form in other parts of the brain and in the spinal cord.

Brain stem glioma: Childhood brain stem gliomas form in the brain stem (the part of the brain connected to the spinal cord).

Central nervous system embryonal tumor: Childhood CNS embryonal tumors form in brain and spinal cord cells when the fetus is beginning to develop. They include the following types of tumors:

- CNS atypical teratoid/rhabdoid tumors
- Ependymoblastoma
- Medulloblastoma
- Medulloepithelioma
- Pineal parenchymal tumors
- Pineoblastoma
- Supratentorial primitive neuroectodermal tumors (SPNET)

Central nervous system germ cell tumor: Childhood CNS germ cell tumors form in germ cells, which are cells that develop into sperm or ova (eggs). There are different types of childhood germ cell tumors. These include germinomas, embryonal yolk sac carcinomas, choriocarcinomas, and teratomas. A mixed germ cell tumor has two types of germ cell tumors in it. Germ cell tumors can be either benign or malignant.

Germ cell brain tumors usually form in the center of the brain, near the pineal gland. The pineal gland is a tiny organ in the brain that makes melatonin, which is a substance that helps control the sleeping and waking cycle. Germ cell tumors can spread to other parts of the brain and spinal cord.

Craniopharyngioma: Childhood craniopharyngiomas are tumors that usually form just above the pituitary gland. The pituitary gland is found in the center of the brain behind the back of the nose. It is about the size of a pea and controls many important body functions including growth. Craniopharyngiomas rarely spread, but may affect important areas of the brain, such as the pituitary gland.

Ependymoma: Childhood ependymomas are slow-growing tumors formed in cells that line the fluid -filled spaces in the brain and spinal cord.

Medulloblastoma: Childhood medulloblastomas form in the cerebellum.

Spinal cord tumors: Tumors of many different cell types may form in the spinal cord. Low-grade spinal cord tumors usually do not spread. High-grade spinal cord tumors may spread to other places in the spinal cord or brain.

Supratentorial primitive neuroectodermal tumor: Childhood supratentorial primitive neuroectodermal tumors (SPNET) form in immature cells in the cerebrum.

Symptoms

The cause of most childhood brain and spinal cord tumors is unknown. The symptoms of childhood brain and spinal cord tumors are not the same in every child.

Headaches and other symptoms may be caused by childhood brain and spinal cord tumors. Other conditions may cause the same symptoms. A doctor should be consulted if any of the following problems occur.

Brain Tumors

- Morning headache or headache that goes away after vomiting
- Frequent nausea and vomiting
- Vision, hearing, and speech problems
- Loss of balance and trouble walking
- Unusual sleepiness or change in activity level
- Unusual changes in personality or behavior
- Seizures
- Increase in the head size (in infants)

Spinal Cord Tumors

- Back pain or pain that spreads from the back towards the arms or legs
- A change in bowel habits or trouble urinating
- Weakness in the legs
- Trouble walking

In addition to these symptoms of brain and spinal cord tumors, some children are unable to reach certain growth and development milestones such as sitting up, walking, and talking in sentences.

Detection

Tests that examine the brain and spinal cord are used to detect (find) childhood brain and spinal cord tumors.

The following tests and procedures may be used:

Physical exam and history: An exam of the body to check general signs of health, including checking for signs of disease, such as lumps or anything else that seems unusual. A history of the patient's health habits and past illnesses and treatments will also be taken.

Neurological exam: A series of questions and tests to check the brain, spinal cord, and nerve function. The exam checks a person's mental status, coordination, and ability to walk normally, and how well the muscles, senses, and reflexes work. This may also be called a neuro exam or a neurologic exam.

Serum tumor marker test: A procedure in which a sample of blood is examined to measure the amounts of certain substances released into the blood by organs, tissues, or tumor cells in the body. Certain substances are linked to specific types of cancer when found in increased levels in the blood. These are called tumor markers.

MRI (magnetic resonance imaging) with gadolinium: A procedure that uses a magnet, radio waves, and a computer to make a series of detailed pictures of the brain and spinal cord. A substance called gadolinium is injected into a vein. The gadolinium collects around the cancer cells so they show up brighter in the picture. This procedure is also called nuclear magnetic resonance imaging (NMRI).

CT scan (CAT scan): A procedure that makes a series of detailed pictures of areas inside the body, taken from different angles. The pictures are made by a computer linked to an x-ray machine. A dye may be injected into a vein or swallowed to help the organs or tissues show up more clearly. This procedure is also called computed tomography, computerized tomography, or computerized axial tomography.

Angiogram: A procedure to look at blood vessels and the flow of blood in the brain. A contrast dye is injected into the blood vessel. As the contrast dye moves through the blood vessel, x-rays are taken to see if there are any blockages.

PET scan (positron emission tomography scan): A procedure to find malignant tumor cells in the body. A small amount of radioactive glucose (sugar) is injected into a vein. The PET scanner rotates around the body and makes a picture of where glucose is being used in the body. Malignant tumor cells show up brighter in the picture because they are more active and take up more glucose than normal cells do.

Diagnosis

Most childhood brain tumors are diagnosed and removed in surgery. If doctors think there might be a brain tumor, a biopsy may be done to remove a sample of tissue. For tumors in the brain, the biopsy is done by removing part of the skull and using a needle to remove a sample of tissue. A pathologist views the tissue under a microscope to look for cancer cells. If cancer cells are found, the doctor may remove as much tumor as safely possible during the same surgery. The pathologist checks the cancer cells to find out the type and grade of brain tumor. The grade of the tumor is based on how abnormal the cancer cells look under a microscope and how quickly the tumor is likely to grow and spread.

The following tests may be done on the sample of tissue that is removed:

Immunohistochemistry study: A laboratory test in which a substance such as an antibody, dye, or radioisotope is added to a sample of cancer tissue to test for certain antigens. This type of study is used to tell the difference between different types of cancer.

Light and electron microscopy: A laboratory test in which cells in a sample of tissue are viewed under regular and high-powered microscopes to look for certain changes in the cells.

Cytogenetic analysis: A laboratory test in which cells in a sample of tissue are viewed under a microscope to look for certain changes in the chromosomes.

Sometimes a biopsy or surgery cannot be done safely because of where the tumor formed in the brain or spinal cord. These tumors are diagnosed based on the results of imaging tests and other procedures.

Prognosis

Certain factors affect prognosis (chance of recovery). The prognosis (chance of recovery) depends on the following:

- Whether there are any cancer cells left after surgery
- The type of tumor
- The location of the tumor
- The child's age

- Whether the tumor has just been diagnosed or has recurred (come back)

Stages of Childhood Brain and Spinal Cord Tumors

In childhood brain and spinal cord tumors, treatment options are based on several factors. Staging is the process used to find how much cancer there is and if cancer has spread within the brain, spinal cord, or to other parts of the body. It is important to know the stage in order to plan cancer treatment.

In childhood brain and spinal cord tumors, there is no standard staging system. Instead, the plan for cancer treatment depends on several factors.

The type of tumor and where the tumor formed in the brain: Whether the tumor is newly diagnosed or recurrent. A newly diagnosed brain or spinal cord tumor is one that has never been treated. A recurrent childhood brain or spinal cord tumor is one that has recurred (come back) after it has been treated. Childhood brain and spinal cord tumors may come back in the same place or in another part of the brain, or spinal cord. Sometimes they come back in another part of the body. The tumor may come back many years after first being treated. Tests and procedures, including biopsy, that were done to diagnose and stage the tumor may be done to find out if the tumor has recurred.

The grade of the tumor: The grade of the tumor is based on how abnormal the cancer cells look under a microscope and how quickly the tumor is likely to grow and spread. It is important to know the grade of the tumor and if there were any cancer cells remaining after surgery in order to plan treatment. The grade of the tumor is not used to plan treatment for all types of brain and spinal cord tumors.

The tumor risk group: Risk groups are either average risk and poor risk or low, intermediate, and high risk. The risk groups are based on the amount of tumor remaining after surgery, the spread of cancer cells within the brain and spinal cord or to other parts of the body, where the tumor has formed, and the age of the child. The risk group is not used to plan treatment for all types of brain and spinal cord tumors.

The information from tests and procedures done to detect (find) childhood brain and spinal cord tumors is used to determine the tumor risk group.

After the tumor is removed in surgery, some of the tests used to detect childhood brain and spinal cord tumors are repeated to help determine the tumor risk group. This is to find out how much tumor remains after surgery. Other tests and procedures may be done to find out if cancer has spread:

Lumbar puncture: A procedure used to collect cerebrospinal fluid from the spinal column. This is done by placing a needle into the spinal column. Lumbar puncture is usually not used to stage childhood spinal cord tumors. This procedure is also called an LP or spinal tap.

Bone scan: A procedure to check if there are rapidly dividing cells, such as cancer cells, in the bone. A very small amount of radioactive material is injected into a vein and travels through the bloodstream. The radioactive material collects in the bones and is detected by a scanner.

Chest x-ray: An x-ray of the organs and bones inside the chest. An x-ray is a type of energy beam that can go through the body and onto film, making a picture of areas inside the body.

Bone marrow aspiration and biopsy: The removal of bone marrow, blood, and a small piece of bone by inserting a hollow needle into the hipbone or breastbone. A pathologist views the bone marrow, blood, and bone under a microscope to look for signs of cancer.

How Cancer Spreads

The three ways that cancer spreads in the body are:

- Through tissue. Cancer invades the surrounding normal tissue.

- Through the lymph system. Cancer invades the lymph system and travels through the lymph vessels to other places in the body.

- Through the blood. Cancer invades the veins and capillaries and travels through the blood to other places in the body.

When cancer cells break away from the primary (original) tumor and travel through the lymph or blood to other places in the body, another (secondary) tumor may form. This process is called metastasis. The secondary (metastatic) tumor is the same type of cancer as the primary tumor. For example, if breast cancer spreads to the bones, the cancer cells in the bones are actually breast cancer cells. The disease is metastatic breast cancer, not bone cancer.

Recurrent Childhood Brain and Spinal Cord Tumors

A recurrent childhood brain or spinal cord tumor is one that has recurred (come back) after it has been treated. Childhood brain and spinal cord tumors may come back in the same place or in another part of the brain. Sometimes they may come back in another part of the body. The tumor may come back many years after first being treated. Diagnostic and staging tests and procedures, including biopsy, may be done to confirm the tumor has recurred.

Treatment Option Overview

Different types of treatment are available for children with brain and spinal cord tumors. Some treatments are standard (the currently used treatment), and some are being tested in clinical trials. A treatment clinical trial is a research study meant to help improve current treatments or obtain information on new treatments for patients with cancer. When clinical trials show that a new treatment is better than the standard treatment, the new treatment may become the standard treatment.

Because cancer in children is rare, taking part in a clinical trial should be considered. Clinical trials are taking place in many parts of the country. Some clinical trials are open only to patients who have not started treatment.

Children with brain or spinal cord tumors should have their treatment planned by a team of health care providers who are experts in treating childhood brain and spinal cord tumors.

Treatment will be overseen by a pediatric oncologist, a doctor who specializes in treating children with cancer. The pediatric oncologist works with other health care providers who are experts in treating children with brain tumors and who specialize in certain areas of medicine. These may include the following specialists:

- Neurosurgeon
- Neurologist
- Neuro-oncologist
- Neuropathologist
- Neuroradiologist
- Radiation oncologist
- Endocrinologist
- Psychologist
- Ophthalmologist
- Rehabilitation specialist
- Social worker
- Nurse specialist

Childhood brain and spinal cord tumors may cause symptoms that continue for months or years. Symptoms caused by the tumor may begin before diagnosis. Symptoms caused by treatment may begin during or right after treatment. Some cancer treatments cause side effects months or years after treatment has ended. These are called late effects. Late effects of cancer treatment may include the following:

- Physical problems

- Changes in mood, feelings, thinking, learning, or memory

- Second cancers (new types of cancer)

Some late effects may be treated or controlled. It is important to talk with your child's doctors about the effects cancer treatment can have on your child.

Three types of standard treatment are used:

Surgery

Surgery may be used to diagnose and treat childhood brain and spinal cord tumors.

Radiation Therapy

Radiation therapy is a cancer treatment that uses high-energy x-rays or other types of radiation to kill cancer cells or keep them from growing. There are two types of radiation therapy. External radiation therapy uses a machine outside the body to send radiation toward the cancer. Internal radiation therapy uses a radioactive substance sealed in needles, seeds, wires, or catheters that are placed directly into or near the cancer.

Radiation therapy to the brain can affect growth and development in young children. For this reason, clinical trials are studying ways of using chemotherapy to delay, reduce, or end the need for radiation therapy. Also, ways of giving radiation therapy that lessen damage to healthy brain tissue are being used. Stereotactic radiosurgery is a type of radiation therapy that uses a rigid head frame attached to the skull to aim high-dose radiation beams directly at the tumors, which causes less damage to nearby healthy tissue. It is also called stereotaxic radiosurgery and radiation surgery. This procedure does not involve surgery.

The way the radiation therapy is given depends on the type and stage of the cancer being treated.

Chemotherapy

Chemotherapy is a cancer treatment that uses drugs to stop the growth of cancer cells, either by killing the cells or by stopping them from dividing. When chemotherapy is taken by mouth or injected into a vein or muscle, the drugs enter the bloodstream and can reach cancer cells throughout the body (systemic chemotherapy). When chemotherapy is placed directly in the spinal column, an organ, or a body cavity such as the abdomen, the drugs mainly affect cancer cells in those areas (regional chemotherapy). The way the chemotherapy is given depends on the type and stage of the cancer being treated.

Anticancer drugs given by mouth or vein to treat brain and spinal cord tumors cannot cross the blood-brain barrier and enter the fluid that surrounds the brain and spinal cord. Instead, an anticancer drug is injected into the fluid-filled space to kill cancer cells there. This is called intrathecal chemotherapy.

Clinical Trials

New types of treatment are being tested in clinical trials. This summary section describes treatments that are being studied in clinical trials. It may not mention every new treatment being studied.

High-dose chemotherapy with stem cell transplant is a way of giving high doses of chemotherapy and replacing blood-forming cells destroyed by the cancer treatment. Stem cells (immature blood cells) are removed from the blood or bone marrow of the patient or a donor and are frozen and stored. After the chemotherapy is completed, the stored stem cells are thawed and given back to the patient through an infusion. These reinfused stem cells grow into (and restore) the body's blood cells.

Patients may want to think about taking part in a clinical trial. For some patients, taking part in a clinical trial may be the best treatment choice. Clinical trials are part of the cancer research process. Clinical trials are done to find out if new cancer treatments are safe and effective or better than the standard treatment.

Many of today's standard treatments for cancer are based on earlier clinical trials. Patients who take part in a clinical trial may receive the standard treatment or be among the first to receive a new treatment.

Patients who take part in clinical trials also help improve the way cancer will be treated in the future. Even when clinical trials do not lead to effective new treatments, they often answer important questions and help move research forward.

Some clinical trials only include patients who have not yet received treatment. Other trials test treatments for patients whose cancer has not gotten better. There are also clinical trials that test new ways to stop cancer from recurring (coming back) or reduce the side effects of cancer treatment.

Clinical trials are taking place in many parts of the country.

Follow-Up Tests

Some of the tests that were done to diagnose the cancer or to find out the stage of the cancer may be repeated. Some tests will be repeated in order to see how well the treatment is working. Decisions about whether to continue, change, or stop treatment may be based on the results of these tests. This is sometimes called re-staging.

Some of the tests will continue to be done from time to time after treatment has ended. The results of these tests can show if your condition has changed or if the cancer has recurred (come back). These tests are sometimes called follow-up tests or check-ups.

Chapter 12

Neuroblastoma

General Information about Neuroblastoma

Neuroblastoma is a disease in which malignant (cancer) cells form in nerve tissue of the adrenal gland, neck, chest, or spinal cord. Neuroblastoma often begins in the nerve tissue of the adrenal glands. There are two adrenal glands, one on top of each kidney in the back of the upper abdomen. The adrenal glands produce important hormones that help control heart rate, blood pressure, blood sugar, and the way the body reacts to stress. Neuroblastoma may also begin in the abdomen, in the chest, in nerve tissue near the spine in the neck, or in the spinal cord.

Neuroblastoma most often begins during early childhood, usually in children younger than five years. It sometimes forms before birth but is usually found later, when the tumor begins to grow and cause symptoms. In rare cases, neuroblastoma may be found before birth by fetal ultrasound.

By the time neuroblastoma is diagnosed, the cancer has usually metastasized (spread), most often to the lymph nodes, bones, bone marrow, liver, and skin.

Neuroblastoma is sometimes caused by a gene mutation passed from the parent to the child. It usually occurs at a younger age than neuroblastoma that is not inherited. There also may be more than one tumor in the adrenal medulla in inherited neuroblastoma.

Excerpted from PDQ® Cancer Information Summary. National Cancer Institute; Bethesda, MD. "Neuroblastoma Treatment (PDQ) - Patient Version." Updated 05/2010. Available at: http://cancer.gov. Accessed June 14, 2010.

Symptoms

Possible signs of neuroblastoma include bone pain and a lump in the abdomen, neck, or chest. The most common symptoms of neuroblastoma are caused by the tumor pressing on nearby tissues as it grows or by cancer spreading to the bone. These and other symptoms may be caused by neuroblastoma. Other conditions may cause the same symptoms. A doctor should be consulted if any of the following problems occur:

- Lump in the abdomen, neck, or chest
- Bulging eyes
- Dark circles around the eyes ("black eyes")
- Bone pain
- Swollen stomach and trouble breathing in infants
- Painless, bluish lumps under the skin in infants
- Weakness or paralysis (loss of ability to move a body part)

Less common signs of neuroblastoma include the following:

- Fever
- Shortness of breath
- Feeling tired
- Easy bruising or bleeding
- Petechiae (flat, pinpoint spots under the skin caused by bleeding)
- High blood pressure
- Severe watery diarrhea
- Jerky muscle movements
- Uncontrolled eye movement
- Swelling of the legs, ankles, feet, or scrotum

Detection and Diagnosis

Tests that examine many different body tissues and fluids are used to detect (find) and diagnose neuroblastoma.

The following tests and procedures may be used:

Physical exam and history: An exam of the body to check general signs of health, including checking for signs of disease, such as lumps or anything else that seems unusual. A history of the patient's health habits and past illnesses and treatments will also be taken.

Twenty-four-hour urine test: A test in which urine is collected for 24 hours to measure the amounts of certain substances. An unusual (higher or lower than normal) amount of a substance can be a sign of disease in the organ or tissue that makes it. A higher than normal amount of the substances homovanillic acid (HMA) and vanillylmandelic acid (VMA) may be a sign of neuroblastoma.

Blood chemistry studies: A procedure in which a blood sample is checked to measure the amounts of certain substances released into the blood by organs and tissues in the body. An unusual (higher or lower than normal) amount of a substance can be a sign of disease in the organ or tissue that makes it. A higher than normal amount of the hormones dopamine and norepinephrine may be a sign of neuroblastoma.

Cytogenetic analysis: A laboratory test in which cells in a sample of tissue are viewed under a microscope to look for certain changes in the chromosomes.

Bone marrow aspiration and biopsy: The removal of bone marrow, blood, and a small piece of bone by inserting a hollow needle into the hipbone or breastbone. A pathologist views the bone marrow, blood, and bone under a microscope to look for signs of cancer.

Biopsy: The removal of cells or tissues so they can be viewed under a microscope by a pathologist to check for signs of cancer.

X-ray: An x-ray is a type of energy beam that can go through the body and onto film, making a picture of areas inside the body.

CT scan (CAT scan): A procedure that makes a series of detailed pictures of areas inside the body, taken from different angles. The pictures are made by a computer linked to an x-ray machine. A dye may be injected into a vein or swallowed to help the organs or tissues show up more clearly. This procedure is also called computed tomography, computerized tomography, or computerized axial tomography.

Neurological exam: A series of questions and tests to check the brain, spinal cord, and nerve function. The exam checks a person's mental status, coordination, and ability to walk normally, and how well the muscles, senses, and reflexes work. This may also be called a neuro exam or a neurologic exam.

Ultrasound exam: A procedure in which high-energy sound waves (ultrasound) are bounced off internal tissues or organs and make echoes. The echoes form a picture of body tissues called a sonogram. The picture can be printed to be looked at later.

Immunohistochemistry study: A laboratory test in which a substance such as an antibody, dye, or radioisotope is added to a sample of cancer tissue to test for certain antigens. This type of study is used to tell the difference between different types of cancer.

MIBG (metaiodobenzylguanidine) scan: A procedure used to find neuroendocrine tumors, such as neuroblastomas and pheochromocytomas. A small amount of radioactive material called MIBG is injected into a vein and travels through the bloodstream. Neuroendocrine tumor cells take up the radioactive material and are detected by a scanner. Scans may be taken over one to three days. An iodine solution may be given before or during the test to prevent the thyroid gland from absorbing too much of the MIBG.

Prognosis

Certain factors affect prognosis (chance of recovery) and treatment options. The prognosis and treatment options depend on the following:

- Age of the child when diagnosed
- Stage of the cancer
- Where the tumor is in the body
- Tumor histology (the shape, function, and structure of the tumor cells)
- Whether there is cancer in the lymph nodes

Prognosis and treatment decisions for neuroblastoma are also affected by tumor biology, which includes:

- The patterns of the tumor cells
- How different the tumor cells are from normal cells
- How fast the tumor cells are growing

The tumor biology is said to be favorable or unfavorable, depending on these factors. A favorable tumor biology means there is a better chance of recovery.

In some infants, neuroblastoma may disappear without treatment. The infant is closely watched for symptoms of neuroblastoma. If symptoms occur, treatment may be needed.

Stages of Neuroblastoma

After neuroblastoma has been diagnosed, tests are done to find out if cancer has spread from where it started to other parts of the body.

The process used to find out the extent or spread of cancer is called staging. The information gathered from the staging process helps determine the stage of the disease. For neuroblastoma, stage is one of the factors used to plan treatment. The following tests and procedures may be used to determine the stage:

Bone marrow aspiration and biopsy: The removal of bone marrow, blood, and a small piece of bone by inserting a hollow needle into the hipbone or breastbone. A pathologist views the bone marrow, blood, and bone under a microscope to look for signs of cancer.

Lymph node biopsy: The removal of all or part of a lymph node. A pathologist views the tissue under a microscope to look for cancer cells. One of the following types of biopsies may be done:

- Excisional biopsy. The removal of an entire lymph node.
- Incisional biopsy. The removal of part of a lymph node.
- Core biopsy. The removal of tissue from a lymph node using a wide needle.
- Fine-needle aspiration (FNA) biopsy. The removal of tissue or fluid from a lymph node using a thin needle.

CT scan (CAT scan): A procedure that makes a series of detailed pictures of areas inside the body, taken from different angles. The pictures are made by a computer linked to an x-ray machine. A dye may be injected into a vein or swallowed to help the organs or tissues show up more clearly. This procedure is also called computed tomography, computerized tomography, or computerized axial tomography.

MRI (magnetic resonance imaging): A procedure that uses a magnet, radio waves, and a computer to make a series of detailed pictures of areas inside the body. This procedure is also called nuclear magnetic resonance imaging (NMRI).

X-rays of the chest, bones, and abdomen: An x-ray is a type of energy beam that can go through the body and onto film, making a picture of areas inside the body.

Ultrasound exam: A procedure in which high-energy sound waves (ultrasound) are bounced off internal tissues or organs and make echoes. The echoes form a picture of body tissues called a sonogram. The picture can be printed to be looked at later.

Radionuclide scan: A procedure to find areas in the body where cells, such as cancer cells, are dividing rapidly. A very small amount of radioactive material is swallowed or injected into a vein and travels through the bloodstream. The radioactive material collects in the bones or other tissues and is detected by a radiation -measuring device.

How Cancer Spreads

There are three ways that cancer spreads in the body. The three ways that cancer spreads in the body are:

- Through tissue. Cancer invades the surrounding normal tissue.

- Through the lymph system. Cancer invades the lymph system and travels through the lymph vessels to other places in the body.

- Through the blood. Cancer invades the veins and capillaries and travels through the blood to other places in the body.

When cancer cells break away from the primary (original) tumor and travel through the lymph or blood to other places in the body, another (secondary) tumor may form. This process is called metastasis. The secondary (metastatic) tumor is the same type of cancer as the primary tumor. For example, if breast cancer spreads to the bones, the cancer cells in the bones are actually breast cancer cells. The disease is metastatic breast cancer, not bone cancer.

Stage 1

In stage 1, the tumor is in only one area and all of the tumor that can be seen is completely removed during surgery.

Stage 2

Stage 2 is divided into stage 2A and 2B.

Stage 2A: The tumor is in only one area and all of the tumor that can be seen cannot be completely removed during surgery.

Stage 2B: The tumor is in only one area and all of the tumor that can be seen may be completely removed during surgery. Cancer cells are found in the lymph nodes near the tumor.

Stage 3

In stage 3, one of the following is true:

- The tumor cannot be completely removed during surgery and has spread from one side of the body to the other side and may also have spread to nearby lymph nodes; or

- The tumor is in only one area, on one side of the body, but has spread to lymph nodes on the other side of the body; or

- The tumor is in the middle of the body and has spread to tissues or lymph nodes on both sides of the body, and the tumor cannot be removed by surgery.

Stage 4

Stage 4 is divided into stage 4 and stage 4S. In stage 4, the tumor has spread to distant lymph nodes, the skin, or other parts of the body. In stage 4S, the following are true:

- The child is younger than one year; and

- The cancer has spread to the skin, liver, and/or bone marrow; and

- The tumor is in only one area and all of the tumor that can be seen may be completely removed during surgery; and/or

- Cancer cells may be found in the lymph nodes near the tumor.

Risk Groups

Treatment of neuroblastoma is based on risk groups. For many types of cancer, stages are used to plan treatment. For neuroblastoma, treatment depends on risk groups. The stage of neuroblastoma is one factor used to determine risk group. Other factors are the age of the child, tumor histology, and tumor biology.

There are three risk groups: low risk, intermediate risk, and high risk.

- Low-risk and intermediate-risk neuroblastoma have a good chance of being cured.

- High-risk neuroblastoma may be difficult to cure.

Progressive/Recurrent Neuroblastoma

Progressive neuroblastoma is cancer that has progressed (continued to grow) during treatment. Recurrent neuroblastoma is cancer that has recurred (come back) after it has been treated. The cancer may come back in the same place or in other parts of the body.

Treatment Option Overview

Different types of treatment are available for patients with neuro-blastoma. Some treatments are standard (the currently used treatment), and some are being tested in clinical trials. A treatment clinical trial is a research study meant to help improve current treatments or obtain information on new treatments for patients with cancer. When clinical trials show that a new treatment is better than the standard treatment, the new treatment may become the standard treatment.

Because cancer in children is rare, taking part in a clinical trial should be considered. Some clinical trials are open only to patients who have not started treatment. Children with neuroblastoma should have their treatment planned by a team of doctors with expertise in treating childhood cancer.

Treatment will be overseen by a pediatric oncologist, a doctor who specializes in treating children with cancer. The pediatric oncologist works with other pediatric doctors who are experts in treating children with neuroblastoma and who specialize in certain areas of medicine. These may include the following specialists:

- Medical oncologist
- Hematologist
- Pediatric surgeon
- Radiation oncologist
- Endocrinologist
- Neurologist
- Neuropathologist
- Neuroradiologist
- Pediatric nurse specialist
- Social worker
- Rehabilitation specialist
- Psychologist

Children who are treated for neuroblastoma may be at higher risk for second cancers.

Some cancer treatments cause side effects that continue or appear years after cancer treatment has ended. These are called late effects. Late effects of cancer treatment may include:

- Physical problems
- Changes in mood, feelings, thinking, learning, or memory
- Second cancers (new types of cancer)

Some late effects may be treated or controlled. It is important that parents of children who are treated for neuroblastoma talk with their doctors about the possible late effects caused by some treatments.

Five types of standard treatment are used.

Surgery

Surgery is usually used to treat neuroblastoma. Depending on where the tumor is and whether it has spread, as much of the tumor as is safely possible will be removed. If the tumor cannot be removed, a biopsy may be done instead.

Radiation Therapy

Radiation therapy is a cancer treatment that uses high-energy x-rays or other types of radiation to kill cancer cells or keep them from growing. There are two types of radiation therapy. External radiation therapy uses a machine outside the body to send radiation toward the cancer. Internal radiation therapy uses a radioactive substance sealed in needles, seeds, wires, or catheters that are placed directly into or near the cancer. The way the radiation therapy is given depends on the type and stage of the cancer being treated.

Chemotherapy

Chemotherapy is a cancer treatment that uses drugs to stop the growth of cancer cells, either by killing the cells or by stopping them from dividing. When chemotherapy is taken by mouth or injected into a vein or muscle, the drugs enter the bloodstream and can reach cancer cells throughout the body (systemic chemotherapy). When chemotherapy is placed directly into the spinal column, an organ, or a body cavity such as the abdomen, the drugs mainly affect cancer cells in those areas (regional chemotherapy). The way the chemotherapy is given depends on the type and stage of the cancer being treated.

The use of two or more anticancer drugs is called combination chemotherapy.

Biologic Therapy

Biologic therapy is a treatment that uses the patient's immune system to fight cancer. Substances made by the body or made in a laboratory are used to boost, direct, or restore the body's natural defenses against cancer. This type of cancer treatment is also called biotherapy or immunotherapy.

Watchful Waiting

Watchful waiting is closely monitoring a patient's condition without giving any treatment until symptoms appear or change.

Clinical Trials

New types of treatment are being tested in clinical trials. This summary section describes treatments that are being studied in clinical trials. It may not mention every new treatment being studied.

Targeted Therapy

Targeted therapy is a type of treatment that uses drugs or other substances to identify and attack specific cancer cells without harming normal cells. Monoclonal antibody therapy is one type of targeted therapy being studied in the treatment of neuroblastoma.

Monoclonal antibody therapy is a cancer treatment that uses antibodies made in the laboratory from a single type of immune system cell. These antibodies can identify substances on cancer cells or normal substances that may help cancer cells grow. The antibodies attach to the substances and kill the cancer cells, block their growth, or keep them from spreading. Monoclonal antibodies are given by infusion. They may be used alone or to deliver drugs, toxins, or radioactive material directly to cancer cells.

High-Dose Chemotherapy and Radiation Therapy with Stem Cell Transplant

High-dose chemotherapy and radiation therapy with stem cell transplant is a way of giving high doses of chemotherapy and radiation therapy and replacing blood -forming cells destroyed by the cancer treatment. Stem cells (immature blood cells) are removed from the blood or bone marrow of the patient or a donor and are frozen and stored. After chemotherapy and radiation therapy are completed, the stored stem cells are thawed and given back to the patient through an infusion. These reinfused stem cells grow into (and restore) the body's blood cells.

Other Drug Therapy

13-cis retinoic acid is a vitamin-like drug that slows the cancer's ability to make more cancer cells and changes how these cells look and act.

Patients may want to think about taking part in a clinical trial. For some patients, taking part in a clinical trial may be the best treatment choice. Clinical trials are part of the cancer research process. Clinical trials are done to find out if new cancer treatments are safe and effective or better than the standard treatment.

Many of today's standard treatments for cancer are based on earlier clinical trials. Patients who take part in a clinical trial may receive the standard treatment or be among the first to receive a new treatment.

Patients who take part in clinical trials also help improve the way cancer will be treated in the future. Even when clinical trials do not lead to effective new treatments, they often answer important questions and help move research forward.

Patients can enter clinical trials before, during, or after starting their cancer treatment.

Some clinical trials only include patients who have not yet received treatment. Other trials test treatments for patients whose cancer has not gotten better. There are also clinical trials that test new ways to stop cancer from recurring (coming back) or reduce the side effects of cancer treatment.

Clinical trials are taking place in many parts of the country.

Follow-Up Tests

Follow-up tests may be needed. Some of the tests that were done to diagnose the cancer or to find out the stage of the cancer may be repeated. Some tests will be repeated in order to see how well the treatment is working. Decisions about whether to continue, change, or stop treatment may be based on the results of these tests. This is sometimes called re-staging.

Some of the tests will continue to be done from time to time after treatment has ended. The results of these tests can show if your condition has changed or if the cancer has recurred (come back). These tests are sometimes called follow-up tests or check-ups.

Chapter 13

Primary Central Nervous System Lymphoma

General Information about Primary CNS Lymphoma

Primary central nervous system (CNS) lymphoma is a disease in which malignant (cancer) cells form in the lymph tissue of the brain and/or spinal cord.

Lymphoma is a disease in which malignant (cancer) cells form in the lymph system. The lymph system is part of the immune system and is made up of the lymph, lymph vessels, lymph nodes, spleen, thymus, tonsils, and bone marrow. Lymphocytes (carried in the lymph) travel in and out of the central nervous system. It is thought that some of these lymphocytes become malignant and cause lymphoma to form in the CNS. Primary CNS lymphoma can start in the brain, spinal cord, or meninges (the layers that form the outer covering of the brain). Because the eye is so close to the brain, primary CNS lymphoma can also start in the eye (called ocular lymphoma).

Having a weakened immune system may increase the risk of developing primary CNS lymphoma. Anything that increases your chance of getting a disease is called a risk factor. Having a risk factor does not mean that you will get cancer; not having risk factors doesn't mean that you will not get cancer. People who think they may be at risk should discuss this with their doctor.

Excerpted from PDQ® Cancer Information Summary. National Cancer Institute; Bethesda, MD. "Primary CNS Lymphoma Treatment (PDQ) - Patient Version." Updated 06/2008. Available at: http://cancer.gov. Accessed January 20, 2010.

Primary CNS lymphoma may occur in patients who have acquired immunodeficiency syndrome (AIDS) or other disorders of the immune system or who have had a kidney transplant.

Detection and Diagnosis

Tests that examine the eyes, brain, and spinal cord are used to detect (find) and diagnose primary CNS lymphoma. The following tests and procedures may be used:

Physical exam and history: An exam of the body to check general signs of health, including checking for signs of disease, such as lumps or anything else that seems unusual. A history of the patient's health habits and past illnesses and treatments will also be taken.

Neurological exam: A series of questions and tests to check the brain, spinal cord, and nerve function. The exam checks a person's mental status, coordination, ability to walk normally, and how well the muscles, senses, and reflexes work. This may also be called a neuro exam or a neurologic exam.

Slit-lamp eye exam: An exam that uses a special microscope with a bright, narrow slit of light to check the outside and inside of the eye.

Vitrectomy: Surgery to remove some or all of the vitreous humor (the gel-like fluid inside the eyeball). The fluid is removed through tiny incisions and then viewed under a microscope by a pathologist to check for cancer cells.

CT scan (CAT scan): A procedure that makes a series of detailed pictures of areas inside the body, taken from different angles. The pictures are made by a computer linked to an x-ray machine. A dye may be injected into a vein or swallowed to help the organs or tissues show up more clearly. This procedure is also called computed tomography, computerized tomography, or computerized axial tomography. For primary CNS lymphoma, a CT scan is done of the chest, abdomen, and pelvis (the part of the body between the hips).

MRI (magnetic resonance imaging): A procedure that uses a magnet, radio waves, and a computer to make a series of detailed pictures of areas inside the brain and spinal cord. A substance called gadolinium is injected into the patient through a vein. The gadolinium collects around the cancer cells so they show up brighter in the picture. This procedure is also called nuclear magnetic resonance imaging (NMRI).

Lumbar puncture: A procedure used to collect cerebrospinal fluid (the fluid in the spaces around the brain and spinal cord) from the spinal column. This is done by placing a needle into the spinal column. This procedure is also called an LP or spinal tap. Laboratory tests to diagnose primary CNS lymphoma may include checking the protein level in the cerebrospinal fluid.

Stereotactic biopsy: A biopsy procedure that uses a computer and a 3-dimensional (3-D) scanning device to find a tumor site and guide the removal of tissue so it can be viewed under a microscope to check for signs of cancer.

Complete blood count (CBC) with differential: A procedure in which a sample of blood is drawn and checked for the following:

- The number of red blood cells and platelets

- The number and type of white blood cells

- The amount of hemoglobin (the protein that carries oxygen) in the red blood cells

- The portion of the blood sample made up of red blood cells

Blood chemistry studies: A procedure in which a blood sample is checked to measure the amounts of certain substances released into the blood by organs and tissues in the body. An unusual (higher or lower than normal) amount of a substance can be a sign of disease in the organ or tissue that makes it.

Prognosis

Certain factors affect prognosis (chance of recovery) and treatment options. The prognosis depends on the following:

- The patient's age and general health

- The level of certain substances in the blood and cerebrospinal fluid (CSF)

- Where the tumor is in the central nervous system

- Whether the patient has AIDS

Treatment

Treatment options depend on the following:

- The stage of the cancer

- Where the tumor is in the central nervous system

- The patient's age and general health

- Whether the cancer has just been diagnosed or has recurred (come back)

Treatment of primary CNS lymphoma works best when the tumor has not spread outside the cerebrum (the largest part of the brain) and the patient is younger than 60 years, able to carry out most daily activities, and does not have AIDS or other diseases that weaken the immune system.

Staging Primary CNS Lymphoma

After primary central nervous system (CNS) lymphoma has been diagnosed, tests are done to find out if cancer cells have spread within the brain and spinal cord or to other parts of the body.

When primary CNS lymphoma continues to grow, it usually does not spread beyond the central nervous system or the eye. The process used to find out if cancer has spread is called staging. The information gathered from the staging process determines the stage of the disease. It is important to know the stage in order to plan treatment. In addition to CT scan, slit-lamp eye exam, and vitrectomy (which are described above with other tests that are also used in detection and diagnosis) bone marrow aspiration and biopsy may be used in the staging process:

Bone marrow aspiration and biopsy: The removal of bone marrow, blood, and a small piece of bone by inserting a hollow needle into the hipbone or breastbone. A pathologist views the bone marrow, blood, and bone under a microscope to look for signs of cancer.

How Cancer Spreads

There are three ways that cancer spreads in the body. The three ways that cancer spreads in the body are:

- Through tissue. Cancer invades the surrounding normal tissue.

- Through the lymph system. Cancer invades the lymph system and travels through the lymph vessels to other places in the body.

- Through the blood. Cancer invades the veins and capillaries and travels through the blood to other places in the body.

When cancer cells break away from the primary (original) tumor and travel through the lymph or blood to other places in the body, another (secondary) tumor may form. This process is called metastasis. The secondary (metastatic) tumor is the same type of cancer as the primary tumor. For example, if breast cancer spreads to the bones, the cancer cells in the bones are actually breast cancer cells. The disease is metastatic breast cancer, not bone cancer.

Recurrent Primary CNS Lymphoma

Recurrent primary central nervous system (CNS) lymphoma is cancer that has recurred (come back) after it has been treated. Primary CNS lymphoma commonly recurs in the brain or the eye.

Treatment Option Overview

Different types of treatment are available for patients with primary central nervous system (CNS) lymphoma. Some treatments are standard (the currently used treatment), and some are being tested in clinical trials. A treatment clinical trial is a research study meant to help improve current treatments or obtain information on new treatments for patients with cancer. When clinical trials show that a new treatment is better than the standard treatment, the new treatment may become the standard treatment. Patients may want to think about taking part in a clinical trial. Some clinical trials are open only to patients who have not started treatment.

Surgery is not used to treat primary CNS lymphoma. Three standard treatments are used.

Radiation Therapy

Radiation therapy is a cancer treatment that uses high-energy x-rays or other types of radiation to kill cancer cells or keep them from growing. There are two types of radiation therapy. External radiation therapy uses a machine outside the body to send radiation toward the cancer. Internal radiation therapy uses a radioactive substance sealed in needles, seeds, wires, or catheters that are placed directly into or near the cancer. The way the radiation therapy is given depends on the type of cancer being treated.

High-dose radiation therapy to the brain can damage healthy tissue and cause disorders that can affect thinking, learning, problem solving, speech, reading, writing, and memory. Clinical trials have tested the use of chemotherapy alone or before radiation therapy to reduce the damage to healthy brain tissue that occurs with the use of radiation therapy.

Chemotherapy

Chemotherapy is a cancer treatment that uses drugs to stop the growth of cancer cells, either by killing the cells or by stopping them from dividing. When chemotherapy is taken by mouth or injected into a vein or muscle, the drugs enter the bloodstream and can reach cancer cells throughout the body (systemic chemotherapy). When chemotherapy is placed directly into the spinal column (intrathecal chemotherapy), an organ, or a body cavity such as the abdomen, the drugs mainly affect cancer cells in those areas (regional chemotherapy). The way the chemotherapy is given depends on the type of cancer being treated. Primary CNS lymphoma may be treated with intrathecal chemotherapy and/or intraventricular chemotherapy, in which anticancer drugs are placed into the ventricles (fluid -filled cavities) of the brain.

A network of blood vessels and tissue, called the blood-brain barrier, protects the brain from harmful substances. This barrier can also keep anticancer drugs from reaching the brain. In order to treat CNS lymphoma, certain drugs may be used to make openings between cells in the blood-brain barrier. This is called blood-brain barrier disruption. Anticancer drugs infused into the bloodstream may then reach the brain.

Steroid Therapy

Steroids are hormones made naturally in the body. They can also be made in a laboratory and used as drugs. Glucocorticoids are steroid drugs that have an anticancer effect in lymphomas.

Clinical Trials

New types of treatment are being tested in clinical trials. This summary section describes treatments that are being studied in clinical trials. It may not mention every new treatment being studied.

High-dose chemotherapy with stem cell transplant is a method of giving high doses of chemotherapy and replacing blood-forming cells destroyed by the cancer treatment. Stem cells (immature blood cells) are removed from the blood or bone marrow of the patient or a donor and are frozen and stored. After the chemotherapy is completed, the stored stem cells are thawed and given back to the patient through an infusion. These reinfused stem cells grow into (and restore) the body's blood cells.

Patients may want to think about taking part in a clinical trial. For some patients, taking part in a clinical trial may be the best treatment choice. Clinical trials are part of the cancer research process. Clinical trials are done to find out if new cancer treatments are safe and effective or better than the standard treatment.

Many of today's standard treatments for cancer are based on earlier clinical trials. Patients who take part in a clinical trial may receive the standard treatment or be among the first to receive a new treatment.

Patients who take part in clinical trials also help improve the way cancer will be treated in the future. Even when clinical trials do not lead to effective new treatments, they often answer important questions and help move research forward.

Patients can enter clinical trials before, during, or after starting their cancer treatment. Some clinical trials only include patients who have not yet received treatment. Other trials test treatments for patients whose cancer has not gotten better. There are also clinical trials that test new ways to stop cancer from recurring (coming back) or reduce the side effects of cancer treatment.

Clinical trials are taking place in many parts of the country.

Follow-Up Tests

Some of the tests that were done to diagnose the cancer or to find out the stage of the cancer may be repeated. Some tests will be repeated in order to see how well the treatment is working. Decisions about whether to continue, change, or stop treatment may be based on the results of these tests. This is sometimes called re-staging.

Some of the tests will continue to be done from time to time after treatment has ended. The results of these tests can show if your condition has changed or if the cancer has recurred (come back). These tests are sometimes called follow-up tests or check-ups.

Chapter 14

Pituitary Tumors

General Information about Pituitary Tumors

A pituitary tumor is a growth of abnormal cells in the tissues of the pituitary gland. Pituitary tumors form in the pituitary gland, a pea-sized organ in the center of the brain, just above the back of the nose. The pituitary gland is sometimes called the "master endocrine gland" because it makes hormones that affect the way many parts of the body work. It also controls hormones made by many other glands in the body. Pituitary tumors are divided into three groups:

- **Benign pituitary adenomas:** Tumors that are not cancer. These tumors grow very slowly and do not spread from the pituitary gland to other parts of the body.

- **Invasive pituitary adenomas:** Benign tumors that may spread to bones of the skull or the sinus cavity below the pituitary gland.

- **Pituitary carcinomas:** Tumors that are malignant (cancer). These pituitary tumors spread into other areas of the central nervous system (brain and spinal cord) or outside of the central nervous system. Very few pituitary tumors are malignant.

Excerpted from PDQ® Cancer Information Summary. National Cancer Institute; Bethesda, MD. "Pituitary Tumors Treatment (PDQ) - Patient Version." Updated 08/2009. Available at: http://cancer.gov. Accessed January 20, 2010.

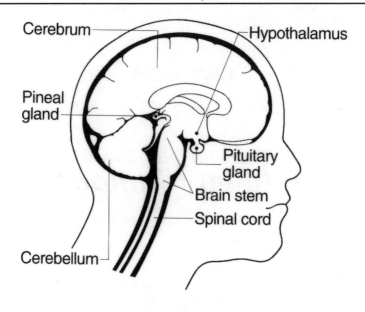

Figure 14.1. *The Pituitary Gland: Located within the Brain (image by the National Cancer Institute, AV-9503-4433).*

Pituitary tumors may be either non-functioning or functioning. Non-functioning pituitary tumors do not make hormones. Functioning pituitary tumors make more than the normal amount of one or more hormones. Most pituitary tumors are functioning tumors. The extra hormones made by pituitary tumors may cause certain signs or symptoms of disease. The pituitary gland hormones control many other glands in the body.

Hormones made by the pituitary gland include the following:

Prolactin: A hormone that causes a woman's breasts to make milk during and after pregnancy.

Adrenocorticotropic hormone (ACTH): A hormone that causes the adrenal glands to make a hormone called cortisol. Cortisol helps control the use of sugar, protein, and fats in the body and helps the body deal with stress.

Growth hormone: A hormone that helps control body growth and the use of sugar and fat in the body. Growth hormone is also called somatotropin.

Thyroid-stimulating hormone: A hormone that causes the thyroid gland to make other hormones that control growth, body temperature, and heart rate. Thyroid-stimulating hormone is also called thyrotropin.

Luteinizing hormone (LH) and follicle-stimulating hormone (FSH): Hormones that control the menstrual cycle in women and the making of sperm in men.

Risk Factors

Having certain genetic conditions increases the risk of developing a pituitary tumor. Anything that increases your risk of getting a disease is called a risk factor. Having a risk factor does not mean that you will get cancer; not having risk factors doesn't mean that you will not get cancer. People who think they may be at risk should discuss this with their doctor. Risk factors for pituitary tumors include having the following hereditary diseases:

- Multiple endocrine neoplasia type 1 (MEN1) syndrome

- Carney complex

- Isolated familial acromegaly

Signs and Symptoms

Possible signs of a pituitary tumor include problems with vision and certain physical changes.

Symptoms can be caused by the growth of the tumor and/or by hormones the tumor makes. Some tumors may not cause symptoms. Conditions other than pituitary tumors can cause the symptoms listed below. A doctor should be consulted if any of these problems occur.

Signs and Symptoms of a Non-Functioning Pituitary Tumor

Sometimes, a pituitary tumor may press on or damage parts of the pituitary gland, causing it to stop making one or more hormones. Too little of a certain hormone will affect the work of the gland or organ that the hormone controls. The following symptoms may occur:

- Headache

- Some loss of vision

- Loss of body hair

- In women, less frequent or no menstrual periods or no milk from the breasts
- In men, loss of facial hair, growth of breast tissue, and impotence
- In women and men, lower sex drive
- In children, slowed growth and sexual development

Most of the tumors that make LH and FSH do not make enough extra hormone to cause symptoms. These tumors are considered to be non-functioning tumors.

Signs and Symptoms of a Functioning Pituitary Tumor

When a functioning pituitary tumor makes extra hormones, the symptoms will depend on the type of hormone being made.

Too much prolactin may cause:

- Headache
- Some loss of vision
- Less frequent or no menstrual periods or menstrual periods with a very light flow
- Trouble becoming pregnant or an inability to become pregnant
- Impotence in men
- Lower sex drive
- Flow of breast milk in a woman who is not pregnant or breast-feeding

Too much ACTH may cause:

- Headache
- Some loss of vision
- Weight gain in the face, neck, and trunk of the body, and thin arms and legs
- A lump of fat on the back of the neck
- Thin skin that may have purple or pink stretch marks on the chest or abdomen
- Easy bruising
- Growth of fine hair on the face, upper back, or arms
- Bones that break easily
- Anxiety, irritability, and depression

Too much growth hormone may cause:

- Headache
- Some loss of vision
- In adults, acromegaly (growth of the bones in the face, hands, and feet). In children, the whole body may grow much taller and larger than normal
- Tingling or numbness in the hands and fingers
- Snoring or pauses in breathing during sleep
- Joint pain
- Sweating more than usual
- Dysmorphophobia (extreme dislike of or concern about one or more parts of the body)

Too much thyroid-stimulating hormone may cause:

- Irregular heartbeat
- Shakiness
- Weight loss
- Trouble sleeping
- Frequent bowel movements
- Sweating

Other general signs and symptoms of pituitary tumors:

- Nausea and vomiting
- Confusion
- Dizziness
- Seizures
- Runny or "drippy" nose (cerebrospinal fluid that surrounds the brain and spinal cord leaks into the nose)

Detection and Diagnosis

Imaging studies and tests that examine the blood and urine are used to detect (find) and diagnose a pituitary tumor.

The following tests and procedures may be used:

Physical exam and history: An exam of the body to check general signs of health, including checking for signs of disease, such as lumps or anything else that seems unusual. A history of the patient's health habits and past illnesses and treatments will also be taken.

Eye exam: An exam to check vision and the general health of the eyes.

Visual field exam: An exam to check a person's field of vision (the total area in which objects can be seen). This test measures both central vision (how much a person can see when looking straight ahead) and peripheral vision (how much a person can see in all other directions while staring straight ahead). The eyes are tested one at a time. The eye not being tested is covered.

Neurological exam: A series of questions and tests to check the brain, spinal cord, and nerve function. The exam checks a person's mental status, coordination, and ability to walk normally, and how well the muscles, senses, and reflexes work. This may also be called a neuro exam or a neurologic exam.

MRI (magnetic resonance imaging) with gadolinium: A procedure that uses a magnet, radio waves, and a computer to make a series of detailed pictures of areas inside the brain and spinal cord. A substance called gadolinium is injected into a vein. The gadolinium collects around the cancer cells so they show up brighter in the picture. This procedure is also called nuclear magnetic resonance imaging (NMRI).

CT scan (CAT scan): A procedure that makes a series of detailed pictures of areas inside the brain, taken from different angles. The pictures are made by a computer linked to an x-ray machine. A dye may be injected into a vein or swallowed to help the organs or tissues show up more clearly. This procedure is also called computed tomography, computerized tomography, or computerized axial tomography.

Blood chemistry study: A procedure in which a blood sample is checked to measure the amounts of certain substances, such as hormones, released into the blood by organs and tissues in the body. An unusual (higher or lower than normal) amount of a substance can be a sign of disease in the organ or tissue that makes it.

Blood tests: Tests to measure the levels of testosterone or estrogen in the blood. A higher or lower than normal amount of these hormones may be a sign of pituitary tumor.

Twenty-four-hour urine test: A test in which urine is collected for 24 hours to measure the amounts of certain substances. An unusual (higher or lower than normal) amount of a substance can be a sign of disease in the organ or tissue that makes it. A higher than normal amount of the hormone cortisol may be a sign of a pituitary tumor.

High-dose dexamethasone suppression test: A test in which one or more high doses of dexamethasone are given. The level of cortisol is checked from a sample of blood or from urine that is collected for three days.

Low-dose dexamethasone suppression test: A test in which one or more small doses of dexamethasone are given. The level of cortisol is checked from a sample of blood or from urine that is collected for three days.

Venous sampling for pituitary tumors: A procedure in which a sample of blood is taken from veins coming from the pituitary gland. The sample is checked to measure the amount of ACTH released into the blood by the gland. Venous sampling may be done if blood tests show there is a tumor making ACTH, but the pituitary gland looks normal in the imaging tests.

Biopsy: The removal of cells or tissues so they can be viewed under a microscope by a pathologist to check for signs of cancer.

Immunohistochemistry study: A laboratory test in which a substance such as an antibody, dye, or radioisotope is added to a sample of cancer tissue to test for certain antigens. This type of study is used to tell the difference between different types of cancer.

Immunocytochemistry study: A laboratory test in which a substance such as an antibody, dye, or radioisotope is added to a sample of cancer cells to test for certain antigens. This type of study is used to tell the difference between different types of cancer.

Light and electron microscopy: A laboratory test in which cells in a sample of tissue are viewed under regular and high-powered microscopes to look for certain changes in the cells.

Prognosis

Certain factors affect prognosis (chance of recovery) and treatment options. The prognosis depends on the type of tumor and whether the tumor has spread into other areas of the central nervous system (brain and spinal cord) or outside of the central nervous system to other parts of the body.

Treatment options depend on the following:

- The type and size of the tumor

- Whether the tumor is making hormones

- Whether the tumor is causing problems with vision or other symptoms

- Whether the tumor has spread into the brain around the pituitary gland or to other parts of the body

- Whether the tumor has just been diagnosed or has recurred (come back)

Stages of Pituitary Tumors

Once a pituitary tumor has been diagnosed, tests are done to find out if it has spread within the central nervous system (brain and spinal cord) or to other parts of the body.

The extent or spread of cancer is usually described as stages. There is no standard staging system for pituitary tumors. Once a pituitary tumor is found, tests are done to find out if the tumor has spread into the brain or to other parts of the body. MRI and CT scan procedures may be used.

Pituitary tumors are described in several ways. Pituitary tumors are described by their size and grade, whether or not they make extra hormones, and whether the tumor has spread to other parts of the body.

The following sizes are used:

- **Microadenoma:** The tumor is smaller than 1 centimeter. Most pituitary adenomas are microadenomas.

- **Macroadenoma:** The tumor is 1 centimeter or larger.

The grade of a pituitary tumor is based on how far it has grown into the surrounding area of the brain, including the sella (the bone at the base of the skull, where the pituitary gland sits).

Recurrent Pituitary Tumors

A recurrent pituitary tumor is cancer that has recurred (come back) after it has been treated. The cancer may come back in the pituitary gland or in other parts of the body.

Treatment Option Overview

Different types of treatments are available for patients with pituitary tumors. Some treatments are standard (the currently used treatment), and some are being tested in clinical trials. A treatment clinical trial is a research study meant to help improve current treatments or obtain information on new treatments for patients with cancer. When clinical trials show that a new treatment is better than the standard treatment, the new treatment may become the standard treatment. Patients may want to think about taking part in a clinical trial. Some clinical trials are open only to patients who have not started treatment.

Four types of standard treatment are used:

Surgery

Many pituitary tumors can be removed by surgery using one of the following operations:

- **Transsphenoidal surgery:** A type of surgery in which the instruments are inserted into part of the brain by going through an incision (cut) made under the upper lip or at the bottom of the nose between the nostrils and then through the sphenoid bone (a butterfly-shaped bone at the base of the skull) to reach the pituitary gland. The pituitary gland lies just above the sphenoid bone.

- **Endoscopic transsphenoidal surgery:** A type of surgery in which an endoscope is inserted through an incision (cut) made at the back of the inside of the nose and then through the sphenoid bone to reach the pituitary gland. An endoscope is a thin, tube-like instrument with a light, a lens for viewing, and a tool for removing tumor tissue.

- **Craniotomy:** Surgery to remove the tumor through an opening made in the skull.

Even if the doctor removes all the cancer that can be seen at the time of the surgery, some patients may be given chemotherapy or radiation therapy after surgery to kill any cancer cells that are left. Treatment given after the surgery, to lower the risk that the cancer will come back, is called adjuvant therapy.

Radiation Therapy

Radiation therapy is a cancer treatment that uses high-energy x-rays or other types of radiation to kill cancer cells or keep them from growing. There are two types of radiation therapy. External radiation therapy uses a machine outside the body to send radiation toward the cancer. Internal radiation therapy uses a radioactive substance sealed in needles, seeds, wires, or catheters that are placed directly into or near the cancer.

Stereotactic radiation surgery uses a rigid head frame attached to the skull to aim a single large dose of radiation directly to a tumor, causing less damage to nearby healthy tissue. It is also called stereotaxic radiosurgery, radiosurgery, and radiation surgery. This procedure does not involve surgery.

The way the radiation therapy is given depends on the type of the cancer being treated.

Drug Therapy

Drugs may be given to stop a functioning pituitary tumor from making too many hormones.

Chemotherapy

Chemotherapy may be used as palliative treatment for pituitary carcinomas, to relieve symptoms and improve the patient's quality of life. Chemotherapy uses drugs to stop the growth of cancer cells, either by killing the cells or by stopping them from dividing. When chemotherapy is taken by mouth or injected into a vein or muscle, the drugs enter the bloodstream and can reach cancer cells throughout the body (systemic chemotherapy). When chemotherapy is placed directly into the spinal column, an organ, or a body cavity such as the abdomen, the drugs mainly affect cancer cells in those areas (regional chemotherapy). The way the chemotherapy is given depends on the type of the cancer being treated.

Clinical Trials

New types of treatment are being tested in clinical trials. Patients may want to think about taking part in a clinical trial.

For some patients, taking part in a clinical trial may be the best treatment choice. Clinical trials are part of the cancer research process. Clinical trials are done to find out if new cancer treatments are safe and effective or better than the standard treatment.

Many of today's standard treatments for cancer are based on earlier clinical trials. Patients who take part in a clinical trial may receive the standard treatment or be among the first to receive a new treatment.

Patients who take part in clinical trials also help improve the way cancer will be treated in the future. Even when clinical trials do not lead to effective new treatments, they often answer important questions and help move research forward.

Patients can enter clinical trials before, during, or after starting their cancer treatment. Some clinical trials only include patients who have not yet received treatment. Other trials test treatments for patients whose cancer has not gotten better. There are also clinical trials that test new ways to stop cancer from recurring (coming back) or reduce the side effects of cancer treatment.

Clinical trials are taking place in many parts of the country.

Follow-Up Tests

Follow-up tests may be needed. Some of the tests that were done to diagnose the cancer or to find out the stage of the cancer may be repeated. Some tests will be repeated in order to see how well the treatment is working. Decisions about whether to continue, change, or stop treatment may be based on the results of these tests. This is sometimes called re-staging.

Some of the tests will continue to be done from time to time after treatment has ended. The results of these tests can show if your condition has changed or if the cancer has recurred (come back). These tests are sometimes called follow-up tests or check-ups.

Chapter 15

Thyroid Cancer

The Thyroid

Your thyroid is a gland at the front of your neck beneath your voice box (larynx). A healthy thyroid is a little larger than a quarter. It usually cannot be felt through the skin. The thyroid has two parts (lobes). A thin piece of tissue (the isthmus) separates the lobes. The thyroid makes hormones:

- **Thyroid hormone:** Thyroid hormone is made by thyroid follicular cells. It affects heart rate, blood pressure, body temperature, and weight.

- **Calcitonin:** Calcitonin is made by C cells in the thyroid. It plays a small role in keeping a healthy level of calcium in the body.

Four or more tiny parathyroid glands are behind the thyroid. They are on its surface. They make parathyroid hormone, which plays a big role in helping the body maintain a healthy level of calcium.

Cancer Cells

Cancer begins in cells, the building blocks that make up tissues. Tissues make up the organs of the body. Normal, healthy cells grow and divide to form new cells as the body needs them. When normal cells grow old or get damaged, they die, and new cells take their place.

Excerpted from "What You Need to Know about Thyroid Cancer," National Cancer Institute (www.cancer.gov), October 26, 2007.

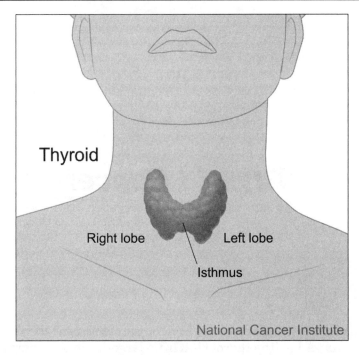

Figure 15.1. *Thyroid Gland (image by Don Bliss, National Cancer Institute).*

Sometimes, this orderly process goes wrong. New cells form when the body does not need them, and old or damaged cells do not die as they should. The build-up of extra cells often forms a mass of tissue called a growth or tumor.

Growths on the thyroid are often called nodules. Most thyroid nodules (more than 90%) are benign (not cancer). Benign nodules are not as harmful as malignant nodules (cancer). Benign nodules are rarely a threat to life. They don't invade the tissues around them and don't spread to other parts of the body. They usually don't need to be removed.

Malignant nodules may sometimes be a threat to life. They can invade nearby tissues and organs and can spread to other parts of the body. Malignant nodules often can be removed or destroyed, but sometimes the cancer returns.

Cancer cells can spread by breaking away from the original tumor. They enter blood vessels or lymph vessels, which branch into all the tissues of the body. The cancer cells attach to other organs and grow to form new tumors that may damage those organs. The spread of cancer is called metastasis.

Types of Thyroid Cancer

There are several types of thyroid cancer:

Papillary thyroid cancer: In the United States, this type makes up about 80% of all thyroid cancers. It begins in follicular cells and grows slowly. If diagnosed early, most people with papillary thyroid cancer can be cured.

Follicular thyroid cancer: This type makes up about 15% of all thyroid cancers. It begins in follicular cells and grows slowly. If diagnosed early, most people with follicular thyroid cancer can be treated successfully.

Medullary thyroid cancer: This type makes up about 3% of all thyroid cancers. It begins in the C cells of the thyroid. Cancer that starts in the C cells can make abnormally high levels of calcitonin. Medullary thyroid cancer tends to grow slowly. It can be easier to control if it's found and treated before it spreads to other parts of the body.

Anaplastic thyroid cancer: This type makes up about 2% of all thyroid cancers. It begins in the follicular cells of the thyroid. The cancer cells tend to grow and spread very quickly. Anaplastic thyroid cancer is very hard to control.

Risk Factors

Doctors often cannot explain why one person develops thyroid cancer and another does not. However, it is clear that no one can catch thyroid cancer from another person.

Research has shown that people with certain risk factors are more likely than others to develop thyroid cancer. A risk factor is something that may increase the chance of developing a disease. Having one or more risk factors does not mean that a person will get thyroid cancer. Most people who have risk factors never develop cancer.

Studies have found the following risk factors for thyroid cancer:

Radiation: People exposed to high levels of radiation are much more likely than others to develop papillary or follicular thyroid cancer. One important source of radiation exposure is treatment with x-rays. Between the 1920s and the 1950s, doctors used high-dose x-rays to treat children who had enlarged tonsils, acne, and other problems affecting the head and neck. Later, scientists found that some people who had received this kind of treatment developed thyroid cancer.

Routine diagnostic x-rays, such as dental x-rays or chest x-rays, use very low doses of radiation. Their benefits usually outweigh their risks. However, repeated exposure could be harmful, so it's a good idea to talk with your dentist and doctor about the need for each x-ray and to ask about the use of shields to protect other parts of the body.

Another source of radiation is radioactive fallout. This includes fallout from atomic weapons testing (such as the testing in the United States and elsewhere in the world, mainly in the 1950s and 1960s), nuclear power plant accidents (such as the Chornobyl [also called Chernobyl] accident in 1986), and releases from atomic weapons production plants (such as the Hanford facility in Washington state in the late 1940s). Such radioactive fallout contains radioactive iodine (I-131) and other radioactive elements. People who were exposed to one or more sources of I-131, especially if they were children at the time of their exposure, may have an increased risk of thyroid diseases. For example, children exposed to radioactive iodine from the Chornobyl accident have an increased risk of thyroid cancer.

Family history of medullary thyroid cancer: Medullary thyroid cancer sometimes runs in families. A change in a gene called RET can be passed from parent to child. Nearly everyone with the changed RET gene develops medullary thyroid cancer. The disease occurs alone as familial medullary thyroid cancer or with other cancers as multiple endocrine neoplasia (MEN) syndrome.

A blood test can detect the changed RET gene. If it's found in a person with medullary thyroid cancer, the doctor may suggest that family members be tested. For those who have the changed gene, the doctor may recommend frequent lab tests or surgery to remove the thyroid before cancer develops.

Family history of goiters or colon growths: A small number of people with a family history of having goiters (swollen thyroids) with multiple thyroid nodules are at risk for developing papillary thyroid cancer. Also, a small number of people with a family history of having multiple growths on the inside of the colon or rectum (familial polyposis) are at risk for developing papillary thyroid cancer.

Personal history: People with a goiter or benign thyroid nodules have an increased risk of thyroid cancer.

Being female: In the United States, women are almost three times more likely than men to develop thyroid cancer.

Age over 45: Most people with thyroid cancer are more than 45 years old. Most people with anaplastic thyroid cancer are more than 60 years old.

Iodine: Iodine is a substance found in shellfish and iodized salt. Scientists are studying iodine as a possible risk factor for thyroid cancer. Too little iodine in the diet may increase the risk of follicular thyroid cancer. However, other studies show that too much iodine in the diet may increase the risk of papillary thyroid cancer. More studies are needed to know whether iodine is a risk factor.

Symptoms

Early thyroid cancer often does not have symptoms. But as the cancer grows, symptoms may include a lump in the front of the neck, hoarseness or voice changes, swollen lymph nodes in the neck, trouble swallowing or breathing, or pain in the throat or neck that does not go away.

Most often, these symptoms are not due to cancer. An infection, a benign goiter, or another health problem is usually the cause of these symptoms. Anyone with symptoms that do not go away in a couple of weeks should see a doctor to be diagnosed and treated as early as possible.

Diagnosis

If you have symptoms that suggest thyroid cancer, your doctor will help you find out whether they are from cancer or some other cause. Your doctor will ask you about your personal and family medical history. You may have one or more of the following tests:

Physical exam: Your doctor feels your thyroid for lumps (nodules). Your doctor also checks your neck and nearby lymph nodes for growths or swelling.

Blood tests: Your doctor may check for abnormal levels of thyroid-stimulating hormone (TSH) in the blood. Too much or too little TSH means the thyroid is not working well. If your doctor thinks you may have medullary thyroid cancer, you may be checked for a high level of calcitonin and have other blood tests.

Ultrasound: An ultrasound device uses sound waves that people cannot hear. The device aims sound waves at the thyroid, and a computer creates a picture of the waves that bounce off the thyroid. The picture can show thyroid nodules that are too small to be felt. The doctor uses the picture to learn the size and shape of each nodule and whether the nodules are solid or filled with fluid. Nodules that are filled with fluid are usually not cancer. Nodules that are solid may be cancer.

Thyroid scan: Your doctor may order a scan of your thyroid. You swallow a small amount of a radioactive substance, and it travels through the bloodstream. Thyroid cells that absorb the radioactive substance can be seen on a scan. Nodules that take up more of the substance than the thyroid tissue around them are called "hot" nodules. Hot nodules are usually not cancer. Nodules that take up less substance than the thyroid tissue around them are called "cold" nodules. Cold nodules may be cancer.

Biopsy: A biopsy is the only sure way to diagnose thyroid cancer. A pathologist checks a sample of tissue for cancer cells with a microscope. Your doctor may take tissue for a biopsy in one of two ways:

- **Fine-needle aspiration:** Most people have this type of biopsy. Your doctor removes a sample of tissue from a thyroid nodule with a thin needle. An ultrasound device can help your doctor see where to place the needle.

- **Surgical biopsy:** If a diagnosis cannot be made from fine-needle aspiration, a surgeon removes the whole nodule during an operation. If the doctor suspects follicular thyroid cancer, surgical biopsy may be needed for diagnosis.

You may want to ask your doctor these questions before having a biopsy:

- Will I have to go to the hospital for the biopsy?

- How long will it take?

- Will I be awake? Will it hurt?

- Are there any risks? What are the chances of infection or bleeding after the biopsy?

- How long will it take me to recover?

- Will I have a scar on my neck?

- How soon will I know the results? Who will explain the results to me?

- If I do have cancer, who will talk to me about the next steps? When?

Staging

To plan the best treatment, your doctor needs to learn the extent (stage) of the disease. Staging is a careful attempt to find out the size of the nodule, whether the cancer has spread, and if so, to what parts of the body.

Thyroid cancer spreads most often to the lymph nodes, lungs, and bones. When cancer spreads from its original place to another part of the body, the new tumor has the same kind of cancer cells and the same name as the original cancer. For example, if thyroid cancer spreads to the lungs, the cancer cells in the lungs are actually thyroid cancer cells. The disease is metastatic thyroid cancer, not lung cancer. For that reason, it's treated as thyroid cancer, not lung cancer. Doctors call the new tumor "distant" or metastatic disease.

Staging may involve one or more of these tests:

Ultrasound: An ultrasound exam of your neck may show whether cancer has spread to lymph nodes or other tissues near your thyroid.

CT scan: An x-ray machine linked to a computer takes a series of detailed pictures of areas inside your body. A CT scan may show whether cancer has spread to lymph nodes, other areas in your neck, or your chest.

MRI: MRI uses a powerful magnet linked to a computer. It makes detailed pictures of tissue. Your doctor can view these pictures on a screen or print them on film. MRI may show whether cancer has spread to lymph nodes or other areas.

Chest x-ray: X-rays of your chest may show whether cancer has spread to the lungs.

Whole body scan: You may have a whole body scan to see if cancer has spread from the thyroid to other parts of the body. You get a small amount of a radioactive substance. The substance travels through the bloodstream. Thyroid cancer cells in other organs or the bones take up the substance. Thyroid cancer that has spread may show up on a whole body scan.

Treatment

People with thyroid cancer have many treatment options. Treatment usually begins within a few weeks after the diagnosis, but you will have time to talk with your doctor about treatment choices and get a second opinion.

The choice of treatment depends on the type of thyroid cancer (papillary, follicular, medullary, or anaplastic), the size of the nodule, your age, and whether the cancer has spread. You and your doctor can work together to develop a treatment plan that meets your needs.

Your doctor may refer you to a specialist who has experience treating thyroid cancer, or you may ask for a referral. An endocrinologist is a doctor who specializes in treating people who have hormone disorders. You may see a thyroidologist, an endocrinologist who specializes in treating diseases of the thyroid.

You may have a team of specialists. Other specialists who treat thyroid cancer include surgeons, medical oncologists, and radiation oncologists . Your health care team may also include an oncology nurse and a registered dietitian.

Your doctor can describe your treatment choices and the expected results. Thyroid cancer may be treated with surgery, thyroid hormone treatment, radioactive iodine therapy, external radiation therapy, or chemotherapy. Most patients receive a combination of treatments. For example, the standard treatment for papillary cancer is surgery, thyroid hormone treatment, and radioactive iodine therapy. Although external radiation therapy and chemotherapy are not often used, when they are, the treatments may be combined.

Surgery and external radiation therapy are local therapies. They remove or destroy cancer in the thyroid. When thyroid cancer has spread to other parts of the body, local therapy may be used to control the disease in those specific areas.

Thyroid hormone treatment, radioactive iodine therapy, and chemotherapy are systemic therapies. Systemic therapies enter the bloodstream and destroy or control cancer throughout the body.

You may want to know about side effects and how treatment may change your normal activities. Because cancer treatments often damage healthy cells and tissues, side effects are common. Side effects depend mainly on the type and extent of the treatment. Side effects may not be the same for each person, and they may change from one treatment session to the next. Before treatment starts, ask your health care team to explain possible side effects and suggest ways to help you manage them.

At any stage of disease, care is available to relieve the side effects of treatment, to control pain and other symptoms, and to help you cope with the feelings that a diagnosis of cancer can bring.

Surgery

Most people with thyroid cancer have surgery. The surgeon removes all or part of the thyroid. The type of surgery depends on the type and stage of thyroid cancer, the size of the nodule, and your age.

- **Total thyroidectomy:** This surgery can be used for all types of thyroid cancer. The surgeon removes all of the thyroid through an incision in the neck. If the surgeon is not able to remove all of the thyroid tissue, it can be destroyed by radioactive iodine therapy later. Nearby lymph nodes also may be removed. If cancer has invaded tissue within the neck, the surgeon may remove nearby tissue. If cancer has spread outside the neck, surgery, radioactive iodine therapy, or external radiation therapy may be used to treat those areas.

- **Lobectomy:** Some people with follicular or papillary thyroid cancer may have only part of the thyroid removed. The surgeon removes one lobe and the isthmus. Some people who have a lobectomy later have a second surgery to remove the rest of the thyroid. Less often, the remaining thyroid tissue is destroyed by radioactive iodine therapy.

The time it takes to heal after surgery is different for each person. You may be uncomfortable for the first few days. Medicine can help control your pain. Before surgery, you should discuss the plan for pain relief with your doctor or nurse. After surgery, your doctor can adjust the plan if you need more pain relief.

Surgery for thyroid cancer removes the cells that make thyroid hormone. After surgery, nearly all people need to take pills to replace the natural thyroid hormone. You will need thyroid hormone pills for the rest of your life.

If the surgeon removes the parathyroid glands, you may need to take calcium and vitamin D pills for the rest of your life.

In a few people, surgery may damage certain nerves or muscles. If this happens, a person may have voice problems or one shoulder may be lower than the other.

You may want to ask your doctor these questions before having surgery:

- Which type of surgery do you suggest for me?

- Do I need any lymph nodes removed? Will the parathyroid glands or other tissues be removed? Why?

- What are the risks of surgery?

- How will I feel after surgery? If I have pain, how will it be controlled?

- How long will I be in the hospital?

- What will my scar look like?

- Will I have any lasting side effects?

- Will I need to take thyroid hormone pills? If so, how soon will I start taking them? Will I need to take them for the rest of my life?

- When can I get back to my normal activities?

Thyroid Hormone Treatment

After surgery to remove part or all of the thyroid, nearly everyone needs to take pills to replace the natural thyroid hormone. However, thyroid hormone pills are also used as part of the treatment for papillary or follicular thyroid cancer. Thyroid hormone slows the growth of thyroid cancer cells left in the body after surgery.

Thyroid hormone pills seldom cause side effects. Your doctor gives you blood tests to make sure you're getting the right dose of thyroid hormone. Too much thyroid hormone may cause you to lose weight and feel hot and sweaty. It may also cause a fast heart rate, chest pain, cramps, and diarrhea. Too little thyroid hormone may cause you to gain weight, feel cold and tired, and have dry skin and hair. If you have side effects, your doctor can adjust your dose of thyroid hormone.

You may want to ask your doctor these questions before taking thyroid hormone:

- Why do I need this treatment?

- What will it do?

- How long will I be on this treatment?

Radioactive Iodine Therapy

Radioactive iodine (I-131) therapy is a treatment for papillary or follicular thyroid cancer. It kills thyroid cancer cells and normal thyroid cells that remain in the body after surgery.

People with medullary thyroid cancer or anaplastic thyroid cancer usually do not receive I-131 therapy. These types of thyroid cancer rarely respond to I-131 therapy.

Even people who are allergic to iodine can take I-131 therapy safely. The therapy is given as a liquid or capsule that you swallow. I-131 goes into the bloodstream and travels to thyroid cancer cells throughout the body. When thyroid cancer cells take in enough I-131, they die.

Many people get I-131 therapy in a clinic or in the outpatient area of a hospital and can go home afterward. Some people have to stay in the hospital for one day or longer. Ask your health care team to explain how to protect family members and coworkers from being exposed to the radiation.

Most radiation from I-131 is gone in about one week. Within three weeks, only traces of I-131 remain in the body.

During treatment, you can help protect your bladder and other healthy tissues by drinking a lot of fluids. Drinking fluids helps I-131 pass out of the body faster.

Some people have mild nausea the first day of I-131 therapy. A few people have swelling and pain in the neck where thyroid cells remain. If thyroid cancer cells have spread outside the neck, those areas may be painful too.

You may have a dry mouth or lose your sense of taste or smell for a short time after I-131 therapy. Chewing sugar-free gum or sucking on sugar-free hard candy may help.

A rare side effect in men who receive a high dose of I-131 is loss of fertility. In women, I-131 may not cause loss of fertility, but some doctors advise women to avoid getting pregnant for one year after a high dose of I-131.

Researchers have reported that a very small number of patients may develop a second cancer years after treatment with a high dose of I-131.

A high dose of I-131 also kills normal thyroid cells, which make thyroid hormone. After radioactive iodine therapy, you need to take thyroid hormone pills to replace the natural hormone.

You may want to ask your doctor these questions before having radioactive iodine therapy:

- Why do I need this treatment?

- What will it do?

- How do I prepare for this treatment? Do I need to avoid foods and medicines that have iodine in them? For how long?

- Will I need to stay in the hospital for this treatment? If so, for how long?

- How do I protect my family members and others from the radiation? For how many days?

- Will the I-131 therapy cause side effects? What can I do about them?

- What is the chance that I will be given I-131 therapy again in the future?

External Radiation Therapy

External radiation therapy (also called radiotherapy) is a treatment for any type of thyroid cancer that can't be treated with surgery or

I-131 therapy. It's also used for cancer that returns after treatment or to treat bone pain from cancer that has spread.

External radiation therapy uses high-energy rays to kill cancer cells. A large machine directs radiation at the neck or other tissues where cancer has spread. Most patients go to the hospital or clinic for their treatment, usually five days a week for several weeks. Each treatment takes only a few minutes.

The side effects depend mainly on how much radiation is given and which part of your body is treated. Radiation to the neck may cause a dry, sore mouth and throat, hoarseness, or trouble swallowing. Your skin in the treated area may become red, dry, and tender.

You are likely to become tired during radiation therapy, especially in the later weeks of treatment. Resting is important, but doctors usually advise patients to try to stay as active as they can.

Although the side effects of radiation therapy can be distressing, your doctor can usually treat or control them. The side effects usually go away after treatment ends.

You may want to ask your doctor these questions about external radiation therapy:

- Why do I need this treatment?
- When will the treatments begin? How often will I have them? When will they end?
- How will I feel during treatment?
- How will we know if the radiation treatment is working?
- What can I do to take care of myself during treatment?
- Can I continue my normal activities?
- Are there any lasting side effects?

Chemotherapy

Chemotherapy is a treatment for anaplastic thyroid cancer. It's sometimes used to relieve symptoms of medullary thyroid cancer or other thyroid cancers.

Chemotherapy uses drugs to kill cancer cells. The drugs are usually given by injection into a vein. They enter the bloodstream and can affect cancer cells all over the body.

You may have treatment in a clinic, at the doctor's office, or at home. Some people may need to stay in the hospital during treatment.

The side effects of chemotherapy depend mainly on which drugs and how much are given. The drugs can harm normal cells that divide rapidly, such as the cells in the mouth. The most common side effects include nausea, vomiting, mouth sores, loss of appetite, and hair loss. Your health care team can suggest ways to control many of these side effects. Most side effects go away after treatment ends.

You may want to ask your doctor these questions about chemo-therapy:

- Why do I need this treatment?

- What will it do?

- Will I have side effects? What can I do about them?

- How long will I be on this treatment?

Second Opinion

Before starting treatment, you might want a second opinion about your diagnosis and treatment plan. Many insurance companies cover a second opinion if you or your doctor requests it. A second opinion can make you feel more confident about the diagnosis and treatment choices.

It may take some time and effort to gather your medical records and see another doctor. In most cases, it's not a problem to take several weeks to get a second opinion. The delay in starting treatment usually will not make treatment less effective. To make sure, you should discuss any delay with your doctor.

There are many ways to find a doctor for a second opinion. You can ask your doctor, a local or state medical society, a nearby hospital, or a medical school for names of specialists.

Follow-Up Care

You need regular checkups after treatment for thyroid cancer. Even when there are no longer any signs of cancer, the disease sometimes returns because cancer cells remained somewhere in the body after treatment.

Your doctor monitors your recovery and checks for return of the cancer with blood tests and imaging tests. If thyroid cancer returns, it is most commonly found in the neck, lungs, or bones.

Also, checkups help detect health problems that can result from cancer treatment. People treated with radioactive iodine therapy or external radiation therapy have an increased chance of developing other cancers later on. If you have any health problems between checkups, you should contact your doctor.

People treated for papillary or follicular thyroid cancer have blood tests to check the levels of TSH and thyroglobulin. Thyroid hormone is normally stored in the thyroid as thyroglobulin. If the whole thyroid has been removed, there should be very little or no thyroglobulin in the blood. A high level of thyroglobulin may mean that thyroid cancer has returned. Your doctor helps you get ready for a thyroglobulin test in one of two ways:

- **You stop taking your thyroid hormone pills for a short time:** About six weeks before the thyroglobulin test, your doctor may change the type of thyroid hormone pill you take. About two weeks before the test, you stop taking any type of thyroid hormone pill. This can cause uncomfortable side effects. You may gain weight and feel very tired. It may be helpful to talk with your doctor or nurse about ways to cope with such problems. After the thyroglobulin test, you can take your usual thyroid hormone pill again.

- **You get a shot of TSH:** Your doctor may give you a shot of TSH. If any cancer cells remain in the body after treatment, TSH causes them to release thyroglobulin. The lab checks the level of thyroglobulin in the blood. People who get this shot don't have to stop taking their thyroid hormone pill.

People treated for medullary thyroid cancer have blood tests to check the level of calcitonin and other substances.

In addition to blood tests, checkups may include one or more of the following imaging tests:

- **Ultrasound:** An ultrasound exam of the neck may show whether cancer has returned there.

- **Whole body scan:** To get ready for the whole body scan, you either stop taking your thyroid hormone pill for several weeks or you get a shot of TSH (as described above for the thyroglobulin test). Most people need to avoid eating shellfish and iodized salt for a week or two before the scan. Your doctor gives you a very small dose of radioactive iodine or another radioactive substance. The radioactive substance is taken up by cancer cells (if any cancer cells are present). Cancer cells show up on the scan.

- **PET scan:** Your doctor uses a PET scan to find cancer that has returned. You receive an injection of a small amount of radioactive sugar. A machine makes computerized pictures of the sugar being used by cells in the body. Cancer cells use sugar faster than normal cells, and areas with cancer look brighter on the pictures.

- **CT scan:** A CT scan may show whether cancer has returned.
- **MRI:** MRI may show whether cancer has returned.

You may want to ask your doctor these questions after you have finished treatment:

- How often will I need checkups?
- Which follow-up tests do you suggest for me? Do I need to avoid iodized salt and other sources of iodine before any of these tests?
- Between checkups, what health problems or symptoms should I tell you about?

Chapter 16

Parathyroid Cancer

General Information about Parathyroid Cancer

Parathyroid cancer is a rare disease in which malignant (cancer) cells form in the tissues of a parathyroid gland. The parathyroid glands are four pea-sized organs found in the neck near the thyroid gland. The parathyroid glands make parathyroid hormone (PTH or parathormone). PTH helps the body use and store calcium to keep the calcium in the blood at normal levels.

A parathyroid gland may become overactive and make too much PTH, a condition called hyperparathyroidism. Hyperparathyroidism can occur when a benign tumor (noncancer), called an adenoma, forms on one of the parathyroid glands, and causes it to grow and become overactive. Sometimes hyperparathyroidism can be caused by parathyroid cancer, but this is very rare.

The extra PTH causes the calcium stored in the bones to move into the blood and the intestines to absorb more calcium from the food we eat. This condition is called hypercalcemia (too much calcium in the blood).

The hypercalcemia caused by hyperparathyroidism is more serious and life-threatening than parathyroid cancer itself and treating hypercalcemia is as important as treating the cancer.

Excerpted from PDQ® Cancer Information Summary. National Cancer Institute; Bethesda, MD. "Parathyroid Cancer Treatment (PDQ) - Patient Version." Updated 06/18/2008. Available at: http://cancer.gov. Accessed January 20, 2010.

Risk Factors

Having certain inherited disorders can increase the risk of developing parathyroid cancer. Anything that increases the chance of getting a disease is called a risk factor. Risk factors for parathyroid cancer include the following rare disorders that are inherited (passed down from parent to child):

- Familial isolated hyperparathyroidism (FIHP)

- Multiple endocrine neoplasia type 1 (MEN1) syndrome

- Treatment with radiation therapy may increase the risk of developing a parathyroid adenoma

Symptoms

Possible signs of parathyroid cancer include weakness, feeling tired, and a lump in the neck. Most parathyroid cancer symptoms are caused by the hypercalcemia that develops. Symptoms of hypercalcemia include the following:

- Weakness

- Feeling very tired

- Nausea and vomiting

- Loss of appetite

- Weight loss for no known reason

- Being much more thirsty than usual

- Urinating much more than usual

- Constipation

- Trouble thinking clearly

Other symptoms of parathyroid cancer include the following:

- Pain in the abdomen, side, or back that doesn't go away

- Pain in the bones

- A broken bone

- A lump in the neck

- Change in voice such as hoarseness

- Trouble swallowing

Other conditions may cause the same symptoms as parathyroid cancer. A doctor should be consulted if any of these problems occur.

Detection and Diagnosis

Tests that examine the neck and blood are used to detect (find) and diagnose parathyroid cancer. Once blood tests are done and hyperparathyroidism is diagnosed, imaging tests may be done to help find which of the parathyroid glands is overactive. Sometimes the parathyroid glands are hard to find and imaging tests are done to find exactly where they are.

Parathyroid cancer may be hard to diagnose because the cells of a benign parathyroid adenoma and a malignant parathyroid cancer look alike. The patient's symptoms, blood levels of calcium and parathyroid hormone, and characteristics of the tumor are also used to make a diagnosis.

The following tests and procedures may be used:

Physical exam and history: An exam of the body to check general signs of health, including checking for signs of disease, such as lumps or anything else that seems unusual. A history of the patient's health habits and past illnesses and treatments will also be taken.

Blood chemistry studies: A procedure in which a blood sample is checked to measure the amounts of certain substances released into the blood by organs and tissues in the body. An unusual (higher or lower than normal) amount of a substance can be a sign of disease in the organ or tissue that makes it. To diagnose parathyroid cancer, the sample of blood is checked for its calcium level.

Parathyroid hormone test: A procedure in which a blood sample is checked to measure the amount of parathyroid hormone released into the blood by the parathyroid glands. A higher than normal amount of parathyroid hormone can be a sign of disease.

Sestamibi scan: A type of radionuclide scan used to find an overactive parathyroid gland. A small amount of a radioactive substance called technetium 99 is injected into a vein and travels through the bloodstream to the parathyroid gland. The radioactive substance will collect in the overactive gland and show up brightly on a special camera that detects radioactivity.

CT scan (CAT scan): A procedure that makes a series of detailed pictures of areas inside the body, taken from different angles. The pictures are made by a computer linked to an x-ray machine. A dye may be injected into a vein or swallowed to help the organs or tissues show up more clearly. This procedure is also called computed tomography, computerized tomography, or computerized axial tomography.

Ultrasound exam: A procedure in which high-energy sound waves (ultrasound) are bounced off internal tissues or organs and make echoes. The echoes form a picture of body tissues called a sonogram.

Angiogram: A procedure to look at blood vessels and the flow of blood. A contrast dye is injected into the blood vessel. As the contrast dye moves through the blood vessel, x-rays are taken to see if there are any blockages.

Venous sampling: A procedure in which a sample of blood is taken from specific veins and checked to measure the amounts of certain substances released into the blood by nearby organs and tissues. If imaging tests do not show which parathyroid gland is overactive, blood samples may be taken from veins near each parathyroid gland to find which one is making too much PTH.

Prognosis

Certain factors affect prognosis (chance of recovery) and treatment options. The prognosis (chance of recovery) and treatment options depend on the following:

- Whether the calcium level in the blood can be controlled
- The stage of the cancer
- Whether the tumor and the capsule around the tumor can be completely removed by surgery
- The patient's general health

Stages of Parathyroid Cancer

After parathyroid cancer has been diagnosed, tests are done to find out if cancer cells have spread to other parts of the body.

The process used to find out if cancer has spread to other parts of the body is called staging. The following imaging tests may be used to determine if cancer has spread to other parts of the body such as the lungs, liver, bone, heart, pancreas, or lymph nodes: CT scan, which is described above with other tests that are used in diagnosis, and MRI (magnetic resonance imaging). MRI is a procedure that uses a magnet, radio waves, and a computer to make a series of detailed pictures of areas inside the body. This procedure is also called nuclear magnetic resonance imaging (NMRI).

How Cancer Spreads

There are three ways that cancer spreads in the body. The three ways that cancer spreads in the body are:

- Through tissue. Cancer invades the surrounding normal tissue.
- Through the lymph system. Cancer invades the lymph system and travels through the lymph vessels to other places in the body.
- Through the blood. Cancer invades the veins and capillaries and travels through the blood to other places in the body.

When cancer cells break away from the primary (original) tumor and travel through the lymph or blood to other places in the body, another (secondary) tumor may form. This process is called metastasis. The secondary (metastatic) tumor is the same type of cancer as the primary tumor. For example, if breast cancer spreads to the bones, the cancer cells in the bones are actually breast cancer cells. The disease is metastatic breast cancer, not bone cancer.

There is no standard staging process for parathyroid cancer.

Parathyroid cancer is described as either localized or metastatic. Localized parathyroid cancer is found in a parathyroid gland and may have spread to nearby tissues. Metastatic parathyroid cancer has spread to other parts of the body, such as the lungs, liver, bone, sac around the heart, pancreas, or lymph nodes.

Recurrent Parathyroid Cancer

Recurrent parathyroid cancer is cancer that has recurred (come back) after it has been treated. More than half of patients have a recurrence. The parathyroid cancer usually recurs between two and five years after the first surgery, but can recur up to 20 years later. It usually comes back in the tissues or lymph nodes of the neck. High blood calcium levels that appear after treatment may be the first sign of recurrence.

Treatment Option Overview

Different types of treatment are available for patients with parathyroid cancer. Some treatments are standard (the currently used treatment), and some are being tested in clinical trials. A treatment clinical trial is a research study meant to help improve current treatments or obtain information on new treatments for patients with cancer. When clinical trials show that a new treatment is better than the standard treatment, the new treatment may become the standard treatment. Patients may want to think about taking part in a clinical trial. Some clinical trials are open only to patients who have not started treatment.

Treatment includes control of hypercalcemia (too much calcium in the blood) in patients who have an overactive parathyroid gland.

In order to reduce the amount of parathyroid hormone that is being made and control the level of calcium in the blood, as much of the tumor as possible is removed in surgery. For patients who cannot have surgery, medication may be used. Four types of standard treatment are used.

Surgery

Surgery (removing the cancer in an operation) is the most common treatment for parathyroid cancer that is in the parathyroid glands or has spread to other parts of the body. Because parathyroid cancer grows very slowly, cancer that has spread to other parts of the body may be removed by surgery in order to cure the patient or control the effects of the disease for a long time. Before surgery, treatment is given to control hypercalcemia.

The following surgical procedures may be used:

En bloc resection: Surgery to remove the entire parathyroid gland and the capsule around it. Sometimes lymph nodes, half of the thyroid gland on the same side of the body as the cancer, and muscles, tissues, and a nerve in the neck are also removed.

Tumor debulking: Surgery to remove as much of the tumor as possible. Sometimes, not all of the tumor can be removed.

Metastasectomy: Surgery to remove any cancer that has spread to distant organs such as the lung.

Surgery for parathyroid cancer sometimes damages nerves of the vocal cords. There are treatments to help with speech problems caused by this nerve damage.

Radiation Therapy

Radiation therapy is a cancer treatment that uses high-energy x-rays or other types of radiation to kill cancer cells or stop them from growing. There are two types of radiation therapy. External radiation therapy uses a machine outside the body to send radiation toward the cancer. Internal radiation therapy uses a radioactive substance sealed in needles, seeds, wires, or catheters that are placed directly into or near the cancer. The way the radiation therapy is given depends on the type and stage of the cancer being treated.

Chemotherapy

Chemotherapy is a cancer treatment that uses drugs to stop the growth of cancer cells, either by killing the cells or by stopping them from dividing. When chemotherapy is taken by mouth or injected into a vein or muscle, the drugs enter the bloodstream and can reach cancer cells throughout the body (systemic chemotherapy). When chemotherapy is placed directly into the spinal column, an organ, or a body cavity such as the abdomen, the drugs mainly affect cancer cells in those areas (regional chemotherapy). The way the chemotherapy is given depends on the type and stage of the cancer being treated.

Supportive Care

Supportive care is given to lessen the problems caused by the disease or its treatment. Supportive care for hypercalcemia caused by parathyroid cancer may include the following:

- Intravenous (IV) fluids

- Drugs that increase how much urine the body makes

- Drugs that stop the body from absorbing calcium from the food we eat

- Drugs that stop the parathyroid gland from making parathyroid hormone

Clinical Trials

New types of treatment are being tested in clinical trials. Patients may want to think about taking part in a clinical trial.

For some patients, taking part in a clinical trial may be the best treatment choice. Clinical trials are part of the cancer research process. Clinical trials are done to find out if new cancer treatments are safe and effective or better than the standard treatment.

Many of today's standard treatments for cancer are based on earlier clinical trials. Patients who take part in a clinical trial may receive the standard treatment or be among the first to receive a new treatment.

Patients who take part in clinical trials also help improve the way cancer will be treated in the future. Even when clinical trials do not lead to effective new treatments, they often answer important questions and help move research forward.

Patients can enter clinical trials before, during, or after starting their cancer treatment.

Some clinical trials only include patients who have not yet received treatment. Other trials test treatments for patients whose cancer has not gotten better. There are also clinical trials that test new ways to stop cancer from recurring (coming back) or reduce the side effects of cancer treatment.

Clinical trials are taking place in many parts of the country.

Follow-Up Tests

Follow-up tests may be needed. Some of the tests that were done to diagnose the cancer or to find out the stage of the cancer may be repeated. Some tests will be repeated in order to see how well the treatment is working. Decisions about whether to continue, change, or stop treatment may be based on the results of these tests. This is sometimes called re-staging.

Some of the tests will continue to be done from time to time after treatment has ended. The results of these tests can show if your condition has changed or if the cancer has recurred (come back). These tests are sometimes called follow-up tests or check-ups.

Parathyroid cancer often recurs. Patients should have regular check-ups for the rest of their lives, to find and treat recurrences early.

Chapter 17

Adrenocortical Carcinoma

General Information about Adrenocortical Carcinoma

Adrenocortical carcinoma is a rare disease in which malignant (cancer) cells form in the outer layer of the adrenal gland.

There are two adrenal glands. The adrenal glands are small and shaped like a triangle. One adrenal gland sits on top of each kidney. Each adrenal gland has two parts. The outer layer of the adrenal gland is the adrenal cortex. The center of the adrenal gland is the adrenal medulla. Cancer that forms in the adrenal medulla is called pheochromocytoma.

The adrenal cortex makes important hormones that balance the water and salt in the body; help keep blood pressure normal; help manage the body's use of protein, fat, and carbohydrates; and cause the body to have masculine or feminine characteristics. The adrenal medulla also makes hormones that help the body react to stress

Adrenocortical carcinoma is also called cancer of the adrenal cortex. A tumor of the adrenal cortex may be functioning (makes more hormones than normal) or nonfunctioning (does not make hormones). The hormones made by functioning tumors may cause certain signs or symptoms of disease.

Excerpted from PDQ® Cancer Information Summary. National Cancer Institute; Bethesda, MD. "Adrenocortical Carcinoma Treatment (PDQ®) - Patient Version." Updated 10/2009. Available at: http://cancer.gov. Accessed January 20, 2010.

Risk Factors, Signs, and Symptoms

Anything that increases your risk of getting a disease is called a risk factor. Having a risk factor does not mean that you will get cancer; not having risk factors doesn't mean that you will not get cancer. People who think they may be at risk should discuss this with their doctor. Risk factors for adrenocortical carcinoma include having the following hereditary diseases:

- Li-Fraumeni syndrome
- Beckwith-Wiedemann syndrome
- Carney complex

Possible signs of adrenocortical carcinoma include pain in the abdomen and certain physical changes. These and other symptoms may be caused by adrenocortical carcinoma:

- A lump in the abdomen
- Pain the abdomen or back
- A nonfunctioning adrenocortical tumor may not cause symptoms in the early stages
- A functioning adrenocortical tumor makes too much of a certain hormone (cortisol, aldosterone testosterone, or estrogen)

Too much cortisol may cause symptoms such as the following:

- Weight gain in the face, neck, and trunk of the body and thin arms and legs
- Growth of fine hair on the face, upper back, or arms
- A round, red, full face
- A lump of fat on the back of the neck
- A deepening of the voice and swelling of the sex organs or breasts in both males and females
- Muscle weakness
- High blood sugar
- High blood pressure

Too much aldosterone may cause high blood pressure, muscle weakness or cramps, frequent urination, or feeling thirsty.

Too much testosterone (in women) may cause growth of fine hair on the face, upper back, or arms, acne, balding, a deepening of the voice, and no menstrual periods. Men who make too much testosterone do not usually have symptoms.

Too much estrogen (in women) may cause irregular menstrual periods in women who have not gone through menopause or menstrual bleeding in women who have gone through menopause. Too much estrogen (in men) may cause growth of breast tissue, lower sex drive, and impotence.

These and other symptoms may be caused by adrenocortical carcinoma. Other conditions may cause the same symptoms. A doctor should be consulted if any of these problems occur.

Detection and Diagnosis

Imaging studies and tests that examine the blood and urine are used to detect (find) and diagnose adrenocortical carcinoma. The tests and procedures used to diagnose adrenocortical carcinoma depend on the patient's symptoms. The following tests and procedures may be used:

Physical exam and history: An exam of the body to check general signs of health, including checking for signs of disease, such as lumps or anything else that seems unusual. A history of the patient's health habits and past illnesses and treatments will also be taken.

Twenty-four-hour urine test: A test in which urine is collected for 24 hours to measure the amounts of cortisol or 17-ketosteroids. A higher than normal amount of these in the urine may be a sign of disease in the adrenal cortex.

Low-dose dexamethasone suppression test: A test in which one or more small doses of dexamethasone is given. The level of cortisol is checked from a sample of blood or from urine that is collected for three days.

High-dose dexamethasone suppression test: A test in which one or more high doses of dexamethasone is given. The level of cortisol is checked from a sample of blood or from urine that is collected for three days.

Blood chemistry study: A procedure in which a blood sample is checked to measure the amounts of certain substances, such as potassium or sodium, released into the blood by organs and tissues in the body. An unusual (higher or lower than normal) amount of a substance can be a sign of disease.

Blood tests: Tests to measure the levels of testosterone or estrogen in the blood. A higher than normal amount of these hormones that may be a sign of adrenocortical carcinoma.

CT scan (CAT scan): A procedure that makes a series of detailed pictures of areas inside the body, taken from different angles. The pictures are made by a computer linked to an x-ray machine. A dye may be injected into a vein or swallowed to help the organs or tissues show up more clearly. This procedure is also called computed tomography, computerized tomography, or computerized axial tomography.

MRI (magnetic resonance imaging): A procedure that uses a magnet, radio waves, and a computer to make a series of detailed pictures of areas inside the body. This procedure is also called nuclear magnetic resonance imaging (NMRI). An MRI of the abdomen is done to diagnose adrenocortical carcinoma.

Adrenal angiography: A procedure to look at the arteries and the flow of blood near the adrenal gland. A contrast dye is injected into the adrenal arteries. As the dye moves through the blood vessel, a series of x-rays are taken to see if any arteries are blocked.

Adrenal venography: A procedure to look at the adrenal veins and the flow of blood near the adrenal gland. A contrast dye is injected into an adrenal vein. As the contrast dye moves through the vein, a series of x-rays are taken to see if any veins are blocked. A catheter (very thin tube) may be inserted into the vein to take a blood sample, which is checked for abnormal hormone levels.

PET scan (positron emission tomography scan): A procedure to find malignant tumor cells in the body. A small amount of radioactive glucose (sugar) is injected into a vein. The PET scanner rotates around the body and makes a picture of where glucose is being used in the body. Malignant tumor cells show up brighter in the picture because they are more active and take up more glucose than normal cells do.

Prognosis

Certain factors affect the prognosis (chance of recovery) and treatment options. The prognosis and treatment options depend on the following:

- The stage of the cancer (the size of the tumor and whether it is in the adrenal gland only or has spread to other places in the body)

- Whether the tumor can be completely removed in surgery

- Whether the cancer has been treated in the past
- The patient's general health

Adrenocortical carcinoma may be cured if treated at an early stage.

Staging Adrenocortical Carcinoma

After adrenocortical carcinoma has been diagnosed, tests are done to find out if cancer cells have spread within the adrenal gland or to other parts of the body. The process used to find out if cancer has spread within the adrenal gland or to other parts of the body is called staging. The information gathered from the staging process determines the stage of the disease. It is important to know the stage in order to plan treatment. Some of the diagnostic tests described above can also be used to help determine stage. Additional tests and procedures used in the staging process may include the following:

MRI (magnetic resonance imaging) with gadolinium: A substance called gadolinium may be injected into a vein. The gadolinium collects around the cancer cells so they show up brighter in the picture. This procedure is also called nuclear magnetic resonance imaging (NMRI).

Cavagram: A procedure to look at the inferior vena cava and the flow of blood through the inferior vena cava. A contrast dye is injected into a blood vessel. As the contrast dye moves through the blood vessel to the inferior vena cava, a series of x-rays are taken to see if there are any changes to the inferior vena cava and the flow of blood through the inferior vena cava.

Ultrasound exam: A procedure in which high-energy sound waves (ultrasound) are bounced off internal tissues or organs, such as the vena cava, and make echoes. The echoes form a picture of body tissues called a sonogram.

Adrenalectomy: A procedure to remove the entire adrenal gland. A tissue sample is viewed under a microscope by a pathologist to check for signs of cancer.

Stages of Adrenocortical Carcinoma

- **Stage I:** In stage I, the tumor is 5 centimeters or smaller and is found only in the adrenal gland.
- **Stage II:** In stage II, the tumor is larger than 5 centimeters and is found only in the adrenal gland.

- **Stage III:** In stage III, the tumor can be any size and may have spread to fat or lymph nodes near the adrenal gland.

- **Stage IV:** In stage IV, the tumor can be any size and has spread to fat or organs and to lymph nodes near the adrenal gland; or to other parts of the body. Adrenocortical carcinoma commonly spreads to the lung, liver, bones, and peritoneum (the tissue that lines the abdominal wall and covers most of the organs in the abdomen).

Recurrent Adrenocortical Carcinoma

Recurrent adrenocortical carcinoma is cancer that has recurred (come back) after it has been treated. The cancer may come back in the adrenal cortex or in other parts of the body.

Treatment Option Overview

Different types of treatments are available for patients with adrenocortical carcinoma. Some treatments are standard (the currently used treatment), and some are being tested in clinical trials. A treatment clinical trial is a research study meant to help improve current treatments or obtain information on new treatments for patients with cancer. When clinical trials show that a new treatment is better than the standard treatment, the new treatment may become the standard treatment. Patients may want to think about taking part in a clinical trial. Some clinical trials are open only to patients who have not started treatment.

Three types of standard treatment are used:

Surgery

Surgery to remove the adrenal gland (adrenalectomy) is often used to treat adrenocortical carcinoma. Sometimes the nearby lymph nodes are also removed.

Radiation Therapy

Radiation therapy is a cancer treatment that uses high-energy x-rays or other types of radiation to kill cancer cells or keep them from growing. There are two types of radiation therapy. External radiation therapy uses a machine outside the body to send radiation toward the cancer. Internal radiation therapy uses a radioactive substance sealed in needles, seeds, wires, or catheters that are placed directly into or near the cancer. The way the radiation therapy is given depends on the type and stage of the cancer being treated.

Chemotherapy

Chemotherapy is a cancer treatment that uses drugs to stop the growth of cancer cells, either by killing the cells or by stopping them from dividing. When chemotherapy is taken by mouth or injected into a vein or muscle, the drugs enter the bloodstream and can reach cancer cells throughout the body (systemic chemotherapy). When chemotherapy is placed directly into the spinal column, an organ, or a body cavity such as the abdomen, the drugs mainly affect cancer cells in those areas (regional chemotherapy). The way the chemotherapy is given depends on the type and stage of the cancer being treated.

Mitotane may be used to treat adrenocortical carcinoma. Mitotane stops the adrenal cortex from making hormones and relieves symptoms caused by the hormones.

Clinical Trials

New types of treatment are being tested in clinical trials. Biologic therapy, for example, is a treatment that uses the patient's immune system to fight cancer. Substances made by the body or made in a laboratory are used to boost, direct, or restore the body's natural defenses against cancer. This type of cancer treatment is also called biotherapy or immunotherapy.

Patients may want to think about taking part in a clinical trial. For some patients, taking part in a clinical trial may be the best treatment choice. Clinical trials are part of the cancer research process. Clinical trials are done to find out if new cancer treatments are safe and effective or better than the standard treatment. Clinical trials are taking place in many parts of the country.

Many of today's standard treatments for cancer are based on earlier clinical trials. Patients who take part in a clinical trial may receive the standard treatment or be among the first to receive a new treatment. Patients who take part in clinical trials also help improve the way cancer will be treated in the future. Even when clinical trials do not lead to effective new treatments, they often answer important questions and help move research forward.

Patients can enter clinical trials before, during, or after starting their cancer treatment. Some clinical trials only include patients who have not yet received treatment. Other trials test treatments for patients whose cancer has not gotten better. There are also clinical trials that test new ways to stop cancer from recurring (coming back) or reduce the side effects of cancer treatment.

Follow-Up Tests

Some of the tests that were done to diagnose the cancer or to find out the stage of the cancer may be repeated. Some tests will be repeated in order to see how well the treatment is working. Decisions about whether to continue, change, or stop treatment may be based on the results of these tests. This is sometimes called re-staging.

Some of the tests will continue to be done from time to time after treatment has ended. The results of these tests can show if your condition has changed or if the cancer has recurred (come back). These tests are sometimes called follow-up tests or check-ups.

Chapter 18

Islet Cell Tumors

General Information about Islet Cell Tumors (Endocrine Pancreas)

Islet cell tumors are abnormal cells that form in the tissues of the pancreas. The pancreas is a gland about six inches long that is shaped like a thin pear lying on its side. The wider end of the pancreas is called the head, the middle section is called the body, and the narrow end is called the tail. The pancreas lies behind the stomach and in front of the spine. There are two kinds of cells in the pancreas:

- Endocrine pancreas cells make several kinds of hormones (chemicals that control the actions of certain cells or organs in the body), such as insulin to control blood sugar. They cluster together in many small groups (islets) throughout the pancreas. Endocrine pancreas cells are also called islet cells or islets of Langerhans. Malignant islet cell tumors are a rare type of pancreatic cancer.

- Exocrine pancreas cells make enzymes that are released into the small intestine to help the body digest food. Most of the pancreas is made of ducts with small sacs at the end of the ducts, which are lined with exocrine cells.

Excerpted from PDQ® Cancer Information Summary. National Cancer Institute; Bethesda, MD. "Islet Cell Tumors (Endocrine Pancreas) Treatment (PDQ) - Patient Version." Updated 03/2010. Available at: http://cancer.gov. Accessed June 21, 2010.

An islet cell tumor may also be called a pancreatic endocrine tumor (PET), pancreatic neuroendocrine tumor, islet cell carcinoma, or pancreatic carcinoid. This summary discusses islet cell tumors of the endocrine pancreas.

Islet cell tumors may or may not cause symptoms. Islet cells make and release hormones into the blood. Islet cell tumors may be functional (the hormones that are released cause symptoms) or nonfunctional (the hormones that are released do not cause symptoms) tumors:

There are different kinds of functional islet cell tumors. Islet cells make different kinds of hormones such as gastrin, insulin, and glucagon. Types of functional islet cell tumors include the following:

- **Gastrinoma:** A tumor that forms in cells that make gastrin. Gastrin is a hormone that causes the stomach to release an acid that helps digest food. Both gastrin and stomach acid are increased by gastrinomas. When increased stomach acid, stomach ulcers, and diarrhea are caused by a tumor that makes gastrin, it is called Zollinger-Ellison syndrome. A gastrinoma usually forms in the head of the pancreas and sometimes forms in the small intestine. Most gastrinomas are malignant (cancer).

- **Insulinoma:** A tumor that forms in cells that make insulin. Insulin is a hormone that controls the amount of glucose (sugar) in the blood. It moves glucose into the cells, where it can be used by the body for energy. Insulinomas are usually slow-growing tumors that rarely spread. An insulinoma forms in the head, body, or tail of the pancreas. Insulinomas are usually benign (not cancer).

- **Glucagonoma:** A tumor that forms in cells that make glucagon. Glucagon is a hormone that increases the amount of glucose in the blood. It causes the liver to break down glycogen. Too much glucagon causes hyperglycemia (high blood sugar). Glucagonomas are often malignant. A glucagonoma usually forms in the tail of the pancreas. Most glucagonomas are malignant (cancer).

- **Other types of tumors:** There are other rare types of functional islet cell tumors that make hormones, including hormones that control the balance of sugar, salt, and water in the body. These other types of tumors are grouped together because they are treated in much the same way. These tumors include VIPomas, which make vasoactive intestinal peptide (VIPoma may also be called Verner-Morrison syndrome) and somatostatinomas, which make somatostatin.

Nonfunctional tumors make hormones that do not cause symptoms. Symptoms are caused by the tumor as it spreads and grows. Most nonfunctional tumors are malignant (cancer).

Risk Factors

Having certain syndromes can increase the risk of developing islet cell tumors. Anything that increases your risk of getting a disease is called a risk factor. Multiple endocrine neoplasia type 1 (MEN1) syndrome is a risk factor for islet cell tumors. Having a risk factor does not mean that you will get cancer; not having risk factors doesn't mean that you will not get cancer. People who think they may be at risk should discuss this with their doctor.

Sign and Symptoms

Different types of islet cell tumors have different signs and symptoms. Symptoms can be caused by the growth of the tumor and/or by hormones the tumor makes. Some tumors may not cause symptoms. Conditions other than islet cell tumors can cause the symptoms listed below. A doctor should be consulted if any of these problems occur.

A non-functioning islet cell tumor may grow for a long time without causing symptoms. It may grow large or spread to other parts of the body before it causes symptoms, such as diarrhea, indigestion, a lump in the abdomen, pain in the abdomen or back, or yellowing of the skin and whites of the eyes. A tumor that makes pancreatic peptides (PPoma) often has no symptoms.

The symptoms of a functioning islet tumor depend on the type of hormone being made:

- Too much gastrin may cause stomach ulcers that keep coming back, pain in the abdomen, which may spread to the back (the pain may come and go and it may go away after taking an antacid), the flow of stomach contents back into the esophagus (gastroesophageal reflux), or diarrhea.

- Too much insulin may cause low blood sugar. This can cause blurred vision, headache, and feeling lightheaded, tired, weak, shaky, nervous, irritable, sweaty, confused, or hungry. It can also cause feeling a fast heartbeat

- Too much glucagon may cause a skin rash on the face, stomach, or legs. It can also cause high blood sugar. This can cause headaches, frequent urination, dry skin and mouth, or feeling hungry, thirsty, tired, or weak. It can cause blood clots in the lung. This can cause shortness of breath, cough or pain in the chest. Blood clots in the arm or leg can cause pain, swelling, warmth, or redness of the arm or leg. Other symptoms can include diarrhea, weight loss for no known reason, or a sore tongue or sores at the corners of the mouth.

- Too much vasoactive intestinal peptide (VIP) may cause very large amounts of watery diarrhea and dehydration. This can cause feeling thirsty, making less urine, dry skin and mouth, feeling tired, headache, or dizziness. It can also cause a low potassium level in the blood. This can cause muscle weakness, aching, or cramps, numbness and tingling, frequent urination, and feeling a fast heartbeat, confused, or thirsty. Another symptom can be weight loss for no known reason.

- Too much somatostatin may cause high blood sugar. This can cause headaches, frequent urination, dry skin and mouth, or feeling hungry, thirsty, tired, or weak. It can also cause diarrhea, steatorrhea (very foul-smelling stool that floats), gallstones, yellowing of the skin and whites of the eyes, or weight loss for no known reason.

Detection and Diagnosis

Lab tests and imaging tests are used to detect (find) and diagnose islet cell tumors. The following tests and procedures may be used:

Physical exam and history: An exam of the body to check general signs of health, including checking for signs of disease, such as lumps or anything else that seems unusual. A history of the patient's health habits and past illnesses and treatments will also be taken.

Blood chemistry studies: A procedure in which a blood sample is checked to measure the amounts of certain substances, such as glucose (sugar), released into the blood by organs and tissues in the body. An unusual (higher or lower than normal) amount of a substance can be a sign of disease in the organ or tissue that makes it.

Serum tumor marker test: A procedure in which a sample of blood is checked to measure the amounts of certain substances released into the blood by organs, tissues, or tumor cells in the body. Certain substances are linked to specific types of cancer when found in increased levels in the blood. These are called tumor markers.

Immunohistochemistry study: A laboratory test in which a substance such as an antibody, dye, or radioisotope is added to a sample of cancer tissue to test for certain antigens. This type of study is used to tell the difference between different types of cancer.

Abdominal CT scan (CAT scan): A procedure that makes a series of detailed pictures of the abdomen, taken from different angles. The pictures are made by a computer linked to an x-ray machine. A dye may be injected into a vein or swallowed to help the organs or tissues show up more clearly. This procedure is also called computed tomography, computerized tomography, or computerized axial tomography.

MRI (magnetic resonance imaging): A procedure that uses a magnet, radio waves, and a computer to make a series of detailed pictures of areas inside the body. This procedure is also called nuclear magnetic resonance imaging (NMRI).

Somatostatin receptor scintigraphy: A type of radionuclide scan that may be used to find small islet cell tumors. A small amount of radioactive octreotide (a hormone that attaches to tumors) is injected into a vein and travels through the blood. The radioactive octreotide attaches to the tumor and a special camera that detects radioactivity is used to show where the tumors are in the body. This procedure is also called octreotide scan and SRS.

Abdominal ultrasound: An ultrasound exam used to make pictures of the inside of the abdomen. The ultrasound transducer is pressed against the skin of the abdomen and directs high-energy sound waves (ultrasound) into the abdomen. The sound waves bounce off the internal tissues and organs and make echoes. The transducer receives the echoes and sends them to a computer, which uses the echoes to make pictures called sonograms. The picture can be printed to be looked at later.

Endoscopic ultrasound (EUS): A procedure in which an endoscope is inserted into the body, usually through the mouth or rectum. An endoscope is a thin, tube-like instrument with a light and a lens for viewing. A probe at the end of the endoscope is used to bounce high-energy sound waves (ultrasound) off internal tissues or organs and make echoes. The echoes form a picture of body tissues called a sonogram. This procedure is also called endosonography.

Angiogram: A procedure to look at blood vessels and the flow of blood. A contrast dye is injected into the blood vessel. As the contrast dye moves through the blood vessel, x-rays are taken to see if there are any blockages.

Laparotomy: A surgical procedure in which an incision (cut) is made in the wall of the abdomen to check the inside of the abdomen for signs of disease. The size of the incision depends on the reason the laparotomy is being done. Sometimes organs are removed or tissue samples are taken and checked under a microscope for signs of disease.

Intraoperative ultrasound: A procedure that uses high-energy sound waves (ultrasound) to create images of internal organs or tissues during surgery. A transducer placed directly on the organ or tissue is used to make the sound waves, which create echoes. The transducer receives the echoes and sends them to a computer, which uses the echoes to make pictures called sonograms.

Biopsy: The removal of cells or tissues so they can be viewed under a microscope by a pathologist to check for signs of cancer. There are several ways to do a biopsy for islet cell tumors. Cells may be removed using a fine or wide needle inserted into the pancreas during an x-ray or ultrasound. Tissue may also be removed during a laparoscopy (a surgical incision made in the wall of the abdomen).

Bone scan: A procedure to check if there are rapidly dividing cells, such as cancer cells, in the bone. A very small amount of radioactive material is injected into a vein and travels through the blood. The radioactive material collects in bones where cancer cells have spread and is detected by a scanner.

Other kinds of lab tests are used to check for the different types of islet cell tumors. The following tests and procedures may be used:

Gastrinoma

Fasting serum gastrin test: A test in which a blood sample is checked to measure the amount of gastrin in the blood. This test is done after the patient has had nothing to eat or drink for at least 8 hours. Conditions other than gastrinoma can cause an increase in the amount of gastrin in the blood.

Gastric acid secretion test: A test to measure the amount of acid made by the stomach. A tube is inserted through the nose or throat, into the stomach. Gastrin or insulin is injected into the patient, which causes the stomach to make stomach secretions (gastric acid). Four samples of gastric acid are taken through the tube 15 minutes apart. These four samples are used to find out the lowest and highest amounts of gastric acid made during the test and the pH level of the gastric secretions.

Secretin stimulation test: If the gastric acid secretion test result is not normal, a secretin stimulation test may be done. The tube is moved into the small intestine and samples are taken from the small intestine after a drug called secretin is injected. Secretin causes the small intestine to make acid. When there is a gastrinoma, the secretin causes an increase in how much gastric acid is made and the level of gastrin in the blood.

Calcium infusion test: A test to measure the amount of gastrin in the blood after a drug called calcium gluconate is infused. Blood samples will be taken to measure the amount of gastrin in the blood at set times.

Somatostatin receptor scintigraphy: A type of radionuclide scan that may be used to find small islet cell tumors. A small amount of radioactive octreotide (a hormone that attaches to tumors) is injected into a vein and travels through the blood. The radioactive octreotide attaches to the tumor and a special camera that detects radioactivity is used to show where the tumors are in the body. This procedure is also called octreotide scan and SRS.

Insulinoma

Fasting serum glucose and insulin test: A test in which a blood sample is checked to measure the amounts of glucose (sugar) and insulin in the blood. The test is done after the patient has had nothing to eat or drink for at least eight hours.

C-peptide suppression test: A test in which a blood sample is checked to measure the amount of C-peptide in the blood. Insulin is injected into a vein to lower the patient's blood sugar. This should decrease the amount of insulin and C-peptide that the body releases into the blood. In patients who have insulinoma, the insulin and C-peptide levels do not drop because the tumor is also releasing insulin and C-peptide into the blood.

Venous sampling after arterial stimulation: A procedure used to help find where a tumor has formed in the pancreas. This is done at the same time as an angiogram. Calcium is injected into an artery that goes to one part of the pancreas (the head, body, and tail are tested one at a time). A blood sample is taken from a vein that comes out of the pancreas and is checked for pancreatic hormones. If there is an islet cell tumor in the area of the pancreas that gets blood from the artery that was injected, there will be an increase in the amount of hormone in the blood sample. If the increase is found after injection into the first artery, the tumor is in the area that gets blood from that artery. If there is no increase, another artery is injected and the test continues.

Anti-insulin antibody test: A test in which a blood sample is checked to see if there are antibodies against insulin in it.

Glucagonoma

Fasting serum glucagon test: A test in which a blood sample is checked to measure the amount of glucagon in the blood. The test is done after the patient has had nothing to eat or drink for at least eight hours.

VIPoma

Serum VIP (vasoactive intestinal peptide) test: A test in which a blood sample is checked to measure the amount of VIP.

Blood chemistry studies: A procedure in which a blood sample is checked to measure the amounts of certain substances released into the blood by organs and tissues in the body. An unusual (higher or lower than normal) amount of a substance can be a sign of disease in the organ or tissue that makes it. In VIPoma, there is a lower than normal amount of potassium.

Stool analysis: A stool sample is checked for a higher than normal sodium (salt) and potassium levels.

Somatostatinoma

Fasting serum somatostatin test: A test in which a blood sample is checked to measure the amount of somatostatin in the blood. The test is done after the patient has had nothing to eat or drink for at least eight hours.

Somatostatin receptor scintigraphy: A type of radionuclide scan that may be used to find small islet cell tumors. A small amount of radioactive octreotide (a hormone that attaches to tumors) is injected into a vein and travels through the blood. The radioactive octreotide attaches to the tumor and a special camera that detects radioactivity is used to show where the tumors are in the body. This procedure is also called octreotide scan and SRS.

PPoma

Fasting serum polypeptide test: A test in which a blood sample is checked to measure the amount of pancreatic polypeptide in the blood.

The test is done after the patient has had nothing to eat or drink for at least eight hours.

Somatostatin receptor scintigraphy: A type of radionuclide scan that may be used to find small islet cell tumors. A small amount of radioactive octreotide (a hormone that attaches to tumors) is injected into a vein and travels through the blood. The radioactive octreotide attaches to the tumor and a special camera that detects radioactivity is used to show where the tumors are in the body. This procedure is also called octreotide scan and SRS.

Atropine suppression test: A test used to help find out if the secretion of a polypeptide (protein) by the pancreas is normal or caused by a tumor. A drug called atropine, which can lessen secretions, is injected into a vein. After the injection, pancreatic polypeptide levels in the blood stay the same in patients with tumors, but drop in patients without tumors.

Immunohistochemistry study: A laboratory test in which a substance such as an antibody, dye, or radioisotope is added to a sample of cancer tissue to test for certain antigens.

Prognosis

Certain factors affect prognosis (chance of recovery) and treatment options. Islet cell tumors can often be cured. The prognosis and treatment options depend on the following:

- The type of cancer cell
- Where the tumor is found in the pancreas
- Whether the tumor has spread to more than one place in the pancreas or to other parts of the body
- Whether the patient has MEN1 syndrome
- The patient's age and general health
- Whether the cancer has just been diagnosed or has recurred (come back)

Stages of Islet Cell Tumors (Endocrine Pancreas)

The extent or spread of cancer is usually described as stages. There is no standard staging system for islet cell cancer. The tumors are treated based on where the cancer is found:

- The cancer is found in one place in the pancreas.

- The cancer is found in several places in the pancreas.

- The cancer has spread to lymph nodes near the pancreas or to other parts of the body such as the liver, lung, peritoneum, or bone.

The type of treatment depends on the results of tests and procedures used to diagnose islet cell tumors. The results of the tests and procedures used to diagnose islet cell tumors and determine whether the cancer has spread help decide the type of treatment that will be used.

Recurrent Islet Cell Tumors (Endocrine Pancreas)

Recurrent islet cell tumors are tumors that have recurred (come back) after being treated. The tumors may come back in the pancreas or in other parts of the body.

Treatment Option Overview

Different types of treatments are available for patients with islet cell tumors. Some treatments are standard (the currently used treatment), and some are being tested in clinical trials.

Surgery

An operation may be done to remove the tumor. One of the following types of surgery may be used:

Enucleation: Surgery to remove the tumor only. This may be done when cancer occurs in one place in the pancreas.

Whipple procedure: A surgical procedure in which the head of the pancreas, the gallbladder, nearby lymph nodes and part of the stomach, small intestine, and bile duct may be removed. Enough of the pancreas is left to make digestive juices and insulin. The organs removed during this procedure depend on the patient's condition.

Distal pancreatectomy: Surgery to remove the body and tail of the pancreas. The spleen may also be removed.

Total gastrectomy: Surgery to remove the whole stomach.

Parietal cell vagotomy: Surgery to cut the nerve that causes stomach cells to make acid.

Liver resection: Surgery to remove part or all of the liver.

Radiofrequency ablation: The use of a special probe with tiny electrodes that kill cancer cells. Sometimes the probe is inserted directly through the skin and only local anesthesia is needed. In other cases, the probe is inserted through an incision in the abdomen. This is done in the hospital with general anesthesia.

Cryosurgical ablation: A procedure in which tissue is frozen to destroy abnormal cells. This is usually done with a special instrument that contains liquid nitrogen or liquid carbon dioxide. The instrument may be used during surgery or laparoscopy or inserted through the skin. This procedure is also called cryoablation.

Chemotherapy

Chemotherapy is a cancer treatment that uses drugs to stop the growth of cancer cells, either by killing the cells or by stopping them from dividing. When chemotherapy is taken by mouth or injected into a vein or muscle, the drugs enter the bloodstream and can reach cancer cells throughout the body (systemic chemotherapy). When chemotherapy is placed directly into the spinal column, an organ, or a body cavity such as the abdomen, the drugs mainly affect cancer cells in those areas (regional chemotherapy). Combination chemotherapy is the use of more than one anticancer drug. The way the chemotherapy is given depends on the type of the cancer being treated.

Hormone Therapy

Hormone therapy is a cancer treatment that removes hormones or blocks their action and stops cancer cells from growing. Hormones are substances made by glands in the body and circulated in the bloodstream. Some hormones can cause certain cancers to grow. If tests show that the cancer cells have places where hormones can attach (receptors), drugs, surgery, or radiation therapy is used to reduce the production of hormones or block them from working.

Hepatic Arterial Occlusion or Chemoembolization

Hepatic arterial occlusion uses drugs, small particles, or other agents to block or reduce the flow of blood to the liver through the hepatic artery (the major blood vessel that carries blood to the liver). This is done to kill cancer cells growing in the liver. The tumor is prevented from getting the oxygen and nutrients it needs to grow. The liver continues to receive blood from the hepatic portal vein, which carries blood from the stomach and intestine.

Chemotherapy delivered during hepatic arterial occlusion is called chemoembolization. The anticancer drug is injected into the hepatic artery through a catheter (thin tube). The drug is mixed with the substance that blocks the artery and cuts off blood flow to the tumor. Most of the anticancer drug is trapped near the tumor and only a small amount of the drug reaches other parts of the body.

The blockage may be temporary or permanent, depending on the substance used to block the artery.

Supportive Care

Supportive care is given to lessen the problems caused by the disease or its treatment. Supportive care for islet cell cancer may include treatment for the following:

- Stomach ulcers may be treated with drug therapy such as proton-pump inhibitor drugs (such as omeprazole, lansoprazole, or pantoprazole), histamine blocking drugs (such as cimetidine, ranitidine, or famotidine), or somatostatin-type drugs (such as octreotide).

- Diarrhea may be treated with intravenous (IV) fluids with electrolytes (such as potassium or chloride) or somatostatin-type drugs (such as octreotide).

- Low blood sugar may be treated by having small, frequent meals or with drug therapy to maintain a normal blood sugar level.

- High blood sugar may be treated with drugs taken by mouth or insulin by injection.

Clinical Trials

Patients may want to think about taking part in a clinical trial. For some patients, taking part in a clinical trial may be the best treatment choice. Clinical trials are part of the cancer research process. Clinical trials are done to find out if new cancer treatments are safe and effective or better than the standard treatment.

Many of today's standard treatments for cancer are based on earlier clinical trials. Patients who take part in a clinical trial may receive the standard treatment or be among the first to receive a new treatment.

Patients who take part in clinical trials also help improve the way cancer will be treated in the future. Even when clinical trials do not lead to effective new treatments, they often answer important questions and help move research forward.

Patients can enter clinical trials before, during, or after starting their cancer treatment. Some clinical trials, however, only include patients who have not yet received treatment. Other trials test treatments for patients whose cancer has not gotten better. There are also clinical trials that test new ways to stop cancer from recurring (coming back) or reduce the side effects of cancer treatment.

Follow-Up Tests

Some of the tests that were done to diagnose the cancer or to find out the stage of the cancer may be repeated. Some tests will be repeated in order to see how well the treatment is working. Decisions about whether to continue, change, or stop treatment may be based on the results of these tests. This is sometimes called re-staging.

Some of the tests will continue to be done from time to time after treatment has ended. The results of these tests can show if your condition has changed or if the cancer has recurred (come back). These tests are sometimes called follow-up tests or check-ups.

Chapter 19

Retinoblastoma

General Information about Retinoblastoma

Retinoblastoma is a disease in which malignant (cancer) cells form in the tissues of the retina. The retina is the nerve tissue that lines the inside of the back of the eye. The retina senses light and sends images to the brain by way of the optic nerve.

Although retinoblastoma may occur at any age, it usually occurs in children younger than five years of age. The tumor may be in one eye or in both eyes. Retinoblastoma rarely spreads from the eye to nearby tissue or other parts of the body. Retinoblastoma is usually found in only one eye and can usually be cured.

Retinoblastoma is sometimes caused by a gene mutation passed from the parent to the child. Retinoblastoma that is caused by an inherited gene mutation is called hereditary retinoblastoma. It usually occurs at a younger age than retinoblastoma that is not inherited. Retinoblastoma that occurs in only one eye is usually not inherited. Retinoblastoma that occurs in both eyes is always inherited. When hereditary retinoblastoma first occurs in only one eye, there is a chance it will develop later in the other eye. After diagnosis of retinoblastoma in one eye, regular follow-up exams of the healthy eye should be done every two to four months for at least 28 months. After treatment for retinoblastoma is finished, it is important that follow-up exams continue until the child is five years of age.

Excerpted from PDQ® Cancer Information Summary. National Cancer Institute; Bethesda, MD. "Retinoblastoma Treatment (PDQ) - Patient Version." Updated 03/2010. Available at: http://cancer.gov. Accessed June 21, 2010.

Treatment for both types of retinoblastoma should include genetic counseling (a discussion with a trained professional about inherited diseases). Brothers and sisters of a child who has retinoblastoma should also have regular exams by an ophthalmologist (a doctor with special training in diseases of the eye) and genetic counseling about the risk of developing the cancer.

Risk Factors

A child who has hereditary retinoblastoma is at risk for developing pineal tumors in the brain. This is called trilateral retinoblastoma. Regular follow-up exams using MRI (magnetic resonance imaging) or CT scans (computerized tomography) to check for this rare condition are important during treatment for retinoblastoma and should be continued until the child is five years of age. Hereditary retinoblastoma also increases the child's risk of developing other types of cancer in later years. Regular follow-up exams are important.

These and other symptoms may be caused by retinoblastoma. Other conditions may cause the same symptoms. A doctor should be consulted if any of the following problems occur:

- Pupil of the eye appears white instead of red when light shines into it. This may be seen in flash photographs of the child.

- Eyes appear to be looking in different directions

- Pain or redness in the eye

Detection and Diagnosis

Tests that examine the retina are used to detect (find) and diagnose retinoblastoma. The following tests and procedures may be used:

Physical exam and history: An exam of the body to check general signs of health, including checking for signs of disease, such as lumps or anything else that seems unusual. A history of the patient's health habits and past illnesses and treatments will also be taken. The doctor will ask if there is a family history of retinoblastoma.

Eye exam with dilated pupil: An exam of the eye in which the pupil is dilated (opened wider) with medicated eyedrops to allow the doctor to look through the lens and pupil to the retina. The inside of the eye, including the retina and the optic nerve, is examined with a light. Depending on the age of the child, this exam may be done under anesthesia.

Ultrasound exam: A procedure in which high-energy sound waves (ultrasound) are bounced off internal tissues or organs and make echoes. The echoes form a picture of body tissues called a sonogram.

CT scan (CAT scan): A procedure that makes a series of detailed pictures of areas inside the body, such as the eye, taken from different angles. The pictures are made by a computer linked to an x-ray machine. A dye may be injected into a vein or swallowed to help the organs or tissues show up more clearly. This procedure is also called computed tomography, computerized tomography, or computerized axial tomography.

MRI (magnetic resonance imaging): A procedure that uses a magnet, radio waves, and a computer to make a series of detailed pictures of areas inside the body, such as the eye. This procedure is also called nuclear magnetic resonance imaging (NMRI).

Biopsy: Retinoblastoma is usually diagnosed without a biopsy (removal of cells or tissues so they can be viewed under a microscope to check for signs of cancer).

Prognosis

Certain factors affect prognosis (chance of recovery) and treatment options. The prognosis and treatment options depend on the stage of the cancer, how likely it is that vision can be saved in one or both eyes, the size and number of tumors, whether the patient has glaucoma, and whether trilateral retinoblastoma occurs.

Stages of Retinoblastoma

After retinoblastoma has been diagnosed, tests are done to find out if cancer cells have spread within the eye or to other parts of the body.

The process used to find out if cancer has spread within the eye or to other parts of the body is called staging. The information gathered from the staging process determines the stage of the disease. It is important to know the stage in order to plan treatment. The diagnostic tests and procedures described above can help determine the stage. A lumbar puncture may also be done if tests show that the cancer may have spread out of the eye. A lumbar puncture is a procedure used to collect cerebrospinal fluid from the spinal column. This is done by placing a needle into the spinal column. This procedure is also called an LP or spinal tap.

There are several staging systems for retinoblastoma. For treatment, retinoblastoma is classified as intraocular (within the eye) or extraocular (outside the eye).

- **Intraocular retinoblastoma:** Cancer is found in the eye but has not spread to tissues around the outside of the eye or to other parts of the body.

- **Extraocular retinoblastoma:** The cancer has spread beyond the eye. It may be found in tissues around the eye or it may have spread to the central nervous system (brain and spinal cord) or to other parts of the body such as the bone marrow or lymph nodes.

Recurrent Retinoblastoma

Recurrent retinoblastoma is cancer that has recurred (come back) after it has been treated. The cancer may recur in the eye, in tissues around the eye, or in other places in the body. Tumors that were not treated with radiation therapy or surgery commonly recur, usually within six months.

Treatment Option Overview

Different types of treatment are available for patients with retinoblastoma. Some treatments are standard (the currently used treatment), and some are being tested in clinical trials.

Children with retinoblastoma should have their treatment planned by a team of health care providers who are experts in treating cancer in children. Treatment will be overseen by a pediatric oncologist, a doctor who specializes in treating children with cancer. The pediatric oncologist works with other health care providers who are experts in treating children with eye cancer and who specialize in certain areas of medicine. These may include a pediatric ophthalmologist (children's eye doctor) who has a lot of experience in treating retinoblastoma and the following specialists:

- Pediatric surgeon
- Pediatric hematologist
- Radiation oncologist
- Neurologist
- Pediatric nurse specialist
- Rehabilitation specialist
- Psychologist
- Social workers
- Geneticist

Six types of standard treatment are used:

Enucleation: Enucleation is surgery to remove the eye and part of the optic nerve. The eye will be checked with a microscope to see if there are any signs that the cancer is likely to spread to other parts of the body. This is done if the tumor is large and there is little or no chance that vision can be saved. The patient will be fitted for an artificial eye after this surgery. Close follow-up is needed for two years or more to check for signs of recurrence in the area around the eye.

Radiation therapy: Radiation therapy is a cancer treatment that uses high-energy x-rays or other types of radiation to kill cancer cells or keep them from growing. There are two types of radiation therapy. External radiation therapy uses a machine outside the body to send radiation toward the cancer. Internal radiation therapy uses a radioactive substance sealed in needles, seeds, wires, plaques, or catheters that are placed directly into or near the cancer. The way the radiation therapy is given depends on the type and stage of the cancer being treated. Methods of radiation therapy used to treat retinoblastoma include the following:

- **Intensity-modulated radiation therapy (IMRT):** A type of three-dimensional (3-D) radiation therapy that uses a computer to make pictures of the size and shape of the tumor. Thin beams of radiation of different intensities (strengths) are aimed at the tumor from many angles. This type of radiation therapy causes less damage to healthy tissue near the tumor.

- **Stereotactic radiation therapy:** Radiation therapy that uses a rigid head frame attached to the skull to aim high-dose radiation beams directly at the tumors, causing less damage to nearby healthy tissue. It is also called stereotactic external-beam radiation and stereotaxic radiation therapy.

- **Proton beam radiation therapy:** Radiation therapy that uses protons made by a special machine. A proton is a type of high-energy radiation that is different from an x-ray.

- **Plaque radiotherapy:** Radioactive seeds are attached to one side of a disk, called a plaque, and placed directly on the outside wall of the eye near the tumor. The side of the plaque with the seeds on it faces the eyeball, aiming radiation at the tumor. The plaque helps protect other nearby tissue from the radiation.

Cryotherapy: Cryotherapy is a treatment that uses an instrument to freeze and destroy abnormal tissue, such as carcinoma in situ. This type of treatment is also called cryosurgery.

Photocoagulation: Photocoagulation is a procedure that uses laser light to destroy blood vessels to the tumor, causing the tumor cells to die. Photocoagulation may be used to treat small tumors. This is also called light coagulation.

Thermotherapy: Thermotherapy is the use of heat to destroy cancer cells. Thermotherapy may be given using a laser beam aimed through the dilated pupil or onto the outside of the eyeball, or using ultrasound, microwaves, or infrared radiation (light that cannot be seen but can be felt as heat).

Chemotherapy: Chemotherapy is a cancer treatment that uses drugs to stop the growth of cancer cells, either by killing the cells or by stopping them from dividing. When chemotherapy is taken by mouth or injected into a vein or muscle, the drugs enter the bloodstream and can reach cancer cells throughout the body (systemic chemotherapy). When chemotherapy is placed directly into the spinal column, an organ (such as the eye), or a body cavity such as the abdomen, the drugs mainly affect cancer cells in those areas (regional chemotherapy). The way the chemotherapy is given depends on the type and stage of the cancer being treated.

A form of chemotherapy called chemoreduction is used to treat retinoblastoma. Chemoreduction reduces the size of the tumor so it may be treated with local treatment (such as radiation therapy, cryotherapy, photocoagulation, or thermotherapy).

Late Side Effects

Side effects from cancer treatment that begin during or after treatment and continue for months or years are called late effects. Late effects of cancer treatment may include physical problems, changes in mood, feelings, thinking, learning, or memory, or second cancers (new types of cancer).

Some late effects may be treated or controlled. It is important to talk with your child's doctors about the effects cancer treatment can have on your child.

Children with the inherited form of retinoblastoma have an increased risk of developing second cancers. Children who have been treated for retinoblastoma with radiation therapy or certain chemotherapy agents also have a risk of developing second cancers. Regular follow-up by health professionals who are expert in finding and treating late effects is important.

Clinical Trials

A treatment clinical trial is a research study meant to help improve current treatments or obtain information on new treatments for patients with cancer. When clinical trials show that a new treatment is better than the standard treatment, the new treatment may become the standard treatment.

Patients may want to think about taking part in a clinical trial. For some patients, taking part in a clinical trial may be the best treatment choice. Clinical trials are part of the cancer research process. Clinical trials are done to find out if new cancer treatments are safe and effective or better than the standard treatment.

Many of today's standard treatments for cancer are based on earlier clinical trials. Patients who take part in a clinical trial may receive the standard treatment or be among the first to receive a new treatment.

Patients who take part in clinical trials also help improve the way cancer will be treated in the future. Even when clinical trials do not lead to effective new treatments, they often answer important questions and help move research forward.

Patients can enter clinical trials before, during, or after starting their cancer treatment. Some clinical trials only include patients who have not yet received treatment. Other trials test treatments for patients whose cancer has not gotten better. There are also clinical trials that test new ways to stop cancer from recurring (coming back) or reduce the side effects of cancer treatment.

Clinical trials are taking place in many parts of the country. This summary section describes treatments that are being studied in clinical trials. It may not mention every new treatment being studied.

Subtenon chemotherapy: Subtenon chemotherapy is the use of drugs injected through the membrane covering the muscles and nerves at the back of the eyeball. This is a type of regional chemotherapy. It is usually combined with systemic chemotherapy and local treatment (such as radiation therapy, cryotherapy, photocoagulation, or thermotherapy).

Ophthalmic arterial infusion therapy: Ophthalmic arterial infusion therapy is a type of regional chemotherapy used to deliver anticancer drugs directly to the eye. A catheter is put into an artery that leads to the eye and the anticancer drug is given through the catheter. During this treatment, a small balloon may be inserted into the artery to block it and keep most of the anticancer drug trapped near the tumor.

High-dose chemotherapy with stem cell transplant: High-dose chemotherapy with stem cell transplant is a way of giving high doses of chemotherapy and replacing blood -forming cells destroyed by the cancer treatment. Stem cells (immature blood cells) are removed from the blood or bone marrow of the patient or a donor and are frozen and stored. After the chemotherapy is completed, the stored stem cells are thawed and given back to the patient through an infusion. These reinfused stem cells grow into (and restore) the body's blood cells.

Biologic therapy: Biologic therapy is a treatment that uses the patient's immune system to fight cancer. Substances made by the body or made in a laboratory are used to boost, direct, or restore the body's natural defenses against cancer. This type of cancer treatment is also called biotherapy or immunotherapy. Clinical trials for retinoblastoma are studying a biologic therapy called gene therapy. This is a treatment that changes a gene to improve the body's ability to fight the disease.

Follow-Up Tests

Some of the tests that were done to diagnose the cancer or to find out the stage of the cancer may be repeated. Some tests will be repeated in order to see how well the treatment is working. Decisions about whether to continue, change, or stop treatment may be based on the results of these tests. This is sometimes called re-staging.

Some of the tests will continue to be done from time to time after treatment has ended. The results of these tests can show if your condition has changed or if the cancer has recurred (come back). These tests are sometimes called follow-up tests or check-ups.

Chapter 20

Oral Cancer

Cancer Cells

Cancer begins in cells, the building blocks that make up tissues. Tissues make up the organs of the body. Normal cells grow and divide to form new cells as the body needs them. When normal cells grow old or get damaged, they die, and new cells take their place. Sometimes, this process goes wrong. New cells form when the body doesn't need them, and old or damaged cells don't die as they should. The buildup of extra cells often forms a mass of tissue called a growth or tumor. Tumors in the mouth or throat can be benign (not cancer) or malignant (cancer).

Almost all oral cancers begin in the flat cells (squamous cells) that cover the surfaces of the mouth, tongue, and lips. These cancers are called squamous cell carcinomas.

Oral cancer cells can spread by breaking away from the original tumor. They enter blood vessels or lymph vessels, which branch into all the tissues of the body. The cancer cells often appear first in nearby lymph nodes in the neck. The cancer cells may attach to other tissues and grow to form new tumors that may damage those tissues. The spread of cancer is called metastasis.

Risk Factors

When you get a diagnosis of cancer, it's natural to wonder what may have caused the disease. Doctors can't always explain why one

Excerpted from "What You Need to Know about Oral Cancer," National Cancer Institute (www.cancer.gov), December 23, 2009.

person gets oral cancer and another doesn't. However, we do know that people with certain risk factors may be more likely than others to develop oral cancer.

A risk factor is something that may increase the chance of getting a disease. The more risk factors that a person has, the greater the chance that oral cancer will develop. However, most people with known risk factors for oral cancer don't develop the disease. Studies have found the following risk factors for oral cancer.

Tobacco use: Tobacco use causes most oral cancers. Smoking cigarettes, cigars, or pipes, or using smokeless tobacco (such as snuff and chewing tobacco) causes oral cancer. The use of other tobacco products (such as bidis and kreteks) may also increase the risk of oral cancer.

Heavy smokers who have smoked tobacco for a long time are most at risk for oral cancer. The risk is even higher for tobacco users who are heavy drinkers of alcohol. In fact, three out of four people with oral cancer have used tobacco, alcohol, or both.

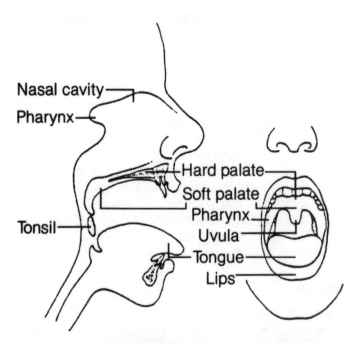

Figure 20.1. Oral Anatomy (image by the National Cancer Institute, AV-0000-4108.

Quitting is important for anyone who uses tobacco. Quitting at any time is beneficial to your health. For people who already have cancer, quitting may reduce the chance of getting another cancer, lung disease, or heart disease caused by tobacco. Quitting can also help cancer treatments work better.

There are many ways to get help:

- Ask your doctor about medicine or nicotine replacement therapy. Your doctor can suggest a number of treatments that help people quit.

- Ask your doctor or dentist to help you find local programs or trained professionals who help people stop using tobacco.

- Call staff at the National Cancer Institute's Smoking Quitline at 877-44U-QUIT (877-448-7848) or instant message them through LiveHelp (http://www.cancer.gov/help). They can tell you about ways to quit smoking, groups that help smokers who want to quit, National Cancer Institute (NCI) publications about quitting smoking, and how to take part in a study of methods to help smokers quit.

- Go online to Smokefree.gov (http://www.smokefree.gov/), a federal government website. It offers a guide to quitting smoking and a list of other resources.

Heavy alcohol use: People who are heavy drinkers are more likely to develop oral cancer than people who don't drink alcohol. The risk increases with the amount of alcohol that a person drinks. The risk increases even more if the person both drinks alcohol and uses tobacco.

HPV infection: Some members of the human papilloma family of viruses (HPV) can infect the mouth and throat. These viruses are passed from person to person through sexual contact. Cancer at the base of the tongue, at the back of the throat, in the tonsils, or in the soft palate is linked with HPV infection.

Sun: Cancer of the lip can be caused by exposure to the sun. Using a lotion or lip balm that has a sunscreen can reduce the risk. Wearing a hat with a brim can also block the sun's harmful rays. The risk of cancer of the lip increases if the person also smokes.

Personal history: People who have had oral cancer are at increased risk of developing another oral cancer. Smoking increases this risk.

Diet: Some studies suggest that not eating enough fruits and vegetables may increase the chance of getting oral cancer.

Betel nut use: Betel nut use is most common in Asia, where millions chew the product. It's a type of palm seed wrapped with a betel leaf and sometimes mixed with spices, sweeteners, and tobacco. Chewing betel nut causes oral cancer. The risk increases even more if the person also drinks alcohol and uses tobacco.

Symptoms

Symptoms of oral cancer may include the following:

- Patches inside your mouth or on your lips. White patches (leukoplakia) are the most common. White patches sometimes become malignant. Mixed red and white patches (erythroleukoplakia) are more likely than white patches to become malignant. Red patches (erythroplakia) are brightly colored, smooth areas that often become malignant.

- A sore on your lip or in your mouth that doesn't heal

- Bleeding in your mouth

- Loose teeth

- Difficulty or pain when swallowing

- Difficulty wearing dentures

- A lump in your neck

- An earache that doesn't go away

- Numbness of lower lip and chin

Most often, these symptoms are not from oral cancer. Another health problem can cause them. Anyone with these symptoms should tell their doctor or dentist so that problems can be diagnosed and treated as early as possible.

Diagnosis

If you have symptoms that suggest oral cancer, your doctor or dentist will check your mouth and throat for red or white patches, lumps, swelling, or other problems. A physical exam includes looking carefully at the roof of your mouth, back of your throat, and insides of your cheeks and lips. Your doctor or dentist also will gently pull out your tongue so it can be checked on the sides and underneath. The floor of your mouth and lymph nodes in your neck will also be checked.

If your doctor or dentist does not find the cause of your symptoms, you may be referred to a specialist. An ear, nose, and throat specialist can see the back of your nose, tongue, and throat by using a small, long-handled mirror or a lighted tube. Sometimes pictures need to be made with a CT scan or MRI to find a hidden tumor.

The removal of a small piece of tissue to look for cancer cells is called a biopsy. Usually, a biopsy is done with local anesthesia. Sometimes, it's done under general anesthesia. A pathologist then looks at the tissue under a microscope to check for cancer cells. A biopsy is the only sure way to know if the abnormal area is cancer.

If you need a biopsy, you may want to ask the doctor or dentist some of the following questions:

- Why do I need a biopsy?

- How much tissue do you expect to remove?

- How long will it take? Will I be awake? Will it hurt?

- How soon will I know the results?

- Are there any risks? What are the chances of infection or bleeding after the biopsy?

- How should I care for the biopsy site afterward? How long will it take to heal?

- Will I be able to eat and drink normally after the biopsy?

- If I do have cancer, who will talk with me about treatment? When?

Staging

If oral cancer is diagnosed, your doctor needs to learn the extent (stage) of the disease to help you choose the best treatment. When oral cancer spreads, cancer cells may be found in the lymph nodes in the neck or in other tissues of the neck. Cancer cells can also spread to the lungs, liver, bones, and other parts of the body.

Doctors describe the stage of oral cancer based on the size of the tumor, whether it has invaded nearby tissues, and whether it has spread to the lymph nodes or other tissues:

Early cancer: Stage I or II oral cancer is usually a small tumor (smaller than a walnut), and no cancer cells are found in the lymph nodes.

Advanced cancer: Stage III or IV oral cancer is usually a large tumor (as big as a lime). The cancer may have invaded nearby tissues or spread to lymph nodes or other parts of the body.

Treatment

People with early oral cancer may be treated with surgery or radiation therapy. People with advanced oral cancer may have a combination of treatments. For example, radiation therapy and chemotherapy are often given at the same time. Another treatment option is targeted therapy. Cetuximab (Erbitux) was the first targeted therapy approved for oral cancer. Cetuximab binds to oral cancer cells and interferes with cancer cell growth and the spread of cancer

The choice of treatment depends mainly on your general health, where in your mouth or throat the cancer began, the size of the tumor, and whether the cancer has spread.

Many doctors encourage people with oral cancer to consider taking part in a clinical trial. Clinical trials are research studies testing new treatments. They are an important option for people with all stages of oral cancer.

Your doctor may refer you to a specialist, or you may ask for a referral. The following specialists may be involved in treating oral cancer:

- Head and neck surgeons

- Dentists who specialize in surgery of the mouth, face, and jaw (oral and maxillofacial surgeons)

- Ear, nose, and throat doctors (otolaryngologists)

- Medical oncologists

- Radiation oncologists

Other health care professionals who work with the specialists as a team may include a dentist, plastic surgeon, reconstructive surgeon, speech pathologist, oncology nurse, registered dietitian, and mental health counselor.

Your health care team can describe your treatment choices, the expected results of each, and the possible side effects. You'll want to consider how treatment may affect eating, swallowing, and talking, and whether treatment will change the way you look. You and your health care team can work together to develop a treatment plan that meets your needs.

Oral cancer and its treatment can lead to other health problems. For example, radiation therapy and chemotherapy for oral cancer can cause dental problems. That's why it's important to get your mouth in good condition before cancer treatment begins. See a dentist for a thorough exam one month, if possible, before starting cancer treatment to give your mouth time to heal after needed dental work.

Before, during, and after cancer treatment, you can have supportive care to control pain and other symptoms, to relieve the side effects of therapy, and to help you cope with the feelings that a diagnosis of cancer can bring.

Second Opinion

Before starting treatment, you might want a second opinion about your diagnosis, the stage of cancer, and the treatment plan. You may even want to talk to several different doctors about all of the treatment options, their side effects, and the expected results. For example, you may wish to discuss your treatment plan with a surgeon, radiation oncologist, and medical oncologist.

Some people worry that the doctor will be offended if they ask for a second opinion. Usually the opposite is true. Most doctors welcome a second opinion. And many health insurance companies will pay for a second opinion if you or your doctor requests it. Some companies require a second opinion.

If you get a second opinion, the second doctor may agree with your first doctor's diagnosis and treatment plan. Or the second doctor may suggest another approach. Either way, you'll have more information and perhaps a greater sense of control. You can feel more confident about the decisions you make, knowing that you've looked at your options.

It may take some time and effort to gather your medical records and see another doctor. In most cases, it's not a problem to take several weeks to get a second opinion. The delay in starting treatment usually will not make treatment less effective. To make sure, you should discuss this delay with your doctor.

There are many ways to find a doctor for a second opinion. You can ask your doctor, a local or state medical society, a nearby hospital, or a medical school for names of specialists. You may want to find a medical center that has a lot of experience treating people with oral cancer.

Nutrition

Your diet is an important part of your treatment for oral cancer. You need the right amount of calories, protein, vitamins, and minerals to maintain your strength and to heal.

However, when you have oral cancer, it may be difficult to eat. You may be uncomfortable or tired, and you may have a dry mouth, have trouble swallowing, or not feel like eating. You also may have nausea, vomiting, constipation, or diarrhea from cancer treatment or pain medicine.

Tell your health care team if you're having any problems eating, drinking, or digesting your food. If you're losing weight, a dietitian can help you choose the foods and nutrition products that will meet your needs.

Here are some tips regarding commonly experienced problems:

Sore mouth: If your mouth is sore, you may find that you want to avoid acidic foods, such as oranges and tomatoes. Also, to protect your mouth during cancer treatment, it helps to avoid sharp, hard foods, such as chips.

Dry mouth: If your mouth is dry, you may find that soft foods moistened with sauces or gravies are easier to eat. Smooth soups, puddings, milkshakes, and blended fruit smoothies often are easier to swallow. Also, meal replacement products (such as instant breakfast, Boost®, or Ensure®) may be helpful.

Keep in mind that a dry mouth puts you at greater risk for tooth decay (cavities). Rinse your mouth often, especially after eating or drinking sweet foods.

Trouble swallowing: If there's a chance that swallowing will become too difficult for you, your dietitian and doctor may recommend another way for you to receive nutrition. For example, after surgery or during radiation therapy for oral cancer, some people need a temporary feeding tube. A feeding tube is a flexible tube that is usually passed into the stomach through an incision in the abdomen. A liquid meal replacement product (such as Boost or Ensure) can be poured through the tube at mealtime. When not in use, the small tube attached to your stomach is not visible to others.

Reconstruction

Some people with oral cancer may need to have plastic or reconstructive surgery to rebuild the bones or tissues of the mouth. Research has led to many advances in the way bones and tissues can be rebuilt.

Some people may need dental implants. Or they may need to have grafts (tissue moved from another part of the body). Skin, muscle, and bone can be moved to the mouth from the chest, arm, or leg. The plastic surgeon uses this tissue for repair.

If you're thinking about reconstruction, you may wish to consult with a plastic or reconstructive surgeon before your treatment for oral cancer begins. You can have reconstructive surgery at the same time as you have the cancer removed, or you can have it later on. Talk with your doctor about which approach is right for you.

Rehabilitation

Your health care team will help you return to normal activities as soon as possible. The goals of rehabilitation depend on the extent of the disease and type of treatment.

If oral cancer or its treatment leads to problems with talking, speech therapy will generally begin as soon as possible. A speech therapist may see you in the hospital to plan therapy and teach speech exercises. Speech therapy may continue after you return home.

Some people will need a prosthesis to help them talk and eat as normally as possible. A prosthesis is an artificial device that replaces the missing teeth or tissues of the mouth. For example, if part of the palate is removed, a dentist with special training (a prosthodontist) may be able to fit you with a plastic device that replaces the missing tissue.

Follow-Up Care

You'll need regular checkups of your mouth, throat, and neck after treatment for oral cancer. Checkups help ensure that any changes in your health are noted and treated if needed. Checkups may include a physical exam, blood tests, chest x-rays, or CT scans. If you have any health problems between checkups, you should contact your doctor.

People who have had oral cancer have a chance of developing a new cancer. A new cancer is especially likely for those who use tobacco or who drink alcohol heavily. Doctors strongly urge people to stop using tobacco and stop drinking alcohol to cut down the risk of a new cancer and other health problems.

Chapter 21

Laryngeal Cancer

The Larynx

The larynx is an organ at the front of your neck. It is also called the voice box. It is about two inches long and two inches wide. It is above the windpipe (trachea). Below and behind the larynx is the esophagus.

The larynx has two bands of muscle that form the vocal cords. The cartilage at the front of the larynx is sometimes called the Adam's apple.

The larynx has three main parts:

- The top part of the larynx is the supraglottis.

- The glottis is in the middle. Your vocal cords are in the glottis.

- The subglottis is at the bottom. The subglottis connects to the windpipe.

The larynx plays a role in breathing, swallowing, and talking. The larynx acts like a valve over the windpipe. The valve opens and closes to allow breathing, swallowing, and speaking.

- **Breathing:** When you breathe, the vocal cords relax and open. When you hold your breath, the vocal cords shut tightly.

- **Swallowing:** The larynx protects the windpipe. When you swallow, a flap called the epiglottis covers the opening of your

Excerpted from "What You Need to Know about Cancer of the Larynx," National Cancer Institute (www.cancer.gov), May 5, 2003. Revised by David A. Cooke, MD, FACP, September 2010.

larynx to keep food out of your lungs. The food passes through the esophagus on its way from your mouth to your stomach.

- **Talking:** The larynx produces the sound of your voice. When you talk, your vocal cords tighten and move closer together. Air from your lungs is forced between them and makes them vibrate. This makes the sound of your voice. Your tongue, lips, and teeth form this sound into words.

Cancer of the larynx also may be called laryngeal cancer. It can develop in any part of the larynx. Most cancers of the larynx begin in the glottis. The inner walls of the larynx are lined with cells called squamous cells. Almost all laryngeal cancers begin in these cells. These cancers are called squamous cell carcinomas.

If cancer of the larynx spreads (metastasizes), the cancer cells often spread to nearby lymph nodes in the neck. The cancer cells can also spread to the back of the tongue, other parts of the throat and neck, the lungs, and other parts of the body. When this happens, the new tumor has the same kind of abnormal cells as the primary tumor in the larynx. For example, if cancer of the larynx spreads to the lungs, the cancer cells in the lungs are actually laryngeal cancer cells. The disease is called metastatic cancer of the larynx, not lung cancer. It is treated as cancer of the larynx, not lung cancer. Doctors sometimes call the new tumor "distant" disease.

Cancer of the Larynx: Who's at Risk?

No one knows the exact causes of cancer of the larynx. Doctors cannot explain why one person gets this disease and another does not. We do know that cancer is not contagious. You cannot "catch" cancer from another person.

People with certain risk factors are more likely to get cancer of the larynx. A risk factor is anything that increases your chance of developing this disease.

Studies have found the following risk factors:

- **Age:** Cancer of the larynx occurs most often in people over the age of 55.

- **Gender:** Men are four times more likely than women to get cancer of the larynx.

- **Race:** African Americans are more likely than whites to be diagnosed with cancer of the larynx.

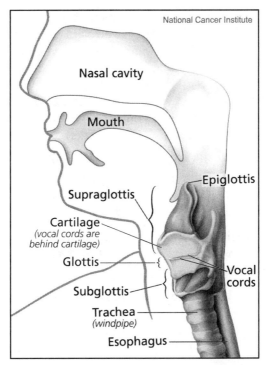

Figure 21.1. *The Larynx and Nearby Structures (image by Alan Hoofring, National Cancer Institute)*

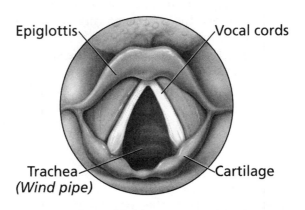

National Cancer Institute

Figure 21.2. *The Larynx, Top View (image by Alan Hoofring, National Cancer Institute)*

- **Smoking:** Smokers are far more likely than nonsmokers to get cancer of the larynx. The risk is even higher for smokers who drink alcohol heavily. People who stop smoking can greatly decrease their risk of cancer of the larynx, as well as cancer of the lung, mouth, pancreas, bladder, and esophagus. Also, quitting smoking reduces the chance that someone with cancer of the larynx will get a second cancer in the head and neck region. (Cancer of the larynx is part of a group of cancers called head and neck cancers.)

- **Alcohol:** People who drink alcohol are more likely to develop laryngeal cancer than people who don't drink. The risk increases with the amount of alcohol that is consumed. The risk also increases if the person drinks alcohol and also smokes tobacco.

- **A personal history of head and neck cancer:** Almost one in four people who have had head and neck cancer will develop a second primary head and neck cancer.

- **Occupation:** Workers exposed to sulfuric acid mist or nickel have an increased risk of laryngeal cancer. Also, working with asbestos can increase the risk of this disease. Asbestos workers should follow work and safety rules to avoid inhaling asbestos fibers.

Recent studies have suggested that infection with human papilloma virus (HPV) in the respiratory tract may be a factor in a significant number of laryngeal cancers. A number of studies are underway to further confirm and understand this association.

Other studies suggest that having certain viruses or a diet low in vitamin A may increase the chance of getting cancer of the larynx. Another risk factor is having gastroesophageal reflux disease (GERD), which causes stomach acid to flow up into the esophagus.

Most people who have these risk factors do not get cancer of the larynx. If you are concerned about your chance of getting cancer of the larynx, you should discuss this concern with your health care provider. Your health care provider may suggest ways to reduce your risk and can plan an appropriate schedule for checkups.

Symptoms

The symptoms of cancer of the larynx depend mainly on the size of the tumor and where it is in the larynx. Symptoms may include the following:

- Hoarseness or other voice changes

- A lump in the neck
- A sore throat or feeling that something is stuck in your throat
- A cough that does not go away
- Problems breathing
- Bad breath
- An earache
- Weight loss

These symptoms may be caused by cancer or by other, less serious problems. Only a doctor can tell for sure.

Diagnosis

If you have symptoms of cancer of the larynx, the doctor may do some or all of the following exams:

Physical exam: The doctor will feel your neck and check your thyroid, larynx, and lymph nodes for abnormal lumps or swelling. To see your throat, the doctor may press down on your tongue.

Indirect laryngoscopy: The doctor looks down your throat using a small, long-handled mirror to check for abnormal areas and to see if your vocal cords move as they should. This test does not hurt. The doctor may spray a local anesthesia in your throat to keep you from gagging. This exam is done in the doctor's office.

Direct laryngoscopy: The doctor inserts a thin, lighted tube called a laryngoscope through your nose or mouth. As the tube goes down your throat, the doctor can look at areas that cannot be seen with a mirror. A local anesthetic eases discomfort and prevents gagging. You may also receive a mild sedative to help you relax. Sometimes the doctor uses general anesthesia to put a person to sleep. This exam may be done in a doctor's office, an outpatient clinic, or a hospital.

CT scan: An x-ray machine linked to a computer takes a series of detailed pictures of the neck area. You may receive an injection of a special dye so your larynx shows up clearly in the pictures. From the CT scan, the doctor may see tumors in your larynx or elsewhere in your neck.

Biopsy: If an exam shows an abnormal area, the doctor may remove a small sample of tissue. Removing tissue to look for cancer cells is called a biopsy. For a biopsy, you receive local or general anesthesia, and the doctor removes tissue samples through a laryngoscope.

A pathologist then looks at the tissue under a microscope to check for cancer cells. A biopsy is the only sure way to know if a tumor is cancerous.

Staging

To plan the best treatment, your doctor needs to know the stage, or extent, of your disease. Staging is a careful attempt to learn whether the cancer has spread and, if so, to what parts of the body. The doctor may use x-rays, CT scans, or magnetic resonance imaging to find out whether the cancer has spread to lymph nodes, other areas in your neck, or distant sites.

Treatment

People with cancer of the larynx often want to take an active part in making decisions about their medical care. It is natural to want to learn all you can about your disease and treatment choices. However, shock and stress after a diagnosis of cancer can make it hard to remember what you want to ask the doctor. Here are some ideas that might help:

- Make a list of questions.
- Take notes at the appointment.
- Ask the doctor if you may use a tape recorder during the appointment.
- Ask a family member or friend to come to the appointment with you.

Your doctor may refer you to a specialist who treats cancer of the larynx, such as a surgeon, otolaryngologist (an ear, nose, and throat doctor), radiation oncologist, or medical oncologist. You can also ask your doctor for a referral. Treatment usually begins within a few weeks of the diagnosis. Usually, there is time to talk to your doctor about treatment choices, get a second opinion, and learn more about the disease before making a treatment decision.

Getting a Second Opinion

Before starting treatment, you might want a second opinion about your diagnosis and treatment plan. Some insurance companies require a second opinion; others may cover a second opinion if you or your doctor requests it. There are a number of ways to find a doctor for a second opinion:

- Your doctor may refer you or you may ask for a referral to one or more specialists. At cancer centers, several specialists often work together as a team. The team may include a surgeon, radiation oncologist, medical oncologist, speech pathologist, and nutritionist. At some cancer centers, you may be able to see them all on the same day.

- The Cancer Information Service, at 800-4-CANCER, can tell you about treatment centers near you.

- A local medical society, a nearby hospital, or a medical school can often provide the names of specialists in your area.

Preparing for Treatment

The doctor can describe your treatment choices and the results you can expect for each treatment option. You will want to consider how treatment may change the way you look, breathe, and talk. You and your doctor can work together to develop a treatment plan that meets your needs and personal values.

The choice of treatment depends on a number of factors, including your general health, where in the larynx the cancer began, the size of the tumor, and whether the cancer has spread.

If you smoke, a good way to prepare for treatment is to stop smoking. Studies show that treatment is more likely to be successful for people who don't smoke. Your doctor or the Cancer Information Service (800-4-CANCER) may be able to suggest ways to help you stop smoking.

You may want to talk with the doctor about taking part in a clinical trial, a research study of new treatment methods. Clinical trials are an important option. Patients who join trials have the first chance to benefit from new treatments that have shown promise in earlier research.

Methods of Treatment

Cancer of the larynx may be treated with radiation therapy, surgery, or chemotherapy. Some patients have a combination of therapies.

Radiation therapy (also called radiotherapy) uses high-energy x-rays to kill cancer cells. The rays are aimed at the tumor and the tissue around it. Radiation therapy is local therapy. It affects cells only in the treated area. Treatments are usually given five days a week for five to eight weeks.

Laryngeal cancer may be treated with radiation therapy alone or in combination with surgery or chemotherapy:

- **Radiation therapy alone:** Radiation therapy is used alone for small tumors or for patients who cannot have surgery.

- **Radiation therapy combined with surgery:** Radiation therapy may be used to shrink a large tumor before surgery or to destroy cancer cells that may remain in the area after surgery. If a tumor grows back after surgery, it is often treated with radiation.

- **Radiation therapy combined with chemotherapy:** Radiation therapy may be used before, during, or after chemotherapy.

After radiation therapy, some people need feeding tubes placed into the abdomen. The feeding tube is usually temporary.

Surgery

Surgery is an operation in which a doctor removes the cancer using a scalpel or laser while the patient is asleep. When patients need surgery, the type of operation depends mainly on the size and exact location of the tumor.

There are several types of laryngectomy (surgery to remove part or all of the larynx):

- **Total laryngectomy:** The surgeon removes the entire larynx.

- **Partial laryngectomy (hemilaryngectomy):** The surgeon removes part of the larynx.

- **Supraglottic laryngectomy:** The surgeon takes out the supraglottis, the top part of the larynx.

- **Cordectomy:** The surgeon removes one or both vocal cords.

Sometimes the surgeon also removes the lymph nodes in the neck. This is called lymph node dissection. The surgeon also may remove the thyroid.

During surgery for cancer of the larynx, the surgeon may need to make a stoma. (This surgery is called a tracheostomy.) The stoma is a new airway through an opening in the front of the neck. Air enters and leaves the windpipe (trachea) and lungs through this opening. A tracheostomy tube, also called a trach ("trake") tube, keeps the new airway open. For many patients, the stoma is temporary. It is needed only until the patient recovers from surgery. After surgery, some people may need a temporary feeding tube.

Chemotherapy

Chemotherapy is the use of drugs to kill cancer cells. Your doctor may suggest one drug or a combination of drugs. The drugs for cancer of the larynx are usually given by injection into the bloodstream. The drugs enter the bloodstream and travel throughout the body. Chemotherapy is used to treat laryngeal cancer in several ways:

- **Before surgery or radiation therapy:** In some cases, drugs are given to try to shrink a large tumor before surgery or radiation therapy.

- **After surgery or radiation therapy:** Chemotherapy may be used after surgery or radiation therapy to kill any cancer cells that may be left. It also may be used for cancers that have spread.

- **Instead of surgery:** Chemotherapy may be used with radiation therapy instead of surgery. The larynx is not removed and the voice is spared.

Chemotherapy may be given in an outpatient part of the hospital, at the doctor's office, or at home. Rarely, a hospital stay may be needed.

Side Effects of Cancer Treatment

Cancer treatments are very powerful. Treatments that remove or destroy cancer cells are likely to damage healthy cells, too. That's why treatments often cause side effects. This section describes some of the side effects of each kind of treatment.

Side effects may not be the same for each person, and they may even change from one treatment session to the next. Before treatment starts, your health care team will explain possible side effects and how they can be managed. It may help to know that although some side effects may not go away completely, most of them become less troubling.

It may also help to talk with other patients. A social worker, nurse, or other member of the medical team can set up a visit with someone who has had the same treatment.

Radiation Therapy

People treated with radiation therapy may have some or all of these side effects:

- **Dry mouth:** Drinking lots of fluids can help. Some patients find artificial saliva helpful. It comes in a spray or squeeze bottle.

301

- **Sore throat or mouth:** Your health care provider may suggest special rinses to numb your throat and mouth and help relieve the soreness.

- **Delayed healing after dental care:** Many doctors recommend having a dental exam and any needed dental work before radiation therapy.

- **Tooth decay:** Good mouth care can help keep your teeth and gums healthy and can help you feel better. If it's hard to floss or brush your teeth in the usual way, you can try using gauze, a soft toothbrush, or a toothbrush that has a spongy tip instead of bristles. A mouthwash made with diluted peroxide, salt water, baking soda, or a combination can keep your mouth fresh and help protect your teeth from decay. It may also be helpful to use fluoride toothpaste or rinse.

- **Changes in sense of taste and smell:** During radiation therapy, food may taste or smell different.

- **Fatigue:** During radiation therapy, you may become very tired, especially in the later weeks of treatment. Resting is important, but doctors usually advise their patients to stay as active as they can.

- **Changes in voice quality:** Your voice may be weak at the end of the day. It may also be affected by changes in the weather. Voice changes and the feeling of a lump in your throat may come from swelling in the larynx caused by the radiation. The doctor may suggest medicine to reduce this swelling.

- **Skin changes in treated area:** The skin in the treated area may become red or dry. Good skin care is important at this time. Try to expose this area to the air but protect it from the sun. Avoid wearing clothes that rub, and do not shave the treated area. You should not put anything on your skin before radiation treatments. Also, you should never use lotion or cream without your doctor's advice. Over time, thickening and hardening of the skin in the radiated area may occur, which may lead to an abnormal texture and appearance.

Surgery

People who have surgery may have any of these side effects:

- **Pain:** You may be uncomfortable for the first few days after surgery. However, medicine can usually control the pain. You should feel free to discuss pain relief with the doctor or nurse.

302

- **Low energy:** It is common to feel tired or weak after surgery. The length of time it takes to recover from an operation is different for each patient.

- **Swelling in the throat:** For a few days after surgery, you won't be able to eat, drink, or swallow. At first, you will receive fluid through an intravenous (IV) tube placed into your arm. Within a day or two, you will get fluids and nutrition through a feeding tube (put in place during surgery) that goes through your nose and throat into your stomach. When the swelling goes away and the area begins to heal, the feeding tube will be removed. Swallowing may be difficult at first, and you may need the help of a nurse or speech pathologist. Soon you will be eating your regular diet. If you need a feeding tube for longer than one week, you may get a tube that goes directly into the abdomen. Most patients slowly return to eating solid foods by mouth, but for a very few patients, the feeding tube may be permanent.

- **Increased mucus production:** After the operation, the lungs and windpipe produce a lot of mucus, also called sputum. To remove it, the nurse applies gentle suction by placing a small plastic tube in the stoma. You will learn to cough and suction mucus through the stoma without the nurse's help.

- **Numbness, stiffness, or weakness:** After a laryngectomy, parts of the neck and throat may be numb because nerves have been cut. Also, the shoulder, neck, and arm may be weak and stiff. You may need physical therapy to improve your strength and flexibility after surgery.

- **Changes in physical appearance:** Your neck will be somewhat smaller, and it will have scars. Some patients find it helpful to wear clothing that covers the neck area.

- **Tracheostomy:** Patients who have surgery will have a stoma. With most supraglottic and partial laryngectomies, the stoma is temporary. After a short recovery period, the tube can be removed, and the stoma closes up. You should then be able to breathe and talk in the usual way. In some people, however, the voice may be hoarse or weak.

After a total laryngectomy, the stoma is permanent. If you have a total laryngectomy, you will need to learn to speak in a new way.

Chemotherapy

The side effects of chemotherapy depend mainly on the specific drugs and the dose. In general, anticancer drugs affect cells that divide rapidly:

- **Blood cells:** These cells fight infection, help your blood to clot, and carry oxygen to all parts of your body. If your blood cells are affected, you are more likely to get infections, may bruise or bleed easily, and may feel very weak and tired.

- **Cells in hair roots:** Chemotherapy can lead to hair loss, but hair will grow back. However, the new hair may be different in color and texture.

- **Cells that line the digestive tract:** Chemotherapy can cause poor appetite, nausea and vomiting, diarrhea, or mouth and lip sores. Many of these side effects can be controlled with new or improved drugs.

Nutrition

Some people who have had treatment for cancer of the larynx may lose their interest in food. Soreness and changes in smell and taste may make eating difficult. Yet good nutrition is important. Eating well means getting enough calories and protein to prevent weight loss, regain strength, and rebuild healthy tissues.

If eating is difficult because your mouth is dry from radiation therapy, you may want to try soft, bland foods moistened with sauces or gravies. Thick soups, puddings, and milkshakes often are easier to swallow. The nurse and the dietitian will help you choose the right foods.

After surgery or radiation therapy, some people need feeding tubes placed into the abdomen. Most people slowly return to a regular diet. Learning to swallow again may take some practice with the help of a nurse or speech pathologist. Some people find liquids easier to swallow; others do better with solid foods. You will find what works best for you.

Living with a Stoma

Learning to live with the changes brought about by cancer of the larynx is a special challenge. The medical team will make every effort to help you return to your normal routine as soon as possible.

If you have a stoma, you will need to learn how to care for it:

- Before leaving the hospital, you will learn to remove and clean the trach tube, suction the trach, and care for the skin around the stoma.

- If the air is too dry, as it may be in heated buildings in the winter, the tissues of the windpipe and lungs may produce extra mucus. Also, the skin around the stoma may get sore. Keeping the skin around the stoma clean and using a humidifier at home or at the office can lessen these problems.

It is very dangerous for water to get into the windpipe and lungs through the stoma. Wearing a special plastic stoma shield or holding a washcloth over the stoma keeps water out when showering or shaving. Other types of stoma covers—such as scarves, neckties, and specially made covers—help keep moisture in and around the stoma. They help filter smoke and dust from the air before it enters the stoma. They also catch any fluids that come out of the windpipe when you cough or sneeze. Many people choose to wear something over their stoma even after the area heals. Stoma covers can be attractive as well as useful.

When shaving, men should keep in mind that the neck may be numb for several months after surgery. To avoid nicks and cuts, it may be best to use an electric shaver until the numbness goes away.

People with stomas work in almost every type of business and can do nearly all of the things they did before. However, they cannot hold their breath, so straining and heavy lifting may be difficult. Also, swimming and water skiing are not possible without special instruction and equipment to keep water from entering the stoma.

Some people may feel self-conscious about the way they look and speak. They may be concerned about how other people feel about them. They may be concerned about how their sexual relationships may be affected. Many people find that talking about these concerns helps them. Counseling or support groups may also be helpful.

Learning to Speak Again

Talking is part of nearly everything we do, so it's natural to be scared if your voice box must be removed. Losing the ability to talk—even for a short time—is hard. Patients and their families and friends need understanding and support during this time.

Within a week or so after a partial laryngectomy, you will be able to talk in the usual way. After a total laryngectomy, however, you must learn to speak in a new way. A speech pathologist usually meets with you before surgery to explain the methods that can be used. In many cases, speech lessons start before you leave the hospital.

Until you begin to talk again, it is important to have other ways to communicate. Here are some ideas that you may find helpful:

- Keep pads of paper and pens or pencils in your pocket or purse.

- Use a typewriter, computer, or other electronic device. Your words can be printed on paper, displayed on a screen, or produced in a male or female voice.

- Carry a small dictionary or a picture book and point to the words you need.

- Write notes on a "magic slate" (a toy with a plastic sheet that covers black wax; lifting the plastic erases the sheet).

The health care team can help patients learn new ways to speak. It takes practice and patience to learn techniques such as esophageal speech or tracheoesophageal puncture speech, and not everyone is successful. How quickly a person learns, how understandable the speech is, and how natural the new voice sounds depend on the extent of the surgery on the larynx.

Esophageal Speech

A speech pathologist can teach you how to force air into the top of your esophagus and then push it out again. The puff of air is like a burp. It vibrates the walls of the throat, making sound for the new voice. The tongue, lips, and teeth form words as the sound passes through the mouth.

This type of speech sounds low pitched and gruff, but it usually sounds more like a natural voice than speech made by a mechanical larynx. There is also no device to carry around, so your hands are free.

Tracheoesophageal Puncture

For tracheoesophageal puncture (TEP), the surgeon makes an opening between the trachea and the esophagus. The opening is made at the time of initial surgery or later. A small plastic or silicone valve fits into this opening. The valve keeps food out of the trachea. After TEP, patients can cover their stoma with a finger and force air into the esophagus through the valve. The air produces sound by making the walls of the throat vibrate. The sound is a lot like natural speech.

Mechanical Speech

You may choose to use a mechanical larynx while you learn esophageal or TEP speech or if you are unable to use these methods. The device may be powered by batteries (electrolarynx) or by air (pneumatic larynx).

Many different mechanical devices are available. The speech pathologist will help you choose the best device for your needs and abilities and will train you to use it.

One kind of electrolarynx looks like a small flashlight. It makes a humming sound. You hold the device against your neck, and the sound travels through your neck to your mouth. Another type of electrolarynx has a flexible plastic tube that carries sound into your mouth from a hand-held device. There are also devices that are built into a denture or retainer and can be worn inside your mouth and operated by a hand-held remote control.

A pneumatic larynx is held over the stoma and uses air from the lungs instead of batteries to make it vibrate. The sound it makes travels to the mouth through a plastic tube.

Follow-Up Care

Follow-up care is important after treatment for cancer of the larynx. Regular checkups ensure that any changes in health are noted. Problems can be found and treated as soon as possible. The doctor will check closely to be sure that the cancer has not returned. Checkups include exams of the stoma, neck, and throat. From time to time, the doctor may do a complete physical exam and take x-rays. If you had radiation therapy or a partial laryngectomy, the doctor will also examine you with a laryngoscope.

Treatments for laryngeal cancer can affect the thyroid. A blood test can tell if the thyroid is making enough thyroid hormone. If the level is low, you may need to take thyroid hormone pills.

People who have laryngeal cancer have a chance of developing a new cancer in the mouth, throat, or other areas of the head and neck. This is especially true for those who are smokers or drink alcohol heavily. Most doctors strongly urge their patients to stop smoking and drinking to cut down the risk of a new cancer and other health problems.

Chapter 22

Lung Cancer: An Overview

The Lungs

Your lungs are a pair of large organs in your chest. They are part of your respiratory system. Air enters your body through your nose or mouth. It passes through your windpipe (trachea) and through each bronchus, and goes into your lungs.

When you breathe in, your lungs expand with air. This is how your body gets oxygen. When you breathe out, air goes out of your lungs. This is how your body gets rid of carbon dioxide.

Your right lung has three parts (lobes). Your left lung is smaller and has two lobes. A thin tissue (the pleura) covers the lungs and lines the inside of the chest. Between the two layers of the pleura is a very small amount of fluid (pleural fluid). Normally, this fluid does not build up.

Risk Factors

Doctors cannot always explain why one person develops lung cancer and another does not. However, we do know that a person with certain risk factors may be more likely than others to develop lung cancer. A risk factor is something that may increase the chance of developing a disease. Studies have found the following risk factors for lung cancer:

Excerpted from "Lung Cancer: An Overview," National Cancer Institute (www .cancer.gov), July 26, 2007. Additional information under the subhead National Lung Screening Trial is excerpted from "National Lung Screening Trial: Questions and Answers," National Cancer Institute, November 4, 2010.

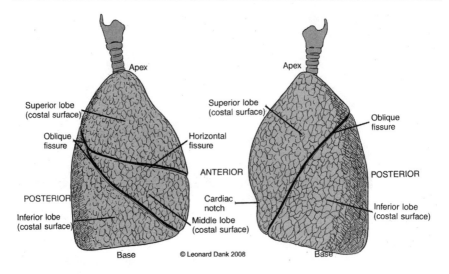

Figure 22.1. Lobes of the Lungs (image by Leonard Dank)

- **Tobacco smoke:** Tobacco smoke causes most cases of lung cancer. It's by far the most important risk factor for lung cancer. Harmful substances in smoke damage lung cells. That's why smoking cigarettes, pipes, or cigars can cause lung cancer and why secondhand smoke can cause lung cancer in nonsmokers.

- **Radon:** Radon is a radioactive gas that you cannot see, smell, or taste. It forms in soil and rocks. People who work in mines may be exposed to radon. In some parts of the country, radon is found in houses. Radon damages lung cells, and people exposed to radon are at increased risk of lung cancer.

- **Asbestos and other substances:** People who have certain jobs (such as those who work in the construction and chemical industries) have an increased risk of lung cancer. Exposure to asbestos, arsenic, chromium, nickel, soot, tar, and other substances can cause lung cancer. The risk is highest for those with years of exposure. The risk of lung cancer from these substances is even higher for smokers.

- **Air pollution:** Air pollution may slightly increase the risk of lung cancer. The risk from air pollution is higher for smokers.

- **Family history of lung cancer:** People with a father, mother, brother, or sister who had lung cancer may be at slightly increased risk of the disease, even if they don't smoke.

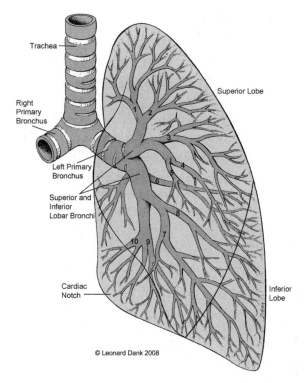

Figure 22.2. Bronchopulmonary Segments (image by Leonard Dank)

- **Personal history of lung cancer:** People who have had lung cancer are at increased risk of developing a second lung tumor.

- **Age over 65:** Most people are older than 65 years when diagnosed with lung cancer.

Researchers have studied other possible risk factors. For example, having certain lung diseases (such as tuberculosis or bronchitis) for many years may increase the risk of lung cancer. It's not yet clear whether having certain lung diseases is a risk factor for lung cancer.

People who think they may be at risk for developing lung cancer should talk to their doctor. The doctor may be able to suggest ways to reduce their risk and can plan an appropriate schedule for checkups. For people who have been treated for lung cancer, it's important to have checkups after treatment. The lung tumor may come back after treatment, or another lung tumor may develop.

311

How to Quit Smoking

Quitting is important for anyone who smokes tobacco—even people who have smoked for many years. For people who already have cancer, quitting may reduce the chance of getting another cancer. Quitting also can help cancer treatments work better. There are many ways to get help:

- Ask your doctor about medicine or nicotine replacement therapy, such as a patch, gum, lozenge, nasal spray, or inhaler. Your doctor can suggest a number of treatments that help people quit.

- Ask your doctor to help you find local programs or trained professionals who help people stop using tobacco.

- Call staff at the National Cancer Institute's Smoking Quitline (877-44U-QUIT) or instant message them through LiveHelp. They can tell you about ways to quit smoking, groups that help smokers who want to quit, NCI publications about quitting smoking, and how to take part in a study of methods to help smokers quit.

- Go online to Smokefree.gov (http://www.smokefree.gov/, a federal government website. It offers a guide to quitting smoking and a list of other resources.

Screening

Several methods of detecting lung cancer have been studied as possible screening tests. The methods under study include tests of sputum (mucus brought up from the lungs by coughing), chest x-rays, or spiral (helical) CT scans.

However, screening tests have risks. For example, an abnormal x-ray result could lead to other procedures (such as surgery to check for cancer cells), but a person with an abnormal test result might not have lung cancer.

You may want to talk with your doctor about your own risk factors and the possible benefits and harms of being screened for lung cancer. Like many other medical decisions, the decision to be screened is a personal one. Your decision may be easier after learning the pros and cons of screening.

National Lung Screening Trial

The National Lung Screening Trial (NLST) is a lung cancer screening trial sponsored by the National Cancer Institute (NCI) and conducted by the American College of Radiology Imaging Network (ACRIN) and the Lung Screening Study group.

Launched in 2002, NLST compared two ways of detecting lung cancer: low-dose helical (spiral) computed tomography (CT) and standard chest X-ray, for their effects on lung cancer death rates in a high-risk population. Both chest X-rays and helical CT scans have been used as a means to find lung cancer early, but the effects of these screening techniques on lung cancer mortality rates had not been determined. Over a 20-month period, more than 53,000 current or former heavy smokers ages 55 to 74 joined NLST at 33 study sites across the United States.

NLST researchers found 20% fewer lung cancer deaths among trial participants screened with low-dose helical CT relative to chest X-ray. This finding was highly significant from a statistical viewpoint.

The NLST participants were a very specific population of men and women ages 55 to 74 who were heavy smokers. They had a smoking history of at least 30 pack-years but no signs or symptoms of lung cancer at the beginning of the trial. Pack-years are calculated by multiplying the average number of packs of cigarettes smoked per day by the number of years a person has smoked. It should also be noted that the population enrolled in this study, while ethnically representative of the high-risk U.S. population of smokers, was a highly motivated and primarily urban group, and these results may not fully translate to other populations.

Men and women in a similar age group and with a similar smoking history should be aware that not all lung cancers found with screening will be early stage. They should also be aware, that at this time, reimbursement for screening CT scans is not provided by most insurance carriers. The current estimated Medicare reimbursement rate for a non-contrast helical diagnostic CT of the lung is $300, but varies by geographic location. A diagnostic CT is done after a person has a sign or symptom of disease, while a screening CT looks for initial signs of disease in healthy people.

The radiation exposures from the screening done in the NLST will be modeled to see how exposure to three low-dose CT scans changed a person's risk for cancer over the remainder of his or her life, but that analysis will take a while to conduct.

Previous studies show that there can be an increased lifetime risk of cancer due to ionizing radiation exposure. It is important to recognize that the low-dose CT used for screening in the NLST delivers a much lower dose of radiation than a regular diagnostic CT. Additionally, the benefit of potentially finding a treatable cancer in current or former heavy smokers, ages 55 to 74, using helical CT appear to outweigh the risk from receiving a low dose of radiation.

313

As with all cancer clinical trials, the NLST provided answers to a set of very specific questions related to a specific population. Whether those answers can be used to provide general recommendations for the entire population must be the subject of future analysis and study. The vast amount of data generated by NLST, which is still being collated and studied, will greatly inform the development of clinical guidelines and policy recommendations.

Symptoms

Early lung cancer often does not cause symptoms. But as the cancer grows, common symptoms may include the following:

- A cough that gets worse or does not go away
- Breathing trouble, such as shortness of breath
- Constant chest pain
- Coughing up blood
- A hoarse voice
- Frequent lung infections, such as pneumonia
- Feeling very tired all the time
- Weight loss with no known cause

Most often these symptoms are not due to cancer. Other health problems can cause some of these symptoms. Anyone with such symptoms should see a doctor to be diagnosed and treated as early as possible.

Diagnosis

If you have a symptom that suggests lung cancer, your doctor must find out whether it's from cancer or something else. Your doctor may ask about your personal and family medical history. Your doctor may order blood tests, and you may have one or more of the following tests:

Physical exam: Your doctor checks for general signs of health, listens to your breathing, and checks for fluid in the lungs. Your doctor may feel for swollen lymph nodes and a swollen liver.

Chest x-ray: X-ray pictures of your chest may show tumors or abnormal fluid.

CT scan: Doctors often use CT scans to take pictures of tissue inside the chest. An x-ray machine linked to a computer takes several pictures.

For a spiral CT scan, the CT scanner rotates around you as you lie on a table. The table passes through the center of the scanner. The pictures may show a tumor, abnormal fluid, or swollen lymph nodes.

Finding Lung Cancer Cells

The only sure way to know if lung cancer is present is for a pathologist to check samples of cells or tissue. The pathologist studies the sample under a microscope and performs other tests. There are many ways to collect samples.

Your doctor may order one or more of the following tests to collect samples:

Sputum cytology: Thick fluid (sputum) is coughed up from the lungs. The lab checks samples of sputum for cancer cells.

Thoracentesis: The doctor uses a long needle to remove fluid (pleural fluid) from the chest. The lab checks the fluid for cancer cells.

Bronchoscopy: The doctor inserts a thin, lighted tube (a bronchoscope) through the nose or mouth into the lung. This allows an exam of the lungs and the air passages that lead to them. The doctor may take a sample of cells with a needle, brush, or other tool. The doctor also may wash the area with water to collect cells in the water.

Fine-needle aspiration: The doctor uses a thin needle to remove tissue or fluid from the lung or lymph node. Sometimes the doctor uses a CT scan or other imaging method to guide the needle to a lung tumor or lymph node.

Thoracoscopy: The surgeon makes several small incisions in your chest and back. The surgeon looks at the lungs and nearby tissues with a thin, lighted tube. If an abnormal area is seen, a biopsy to check for cancer cells may be needed.

Thoracotomy: The surgeon opens the chest with a long incision. Lymph nodes and other tissue may be removed.

Mediastinoscopy: The surgeon makes an incision at the top of the breastbone. A thin, lighted tube is used to see inside the chest. The surgeon may take tissue and lymph node samples.

Types of Lung Cancer

The pathologist checks the sputum, pleural fluid, tissue, or other samples for cancer cells. If cancer is found, the pathologist reports the type.

The types of lung cancer are treated differently. The most common types are named for how the lung cancer cells look under a microscope:

Small cell lung cancer: About 13% of lung cancers are small cell lung cancers. This type tends to spread quickly. For additional information about this type of lung cancer, including facts about its treatment, see chapter 23.

Non-small cell lung cancer: Most lung cancers (about 87%) are non-small cell lung cancers. This type spreads more slowly than small cell lung cancer. For additional information about this type of lung cancer, including facts about its treatment, see chapter 24.

Second Opinion

Before starting treatment, you might want a second opinion about your diagnosis and treatment plan. Many insurance companies cover a second opinion if you or your doctor requests it.

It may take some time and effort to gather your medical records and see another doctor. In most cases, a brief delay in starting treatment will not make treatment less effective. To make sure, you should discuss this delay with your doctor. Sometimes people with lung cancer need treatment right away. For example, a doctor may advise a person with small cell lung cancer not to delay treatment more than a week or two.

There are many ways to find a doctor for a second opinion. You can ask your doctor, a local or state medical society, a nearby hospital, or a medical school for names of specialists. Also, your nearest cancer center can tell you about doctors who work there.

Comfort Care

Lung cancer and its treatment can lead to other health problems. You may need comfort care to prevent or control these problems. Comfort care is available both during and after treatment. It can improve your quality of life.

Your health care team can tell you more about the following problems and how to control them:

Pain: Your doctor or a pain control specialist can suggest ways to relieve or reduce pain.

Shortness of breath or trouble breathing: People with lung cancer often have trouble breathing. Your doctor may refer you to a lung specialist or respiratory therapist. Some people are helped by oxygen therapy, photodynamic therapy, laser surgery, cryotherapy, or stents.

Fluid in or around lungs: Advanced cancer can cause fluid to collect in or around the lungs. The fluid can make it hard to breathe. Your health care team can remove fluid when it builds up. In some cases, a procedure can be done that may prevent fluid from building up again. Some people may need chest tubes to drain the fluid.

Pneumonia: You may have chest x-rays to check for lung infections. Your doctor can treat infections.

Cancer that spreads to the brain: Lung cancer can spread to the brain. The symptoms may include headache, seizures, trouble walking, and problems with balance. Medicine to relieve swelling, radiation therapy, or sometimes surgery can help. People with small cell lung cancer may receive radiation therapy to the brain to try to prevent brain tumors from forming. This is called prophylactic cranial irradiation.

Cancer that spreads to the bone: Lung cancer that spreads to the bone can be painful and can weaken bones. You can ask for pain medicine, and the doctor may suggest external radiation therapy. Your doctor also may give you drugs to help lower your risk of breaking a bone.

Sadness and other feelings: It's normal to feel sad, anxious, or confused after a diagnosis of a serious illness. Some people find it helpful to talk about their feelings.

Nutrition

It's important for you to take care of yourself by eating well. You need the right amount of calories to maintain a good weight. You also need enough protein to keep up your strength. Eating well may help you feel better and have more energy.

Sometimes, especially during or soon after treatment, you may not feel like eating. You may be uncomfortable or tired. You may find that foods don't taste as good as they used to. In addition, the side effects of treatment (such as poor appetite, nausea, vomiting, or mouth sores) can make it hard to eat well.

Your doctor, a registered dietitian, or another health care provider can suggest ways to deal with these problems.

Follow-Up Care

You'll need regular checkups after treatment for lung cancer. Even when there are no longer any signs of cancer, the disease sometimes returns because undetected cancer cells remained somewhere in your body after treatment.

Checkups help ensure that any changes in your health are noted and treated if needed. Checkups may include a physical exam, blood tests, chest x-rays, CT scans, and bronchoscopy.

If you have any health problems between checkups, contact your doctor.

Chapter 23

Small Cell Lung Cancer

General Information about Small Cell Lung Cancer

Small cell lung cancer is a disease in which malignant (cancer) cells form in the tissues of the lung. There are two types of small cell lung cancer. These two types include many different types of cells. The cancer cells of each type grow and spread in different ways. The types of small cell lung cancer are named for the kinds of cells found in the cancer and how the cells look when viewed under a microscope:

- Small cell carcinoma (oat cell cancer)

- Combined small cell carcinoma

Staging Small Cell Lung Cancer

After small cell lung cancer has been diagnosed, tests are done to find out if cancer cells have spread within the chest or to other parts of the body.

The process used to find out if cancer has spread within the chest or to other parts of the body is called staging. The information gathered from the staging process determines the stage of the disease. It is important to know the stage in order to plan treatment. Some of the tests used to diagnose small cell lung cancer are also used to stage the

Excerpted from PDQ® Cancer Information Summary. National Cancer Institute; Bethesda, MD. "Small Cell Lung Cancer Treatment (PDQ) - Patient Version." Updated 08/2009. Available at: http://cancer.gov. Accessed January 20, 2010.

disease. Other tests and procedures that may be used in the staging process include the following:

Laboratory tests: Medical procedures that test samples of tissue, blood, urine, or other substances in the body. These tests help to diagnose disease, plan and check treatment, or monitor the disease over time.

Bone marrow aspiration and biopsy: The removal of bone marrow, blood, and a small piece of bone by inserting a hollow needle into the hipbone or breastbone. A pathologist views the bone marrow, blood, and bone under a microscope to look for signs of cancer.

MRI (magnetic resonance imaging) of the brain: A procedure that uses a magnet, radio waves, and a computer to make a series of detailed pictures of areas inside the body. This procedure is also called nuclear magnetic resonance imaging (NMRI).

Endoscopic ultrasound (EUS): A procedure in which an endoscope is inserted into the body. An endoscope is a thin, tube-like instrument with a light and a lens for viewing. A probe at the end of the endoscope is used to bounce high-energy sound waves (ultrasound) off internal tissues or organs and make echoes. The echoes form a picture of body tissues called a sonogram. This procedure is also called endosonography. EUS may be used to guide fine-needle aspiration (FNA) biopsy of the lung, lymph nodes, or other areas.

Lymph node biopsy: The removal of all or part of a lymph node. A pathologist views the tissue under a microscope to look for cancer cells.

Radionuclide bone scan: A procedure to check if there are rapidly dividing cells, such as cancer cells, in the bone. A very small amount of radioactive material is injected into a vein and travels through the bloodstream. The radioactive material collects in the bones and is detected by a scanner.

Stages Used to Describe Small Cell Lung Cancer

Limited-stage small cell lung cancer: In limited-stage, cancer is found in one lung, the tissues between the lungs, and nearby lymph nodes only.

Extensive-stage small cell lung cancer: In extensive-stage, cancer has spread outside of the lung in which it began or to other parts of the body.

Recurrent small cell lung cancer: Recurrent small cell lung cancer is cancer that has recurred (come back) after it has been treated. The cancer may come back in the chest, central nervous system, or in other parts of the body.

Treatment Option Overview

Different types of treatment are available for patients with small cell lung cancer. Some treatments are standard (the currently used treatment), and some are being tested in clinical trials. Five types of standard treatment are used.

Surgery

Surgery may be used if the cancer is found in one lung and in nearby lymph nodes only. Because this type of lung cancer is usually found in both lungs, surgery alone is not often used. Occasionally, surgery may be used to help determine the patient's exact type of lung cancer. During surgery, the doctor will also remove lymph nodes to see if they contain cancer.

Even if the doctor removes all the cancer that can be seen at the time of the operation, some patients may be given chemotherapy or radiation therapy after surgery to kill any cancer cells that are left. Treatment given after the surgery, to lower the risk that the cancer will come back, is called adjuvant therapy.

Chemotherapy

Chemotherapy is a cancer treatment that uses drugs to stop the growth of cancer cells, either by killing the cells or by stopping them from dividing. When chemotherapy is taken by mouth or injected into a vein or muscle, the drugs enter the bloodstream and can reach cancer cells throughout the body (systemic chemotherapy). When chemotherapy is placed directly into the spinal column, an organ, or a body cavity such as the abdomen, the drugs mainly affect cancer cells in those areas (regional chemotherapy). The way the chemotherapy is given depends on the type and stage of the cancer being treated.

Radiation Therapy

Radiation therapy is a cancer treatment that uses high-energy x-rays or other types of radiation to kill cancer cells or keep them from growing. There are two types of radiation therapy. External radiation therapy uses a machine outside the body to send radiation toward the cancer. Internal radiation therapy uses a radioactive substance sealed in needles, seeds, wires, or catheters that are placed directly into or near the cancer. Prophylactic cranial irradiation (radiation therapy to the brain to reduce the risk that cancer will spread to the brain) may also be given. The way the radiation therapy is given depends on the type and stage of the cancer being treated.

Laser Therapy

Laser therapy is a cancer treatment that uses a laser beam (a narrow beam of intense light) to kill cancer cells.

Endoscopic Stent Placement

An endoscope is a thin, tube-like instrument used to look at tissues inside the body. An endoscope has a light and a lens for viewing and may be used to place a stent in a body structure to keep the structure open. Endoscopic stent placement can be used to open an airway blocked by abnormal tissue.

Clinical Trials

A treatment clinical trial is a research study meant to help improve current treatments or obtain information on new treatments for patients with cancer. When clinical trials show that a new treatment is better than the standard treatment, the new treatment may become the standard treatment. Patients may want to think about taking part in a clinical trial. Some clinical trials are open only to patients who have not started treatment.

Patients may want to think about taking part in a clinical trial. For some patients, taking part in a clinical trial may be the best treatment choice. Clinical trials are part of the cancer research process. Clinical trials are done to find out if new cancer treatments are safe and effective or better than the standard treatment.

Many of today's standard treatments for cancer are based on earlier clinical trials. Patients who take part in a clinical trial may receive the standard treatment or be among the first to receive a new treatment.

Patients who take part in clinical trials also help improve the way cancer will be treated in the future. Even when clinical trials do not lead to effective new treatments, they often answer important questions and help move research forward.

Patients can enter clinical trials before, during, or after starting their cancer treatment. Some clinical trials only include patients who have not yet received treatment. Other trials test treatments for patients whose cancer has not gotten better. There are also clinical trials that test new ways to stop cancer from recurring (coming back) or reduce the side effects of cancer treatment.

Clinical trials are taking place in many parts of the country

Follow-Up Tests

Some of the tests that were done to diagnose the cancer or to find out the stage of the cancer may be repeated. Some tests will be repeated in order to see how well the treatment is working. Decisions about whether to continue, change, or stop treatment may be based on the results of these tests. This is sometimes called re-staging.

Some of the tests will continue to be done from time to time after treatment has ended. The results of these tests can show if your condition has changed or if the cancer has recurred (come back). These tests are sometimes called follow-up tests or check-ups.

Chapter 24

Non-Small Cell Lung Cancer

General Information about Non-Small Cell Lung Cancer

There are two main types of lung cancer: non-small cell lung cancer and small cell lung cancer. Non-small cell lung cancer is a disease in which malignant (cancer) cells form in the tissues of the lung.

There are several types of non-small cell lung cancer. Each type of non-small cell lung cancer has different kinds of cancer cells. The cancer cells of each type grow and spread in different ways. The types of non-small cell lung cancer are named for the kinds of cells found in the cancer and how the cells look under a microscope:

- **Squamous cell carcinoma:** Cancer that begins in squamous cells, which are thin, flat cells that look like fish scales. This is also called epidermoid carcinoma.

- **Large cell carcinoma:** Cancer that may begin in several types of large cells.

- **Adenocarcinoma:** Cancer that begins in the cells that line the alveoli and make substances such as mucus.

Other less common types of non-small cell lung cancer are: pleomorphic, carcinoid tumor, salivary gland carcinoma, and unclassified carcinoma.

Excerpted from PDQ® Cancer Information Summary. National Cancer Institute; Bethesda, MD. Non-Small Cell Lung Cancer Treatment (PDQ) - Patient Version. Updated 01/2010. Available at: http://cancer.gov. Accessed June 21, 2010.

Risk Factors

Smoking can increase the risk of developing non-small cell lung cancer. Smoking cigarettes, pipes, or cigars is the most common cause of lung cancer. The earlier in life a person starts smoking, the more often a person smokes, and the more years a person smokes, the greater the risk. If a person has stopped smoking, the risk becomes lower as the years pass.

Anything that increases a person's chance of developing a disease is called a risk factor. Having a risk factor does not mean that you will get cancer; not having risk factors doesn't mean that you will not get cancer. People who think they may be at risk should discuss this with their doctor. Risk factors for lung cancer include the following:

- Smoking cigarettes, pipes, or cigars, now or in the past
- Being exposed to second-hand smoke
- Being treated with radiation therapy to the breast or chest
- Being exposed to asbestos, radon, chromium, nickel, arsenic, soot, or tar
- Living where there is air pollution

When smoking is combined with other risk factors, the risk of developing lung cancer is increased.

Detection and Diagnosis

Tests that examine the lungs are used to detect (find), diagnose, and stage non-small cell lung cancer. Tests and procedures to detect, diagnose, and stage non-small cell lung cancer are often done at the same time. The following tests and procedures may be used:

Physical exam and history: An exam of the body to check general signs of health, including checking for signs of disease, such as lumps or anything else that seems unusual. A history of the patient's health habits, including smoking, and past jobs, illnesses, and treatments will also be taken.

Laboratory tests: Medical procedures that test samples of tissue, blood, urine, or other substances in the body. These tests help to diagnose disease, plan and check treatment, or monitor the disease over time.

Chest x-ray: An x-ray of the organs and bones inside the chest. An x-ray is a type of energy beam that can go through the body and onto film, making a picture of areas inside the body.

CT scan (CAT scan): A procedure that makes a series of detailed pictures of areas inside the body, such as the chest, taken from different angles. The pictures are made by a computer linked to an x-ray machine. A dye may be injected into a vein or swallowed to help the organs or tissues show up more clearly. This procedure is also called computed tomography, computerized tomography, or computerized axial tomography.

PET scan (positron emission tomography scan): A procedure to find malignant tumor cells in the body. A small amount of radioactive glucose (sugar) is injected into a vein. The PET scanner rotates around the body and makes a picture of where glucose is being used in the body. Malignant tumor cells show up brighter in the picture because they are more active and take up more glucose than normal cells do.

Sputum cytology: A procedure in which a pathologist views a sample of sputum (mucus coughed up from the lungs) under a microscope, to check for cancer cells.

Fine-needle aspiration (FNA) biopsy of the lung: The removal of tissue or fluid from the lung using a thin needle. A CT scan, ultrasound, or other imaging procedure is used to locate the abnormal tissue or fluid in the lung. A small incision may be made in the skin where the biopsy needle is inserted into the abnormal tissue or fluid. A sample is removed with the needle and sent to the laboratory. A pathologist then views the sample under a microscope to look for cancer cells. A chest x-ray is done after the procedure to make sure no air is leaking from the lung into the chest.

Bronchoscopy: A procedure to look inside the trachea and large airways in the lung for abnormal areas. A bronchoscope is inserted through the nose or mouth into the trachea and lungs. A bronchoscope is a thin, tube-like instrument with a light and a lens for viewing. It may also have a tool to remove tissue samples, which are checked under a microscope for signs of cancer.

Thoracoscopy: A surgical procedure to look at the organs inside the chest to check for abnormal areas. An incision (cut) is made between two ribs, and a thoracoscope is inserted into the chest. A thoracoscope is a thin, tube-like instrument with a light and a lens for viewing. It may also have a tool to remove tissue or lymph node samples, which are checked under a microscope for signs of cancer. In some cases, this procedure is used to remove part of the esophagus or lung. If certain tissues, organs, or lymph nodes can't be reached, a thoracotomy may be done. In this procedure, a larger incision is made between the ribs and the chest is opened.

Thoracentesis: The removal of fluid from the space between the lining of the chest and the lung, using a needle. A pathologist views the fluid under a microscope to look for cancer cells.

Light and electron microscopy: A laboratory test in which cells in a sample of tissue are viewed under regular and high-powered microscopes to look for certain changes in the cells.

Immunohistochemistry study: A laboratory test in which a substance such as an antibody, dye, or radioisotope is added to a sample of cancer tissue to test for certain antigens. This type of study is used to tell the difference between different types of cancer.

Prognosis

Certain factors affect prognosis (chance of recovery) and treatment options. The prognosis and treatment options depend on the following:

- The stage of the cancer (the size of the tumor and whether it is in the lung only or has spread to other places in the body).
- The type of lung cancer.
- Whether there are symptoms such as coughing or trouble breathing.
- The patient's general health.

For most patients with non-small cell lung cancer, current treatments do not cure the cancer. If lung cancer is found, taking part in one of the many clinical trials being done to improve treatment should be considered. Clinical trials are taking place in most parts of the country for patients with all stages of non-small cell lung cancer. Information about ongoing clinical trials is available from the National Cancer Institute's website (www.cancer.gov).

Stages of Non-Small Cell Lung Cancer

After lung cancer has been diagnosed, tests are done to find out if cancer cells have spread within the lungs or to other parts of the body.

The process used to find out if cancer has spread within the lungs or to other parts of the body is called staging. The information gathered from the staging process determines the stage of the disease. It is important to know the stage in order to plan treatment. Some of the tests used to diagnose non-small cell lung cancer are also used to stage the disease. Other tests and procedures that may be used in the staging process include the following:

MRI (magnetic resonance imaging): A procedure that uses a magnet, radio waves, and a computer to make a series of detailed pictures of areas inside the body, such as the brain. This procedure is also called nuclear magnetic resonance imaging (NMRI).

Radionuclide bone scan: A procedure to check if there are rapidly dividing cells, such as cancer cells, in the bone. A very small amount of radioactive material is injected into a vein and travels through the bloodstream. The radioactive material collects in the bones and is detected by a scanner.

Endoscopic ultrasound (EUS): A procedure in which an endoscope is inserted into the body. An endoscope is a thin, tube-like instrument with a light and a lens for viewing. A probe at the end of the endoscope is used to bounce high-energy sound waves (ultrasound) off internal tissues or organs and make echoes. The echoes form a picture of body tissues called a sonogram. This procedure is also called endosonography. EUS may be used to guide fine needle aspiration (FNA) biopsy of the lung, lymph nodes, or other areas.

Lymph node biopsy: The removal of all or part of a lymph node. A pathologist views the tissue under a microscope to look for cancer cells.

Mediastinoscopy: A surgical procedure to look at the organs, tissues, and lymph nodes between the lungs for abnormal areas. An incision (cut) is made at the top of the breastbone and a mediastinoscope is inserted into the chest. A mediastinoscope is a thin, tube-like instrument with a light and a lens for viewing. It may also have a tool to remove tissue or lymph node samples, which are checked under a microscope for signs of cancer.

Anterior mediastinotomy: A surgical procedure to look at the organs and tissues between the lungs and between the breastbone and heart for abnormal areas. An incision (cut) is made next to the breastbone and a mediastinoscope is inserted into the chest. A mediastinoscope is a thin, tube-like instrument with a light and a lens for viewing. It may also have a tool to remove tissue or lymph node samples, which are checked under a microscope for signs of cancer. This is also called the Chamberlain procedure.

Occult (Hidden) Stage

In the occult (hidden) stage, cancer cells are found in sputum (mucus coughed up from the lungs), but no tumor can be found in the lung by imaging or bronchoscopy, or the primary tumor is too small to be checked.

Stage 0 (Carcinoma in Situ)

In stage 0, abnormal cells are found in the innermost lining of the lung. These abnormal cells may become cancer and spread into nearby normal tissue. Stage 0 is also called carcinoma in situ.

Stage I

In stage I, cancer has formed. Stage I is divided into stages IA and IB:

Stage IA: The tumor is in the lung only and is three centimeters or smaller.

Stage IB: One or more of the following is true:

- The tumor is larger than three centimeters
- Cancer has spread to the main bronchus of the lung, and is at least 2 centimeters from the carina (where the trachea joins the bronchi)
- Cancer has spread to the innermost layer of the membrane that covers the lungs
- The tumor partly blocks the bronchus or bronchioles and part of the lung has collapsed or developed pneumonitis (inflammation of the lung)

Stage II

Stage II is divided into stages IIA and IIB:

Stage IIA: The tumor is three centimeters or smaller and cancer has spread to nearby lymph nodes on the same side of the chest as the tumor.

Stage IIB: Cancer has spread to nearby lymph nodes on the same side of the chest as the tumor and one or more of the following is true:

- The tumor is larger than three centimeters
- Cancer has spread to the main bronchus of the lung and is two centimeters or more from the carina (where the trachea joins the bronchi)
- Cancer has spread to the innermost layer of the membrane that covers the lungs
- The tumor partly blocks the bronchus or bronchioles and part of the lung has collapsed or developed pneumonitis (inflammation of the lung)

Or cancer has not spread to lymph nodes and one or more of the following is true:

- The tumor may be any size and cancer has spread to the chest wall, or the diaphragm, or the pleura between the lungs, or membranes surrounding the heart.

- Cancer has spread to the main bronchus of the lung and is no more than two centimeters from the carina (where the trachea meets the bronchi), but has not spread to the trachea.

- Cancer blocks the bronchus or bronchioles and the whole lung has collapsed or developed pneumonitis (inflammation of the lung).

Stage IIIA

In stage IIIA, cancer has spread to lymph nodes on the same side of the chest as the tumor. Also the following characteristics are observed:

- The tumor may be any size.

- Cancer may have spread to the main bronchus, the chest wall, the diaphragm, the pleura around the lungs, or the membrane around the heart, but has not spread to the trachea.

- Part or all of the lung may have collapsed or developed pneumonitis (inflammation of the lung).

Stage IIIB

In stage IIIB, the tumor may be any size and has spread to lymph nodes above the collarbone or in the opposite side of the chest from the tumor; and/or to any of the following:

- Heart
- Major blood vessels that lead to or from the heart
- Chest wall
- Diaphragm
- Trachea
- Esophagus
- Sternum (chest bone) or backbone
- More than one place in the same lobe of the lung
- The fluid of the pleural cavity surrounding the lung

Stage IV

Stage IV non-small cell lung cancer. The cancer has spread to another lobe of the same lung, to the other lung, and/or to one or more other parts of the body. In stage IV, cancer may have spread to lymph nodes and has spread to another lobe of the lungs or to other parts of the body, such as the brain, liver, adrenal glands, kidneys, or bone.

Recurrent Non-Small Cell Lung Cancer

Recurrent non-small cell lung cancer is cancer that has recurred (come back) after it has been treated. The cancer may come back in the brain, lung, or other parts of the body.

Treatment Option Overview

Different types of treatments are available for patients with non-small cell lung cancer. Some treatments are standard (the currently used treatment), and some are being tested in clinical trials. Nine types of standard treatment are used.

Surgery

Four types of surgery are used:

- **Wedge resection:** Surgery to remove a tumor and some of the normal tissue around it. When a slightly larger amount of tissue is taken, it is called a segmental resection.

- **Lobectomy:** Surgery to remove a whole lobe (section) of the lung.

- **Pneumonectomy:** Surgery to remove one whole lung.

- **Sleeve resection:** Surgery to remove part of the bronchus.

Even if the doctor removes all the cancer that can be seen at the time of the surgery, some patients may be given chemotherapy or radiation therapy after surgery to kill any cancer cells that are left. Treatment given after the surgery, to lower the risk that the cancer will come back, is called adjuvant therapy.

Radiation Therapy

Radiation therapy is a cancer treatment that uses high-energy x-rays or other types of radiation to kill cancer cells or keep them from growing. There are two types of radiation therapy. External radiation therapy uses a machine outside the body to send radiation toward the cancer. Internal radiation therapy uses a radioactive substance sealed in needles, seeds, wires, or catheters that are placed directly into or near the cancer.

Radiosurgery is a method of delivering radiation directly to the tumor with little damage to healthy tissue. It does not involve surgery and may be used to treat certain tumors in patients who cannot have surgery.

The way the radiation therapy is given depends on the type and stage of the cancer being treated.

Chemotherapy

Chemotherapy is a cancer treatment that uses drugs to stop the growth of cancer cells, either by killing the cells or by stopping them from dividing. When chemotherapy is taken by mouth or injected into a vein or muscle, the drugs enter the bloodstream and can reach cancer cells throughout the body (systemic chemotherapy). When chemotherapy is placed directly into the spinal column, an organ, or a body cavity such as the abdomen, the drugs mainly affect cancer cells in those areas (regional chemotherapy). The way the chemotherapy is given depends on the type and stage of the cancer being treated.

Targeted Therapy

Targeted therapy is a type of treatment that uses drugs or other substances to identify and attack specific cancer cells without harming normal cells. Monoclonal antibodies and tyrosine kinase inhibitors are two types of targeted therapy being used in the treatment of non-small cell lung cancer.

Monoclonal antibody therapy is a cancer treatment that uses antibodies made in the laboratory from a single type of immune system cell. These antibodies can identify substances on cancer cells or normal substances that may help cancer cells grow. The antibodies attach to the substances and kill the cancer cells, block their growth, or keep them from spreading. Monoclonal antibodies are given by infusion. They may be used alone or to carry drugs, toxins, or radioactive material directly to cancer cells.

Tyrosine kinase inhibitors are targeted therapy drugs that block signals needed for tumors to grow. Tyrosine kinase inhibitors may be used with other anticancer drugs as adjuvant therapy.

Laser Therapy

Laser therapy is a cancer treatment that uses a laser beam (a narrow beam of intense light) to kill cancer cells.

Photodynamic Therapy (PDT)

Photodynamic therapy (PDT) is a cancer treatment that uses a drug and a certain type of laser light to kill cancer cells. A drug that is not active until it is exposed to light is injected into a vein. The drug collects more in cancer cells than in normal cells. Fiberoptic tubes are then used to carry the laser light to the cancer cells, where the drug becomes active and kills the cells. Photodynamic therapy causes little damage to healthy tissue. It is used mainly to treat tumors on or just under the skin or in the lining of internal organs.

Cryosurgery

Cryosurgery is a treatment that uses an instrument to freeze and destroy abnormal tissue, such as carcinoma in situ. This type of treatment is also called cryotherapy.

Electrocautery

Electrocautery is a treatment that uses a probe or needle heated by an electric current to destroy abnormal tissue.

Watchful Waiting

Watchful waiting is closely monitoring a patient's condition without giving any treatment until symptoms appear or change. This may be done in certain rare cases of non-small cell lung cancer.

Clinical Trials

New types of treatment are being tested in clinical trials. Chemoprevention, for example, is the use of drugs, vitamins, or other substances to reduce the risk of developing cancer or to reduce the risk cancer will recur (come back). New combinations of treatments are also being studied in clinical trials.

A treatment clinical trial is a research study meant to help improve current treatments or obtain information on new treatments for patients with cancer. When clinical trials show that a new treatment is better than the standard treatment, the new treatment may become the standard treatment. Patients may want to think about taking part in a clinical trial. Some clinical trials are open only to patients who have not started treatment.

Patients may want to think about taking part in a clinical trial. For some patients, taking part in a clinical trial may be the best treatment choice. Clinical trials are part of the cancer research process. Clinical trials are done to find out if new cancer treatments are safe and effective or better than the standard treatment. Many of today's standard treatments for cancer are based on earlier clinical trials. Patients who take part in a clinical trial may receive the standard treatment or be among the first to receive a new treatment. Patients who take part in clinical trials also help improve the way cancer will be treated in the future. Even when clinical trials do not lead to effective new treatments, they often answer important questions and help move research forward.

Follow-Up Tests

Some of the tests that were done to diagnose the cancer or to find out the stage of the cancer may be repeated. Some tests will be repeated in order to see how well the treatment is working. Decisions about whether to continue, change, or stop treatment may be based on the results of these tests. This is sometimes called re-staging.

Some of the tests will continue to be done from time to time after treatment has ended. The results of these tests can show if your condition has changed or if the cancer has recurred (come back). These tests are sometimes called follow-up tests or check-ups.

Chapter 25

Malignant Mesothelioma

General Information about Malignant Mesothelioma

Malignant mesothelioma is a disease in which malignant (cancer) cells are found in the pleura (the thin layer of tissue that lines the chest cavity and covers the lungs) or the peritoneum (the thin layer of tissue that lines the abdomen and covers most of the organs in the abdomen). This summary is about malignant mesothelioma of the pleura.

Risk Factors and Signs

Anything that increases your chance of getting a disease is called a risk factor. Having a risk factor does not mean that you will get cancer; not having risk factors doesn't mean that you will not get cancer. People who think they may be at risk should discuss this with their doctor.

Many people with malignant mesothelioma have worked or lived in places where they inhaled or swallowed asbestos. After being exposed to asbestos, it usually takes a long time for malignant mesothelioma to occur. Other risk factors for malignant mesothelioma include living with a person who works near asbestos and being exposed to a certain virus.

Possible signs of malignant mesothelioma include shortness of breath and pain under the rib cage. Sometimes the cancer causes fluid to collect around the lung or in the abdomen. These symptoms may be

Excerpted from PDQ® Cancer Information Summary. National Cancer Institute; Bethesda, MD. "Malignant Mesothelioma Treatment (PDQ) - Patient Version. Updated 08/2009. Available at: http://cancer.gov. Accessed January 20, 2010.

caused by the fluid or malignant mesothelioma. Other conditions may cause the same symptoms. A doctor should be consulted if any of the following problems occur:

- Trouble breathing
- Pain under the rib cage
- Pain or swelling in the abdomen
- Lumps in the abdomen
- Weight loss for no known reason

Detection and Diagnosis

Tests that examine the inside of the chest and abdomen are used to detect (find) and diagnose malignant mesothelioma. Sometimes it is hard to tell the difference between malignant mesothelioma and lung cancer. The following tests and procedures may be used:

Physical exam and history: An exam of the body to check general signs of health, including checking for signs of disease, such as lumps or anything else that seems unusual. A history of the patient's health habits, exposure to asbestos, past illnesses and treatments will also be taken.

Chest x-ray: An x-ray of the organs and bones inside the chest. An x-ray is a type of energy beam that can go through the body and onto film, making a picture of areas inside the body.

Complete blood count (CBC): A procedure in which a sample of blood is drawn and checked for the number of red blood cells, white blood cells, and platelets; the amount of hemoglobin (the protein that carries oxygen) in the red blood cells; and the portion of the blood sample made up of red blood cells.

Sedimentation rate: A procedure in which a sample of blood is drawn and checked for the rate at which the red blood cells settle to the bottom of the test tube.

Biopsy: The removal of cells or tissues from the pleura or peritoneum so they can be viewed under a microscope by a pathologist to check for signs of cancer.

Fine-needle (FNA) aspiration biopsy of the lung: The removal of tissue or fluid using a thin needle. An imaging procedure is used to locate the abnormal tissue or fluid in the lung. A small incision may be made in the skin where the biopsy needle is inserted into the abnormal tissue or fluid, and a sample is removed.

Thoracoscopy: An incision (cut) is made between two ribs and a thoracoscope (a thin, tube-like instrument with a light and a lens for viewing) is inserted into the chest.

Peritoneoscopy: An incision is made in the abdominal wall and a peritoneoscope (a thin, tube-like instrument with a light and a lens for viewing) is inserted into the abdomen.

Laparotomy: An incision is made in the wall of the abdomen to check the inside of the abdomen for signs of disease.

Thoracotomy: An incision is made between two ribs to check inside the chest for signs of disease.

Bronchoscopy: A procedure to look inside the trachea and large airways in the lung for abnormal areas. A bronchoscope is inserted through the nose or mouth into the trachea and lungs. A bronchoscope is a thin, tube-like instrument with a light and a lens for viewing. It may also have a tool to remove tissue samples, which are checked under a microscope for signs of cancer.

Cytologic exam: An exam of cells under a microscope (by a pathologist) to check for anything abnormal. For mesothelioma, fluid is taken from around the lungs or from the abdomen. A pathologist checks the cells in the fluid.

Prognosis

Certain factors affect prognosis (chance of recovery) and treatment options. The prognosis and treatment options depend on the following:

- The stage of the cancer
- The size of the tumor
- Whether the tumor can be removed completely by surgery
- The amount of fluid in the chest or abdomen
- The patient's age and general health, including lung and heart health
- The type of mesothelioma cancer cells and how they look under a microscope
- Whether the cancer has just been diagnosed or has recurred (come back)

Stages of Malignant Mesothelioma

After malignant mesothelioma has been diagnosed, tests are done to find out if cancer cells have spread to other parts of the body. The process used to find out if cancer has spread outside the pleura or peritoneum is called staging. The information gathered from the staging process determines the stage of the disease. It is important to know the spread of the cancer in order to plan treatment. Chest x-rays, which can be used in diagnosis, can also be used in the staging process. Other tests that may be used include the following:

CT scan (CAT scan): A procedure that makes a series of detailed pictures of the chest and abdomen, taken from different angles. The pictures are made by a computer linked to an x-ray machine. A dye may be injected into a vein or swallowed to help the organs or tissues show up more clearly. This procedure is also called computed tomography, computerized tomography, or computerized axial tomography.

MRI (magnetic resonance imaging): A procedure that uses a magnet, radio waves, and a computer to make a series of detailed pictures of the chest or abdomen. This procedure is also called nuclear magnetic resonance imaging (NMRI).

Endoscopic ultrasound (EUS): A procedure in which an endoscope is inserted into the body. An endoscope is a thin, tube-like instrument with a light and a lens for viewing. A probe at the end of the endoscope is used to bounce high-energy sound waves (ultrasound) off internal tissues or organs and make echoes. The echoes form a picture of body tissues called a sonogram. This procedure is also called endosonography. EUS may be used to guide fine-needle aspiration (FNA) biopsy of the lung, lymph nodes, or other areas.

Stage Groups

The stages of malignant mesothelioma are divided into two groups: localized and advanced.

Localized malignant mesothelioma (stage I): In localized malignant mesothelioma, cancer is found in the lining of the chest wall and may also be found in the lining of the lung, the lining of the diaphragm, or the lining of the sac that covers the heart on the same side of the chest.

Advanced malignant mesothelioma (stage II, stage III, and stage IV): In stage II, cancer is found in the lining of the chest wall and the lymph nodes on the same side of the chest. Cancer may also be found in the lining of the lung, the lining of the diaphragm, or the lining of the sac that covers the heart on the same side of the chest.

In stage III, cancer has spread to any of the following areas:

- The chest wall
- The mediastinum
- The heart
- Beyond the diaphragm
- The peritoneum

Cancer may have also spread to lymph nodes on the other side of the chest or outside the chest. In stage IV, cancer has spread to distant organs or tissues.

Recurrent Malignant Mesothelioma

Recurrent malignant mesothelioma is cancer that has recurred (come back) after it has been treated. The cancer may come back in the chest or abdomen or in other parts of the body.

Treatment Option Overview

Different types of treatments are available for patients with malignant mesothelioma. Some treatments are standard (the currently used treatment), and some are being tested in clinical trials. Three types of standard treatment are used.

Surgery

The following surgical treatments may be used for malignant mesothelioma:

- **Wide local excision:** Surgery to remove the cancer and some of the healthy tissue around it.
- **Pleurectomy and decortication:** Surgery to remove part of the covering of the lungs and lining of the chest and part of the outside surface of the lungs.
- **Extrapleural pneumonectomy:** Surgery to remove one whole lung and part of the lining of the chest, the diaphragm, and the lining of the sac around the heart.
- **Pleurodesis:** A surgical procedure that uses chemicals or drugs to make a scar in the space between the layers of the pleura.

Fluid is first drained from the space using a catheter or chest tube and the chemical or drug is put into the space. The scarring stops the build-up of fluid in the pleural cavity.

Even if the doctor removes all the cancer that can be seen at the time of the surgery, some patients may be given chemotherapy or radiation therapy after surgery to kill any cancer cells that are left. Treatment given after surgery, to lower the risk that the cancer will come back, is called adjuvant therapy.

Radiation Therapy

Radiation therapy is a cancer treatment that uses high-energy x-rays or other types of radiation to kill cancer cells or keep them from growing. There are two types of radiation therapy. External radiation therapy uses a machine outside the body to send radiation toward the cancer. Internal radiation therapy uses a radioactive substance sealed in needles, seeds, wires, or catheters that are placed directly into or near the cancer. The way the radiation therapy is given depends on the type and stage of the cancer being treated.

Chemotherapy

Chemotherapy is a cancer treatment that uses drugs to stop the growth of cancer cells, either by killing the cells or by stopping them from dividing. When chemotherapy is taken by mouth or injected into a vein or muscle, the drugs enter the bloodstream and can reach cancer cells throughout the body (systemic chemotherapy). When chemotherapy is placed directly into the spinal column, an organ, or a body cavity such as the abdomen, the drugs mainly affect cancer cells in those areas (regional chemotherapy). Combination chemotherapy is the use of more than one anticancer drug. The way the chemotherapy is given depends on the type and stage of the cancer being treated.

Clinical Trials

New types of treatment are being tested in clinical trials. A treatment clinical trial is a research study meant to help improve current treatments or obtain information on new treatments for patients with cancer. When clinical trials show that a new treatment is better than the standard treatment, the new treatment may become the standard treatment. Patients may want to think about taking part in a clinical trial. Some clinical trials are open only to patients who have not started treatment.

Biologic therapy, for example, is a treatment that uses the patient's immune system to fight cancer. Substances made by the body or made in a laboratory are used to boost, direct, or restore the body's natural defenses against cancer. This type of cancer treatment is also called biotherapy or immunotherapy.

Follow-Up Tests

Some of the tests that were done to diagnose the cancer or to find out the stage of the cancer may be repeated. Some tests will be repeated in order to see how well the treatment is working. Decisions about whether to continue, change, or stop treatment may be based on the results of these tests. This is sometimes called re-staging.

Some of the tests will continue to be done from time to time after treatment has ended. The results of these tests can show if your condition has changed or if the cancer has recurred (come back). These tests are sometimes called follow-up tests or check-ups.

Chapter 26

Esophageal Cancer

The Esophagus

The esophagus is in the chest. It's about 10 inches long. This organ is part of the digestive tract. Food moves from the mouth through the esophagus to the stomach. The esophagus is a muscular tube. The wall of the esophagus has several layers:

- **Inner layer or lining (mucosa):** The lining of the esophagus is moist so that food can pass to the stomach.

- **Submucosa:** The glands in this layer make mucus. Mucus keeps the esophagus moist.

- **Muscle layer:** The muscles push the food down to the stomach.

- **Outer layer:** The outer layer covers the esophagus.

Types of Esophageal Cancer

There are two main types of esophageal cancer. Both types are diagnosed, treated, and managed in similar ways. The two most common types are named for how the cancer cells look under a microscope. Both types begin in cells in the inner lining of the esophagus:

- **Adenocarcinoma of the esophagus:** This type is usually found in the lower part of the esophagus, near the stomach. In

Excerpted from "What You Need to Know about Cancer of the Esophagus," National Cancer Institute (www.cancer.gov), November 11, 2008.

the United States, adenocarcinoma is the most common type of esophageal cancer. It's been increasing since the 1970s.

- **Squamous cell carcinoma of the esophagus:** This type is usually found in the upper part of the esophagus. This type is becoming less common among Americans. Around the world, however, squamous cell carcinoma is the most common type.

Risk Factors

Doctors can seldom explain why one person develops esophageal cancer and another doesn't. However, we do know that people with certain risk factors are more likely than others to develop esophageal cancer. A risk factor is something that may increase the chance of getting a disease. Studies have found the following risk factors for esophageal cancer:

- **Age 65 or older:** Age is the main risk factor for esophageal cancer. The chance of getting this disease goes up as you get older. In the United States, most people are 65 years of age or older when they are diagnosed with esophageal cancer.

- **Being male:** In the United States, men are more than three times as likely as women to develop esophageal cancer.

- **Smoking:** People who smoke are more likely than people who don't smoke to develop esophageal cancer.

- **Heavy drinking:** People who have more than three alcoholic drinks each day are more likely than people who don't drink to develop squamous cell carcinoma of the esophagus. Heavy drinkers who smoke are at a much higher risk than heavy drinkers who don't smoke. In other words, these two factors act together to increase the risk even more.

- **Diet:** Studies suggest that having a diet that's low in fruits and vegetables may increase the risk of esophageal cancer. However, results from diet studies don't always agree, and more research is needed to better understand how diet affects the risk of developing esophageal cancer.

- **Obesity:** Being obese increases the risk of adenocarcinoma of the esophagus.

- **Acid reflux:** Acid reflux is the abnormal backward flow of stomach acid into the esophagus. Reflux is very common. A symptom

346

of reflux is heartburn, but some people don't have symptoms. The stomach acid can damage the tissue of the esophagus. After many years of reflux, this tissue damage may lead to adenocarcinoma of the esophagus in some people.

- **Barrett esophagus:** Acid reflux may damage the esophagus and over time cause a condition known as Barrett esophagus. The cells in the lower part of the esophagus are abnormal. Most people who have Barrett esophagus don't know it. The presence of Barrett esophagus increases the risk of adenocarcinoma of the esophagus. It's a greater risk factor than acid reflux alone.

Many other possible risk factors (such as smokeless tobacco) have been studied. Researchers continue to study these possible risk factors. Having a risk factor doesn't mean that a person will develop cancer of the esophagus. Most people who have risk factors never develop esophageal cancer.

Symptoms

Early esophageal cancer may not cause symptoms. As the cancer grows, the most common symptoms are:

- Food gets stuck in the esophagus, and food may come back up
- Pain when swallowing
- Pain in the chest or back
- Weight loss
- Heartburn
- A hoarse voice or cough that doesn't go away within two weeks

These symptoms may be caused by esophageal cancer or other health problems. If you have any of these symptoms, you should tell your doctor so that problems can be diagnosed and treated as early as possible.

Diagnosis

If you have a symptom that suggests esophageal cancer, your doctor must find out whether it's really due to cancer or to some other cause. The doctor gives you a physical exam and asks about your personal and family health history. You may have blood tests. You also may have other tests such as the following:

Barium swallow: After you drink a barium solution, you have x-rays taken of your esophagus and stomach. The barium solution makes your esophagus show up more clearly on the x-rays. This test is also called an upper GI series.

Endoscopy: The doctor uses a thin, lighted tube (endoscope) to look down your esophagus. The doctor first numbs your throat with an anesthetic spray, and you may also receive medicine to help you relax. The tube is passed through your mouth or nose to the esophagus. The doctor may also call this procedure upper endoscopy, EGD, or esophagoscopy.

Biopsy: Usually, cancer begins in the inner layer of the esophagus. The doctor uses an endoscope to remove tissue from the esophagus. A pathologist checks the tissue under a microscope for cancer cells. A biopsy is the only sure way to know if cancer cells are present.

The Staging Process

If the biopsy shows that you have cancer, your doctor needs to learn the extent (stage) of the disease to help you choose the best treatment. Staging is a careful attempt to find out how deeply the cancer invades the walls of the esophagus, whether the cancer invades nearby tissues, and whether the cancer has spread, and if so, to what parts of the body .

When esophageal cancer spreads, it's often found in nearby lymph nodes. If cancer has reached these nodes, it may also have spread to other lymph nodes, the bones, or other organs. Also, esophageal cancer may spread to the liver and lungs.

Your doctor may order one or more of the following staging tests:

- **Endoscopic ultrasound:** The doctor passes a thin, lighted tube (endoscope) down your throat, which has been numbed with anesthetic. A probe at the end of the tube sends out sound waves that you can't hear. The waves bounce off tissues in your esophagus and nearby organs. A computer creates a picture from the echoes. The picture can show how deeply the cancer has invaded the wall of the esophagus. The doctor may use a needle to take tissue samples of lymph nodes.

- **CT scan:** An x-ray machine linked to a computer takes a series of detailed pictures of your chest and abdomen. Doctors use CT scans to look for esophageal cancer that has spread to lymph nodes and other areas. You may receive contrast material by mouth or by injection into a blood vessel. The contrast material makes abnormal areas easier to see.

- **MRI:** A strong magnet linked to a computer is used to make detailed pictures of areas inside your body. An MRI can show whether cancer has spread to lymph nodes or other areas. Sometimes contrast material is given by injection into your blood vessel. The contrast material makes abnormal areas show up more clearly on the picture.

- **PET scan:** You receive an injection of a small amount of radioactive sugar. The radioactive sugar gives off signals that the PET scanner picks up. The PET scanner makes a picture of the places in your body where the sugar is being taken up. Cancer cells show up brighter in the picture because they take up sugar faster than normal cells do. A PET scan shows whether esophageal cancer may have spread.

- **Bone scan:** You get an injection of a small amount of a radioactive substance. It travels through the bloodstream and collects in the bones. A machine called a scanner detects and measures the radiation. The scanner makes pictures of the bones. The pictures may show cancer that has spread to the bones.

- **Laparoscopy:** After you are given general anesthesia, the surgeon makes small incisions (cuts) in your abdomen. The surgeon inserts a thin, lighted tube (laparoscope) into the abdomen. Lymph nodes or other tissue samples may be removed to check for cancer cells.

Sometimes staging is not complete until after surgery to remove the cancer and nearby lymph nodes.

When cancer spreads from its original place to another part of the body, the new tumor has the same kind of abnormal cells and the same name as the primary tumor. For example, if esophageal cancer spreads to the liver, the cancer cells in the liver are actually esophageal cancer cells. The disease is metastatic esophageal cancer, not liver cancer. For that reason, it's treated as esophageal cancer, not liver cancer. Doctors call the new tumor "distant" or metastatic disease.

Stages of Esophageal Cancer

Stage 0: Abnormal cells are found only in the inner layer of the esophagus. It's called carcinoma in situ.

Stage I: The cancer has grown through the inner layer to the submucosa. (The picture shows the submucosa and other layers.)

Stage II: Stage II is one of the following: The cancer has grown through the inner layer to the submucosa, and cancer cells have spread to lymph nodes. Or, the cancer has invaded the muscle layer. Cancer cells may be found in lymph nodes. Or, the cancer has grown through the outer layer of the esophagus.

Stage III: Stage III is one of the following: The cancer has grown through the outer layer, and cancer cells have spread to lymph nodes. Or, the cancer has invaded nearby structures, such as the airways. Cancer cells may have spread to lymph nodes.

Stage IV: Cancer cells have spread to distant organs, such as the liver.

Treatment

People with esophageal cancer have several treatment options. The options are surgery, radiation therapy, chemotherapy, or a combination of these treatments. For example, radiation therapy and chemotherapy may be given before or after surgery.

The treatment that's right for you depends mainly on where the cancer is located within the esophagus, whether the cancer has invaded nearby structures, whether the cancer has spread to lymph nodes or other organs, your symptoms, and your general health.

Esophageal cancer is hard to control with current treatments. For that reason, many doctors encourage people with this disease to consider taking part in a clinical trial, a research study of new treatment methods. Clinical trials are an important option for people with all stages of esophageal cancer.

You may have a team of specialists to help plan your treatment. Your doctor may refer you to specialists, or you may ask for a referral. You may want to see a gastroenterologist, a doctor who specializes in treating problems of the digestive organs. Other specialists who treat esophageal cancer include thoracic (chest) surgeons, thoracic surgical oncologists, medical oncologists, and radiation oncologists. Your health care team may also include an oncology nurse and a registered dietitian. If your airways are affected by the cancer, you may have a respiratory therapist as part of your team. If you have trouble swallowing, you may see a speech pathologist.

Your health care team can describe your treatment choices, the expected results of each, and the possible side effects. Because cancer therapy often damages healthy cells and tissues, side effects are common. Before treatment starts, ask your health care team about possible side effects and how treatment may change your normal activities. You and your health care team can work together to develop a treatment plan that meets your needs.

You may want to ask your doctor these questions before your treatment begins:

- What is the stage of the disease? Has the cancer spread? Do any lymph nodes show signs of cancer?

- What is the goal of treatment? What are my treatment choices? Which do you recommend for me? Why?

- Will I have more than one kind of treatment?

- What can I do to prepare for treatment?

- Will I need to stay in the hospital? If so, for how long?

- What are the risks and possible side effects of each treatment? For example, am I likely to have eating problems during or after treatment? How can side effects be managed?

- What will the treatment cost? Will my insurance cover it?

- Would a research study (clinical trial) be appropriate for me?

- Can you recommend other doctors who could give me a second opinion about my treatment options?

- How often should I have checkups?

Surgery

There are several types of surgery for esophageal cancer. The type depends mainly on where the cancer is located. The surgeon may remove the whole esophagus or only the part that has the cancer. Usually, the surgeon removes the section of the esophagus with the cancer, lymph nodes, and nearby soft tissues. Part or all of the stomach may also be removed. You and your surgeon can talk about the types of surgery and which may be right for you.

The surgeon makes incisions into your chest and abdomen to remove the cancer. In most cases, the surgeon pulls up the stomach and joins it to the remaining part of the esophagus. Or a piece of intestine may be used to connect the stomach to the remaining part of the esophagus. The surgeon may use either a piece of small intestine or large intestine. If the stomach was removed, a piece of intestine is used to join the remaining part of the esophagus to the small intestine.

During surgery, the surgeon may place a feeding tube into your small intestine. This tube helps you get enough nutrition while you heal.

You may have pain for the first few days after surgery. However, medicine will help control the pain. Before surgery, you should discuss the plan for pain relief with your health care team. After surgery, your team can adjust the plan if you need more relief.

Your health care team will watch for signs of food leaking from the newly joined parts of your digestive tract. They will also watch for pneumonia or other infections, breathing problems, bleeding, or other problems that may require treatment.

The time it takes to heal after surgery is different for everyone and depends on the type of surgery. You may be in the hospital for at least one week.

Radiation Therapy

Radiation therapy (also called radiotherapy) uses high-energy rays to kill cancer cells. It affects cells only in the treated area. Radiation therapy may be used before or after surgery. Or it may be used instead of surgery. Radiation therapy is usually given with chemotherapy to treat esophageal cancer.

Doctors use two types of radiation therapy to treat esophageal cancer. Some people receive both types:

- **External radiation therapy:** The radiation comes from a large machine outside the body. The machine aims radiation at your cancer. You may go to a hospital or clinic for treatment. Treatments are usually five days a week for several weeks.

- **Internal radiation therapy (brachytherapy):** The doctor numbs your throat with an anesthetic spray and gives you medicine to help you relax. The doctor puts a tube into your esophagus. The radiation comes from the tube. Once the tube is removed, no radioactivity is left in your body. Usually, only a single treatment is done.

Side effects depend mainly on the dose and type of radiation. External radiation therapy to the chest and abdomen may cause a sore throat, pain similar to heartburn, or pain in the stomach or the intestine. You may have nausea and diarrhea. Your health care team can give you medicines to prevent or control these problems.

Also, your skin in the treated area may become red, dry, and tender. You may lose hair in the treated area. A much less common side effect of radiation therapy aimed at the chest is harm to the lung, heart, or spinal cord.

You are likely to be very tired during radiation therapy, especially in the later weeks of external radiation therapy. You may also continue to feel very tired for a few weeks after radiation therapy is completed. Resting is important, but doctors usually advise patients to try to stay as active as they can.

Radiation therapy can lead to problems with swallowing. For example, sometimes radiation therapy can harm the esophagus and make it painful for you to swallow. Or, the radiation may cause the esophagus to narrow. Before radiation therapy, a plastic tube may be inserted into the esophagus to keep it open. If radiation therapy leads to a problem with swallowing, it may be hard to eat well. Ask your health care team for help getting good nutrition.

Chemotherapy

Most people with esophageal cancer get chemotherapy. Chemotherapy uses drugs to destroy cancer cells. The drugs for esophageal cancer are usually given through a vein (intravenous). You may have your treatment in a clinic, at the doctor's office, or at home. Some people need to stay in the hospital for treatment.

Chemotherapy is usually given in cycles. Each cycle has a treatment period followed by a rest period.

The side effects depend mainly on which drugs are given and how much. Chemotherapy kills fast-growing cancer cells, but the drug can also harm normal cells that divide rapidly:

- **Blood cells:** When chemotherapy lowers the levels of healthy blood cells, you're more likely to get infections, bruise or bleed easily, and feel very weak and tired. Your health care team will check for low levels of blood cells. If your levels are low, your health care team may stop the chemotherapy for a while or reduce the dose of drug. There also are medicines that can help your body make new blood cells.

- **Cells in hair roots:** Chemotherapy may cause hair loss. If you lose your hair, it will grow back, but it may change in color and texture.

- **Cells that line the digestive tract:** Chemotherapy can cause poor appetite, nausea and vomiting, diarrhea, or mouth and lip sores. Your health care team can give you medicines and suggest other ways to help with these problems.

Other possible side effects include a skin rash, joint pain, tingling or numbness in your hands and feet, hearing problems, or swollen feet or legs. Your healthcare team can suggest ways to control many of these problems. Most go away when treatment ends.

Getting a Second Opinion

Before starting treatment, you might want a second opinion about your diagnosis and treatment plan. You may want to find a medical center that has a lot of experience with treating esophageal cancer. You may even want to talk to several different doctors about all of the treatment options, their side effects, and the expected results.

Some people worry that the doctor will be offended if they ask for a second opinion. Usually the opposite is true. Most doctors welcome a second opinion. And many health insurance companies will pay for a second opinion if you or your doctor requests it.

If you get a second opinion, the second doctor may agree with your first doctor's diagnosis and treatment plan. Or the second doctor may suggest another approach. Either way, you have more information and perhaps a greater sense of control. You can feel more confident about the decisions you make, knowing that you've looked at your options.

It may take some time and effort to gather your medical records and see another doctor. In most cases, it's not a problem to take several weeks to get a second opinion. The delay in starting treatment usually will not make treatment less effective. To make sure, you should discuss this delay with your doctor.

There are many ways to find a doctor for a second opinion. You can ask your doctor, a local or state medical society, a nearby hospital, or a medical school for names of specialists. The National Cancer Institute's Cancer Information Service at 800-4-CANCER can tell you about nearby treatment centers.

Supportive Care

Esophageal cancer and its treatment can lead to other health problems. You can have supportive care before, during, or after cancer treatment.

Supportive care is treatment to control pain and other symptoms, to relieve the side effects of therapy, and to help you cope with the feelings that a diagnosis of cancer can bring. You may receive supportive care to prevent or control these problems and to improve your comfort and quality of life during treatment.

Pain

Cancer and its treatments may cause pain. It may be painful to swallow, or you may have pain in your chest from the cancer or from a stent. Your health care team or a pain control specialist can suggest ways to relieve or reduce pain.

Sadness and Other Feelings

It's normal to feel sad, anxious, or confused after a diagnosis of a serious illness. Some people find it helpful to talk about their feelings.

Cancer Blocks the Esophagus

You may have trouble swallowing because the cancer blocks the esophagus. Not being able to swallow makes it hard or impossible to eat. It also increases the risk of food getting in your airways. This can lead to a lung infection like pneumonia. Also, not being able to swallow liquids or saliva can be very distressing.

Your health care team may suggest one or more of the following options:

Stent: You get an injection of a medicine to help you relax. The doctor places a stent (a tube made of metal mesh or plastic) in your esophagus. Food and liquid can pass through the center of the tube. However, solid foods need to be chewed well before swallowing. A large swallow of food could get stuck in the stent.

Laser therapy: A laser is a concentrated beam of intense light that kills tissue with heat. The doctor uses the laser to destroy the cancer cells blocking the esophagus. Laser therapy may make swallowing easier for a while, but you may need to repeat the treatment several weeks later.

Photodynamic therapy: You get an injection, and the drug collects in the esophageal cancer cells. Two days after the injection, the doctor uses an endoscope to shine a special light (such as a laser) on the cancer. The drug becomes active when exposed to light. Two or three days later, the doctor may check to see if the cancer cells have been killed. People getting this drug must avoid sunlight for one month or longer. Also, you may need to repeat the treatment several weeks later.

Radiation therapy: Radiation therapy helps shrink the tumor. If the tumor blocks the esophagus, internal radiation therapy or sometimes external radiation therapy can be used to help make swallowing easier.

Balloon dilation: The doctor inserts a tube through the blocked part of the esophagus. A balloon helps widen the opening. This method helps improve swallowing for a few days.

Other ways to get nutrition: See the nutrition information below for ways to get food when eating becomes difficult.

Nutrition

It's important to meet your nutrition needs before, during, and after cancer treatment. You need the right amount of calories, protein, vitamins, and minerals. Getting the right nutrition can help you feel better and have more energy.

However, when you have esophageal cancer, it may be hard to eat for many reasons. You may be uncomfortable or tired, and you may not feel like eating. Also, the cancer may make it hard to swallow food. If you're getting chemotherapy, you may find that foods don't taste as good as they used to. You also may have side effects of treatment such as poor appetite, nausea, vomiting, or diarrhea.

If you develop problems with eating, there are a number of ways to meet your nutrition needs. A registered dietitian can help you figure out a way to get enough calories, protein, vitamins, and minerals:

- A dietitian may suggest a change in the types of foods you eat. Sometimes changing the texture, fiber, and fat content of your foods can lessen your discomfort. A dietitian may also suggest a change in the portion size and meal times.

- A dietitian may recommend liquid meals, such as canned nutrition beverages, milk shakes, or smoothies.

- If swallowing becomes too difficult, your dietitian and your doctor may recommend that you receive nutrition through a feeding tube.

- Sometimes, nutrition is provided directly into the bloodstream with intravenous nutrition.

Nutrition after Surgery

A registered dietitian can help you plan a diet that will meet your nutrition needs. A plan that describes the type and amount of food to eat after surgery can help you prevent weight loss and discomfort with eating.

If your stomach is removed during surgery, you may develop a problem afterward known as the dumping syndrome. This problem occurs when food or liquid enters the small intestine too fast. It can cause cramps, nausea, bloating, diarrhea, and dizziness. There are steps you can take to help control dumping syndrome:

- Eat smaller meals.

- Drink liquids before or after eating solid meals.

- Limit very sweet foods and drinks, such as cookies, candy, soda, and juices.

Your health care team may suggest medicine to control the symptoms. Also, after surgery, you may need to take daily supplements of vitamins and minerals, such as calcium, and you may need injections of vitamin B12.

You may want to ask a registered dietitian these questions about nutrition:

- How do I keep from losing too much weight? How do I know whether I'm getting enough calories and protein?

- What are some sample meals that would meet my needs?

- How can I include my favorite foods without causing or worsening digestive problems?

- Are there foods or drinks that I should avoid?

- What vitamins and minerals might I need to take?

Follow-Up Care

You'll need checkups after treatment for esophageal cancer. Checkups help ensure that any changes in your health are noted and treated if needed. If you have any health problems between checkups, you should contact your doctor.

Checkups may include a physical exam, blood tests, chest x-ray, CT scans, endoscopy, or other tests. You may want to ask your doctor these questions after you have finished treatment:

- How often will I need checkups?

- Which follow-up tests do you suggest for me?

- Between checkups, what health problems or symptoms should I tell you about?

Chapter 27

Stomach Cancer

The Stomach

The stomach is a hollow organ in the upper abdomen, under the ribs. It's part of the digestive system. Food moves from the mouth through the esophagus to the stomach. In the stomach, the food becomes liquid. Muscles in the stomach wall push the liquid into the small intestine.

The wall of the stomach has five layers:

- **Inner layer or lining (mucosa):** Juices made by glands in the inner layer help digest food. Most stomach cancers begin in this layer.

- **Submucosa:** This is the support tissue for the inner layer.

- **Muscle layer:** Muscles in this layer contract to mix and mash the food.

- **Subserosa:** This is the support tissue for the outer layer.

- **Outer layer (serosa):** The outer layer covers the stomach. It holds the stomach in place.

Stomach cancer usually begins in cells in the inner layer of the stomach. Over time, the cancer may invade more deeply into the stomach wall. A stomach tumor can grow through the stomach's outer layer into nearby organs, such as the liver, pancreas, esophagus, or intestine.

Excerpted from "What You Need to Know about Stomach Cancer," National Cancer Institute (www.cancer.gov), October 15, 2009.

Stomach cancer cells can spread by breaking away from the original tumor. They enter blood vessels or lymph vessels, which branch into all the tissues of the body. The cancer cells may be found in lymph nodes near the stomach. The cancer cells may attach to other tissues and grow to form new tumors that may damage those tissues.

The spread of cancer is called metastasis.

Risk Factors

When you're told that you have stomach cancer, it's natural to wonder what may have caused the disease. But no one knows the exact causes of stomach cancer. Doctors seldom know why one person develops stomach cancer and another doesn't.

Doctors do know that people with certain risk factors are more likely than others to develop stomach cancer. A risk factor is something that may increase the chance of getting a disease.

Studies have found the following risk factors for stomach cancer:

- ***Helicobacter pylori* infection:** *H. pylori* is a bacterium that commonly infects the inner lining (the mucosa) of the stomach. Infection with *H. pylori* can cause stomach inflammation and peptic ulcers. It also increases the risk of stomach cancer, but only a small number of infected people develop stomach cancer.

- **Long-term inflammation of the stomach:** People who have conditions associated with long-term stomach inflammation (such as the blood disease pernicious anemia) are at increased risk of stomach cancer. Also, people who have had part of their stomach removed may have long-term stomach inflammation and increased risk of stomach cancer many years after their surgery.

- **Smoking:** Smokers are more likely than nonsmokers to develop stomach cancer. Heavy smokers are most at risk.

- **Family history:** Close relatives (parents, brothers, sisters, or children) of a person with a history of stomach cancer are somewhat more likely to develop the disease themselves. If many close relatives have a history of stomach cancer, the risk is even greater.

- **Poor diet, lack of physical activity, or obesity:** Studies suggest that people who eat a diet high in foods that are smoked, salted, or pickled have an increased risk for stomach cancer. On the other hand, people who eat a diet high in fresh fruits and vegetables may have a lower risk of this disease. A lack of physical activity may increase the risk of stomach cancer. Also, people who are obese may have an increased risk of cancer developing in the upper part of the stomach.

Most people who have known risk factors do not develop stomach cancer. For example, many people have an *H. pylori* infection but never develop cancer. On the other hand, people who do develop the disease sometimes have no known risk factors.

Symptoms

Early stomach cancer often does not cause symptoms. As the cancer grows, the most common symptoms are the following:

- Discomfort or pain in the stomach area
- Difficulty swallowing
- Nausea and vomiting
- Weight loss
- Feeling full or bloated after a small meal
- Vomiting blood or having blood in the stool

Most often, these symptoms are not due to cancer. Other health problems, such as an ulcer or infection, can cause the same symptoms. Anyone who has these symptoms should tell their doctor so that problems can be diagnosed and treated as early as possible.

Diagnosis

If you have symptoms that suggest stomach cancer, your doctor will check to see whether they are due to cancer or to some other cause. Your doctor may refer you to a gastroenterologist, a doctor whose specialty is diagnosing and treating digestive problems.

Your doctor will ask about your personal and family health history. You may have blood or other lab tests. You also may have these tests:

Physical exam: Your doctor feels your abdomen for fluid, swelling, or other changes. Your doctor also will check for swollen lymph nodes.

Endoscopy: Your doctor uses a thin, lighted tube (endoscope) to look into your stomach. Your doctor first numbs your throat with an anesthetic spray. You also may receive medicine to help you relax. The tube is passed through your mouth and esophagus to the stomach.

Biopsy: An endoscope has a tool for removing tissue. Your doctor uses the endoscope to remove tissue from the stomach. A pathologist checks the tissue under a microscope for cancer cells. A biopsy is the only sure way to know if cancer cells are present.

You may want to ask your doctor these questions before having a biopsy:

- How will the biopsy be done?
- Will it hurt?
- Are there any risks? What are the chances of infection or bleeding after the biopsy?
- When can I resume my normal diet?
- How soon will I know the results?
- If I do have cancer, who will talk with me about the next steps? When?

Staging

If the biopsy shows that you have stomach cancer, your doctor needs to learn the stage (extent) of the disease to help you choose the best treatment. Staging is a careful attempt to find out how deeply the tumor invades the wall of the stomach, whether the stomach tumor has invaded nearby tissues, and whether the cancer has spread and, if so, to what parts of the body. When stomach cancer spreads, cancer cells may be found in nearby lymph nodes, the liver, the pancreas, esophagus, intestine, or other organs. Your doctor may order blood tests and other tests to check these areas.

- **Chest x-ray:** An x-ray of your chest can show whether cancer has spread to the lungs.

- **CT scan:** An x-ray machine linked to a computer takes a series of detailed pictures of your organs. You may receive an injection of dye. The dye makes abnormal areas easier to see. Tumors in your liver, pancreas, or elsewhere in the body can show up on a CT scan.

- **Endoscopic ultrasound:** Your doctor passes a thin, lighted tube (endoscope) down your throat. A probe at the end of the tube sends out sound waves that you cannot hear. The waves bounce off tissues in your stomach and other organs. A computer creates a picture from the echoes. The picture can show how deeply the cancer has invaded the wall of the stomach. Your doctor may use a needle to take tissue samples of lymph nodes.

- **Laparoscopy:** A surgeon makes small incisions (cuts) in your abdomen. The surgeon inserts a thin, lighted tube (laparoscope) into the abdomen. The surgeon may remove lymph nodes or take tissue samples for biopsy.

Sometimes staging is not complete until after surgery to remove the tumor and nearby lymph nodes.

When stomach cancer spreads from its original place to another part of the body, the new tumor has the same kind of abnormal cells and the same name as the primary (original) tumor. For example, if stomach cancer spreads to the liver, the cancer cells in the liver are actually stomach cancer cells. The disease is metastatic stomach cancer, not liver cancer. For that reason, it is treated as stomach cancer, not liver cancer. Doctors call the new tumor "distant" or metastatic disease.

These are the stages of stomach cancer:

Stage 0: The tumor is found only in the inner layer of the stomach. Stage 0 is also called carcinoma in situ.

Stage I is one of the following:

- The tumor has invaded only the submucosa. Cancer cells may be found in up to six lymph nodes.

- Or, the tumor has invaded the muscle layer or subserosa. Cancer cells have not spread to lymph nodes or other organs.

Stage II is one of the following:

- The tumor has invaded only the submucosa. Cancer cells have spread to seven to 15 lymph nodes.

- Or, the tumor has invaded the muscle layer or subserosa. Cancer cells have spread to one to six lymph nodes.

- Or, the tumor has penetrated the outer layer of the stomach. Cancer cells have not spread to lymph nodes or other organs.

Stage III is one of the following:

- The tumor has invaded the muscle layer or subserosa. Cancer cells have spread to seven to 15 lymph nodes.

- Or, the tumor has penetrated the outer layer. Cancer cells have spread to one to 15 lymph nodes.

- Or, the tumor has invaded nearby organs, such as the liver, co-lon, or spleen. Cancer cells have not spread to lymph nodes or to distant organs.

Stage IV is one of the following:

- Cancer cells have spread to more than 15 lymph nodes.
- Or, the tumor has invaded nearby organs and at least one lymph node.
- Or, cancer cells have spread to distant organs.

Treatment

The choice of treatment depends mainly on the size and location of the tumor, the stage of disease, and your general health.

Treatment for stomach cancer may involve surgery, chemotherapy, or radiation therapy. You'll probably receive more than one type of treatment. For example, chemotherapy may be given before or after surgery. It's often given at the same time as radiation therapy.

You may want to talk with your doctor about taking part in a clinical trial, a research study of new treatment methods. Clinical trials are an important option for people at any stage of stomach cancer.

You may have a team of specialists to help plan your treatment. Your doctor may refer you to a specialist, or you may ask for a referral. Specialists who treat stomach cancer include gastroenterologists, surgeons, medical oncologists, and radiation oncologists. Your health care team may also include an oncology nurse and a registered dietitian.

Your health care team can describe your treatment choices, the expected results, and the possible side effects. Because cancer therapy often damages healthy cells and tissues, side effects are common. Before treatment starts, ask your health care team about possible side effects, how to prevent or reduce these effects, and how treatment may change your normal activities. You and your health care team can work together to make a treatment plan that meets your needs.

Surgery

The type of surgery for stomach cancer depends mainly on where the cancer is located. The surgeon may remove the whole stomach or only the part that has the cancer. You and your surgeon can talk about the types of surgery and which may be right for you:

- **Partial (subtotal) gastrectomy for tumors at the lower part of the stomach:** The surgeon removes the lower part of the stomach with the cancer. The surgeon attaches the remaining part of the stomach to the intestine. Nearby lymph nodes and other tissues may also be removed.

- **Total gastrectomy for tumors at the upper part of the stomach:** The surgeon removes the entire stomach, nearby lymph nodes, parts of the esophagus and small intestine, and other tissues near the tumor. Rarely, the spleen also may be removed. The surgeon then connects the esophagus directly to the small intestine.

The time it takes to heal after surgery is different for each person, and you may be in the hospital for a week or longer. You may have pain for the first few days. Medicine can help control your pain. Before surgery, you should discuss the plan for pain relief with your doctor or nurse. After surgery, your doctor can adjust the plan if you need more pain relief.

Many people who have stomach surgery feel tired or weak for a while. Your health care team will watch for signs of bleeding, infection, or other problems that may require treatment.

The surgery can also cause constipation or diarrhea. These symptoms usually can be controlled with diet changes and medicine.

You may want to ask your doctor these questions before having surgery:

- What kind of surgery do you recommend for me? Why?

- Will you remove lymph nodes? Will you remove other tissue? Why?

- How will I feel after surgery?

- Will I need a special diet?

- If I have pain, how will you control it?

- How long will I be in the hospital?

- Am I likely to have eating problems?

- Will I have any long-term side effects?

Chemotherapy

Most people with stomach cancer get chemotherapy. Chemotherapy uses drugs to kill cancer cells. It may be given before or after surgery. After surgery, radiation therapy may be given along with chemotherapy.

The drugs that treat stomach cancer are usually given through a vein (intravenous). You'll probably receive a combination of drugs.

You may receive chemotherapy in an outpatient part of the hospital, at the doctor's office, or at home. Some people need to stay in the hospital during treatment.

The side effects depend mainly on which drugs are given and how much. Chemotherapy kills fast-growing cancer cells, but the drugs can also harm normal cells that divide rapidly:

- **Blood cells:** When drugs lower the levels of healthy blood cells, you're more likely to get infections, bruise or bleed easily, and feel very weak and tired. Your health care team will check for low levels of blood cells. If your levels are low, your health care team may stop the chemotherapy for a while or reduce the dose of the drug. There are also medicines that can help your body make new blood cells.

- **Cells in hair roots:** Chemotherapy may cause hair loss. If you lose your hair, it will grow back after treatment, but the color and texture may be changed.

- **Cells that line the digestive tract:** Chemotherapy can cause a poor appetite, nausea and vomiting, diarrhea, or mouth and lip sores. Your health care team can give you medicines and suggest other ways to help with these problems. They usually go away when treatment ends.

Some drugs used for stomach cancer also may cause a skin rash, hearing loss, and tingling or numbness in your hands and feet. Your health care team can suggest ways to control many of these side effects.

You may want to ask your doctor these questions before having chemotherapy:

- Why do I need this treatment?
- Which drug or drugs will I have?
- How do the drugs work?
- When will treatment start? When will it end?
- Will I have any long-term side effects?

Radiation Therapy

Radiation therapy (also called radiotherapy) uses high-energy rays to kill cancer cells. It affects cells only in the part of the body that is treated. Radiation therapy is usually given with chemotherapy to treat stomach cancer.

The radiation comes from a large machine outside the body. You'll go to a hospital or clinic for treatment. Treatments are usually five days a week for several weeks.

Side effects depend mainly on the dose and type of radiation. External radiation therapy to the chest and abdomen may cause a sore throat, pain similar to heartburn, or pain in the stomach or the intestine. You may have nausea and diarrhea. Your health care team can give you medicines to prevent or control these problems.

It's common for the skin in the treated area to become red, dry, tender, and itchy.

You're likely to become very tired during radiation therapy, especially in the later weeks of treatment. Resting is important, but doctors usually advise patients to try to stay active, unless it leads to pain or other problems.

Although the side effects of radiation therapy can be distressing, your doctor can usually treat or control them. Also, side effects usually go away after treatment ends.

You may want to ask your doctor these questions before having radiation therapy:

- Why do I need this treatment?
- When will the treatments begin? When will they end?
- How will I feel during treatment?
- How will we know if the radiation treatment is working?
- Will I have any long-term side effects?

Second Opinion

Before starting treatment, you might want a second opinion from another doctor about your diagnosis and treatment plan. Some people worry that their doctor will be offended if they ask for a second opinion. Usually the opposite is true. Most doctors welcome a second opinion. And many health insurance companies will pay for a second opinion if you or your doctor requests it. Some companies require a second opinion.

If you get a second opinion, the doctor may agree with your first doctor's diagnosis and treatment plan. Or the second doctor may suggest another approach. Either way, you'll have more information and perhaps a greater sense of control. You may also feel more confident about the decisions you make, knowing that you've looked carefully at your options.

It may take some time and effort to gather your medical records and see another doctor. Usually it's not a problem if it takes you several weeks to get a second opinion. In most cases, the delay in starting treatment will not make treatment less effective. To make sure, you should discuss this possible delay with your doctor. Some people with stomach cancer need treatment right away.

There are many ways to find a doctor for a second opinion. You can ask your doctor, a local or state medical society, a nearby hospital, or a medical school for names of specialists. Also, you can request a consultation with specialists at the National Institutes of Health Clinical Center in Bethesda, Maryland. Specialists in the NCI Surgery Branch provide consultations and surgical care for people with stomach cancer. The telephone number is 301-496-4164. The website is located at http:// ccr.cancer.gov/labs/lab.asp?labid=93.

The NCI Cancer Information Service at 800-4-CANCER (800-422-6237) or at LiveHelp (http://www.cancer.gov/help) can tell you about nearby treatment centers.

Nutrition

Nutrition is an important part of your treatment for stomach cancer. You need the right amount of calories, protein, vitamins, and minerals to maintain your strength and to heal. However, when you have stomach cancer, it may be difficult to eat. You may be uncomfortable or tired, and you may not feel like eating. You also may have nausea, vomiting, constipation, or diarrhea from cancer treatment or pain medicine.

Tell your health care team if you're losing weight or having any problems digesting your food. A dietitian can help you choose the foods and nutrition products that will meet your needs. Some people with stomach cancer are helped by receiving nutrition by IV (intravenous). A temporary feeding tube is rarely needed.

Nutrition after Stomach Surgery

A registered dietitian can help you plan a diet that will meet your nutrition needs. A plan that describes the type and amount of food to eat after surgery can help you prevent weight loss and discomfort with eating.

After stomach surgery, you may need to take daily supplements of vitamins and minerals, such as vitamin D, calcium, and iron. You may also need vitamin B12 shots.

Some people have problems eating and drinking after stomach surgery. Liquids may pass into the small intestine too fast, which causes dumping syndrome. The symptoms are cramps, nausea, bloating, diarrhea, and dizziness. To prevent these symptoms, it may help to make the following changes:

- Plan to have smaller, more frequent meals (some doctors suggest six meals per day)

- Drink liquids before or after meals
- Cut down on very sweet foods and drinks (such as cookies, candy, soda, and juices)
- Ask your health care team if they can suggest medicine to control the symptoms

You may want to ask a dietitian these questions about nutrition:

- What foods are best soon after surgery?
- How can I avoid dumping syndrome?
- Are there foods or drinks that I should avoid?

Supportive Care

Stomach cancer and its treatment can lead to other health problems. You can have supportive care before, during, and after cancer treatment.

Supportive care is treatment to control pain and other symptoms, to relieve the side effects of therapy, and to help you cope with the feelings that a diagnosis of cancer can bring. You may receive supportive care to prevent or control these problems and to improve your comfort and quality of life during treatment.

Cancer That Blocks the Digestive Tract

People with advanced stomach cancer may develop a tumor that blocks the passage of food through the digestive tract. Your health care team may suggest one or more of the following options:

Stent: The doctor uses an endoscope to place a stent (a tube made of metal mesh or plastic) in your intestine. Food and liquid can pass through the center of the tube.

Radiation therapy: Radiation therapy may help shrink the tumor that is blocking the intestine.

Laser therapy: A laser is a concentrated beam of intense light that kills tissue with heat. The doctor uses an endoscope to place the laser in your digestive tract. The laser destroys the cancer cells blocking the digestive tract.

Pain

Cancer and its treatments may cause pain. Your health care team or a pain control specialist can suggest ways to relieve or reduce pain. Radiation therapy and pain medicine may help.

Follow-Up Care

You'll need regular checkups after treatment for stomach cancer. Checkups help ensure that any changes in your health are noted and treated if needed. If you have any health problems between checkups, you should contact your doctor.

Your doctor will check for return of the cancer. Also, checkups help detect health problems that can result from cancer treatment.

Checkups may include a physical exam, blood tests, x-rays, CT scans, endoscopy, or other tests. If you had surgery on the stomach, your doctor may order blood tests to check the levels of certain vitamins and minerals, such as vitamin B12, calcium, and iron.

Chapter 28

Gallbladder Cancer

General Information about Gallbladder Cancer

Gallbladder cancer is a rare disease in which malignant (cancer) cells are found in the tissues of the gallbladder. The gallbladder is a pear-shaped organ that lies just under the liver in the upper abdomen. The gallbladder stores bile, a fluid made by the liver to digest fat. When food is being broken down in the stomach and intestines, bile is released from the gallbladder through a tube called the common bile duct, which connects the gallbladder and liver to the first part of the small intestine.

The wall of the gallbladder has three main layers of tissue: mucosal (innermost) layer; muscularis (middle, muscle) layer; and serosal (outer) layer. Between these layers is supporting connective tissue. Primary gallbladder cancer starts in the innermost layer and spreads through the outer layers as it grows.

Risk Factors

Anything that increases your chance of getting a disease is called a risk factor. Risk factors for gallbladder cancer include being female and being Native American.

Excerpted from PDQ® Cancer Information Summary. National Cancer Institute; Bethesda, MD. "Gallbladder Cancer Treatment (PDQ) - Patient Version." Updated 04/2010. Available at: http://cancer.gov. Accessed June 21, 2010.

Signs and Symptoms

Possible signs of gallbladder cancer include jaundice, pain, and fever. These and other symptoms may be caused by gallbladder cancer. Other conditions may cause the same symptoms. A doctor should be consulted if any of the following problems occur:

- Jaundice (yellowing of the skin and whites of the eyes)
- Pain above the stomach
- Fever
- Nausea and vomiting
- Bloating
- Lumps in the abdomen

Detection and Diagnosis

Gallbladder cancer is difficult to detect (find) and diagnose early. Gallbladder cancer is difficult to detect and diagnose for the following reasons:

- There aren't any noticeable signs or symptoms in the early stages of gallbladder cancer
- The symptoms of gallbladder cancer, when present, are like the symptoms of many other illnesses
- The gallbladder is hidden behind the liver

Gallbladder cancer is sometimes found when the gallbladder is removed for other reasons. Patients with gallstones rarely develop gallbladder cancer.

Tests that examine the gallbladder and nearby organs are used to detect (find), diagnose, and stage gallbladder cancer. Procedures that create pictures of the gallbladder and the area around it help diagnose gallbladder cancer and show how far the cancer has spread. The process used to find out if cancer cells have spread within and around the gallbladder is called staging.

In order to plan treatment, it is important to know if the gallbladder cancer can be removed by surgery. Tests and procedures to detect, diagnose, and stage gallbladder cancer are usually done at the same time. The following tests and procedures may be used:

Physical exam and history: An exam of the body to check general signs of health, including checking for signs of disease, such as lumps or anything else that seems unusual. A history of the patient's health habits and past illnesses and treatments will also be taken.

Ultrasound exam: A procedure in which high-energy sound waves (ultrasound) are bounced off internal tissues or organs and make echoes. The echoes form a picture of body tissues called a sonogram. An abdominal ultrasound is done to diagnose gallbladder cancer.

Liver function tests: A procedure in which a blood sample is checked to measure the amounts of certain substances released into the blood by the liver. A higher than normal amount of a substance can be a sign of liver disease that may be caused by gallbladder cancer.

Carcinoembryonic antigen (CEA) assay: A test that measures the level of CEA in the blood. CEA is released into the bloodstream from both cancer cells and normal cells. When found in higher than normal amounts, it can be a sign of gallbladder cancer or other conditions.

CA 19-9 assay: A test that measures the level of CA 19-9 in the blood. CA 19-9 is released into the bloodstream from both cancer cells and normal cells. When found in higher than normal amounts, it can be a sign of gallbladder cancer or other conditions.

CT scan (CAT scan): A procedure that makes a series of detailed pictures of areas inside the body, taken from different angles. The pictures are made by a computer linked to an x-ray machine. A dye may be injected into a vein or swallowed to help the organs or tissues show up more clearly. This procedure is also called computed tomography, computerized tomography, or computerized axial tomography.

Blood chemistry studies: A procedure in which a blood sample is checked to measure the amounts of certain substances released into the blood by organs and tissues in the body. An unusual (higher or lower than normal) amount of a substance can be a sign of disease in the organ or tissue that produces it.

Chest x-ray: An x-ray of the organs and bones inside the chest. An x-ray is a type of energy beam that can go through the body and onto film, making a picture of areas inside the body.

MRI (magnetic resonance imaging): A procedure that uses a magnet, radio waves, and a computer to make a series of detailed pictures of areas inside the body. This procedure is also called nuclear magnetic resonance imaging (NMRI). A dye may be injected into the gallbladder area so the ducts (tubes) that carry bile from the liver to the gallbladder and from the gallbladder to the small intestine will show up better in the image. This procedure is called MRCP (magnetic resonance cholangiopancreatography). To create detailed pictures of blood vessels near the gallbladder, the dye is injected into a vein. This procedure is called MRA (magnetic resonance angiography).

ERCP (endoscopic retrograde cholangiopancreatography): A procedure used to x-ray the ducts (tubes) that carry bile from the liver to the gallbladder and from the gallbladder to the small intestine. Sometimes gallbladder cancer causes these ducts to narrow and block or slow the flow of bile, causing jaundice. An endoscope (a thin, lighted tube) is passed through the mouth, esophagus, and stomach into the first part of the small intestine. A catheter (a smaller tube) is then inserted through the endoscope into the bile ducts. A dye is injected through the catheter into the ducts and an x-ray is taken. If the ducts are blocked by a tumor, a fine tube may be inserted into the duct to unblock it. This tube (or stent) may be left in place to keep the duct open. Tissue samples may also be taken.

Biopsy: The removal of cells or tissues so they can be viewed under a microscope by a pathologist to check for signs of cancer. The biopsy may be done after surgery to remove the tumor. If the tumor clearly cannot be removed by surgery, the biopsy may be done using a fine needle to remove cells from the tumor.

Laparoscopy: A surgical procedure to look at the organs inside the abdomen to check for signs of disease. Small incisions (cuts) are made in the wall of the abdomen and a laparoscope (a thin, lighted tube) is inserted into one of the incisions. Other instruments may be inserted through the same or other incisions to perform procedures such as removing organs or taking tissue samples for biopsy. The laparoscopy helps to determine if the cancer is within the gallbladder only or has spread to nearby tissues and if it can be removed by surgery.

PTC (percutaneous transhepatic cholangiography): A procedure used to x-ray the liver and bile ducts. A thin needle is inserted through the skin below the ribs and into the liver. Dye is injected into the liver or bile ducts and an x-ray is taken. If a blockage is found, a thin, flexible tube called a stent is sometimes left in the liver to drain bile into the small intestine or a collection bag outside the body.

Prognosis

Certain factors affect the prognosis (chance of recovery) and treatment options. The prognosis and treatment options depend on the following:

- The stage of the cancer (whether the cancer has spread from the gallbladder to other places in the body).

- Whether the cancer can be completely removed by surgery.

- The type of gallbladder cancer (how the cancer cell looks under a microscope).

- Whether the cancer has just been diagnosed or has recurred (come back).

Treatment may also depend on the age and general health of the patient and whether the cancer is causing symptoms.

Gallbladder cancer can be cured only if it is found before it has spread, when it can be removed by surgery. If the cancer has spread, palliative treatment can improve the patient's quality of life by controlling the symptoms and complications of this disease.

Taking part in one of the clinical trials being done to improve treatment should be considered.

Stages of Gallbladder Cancer

Tests and procedures to stage gallbladder cancer are usually done at the same time as diagnosis. See the section above for a description of tests and procedures used to detect, diagnose, and stage gallbladder cancer.

Stage 0 (Carcinoma in Situ)

In stage 0, abnormal cells are found in the innermost (mucosal) layer of the gallbladder. These abnormal cells may become cancer and spread into nearby normal tissue. Stage 0 is also called carcinoma in situ.

Stage I

In stage I, cancer has formed. Stage I is divided into stage IA and stage IB.

Stage IA: Cancer has spread beyond the innermost (mucosal) layer to the connective tissue or to the muscle (muscularis) layer.

Stage IB: Cancer has spread beyond the muscle layer to the connective tissue around the muscle.

Stage II

Stage II is divided into stage IIA and stage IIB.

Stage IIA: Cancer has spread beyond the visceral peritoneum (tissue that covers the gallbladder) and/or to the liver and/or one nearby organ (such as the stomach, small intestine, colon, pancreas, or bile ducts outside the liver).

Stage IIB: Cancer has spread:

- beyond the innermost layer to the connective tissue and to nearby lymph nodes; or

- to the muscle layer and nearby lymph nodes; or

- beyond the muscle layer to the connective tissue around the muscle and to nearby lymph nodes; or

- through the visceral peritoneum (tissue that covers the gallbladder) and/or to the liver and/or to one nearby organ (such as the stomach, small intestine, colon, pancreas, or bile ducts outside the liver), and to nearby lymph nodes.

Stage III

In stage III, cancer has spread to a main blood vessel in the liver or to nearby organs and may have spread to nearby lymph nodes.

Stage IV

In stage IV, cancer has spread to nearby lymph nodes and/or to organs far away from the gallbladder.

Treatment Groups

For gallbladder cancer, stages are also grouped according to how the cancer may be treated. There are two treatment groups:

Localized (Stage I): Cancer is found in the wall of the gallbladder and can be completely removed by surgery.

Unresectable (Stage II, Stage III, and Stage IV): Cancer has spread through the wall of the gallbladder to surrounding tissues or organs or throughout the abdominal cavity. Except in patients whose cancer has spread only to lymph nodes, the cancer is unresectable (cannot be completely removed by surgery).

Recurrent Gallbladder Cancer

Recurrent gallbladder cancer is cancer that has recurred (come back) after it has been treated. The cancer may come back in the gallbladder or in other parts of the body.

Treatment Option Overview

Different types of treatments are available for patients with gallbladder cancer. Some treatments are standard (the currently used treatment), and some are being tested in clinical trials. Three types of standard treatment are used.

Surgery

Gallbladder cancer may be treated with a cholecystectomy, surgery to remove the gallbladder and some of the tissues around it. Nearby lymph nodes may be removed. A laparoscope is sometimes used to guide gallbladder surgery. The laparoscope is attached to a video camera and inserted through an incision (port) in the abdomen. Surgical instruments are inserted through other ports to perform the surgery. Because there is a risk that gallbladder cancer cells may spread to these ports, tissue surrounding the port sites may also be removed.

If the cancer has spread and cannot be removed, the following types of palliative surgery may relieve symptoms:

Surgical biliary bypass: If the tumor is blocking the small intestine and bile is building up in the gallbladder, a biliary bypass may be done. During this operation, the gallbladder or bile duct will be cut and sewn to the small intestine to create a new pathway around the blocked area.

Endoscopic stent placement: If the tumor is blocking the bile duct, surgery may be done to put in a stent (a thin, flexible tube) to drain bile that has built up in the area. The stent may be placed through a catheter that drains to the outside of the body or the stent may go around the blocked area and drain the bile into the small intestine.

Percutaneous transhepatic biliary drainage: A procedure done to drain bile when there is a blockage and endoscopic stent placement is not possible. An x-ray of the liver and bile ducts is done to locate the blockage. Images made by ultrasound are used to guide placement of a stent, which is left in the liver to drain bile into the small intestine or a collection bag outside the body. This procedure may be done to relieve jaundice before surgery.

Radiation Therapy

Radiation therapy is a cancer treatment that uses high-energy x-rays or other types of radiation to kill cancer cells. There are two types of radiation therapy. External radiation therapy uses a machine outside the body to send radiation toward the cancer. Internal radiation therapy uses a radioactive substance sealed in needles, seeds, wires, or catheters that are placed directly into or near the cancer. The way the radiation therapy is given depends on the type and stage of the cancer being treated.

Chemotherapy

Chemotherapy is a cancer treatment that uses drugs to stop the growth of cancer cells, either by killing the cells or by stopping the cells from dividing. When chemotherapy is taken by mouth or injected into a vein or muscle, the drugs enter the bloodstream and can reach cancer cells throughout the body (systemic chemotherapy). When chemotherapy is placed directly into the spinal column, an organ, or a body cavity such as the abdomen, the drugs mainly affect cancer cells in those areas (regional chemotherapy). The way the chemotherapy is given depends on the type and stage of the cancer being treated.

Clinical Trials

A treatment clinical trial is a research study meant to help improve current treatments or obtain information on new treatments for patients with cancer. When clinical trials show that a new treatment is better than the standard treatment, the new treatment may become the standard treatment. Patients may want to think about taking part in a clinical trial. Some clinical trials are open only to patients who have not started treatment.

New types of treatment are being tested in clinical trials. Radiosensitizers, for example, are drugs that make tumor cells more sensitive to radiation therapy. Combining radiation therapy with radiosensitizers may kill more tumor cells.

Follow-Up Tests

Some of the tests that were done to diagnose the cancer or to find out the stage of the cancer may be repeated. Some tests will be repeated in order to see how well the treatment is working. Decisions about whether to continue, change, or stop treatment may be based on the results of these tests. This is sometimes called re-staging.

Some of the tests will continue to be done from time to time after treatment has ended. The results of these tests can show if your condition has changed or if the cancer has recurred (come back). These tests are sometimes called follow-up tests or check-ups.

Chapter 29

Pancreatic Cancer

General Information about Pancreatic Cancer

Pancreatic cancer is a disease in which malignant (cancer) cells form in the tissues of the pancreas. The pancreas is a gland about six inches long that is shaped like a thin pear lying on its side. The wider end of the pancreas is called the head, the middle section is called the body, and the narrow end is called the tail. The pancreas lies behind the stomach and in front of the spine.

The pancreas has two main jobs in the body: To produce juices that help digest (break down) food, and to produce hormones, such as insulin and glucagon, that help control blood sugar levels. Both of these hormones help the body use and store the energy it gets from food.

The digestive juices are produced by exocrine pancreas cells and the hormones are produced by endocrine pancreas cells. About 95% of pancreatic cancers begin in exocrine cells. This chapter provides information on exocrine pancreatic cancer. For information about endocrine pancreatic cancer (islet cell tumors), see chapter 18.

Risk Factors and Signs

Anything that increases your risk of getting a disease is called a risk factor. Having a risk factor does not mean that you will get cancer; not

Excerpted from PDQ® Cancer Information Summary. National Cancer Institute; Bethesda, MD. "Pancreatic Cancer Treatment (PDQ) - Patient Version." Updated 07/2010. Available at: http://cancer.gov. Accessed September 28, 2010.

having risk factors doesn't mean that you will not get cancer. People who think they may be at risk should discuss this with their doctor. Risk factors for pancreatic cancer include smoking, long-standing diabetes, chronic pancreatitis, and certain hereditary conditions, such as hereditary pancreatitis, multiple endocrine neoplasia type 1 syndrome, hereditary nonpolyposis colon cancer (HNPCC; Lynch syndrome), von Hippel-Lindau syndrome, ataxia-telangiectasia, and the familial atypical multiple mole melanoma syndrome (FAMMM).

Possible signs of pancreatic cancer include jaundice, pain, and weight loss. These and other symptoms may be caused by pancreatic cancer. Other conditions may cause the same symptoms. A doctor should be consulted if any of the following problems occur:

- Jaundice (yellowing of the skin and whites of the eyes)
- Pain in the upper or middle abdomen and back
- Unexplained weight loss
- Loss of appetite
- Fatigue

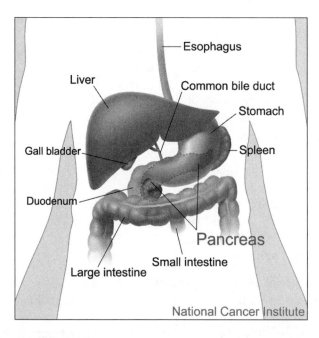

Figure 29.1. The Pancreas and Nearby Organs (image by Don Bliss, National Cancer Institute)

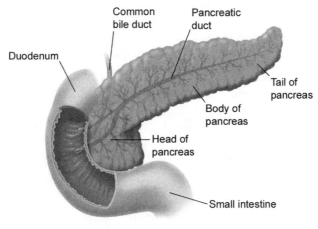

National Cancer Institute

Figure 29.2. *Anatomy of the Pancreas (image by Don Bliss, National Cancer Institute)*

Detection and Diagnosis

Pancreatic cancer is difficult to detect and diagnose for the following reasons:

- There aren't any noticeable signs or symptoms in the early stages of pancreatic cancer.

- The signs of pancreatic cancer, when present, are like the signs of many other illnesses.

- The pancreas is hidden behind other organs such as the stomach, small intestine, liver, gallbladder, spleen, and bile ducts.

Pancreatic cancer is usually diagnosed with tests and procedures that produce pictures of the pancreas and the area around it. The process used to find out if cancer cells have spread within and around the pancreas is called staging. Tests and procedures to detect, diagnose, and stage pancreatic cancer are usually done at the same time. In order to plan treatment, it is important to know the stage of the disease and whether or not the pancreatic cancer can be removed by surgery. The following tests and procedures may be used:

Chest x-ray: An x-ray of the organs and bones inside the chest. An x-ray is a type of energy beam that can go through the body and onto film, making a picture of areas inside the body.

Physical exam and history: An exam of the body to check general signs of health, including checking for signs of disease, such as lumps or anything else that seems unusual. A history of the patient's health habits and past illnesses and treatments will also be taken.

CT scan (CAT scan): A procedure that makes a series of detailed pictures of areas inside the body, taken from different angles. The pictures are made by a computer linked to an x-ray machine. A dye may be injected into a vein or swallowed to help the organs or tissues show up more clearly. This procedure is also called computed tomography, computerized tomography, or computerized axial tomography. A spiral or helical CT scan makes a series of very detailed pictures of areas inside the body using an x-ray machine that scans the body in a spiral path.

MRI (magnetic resonance imaging): A procedure that uses a magnet, radio waves, and a computer to make a series of detailed pictures of areas inside the body. This procedure is also called nuclear magnetic resonance imaging (NMRI).

PET scan (positron emission tomography scan): A procedure to find malignant tumor cells in the body. A small amount of radionuclide glucose (sugar) is injected into a vein. The PET scanner rotates around the body and makes a picture of where glucose is being used in the body. Malignant tumor cells show up brighter in the picture because they are more active and take up more glucose than normal cells do.

Endoscopic ultrasound (EUS): A procedure in which an endoscope is inserted into the body, usually through the mouth or rectum. An endoscope is a thin, tube-like instrument with a light and a lens for viewing. A probe at the end of the endoscope is used to bounce high-energy sound waves (ultrasound) off internal tissues or organs and make echoes. The echoes form a picture of body tissues called a sonogram. This procedure is also called endosonography.

Laparoscopy: A surgical procedure to look at the organs inside the abdomen to check for signs of disease. Small incisions (cuts) are made in the wall of the abdomen and a laparoscope (a thin, lighted tube) is inserted into one of the incisions. Other instruments may be inserted through the same or other incisions to perform procedures such as removing organs or taking tissue samples for biopsy.

Endoscopic retrograde cholangiopancreatography (ERCP): A procedure used to x-ray the ducts (tubes) that carry bile from the liver to the gallbladder and from the gallbladder to the small intestine. Sometimes pancreatic cancer causes these ducts to narrow and block or slow the flow of bile, causing jaundice. An endoscope (a thin, lighted tube) is passed through the mouth, esophagus, and stomach into the first part of the small intestine. A catheter (a smaller tube) is then inserted through the endoscope into the pancreatic ducts. A dye is injected through the catheter into the ducts and an x-ray is taken. If the ducts are blocked by a tumor, a fine tube may be inserted into the duct to unblock it. This tube (or stent) may be left in place to keep the duct open. Tissue samples may also be taken.

Percutaneous transhepatic cholangiography (PTC): A procedure used to x-ray the liver and bile ducts. A thin needle is inserted through the skin below the ribs and into the liver. Dye is injected into the liver or bile ducts and an x-ray is taken. If a blockage is found, a thin, flexible tube called a stent is sometimes left in the liver to drain bile into the small intestine or a collection bag outside the body. This test is done only if ERCP cannot be done.

Biopsy: The removal of cells or tissues so they can be viewed under a microscope by a pathologist to check for signs of cancer. There are several ways to do a biopsy for pancreatic cancer. A fine needle may be inserted into the pancreas during an x-ray or ultrasound to remove cells. Tissue may also be removed during a laparoscopy (a surgical incision made in the wall of the abdomen).

Prognosis

The prognosis (chance of recovery) and treatment options depend on whether or not the tumor can be removed by surgery, the stage of the cancer (the size of the tumor and whether the cancer has spread outside the pancreas to nearby tissues or lymph nodes or to other places in the body), the patient's general health, and whether the cancer has just been diagnosed or has recurred (come back).

Pancreatic cancer can be controlled only if it is found before it has spread, when it can be removed by surgery. If the cancer has spread, palliative treatment can improve the patient's quality of life by controlling the symptoms and complications of this disease.

Stages of Pancreatic Cancer

The following stages are used for pancreatic cancer:

Stage 0 (Carcinoma in Situ)

In stage 0, abnormal cells are found in the lining of the pancreas. These abnormal cells may become cancer and spread into nearby normal tissue. Stage 0 is also called carcinoma in situ.

Stage I

In stage I, cancer has formed and is found in the pancreas only. Stage I is divided into stage IA and stage IB, based on the size of the tumor.

- **Stage IA:** The tumor is two centimeters or smaller.
- **Stage IB:** The tumor is larger than two centimeters.

Stage II

In stage II, cancer may have spread to nearby tissue and organs, and may have spread to lymph nodes near the pancreas. Stage II is divided into stage IIA and stage IIB, based on where the cancer has spread.

- **Stage IIA:** Cancer has spread to nearby tissue and organs but has not spread to nearby lymph nodes.
- **Stage IIB:** Cancer has spread to nearby lymph nodes and may have spread to nearby tissue and organs.

Stage III

In stage III, cancer has spread to the major blood vessels near the pancreas and may have spread to nearby lymph nodes.

Stage IV

In stage IV, cancer may be of any size and has spread to distant organs, such as the liver, lung, and peritoneal cavity. It may have also spread to organs and tissues near the pancreas or to lymph nodes.

Recurrent Pancreatic Cancer

Recurrent pancreatic cancer is cancer that has recurred (come back) after it has been treated. The cancer may come back in the pancreas or in other parts of the body.

Treatment Option Overview

Different types of treatment are available for patients with pancreatic cancer. Some treatments are standard (the currently used treatment), and some are being tested in clinical trials. Three types of standard treatment are used: surgery, radiation therapy, and chemotherapy.

Surgery

One of the following types of surgery may be used to take out the tumor:

- **Whipple procedure:** A surgical procedure in which the head of the pancreas, the gallbladder, part of the stomach, part of the small intestine, and the bile duct are removed. Enough of the pancreas is left to produce digestive juices and insulin.

- **Total pancreatectomy:** This operation removes the whole pancreas, part of the stomach, part of the small intestine, the common bile duct, the gallbladder, the spleen, and nearby lymph nodes.

- **Distal pancreatectomy:** The body and the tail of the pancreas and usually the spleen are removed.

If the cancer has spread and cannot be removed, the following types of palliative surgery may be done to relieve symptoms:

- **Surgical biliary bypass:** If cancer is blocking the small intestine and bile is building up in the gallbladder, a biliary bypass may be done. During this operation, the doctor will cut the gallbladder or bile duct and sew it to the small intestine to create a new pathway around the blocked area.

- **Endoscopic stent placement:** If the tumor is blocking the bile duct, surgery may be done to put in a stent (a thin tube) to drain bile that has built up in the area. The doctor may place the stent through a catheter that drains to the outside of the body or the stent may go around the blocked area and drain the bile into the small intestine.

- **Gastric bypass:** If the tumor is blocking the flow of food from the stomach, the stomach may be sewn directly to the small intestine so the patient can continue to eat normally.

Radiation Therapy

Radiation therapy is a cancer treatment that uses high-energy x-rays or other types of radiation to kill cancer cells or keep them from growing. There are two types of radiation therapy. External radiation therapy uses a machine outside the body to send radiation toward the cancer. Internal radiation therapy uses a radioactive substance sealed in needles, seeds, wires, or catheters that are placed directly into or near the cancer. The way the radiation therapy is given depends on the type and stage of the cancer being treated.

Chemotherapy

Chemotherapy is a cancer treatment that uses drugs to stop the growth of cancer cells, either by killing the cells or by stopping them from dividing. When chemotherapy is taken by mouth or injected into a vein or muscle, the drugs enter the bloodstream and can reach cancer cells throughout the body (systemic chemotherapy). When chemotherapy is placed directly into the cerebrospinal fluid, an organ, or a body cavity such as the abdomen, the drugs mainly affect cancer cells in those areas (regional chemotherapy). The way the chemotherapy is given depends on the type and stage of the cancer being treated.

Treating Pain

Pain can occur when the tumor presses on nerves or other organs near the pancreas. When pain medicine is not enough, there are treatments that act on nerves in the abdomen to relieve the pain. The doctor may inject medicine into the area around affected nerves or may cut the nerves to block the feeling of pain. Radiation therapy with or without chemotherapy can also help relieve pain by shrinking the tumor.

Nutritional Needs

Surgery to remove the pancreas may interfere with the production of pancreatic enzymes that help to digest food. As a result, patients may have problems digesting food and absorbing nutrients into the body. To prevent malnutrition, the doctor may prescribe medicines that replace these enzymes.

Clinical Trials

A treatment clinical trial is a research study meant to help improve current treatments or obtain information on new treatments for patients with cancer. When clinical trials show that a new treatment is better than the standard treatment, the new treatment may become the standard treatment. Patients may want to think about taking part in a clinical trial. Some clinical trials are open only to patients who have not started treatment.

Biologic therapy is a treatment that uses the patient's immune system to fight cancer. Substances made by the body or made in a laboratory are used to boost, direct, or restore the body's natural defenses against cancer. This type of cancer treatment is also called biotherapy or immunotherapy.

There may be other treatments that are being studied in clinical trials. Information about clinical trials is available from the NCI website (www.cancer.gov).

Follow-Up Tests

Some of the tests that were done to diagnose the cancer or to find out the stage of the cancer may be repeated. Some tests will be repeated in order to see how well the treatment is working. Decisions about whether to continue, change, or stop treatment may be based on the results of these tests. This is sometimes called re-staging.

Some of the tests will continue to be done from time to time after treatment has ended. The results of these tests can show if your condition has changed or if the cancer has recurred (come back). These tests are sometimes called follow-up tests or check-ups.

Chapter 30

Liver Cancer

The Liver

The liver is the largest organ inside your abdomen. It's found behind your ribs on the right side of your body. The liver does important work to keep you healthy:

- It removes harmful substances from the blood.
- It makes enzymes and bile that help digest food.
- It also converts food into substances needed for life and growth.

The liver gets its supply of blood from two vessels. Most of its blood comes from the hepatic portal vein. The rest comes from the hepatic artery.

Most primary liver cancers begin in hepatocytes (liver cells). This type of cancer is called hepatocellular carcinoma or malignant hepatoma.

Liver cancer cells can spread by breaking away from the original tumor. They mainly spread by entering blood vessels, but liver cancer cells can also be found in lymph nodes. The cancer cells may attach to other tissues and grow to form new tumors that may damage those tissues.

Risk Factors

When you get a diagnosis of cancer, it's natural to wonder what may have caused the disease. Doctors can't always explain why one

Excerpted from, "What You Need to Know about Liver Cancer," National Cancer Institute (www.cancer.gov), April 2009.

person gets liver cancer and another doesn't. However, we do know that people with certain risk factors may be more likely than others to develop liver cancer. A risk factor is something that may increase the chance of getting a disease.

The more risk factors a person has, the greater the chance that liver cancer will develop. However, many people with known risk factors for liver cancer don't develop the disease. Studies have found the following risk factors for liver cancer:

Hepatitis: Liver cancer can develop after many years of infection with hepatitis B virus (HBV) or hepatitis C virus (HCV). Around the world, infection with HBV or HCV is the main cause of liver cancer. HBV and HCV can be passed from person to person through blood (such as by sharing needles) or sexual contact. An infant may catch these viruses from an infected mother. Although HBV and HCV infections are contagious diseases, liver cancer is not. You can't catch liver cancer from another person. HBV and HCV infections may not cause symptoms, but blood tests can show whether either virus is present. If so, the doctor may suggest treatment. Also, the doctor may discuss ways to avoid infecting other people. In people who are not already infected with HBV, hepatitis B vaccine can prevent HBV infection. Researchers are working to develop a vaccine to prevent HCV infection.

Heavy alcohol use: Having more than two drinks of alcohol each day for many years increases the risk of liver cancer and certain other cancers. The risk increases with the amount of alcohol that a person drinks.

Aflatoxin: Liver cancer can be caused by aflatoxin, a harmful substance made by certain types of mold. Aflatoxin can form on peanuts, corn, and other nuts and grains. In parts of Asia and Africa, levels of aflatoxin are high. However, the United States has safety measures limiting aflatoxin in the food supply.

Iron storage disease: Liver cancer may develop among people with a disease that causes the body to store too much iron in the liver and other organs.

Cirrhosis: Cirrhosis is a serious disease that develops when liver cells are damaged and replaced with scar tissue. Many exposures cause cirrhosis, including HBV or HCV infection, heavy alcohol use, too much iron stored in the liver, certain drugs, and certain parasites. Almost all cases of liver cancer in the United States occur in people who first had cirrhosis, usually resulting from hepatitis B or C infection, or from heavy alcohol use.

Obesity and diabetes: Studies have shown that obesity and diabetes may be important risk factors for liver cancer.

Symptoms

Early liver cancer often doesn't cause symptoms. When the cancer grows larger, people may notice one or more of these common symptoms:

- Pain in the upper abdomen on the right side
- A lump or a feeling of heaviness in the upper abdomen
- Swollen abdomen (bloating)
- Loss of appetite and feelings of fullness
- Weight loss
- Weakness or feeling very tired
- Nausea and vomiting
- Yellow skin and eyes, pale stools, and dark urine from jaundice
- Fever

These symptoms may be caused by liver cancer or other health problems. If you have any of these symptoms, you should tell your doctor so that problems can be diagnosed and treated as early as possible.

Diagnosis

If you have symptoms that suggest liver cancer, your doctor will try to find out what's causing the problems. You may have one or more of the following tests:

Physical exam: Your doctor feels your abdomen to check the liver, spleen, and other nearby organs for any lumps or changes in their shape or size. Your doctor also checks for ascites, an abnormal buildup of fluid in the abdomen. Also, your skin and eyes may be checked for signs of jaundice.

Blood tests: Many blood tests may be used to check for liver problems. One blood test detects alpha-fetoprotein (AFP). High AFP levels could be a sign of liver cancer. Other blood tests can show how well the liver is working.

CT scan: An x-ray machine linked to a computer takes a series of detailed pictures of your liver and other organs and blood vessels in your abdomen. You may receive an injection of contrast material so that your liver shows up clearly in the pictures. On the CT scan, your doctor may see tumors in the liver or elsewhere in the abdomen.

MRI: A large machine with a strong magnet linked to a computer is used to make detailed pictures of areas inside your body. Sometimes contrast material makes abnormal areas show up more clearly on the picture.

Ultrasound test: The ultrasound device uses sound waves that can't be heard by humans. The sound waves produce a pattern of echoes as they bounce off internal organs. The echoes create a picture (sonogram) of your liver and other organs in the abdomen. Tumors may produce echoes that are different from the echoes made by healthy tissues.

Biopsy

A biopsy usually is not needed to diagnose liver cancer, but in some cases, the doctor may remove a sample of tissue. A pathologist uses a microscope to look for cancer cells in the tissue. The doctor may obtain tissue in one of several ways:

- **A needle through the skin:** The doctor inserts a thin needle into the liver to remove a small amount of tissue. CT or ultrasound may be used to guide the needle.

- **Laparoscopic surgery:** The surgeon makes a few small incisions in your abdomen. A thin, lighted tube (laparoscope) is inserted through the incision. The laparoscope has a tool to remove tissue from the liver.

- **Open surgery:** The surgeon can remove tissue from the liver through a large incision.

You may want to ask the doctor these questions before having a biopsy:

- How will the biopsy results affect my treatment plan?

- What kind of biopsy will I have?

- How long will it take? Will I be awake? Will it hurt?

- Is there a risk that a needle biopsy procedure will cause the cancer to spread? What are the chances of infection or bleeding after the biopsy? Are there any other risks?

- How soon will I know the results? How do I get a copy of the pathology report?

- If I do have cancer, who will talk with me about treatment? When?

Staging

If liver cancer is diagnosed, your doctor needs to learn the extent (stage) of the disease to help you choose the best treatment. Staging is an attempt to find out whether the cancer has spread, and if so, to what parts of the body.

When liver cancer spreads, the cancer cells may be found in the lungs. Cancer cells also may be found in the bones and in lymph nodes near the liver.

When cancer spreads from its original place to another part of the body, the new tumor has the same kind of abnormal cells and the same name as the primary tumor. For example, if liver cancer spreads to the bones, the cancer cells in the bones are actually liver cancer cells. The disease is metastatic liver cancer, not bone cancer. It's treated as liver cancer, not bone cancer. Doctors sometimes call the new tumor "distant" or metastatic disease.

To learn whether the liver cancer has spread, your doctor may order one or more of the following tests:

CT scan of the chest: A CT scan often can show whether liver cancer has spread to the lungs.

Bone scan: The doctor injects a small amount of a radioactive substance into your blood vessel. It travels through the bloodstream and collects in the bones. A machine called a scanner detects and measures the radiation. The scanner makes pictures of the bones. The pictures may show cancer that has spread to the bones.

PET scan: You receive an injection of a small amount of radioactive sugar. The radioactive sugar gives off signals that the PET scanner picks up. The PET scanner makes a picture of the places in your body where the sugar is being taken up. Cancer cells show up brighter in the picture because they take up sugar faster than normal cells do. A PET scan shows whether liver cancer may have spread.

Treatment Overview

Treatment options for people with liver cancer are surgery (including a liver transplant), ablation, embolization, targeted therapy, radiation therapy, and chemotherapy. You may have a combination of treatments.

The treatment that's right for you depends mainly on the number, size, and location of tumors in your liver; how well your liver is working and whether you have cirrhosis; and whether the cancer has spread outside your liver. Other factors to consider include your age, general health, and concerns about the treatments and their possible side effects.

At this time, liver cancer can be cured only when it's found at an early stage (before it has spread) and only if people are healthy enough to have surgery. For people who can't have surgery, other treatments may be able to help them live longer and feel better. Many doctors encourage people with liver cancer to consider taking part in a clinical trial. Clinical trials are research studies testing new treatments. They are an important option for people with all stages of liver cancer.

Your doctor may refer you to a specialist, or you may ask for a referral. Specialists who treat liver cancer include surgeons (especially hepatobiliary surgeons, surgical oncologists, and transplant surgeons), gastroenterologists, medical oncologists, and radiation oncologists. Your health care team may also include an oncology nurse and a registered dietitian.

Your health care team can describe your treatment choices, the expected results of each, and the possible side effects. Because cancer therapy often damages healthy cells and tissues, side effects are common. Before treatment starts, ask your health care team about possible side effects and how treatment may change your normal activities. You and your health care team can work together to develop a treatment plan that meets your needs.

Liver Surgeries and Other Therapies

Surgery is an option for people with an early stage of liver cancer. The surgeon may remove the whole liver or only the part that has cancer. If the whole liver is removed, it's replaced with healthy liver tissue from a donor. You and your surgeon can talk about the types of surgery and which may be right for you.

Removal of Part of the Liver

Surgery to remove part of the liver is called partial hepatectomy. A person with liver cancer may have part of the liver removed if lab tests show that the liver is working well and if there is no evidence that the cancer has spread to nearby lymph nodes or to other parts of the body.

The surgeon removes the tumor along with a margin of normal liver tissue around the tumor. The extent of the surgery depends on the size, number, and location of the tumors. It also depends on how well the liver is working.

As much as 80% of the liver may be removed. The surgeon leaves behind normal liver tissue. The remaining healthy tissue takes over the work of the liver. Also, the liver can regrow the missing part. The new cells grow over several weeks.

It takes time to heal after surgery, and the time needed to recover is different for each person. You may have pain or discomfort for the first few days. Medicine can help control your pain. Before surgery, you should discuss the plan for pain relief with your doctor or nurse. After surgery, your doctor can adjust the plan if you need more pain control.

It's common to feel tired or weak for a while. Also, you may have diarrhea and a feeling of fullness in the abdomen.

The health care team will watch you for signs of bleeding, infection, liver failure, or other problems.

Liver Transplant

A liver transplant is an option if the tumors are small, the disease has not spread outside the liver, and suitable donated liver tissue can be found.

Donated liver tissue comes from a deceased person or a live donor. If the donor is living, the tissue is part of a liver, rather than a whole liver.

While you wait for donated liver tissue to become available, the health care team monitors your health and provides other treatments.

When healthy liver tissue from a donor is available, the transplant surgeon removes your entire liver (total hepatectomy) and replaces it with the donated tissue. After surgery, your health care team will give you medicine to help control your pain. You may need to stay in the hospital for several weeks. During that time, your health care team monitors how well your body is accepting the new liver tissue. You'll take medicine to prevent your body's immune system from rejecting the new liver. These drugs may cause puffiness in your face, high blood pressure, or an increase in body hair.

Ablation

Methods of ablation destroy the cancer in the liver. They are treatments to control liver cancer and extend life. They may be used for people waiting for a liver transplant. Or they may be used for people who can't have surgery or a liver transplant. Surgery to remove the tumor may not be possible because of cirrhosis or other conditions that cause poor liver function, the location of the tumor within the liver, or other health problems.

Methods of ablation include the following:

Radiofrequency ablation: The doctor uses a special probe that contains tiny electrodes to kill the cancer cells with heat. Ultrasound, CT, or MRI may be used to guide the probe to the tumor. Usually, the doctor can insert the probe directly through your skin, and only local anesthesia is needed.

Sometimes, surgery under general anesthesia is needed. The doctor inserts the probe through a small incision in your abdomen (using a laparoscope) or through a wider incision that opens your abdomen.

Some people have pain or a slight fever after this procedure. Staying overnight in the hospital is not usually needed.

Radiofrequency ablation is a type of hyperthermia therapy. Other therapies that use heat to destroy liver tumors include laser or microwave therapy. They are used less often than radiofrequency ablation.

Percutaneous ethanol injection: The doctor uses ultrasound to guide a thin needle into the liver tumor. Alcohol (ethanol) is injected directly into the tumor and kills cancer cells. The procedure may be performed once or twice a week. Usually local anesthesia is used, but if you have many tumors in the liver, general anesthesia may be needed.

You may have fever and pain after the injection. Your doctor can suggest medicines to relieve these problems.

Embolization

For those who can't have surgery or a liver transplant, embolization or chemoembolization may be an option. The doctor inserts a tiny catheter into an artery in your leg and moves the catheter into the hepatic artery. For embolization, the doctor injects tiny sponges or other particles into the catheter. The particles block the flow of blood through the artery. Depending on the type of particles used, the blockage may be temporary or permanent.

Without blood flow from the hepatic artery, the tumor dies. Although the hepatic artery is blocked, healthy liver tissue continues to receive blood from the hepatic portal vein.

For chemoembolization, the doctor injects an anticancer drug (chemotherapy) into the artery before injecting the tiny particles that block blood flow. Without blood flow, the drug stays in the liver longer. You'll need to be sedated for this procedure, but general anesthesia is not usually needed. You'll probably stay in the hospital for two to three days after the treatment.

Embolization often causes abdominal pain, nausea, vomiting, and fever. Your doctor can give you medicine to help lessen these problems. Some people may feel very tired for several weeks after the treatment.

Targeted Therapy

People with liver cancer who can't have surgery or a liver transplant may receive a drug called targeted therapy. Sorafenib (Nexavar) tablets were the first targeted therapy approved for liver cancer.

Targeted therapy slows the growth of liver tumors. It also reduces their blood supply. The drug is taken by mouth.

Side effects include nausea, vomiting, mouth sores, and loss of appetite. Sometimes, a person may have chest pain, bleeding problems, or blisters on the hands or feet. The drug can also cause high blood pressure. The health care team will check your blood pressure often during the first six weeks of treatment.

Radiation Therapy

Radiation therapy uses high-energy rays to kill cancer cells. It may be an option for a few people who can't have surgery. Sometimes it's used with other approaches. Radiation therapy also may be used to help relieve pain from liver cancer that has spread to the bones.

Doctors use two types of radiation therapy to treat liver cancer:

- External radiation therapy: The radiation comes from a large machine. The machine aims beams of radiation at the chest and abdomen.

- Internal radiation therapy: The radiation comes from tiny radioactive spheres. A doctor uses a catheter to inject the tiny spheres into your hepatic artery. The spheres destroy the blood supply to the liver tumor.

The side effects from radiation therapy include nausea, vomiting, or diarrhea. Your health care team can suggest ways to treat or control the side effects.

Chemotherapy

Chemotherapy, the use of drugs to kill cancer cells, is sometimes used to treat liver cancer. Drugs are usually given by vein (intravenous). The drugs enter the bloodstream and travel throughout your body.

Chemotherapy may be given in an outpatient part of the hospital, at the doctor's office, or at home. Rarely, you may need to stay in the hospital.

The side effects of chemotherapy depend mainly on which drugs are given and how much. Common side effects include nausea and vomiting, loss of appetite, headache, fever and chills, and weakness.

Some drugs lower the levels of healthy blood cells, and you're more likely to get infections, bruise or bleed easily, and feel very weak and tired. Your health care team will check for low levels of blood cells. Some side effects may be relieved with medicine.

Second Opinion

Before starting treatment, you may want a second opinion about your diagnosis, the stage of cancer, and the treatment plan. You may also want to find a medical center that has a lot of experience with treating people with liver cancer. You may even want to talk to several different doctors about all of the treatment options, their side effects, and the expected results. For example, you could discuss your treatment plan with a hepatobiliary surgeon, radiation oncologist, and medical oncologist.

Some people worry that the doctor will be offended if they ask for a second opinion. Usually the opposite is true. Most doctors welcome a second opinion. And many health insurance companies will pay for a second opinion if you or your doctor requests it. Some companies require a second opinion.

If you get a second opinion, the second doctor may agree with your first doctor's diagnosis and treatment plan. Or the second doctor may suggest another approach. Either way, you have more information and perhaps a greater sense of control. You can feel more confident about the decisions you make, knowing that you've looked at your options.

It may take some time and effort to gather your medical records and see another doctor. In most cases, it's not a problem to take several weeks to get a second opinion. The delay in starting treatment usually will not make treatment less effective. To make sure, you should discuss this delay with your doctor.

There are many ways to find a doctor for a second opinion. You can ask your doctor, a local or state medical society, a nearby hospital, or a medical school for names of specialists. Also, you can request a consultation with specialists at the National Institutes of Health Clinical Center in Bethesda, Maryland. Specialists in the NCI Surgery Branch provide consultations and surgical care for people with liver cancer. The telephone number is 301-496-4164. The website is located at http://ccr.cancer.gov/labs/lab.asp?labid=93.

The NCI Cancer Information Service at 800-4-CANCER (800-422-6237) can tell you about nearby treatment centers.

Supportive Care

Supportive care is treatment to control pain and other symptoms, to relieve the side effects of therapy, and to help you cope with the feelings that a diagnosis of cancer can bring. You may receive supportive care to prevent or control these problems and to improve your comfort and quality of life during treatment.

Pain Control

Liver cancer and its treatment may lead to pain. Your doctor or a specialist in pain control can suggest several ways to relieve or reduce pain:

- **Pain medicine:** Medicines often can relieve pain. (These medicines may make people drowsy and constipated, but resting and taking laxatives can help.)

- **Radiation therapy:** Radiation therapy can help relieve pain by shrinking the cancer.

- **Nerve block:** The doctor may inject alcohol into the area around certain nerves in the abdomen to block the pain.

The health care team may suggest other ways to relieve or reduce pain. For example, massage, acupuncture, or acupressure may be used along with other approaches. Also, you may learn to relieve pain through relaxation techniques such as listening to slow music or breathing slowly and comfortably.

Sadness and Other Feelings

It's normal to feel sad, anxious, or confused after a diagnosis of a serious illness. Some people find it helpful to talk about their feelings.

Nutrition

It's important to meet your nutrition needs before, during, and after cancer treatment. You need the right amount of calories, protein, vitamins, and minerals. Getting the right nutrition can help you feel better and have more energy.

However, you may be uncomfortable or tired, and you may not feel like eating. You also may have side effects of treatment such as poor appetite, nausea, vomiting, or diarrhea. Your doctor, a registered dietitian, or another health care provider can advise you about ways to have a healthy diet.

Careful planning and checkups are important. Liver cancer and its treatment may make it hard for you to digest food and maintain your weight. Your doctor will check you for weight loss, weakness, and lack of energy.

Follow-Up Care

You'll need regular checkups (such as every three months) after treatment for liver cancer. Checkups help ensure that any changes in your health are noted and treated if needed. If you have any health problems between checkups, you should contact your doctor.

Sometimes liver cancer comes back after treatment. Your doctor will check for return of cancer. Checkups may include a physical exam, blood tests, ultrasound, CT scans, or other tests.

For people who have had a liver transplant, the doctor will test how well the new liver is working. The doctor also will watch you closely to make sure the new liver isn't being rejected. People who have had a liver transplant may want to discuss with the doctor the type and schedule of follow-up tests that will be needed.

Chapter 31

Extrahepatic
Bile Duct Cancer

General Information about Extrahepatic Bile Duct Cancer

Extrahepatic bile duct cancer is a rare disease in which malignant (cancer) cells form in the part of bile duct that is outside the liver.

A network of bile ducts (tubes) connects the liver and the gallbladder to the small intestine. This network begins in the liver where many small ducts collect bile, a fluid made by the liver to break down fats during digestion. The small ducts come together to form the right and left hepatic bile ducts, which lead out of the liver. The two ducts join outside the liver to become the common hepatic duct. The part of the common hepatic duct that is outside the liver is called the extrahepatic bile duct. The extrahepatic bile duct is joined by a duct from the gallbladder (which stores bile) to form the common bile duct. Bile is released from the gallbladder through the common bile duct into the small intestine when food is being digested.

Risk Factors and Signs

Anything that increases your risk of getting a disease is called a risk factor. Having a risk factor does not mean that you will get cancer; not having risk factors doesn't mean that you will not get cancer. People who think they may be at risk should discuss this with their doctor. Risk factors include having any of the following disorders:

Excerpted from PDQ® Cancer Information Summary. National Cancer Institute; Bethesda, MD. "Extrahepatic Bile Duct Cancer Treatment (PDQ) - Patient Version." Updated 04/2010. Available at: http://cancer.gov. Accessed June 21, 2010.

- Primary sclerosing cholangitis
- Chronic ulcerative colitis
- Choledochal cysts
- Infection with a Chinese liver fluke parasite

Possible signs of extrahepatic bile duct cancer include jaundice and pain. These and other symptoms may be caused by extrahepatic bile duct cancer or by other conditions. A doctor should be consulted if any of the following problems occur:

- Jaundice (yellowing of the skin or whites of the eyes)
- Pain in the abdomen
- Fever
- Itchy skin

Detection and Diagnosis

Tests that examine the bile duct and liver are used to detect (find) and diagnose extrahepatic bile duct cancer. The following tests and procedures may be used:

Physical exam and history: An exam of the body to check general signs of health, including checking for signs of disease, such as lumps or anything else that seems unusual. A history of the patient's health habits and past illnesses and treatments will also be taken.

Ultrasound exam: A procedure in which high-energy sound waves (ultrasound) are bounced off internal tissues or organs and make echoes. The echoes form a picture of body tissues called a sonogram. The picture can be printed to be looked at later.

CT scan (CAT scan): A procedure that makes a series of detailed pictures of areas inside the body, taken from different angles. The pictures are made by a computer linked to an x-ray machine. A dye may be injected into a vein or swallowed to help the organs or tissues show up more clearly. This procedure is also called computed tomography, computerized tomography, or computerized axial tomography. A spiral or helical CT scan makes detailed pictures of areas inside the body using an x-ray machine that scans the body in a spiral path.

MRI (magnetic resonance imaging): A procedure that uses a magnet, radio waves, and a computer to make a series of detailed pictures of areas inside the body. This procedure is also called nuclear magnetic resonance imaging (NMRI).

ERCP (endoscopic retrograde cholangiopancreatography): A procedure used to x-ray the ducts (tubes) that carry bile from the liver to the gallbladder and from the gallbladder to the small intestine. Sometimes bile duct cancer causes these ducts to narrow and block or slow the flow of bile, causing jaundice. An endoscope is passed through the mouth, esophagus, and stomach into the first part of the small intestine. An endoscope is a thin, tube-like instrument with a light and a lens for viewing. A catheter (a smaller tube) is then inserted through the endoscope into the pancreatic ducts. A dye is injected through the catheter into the ducts and an x-ray is taken. If the ducts are blocked by a tumor, a fine tube may be inserted into the duct to unblock it. This tube (or stent) may be left in place to keep the duct open. Tissue samples may also be taken and checked under a microscope for signs of cancer.

PTC (percutaneous transhepatic cholangiography): A procedure used to x-ray the liver and bile ducts. A thin needle is inserted through the skin below the ribs and into the liver. Dye is injected into the liver or bile ducts and an x-ray is taken. If a blockage is found, a thin, flexible tube called a stent is sometimes left in the liver to drain bile into the small intestine or a collection bag outside the body.

Biopsy: The removal of cells or tissues so they can be viewed under a microscope to check for signs of cancer. The sample may be taken using a thin needle inserted into the duct during an x-ray or ultrasound. This is called a fine-needle aspiration (FNA) biopsy. The biopsy is usually done during PTC or ERCP. Tissue may also be removed during surgery.

Liver function tests: A procedure in which a blood sample is checked to measure the amounts of certain substances released into the blood by the liver. A higher than normal amount of a substance can be a sign of liver disease that may be caused by extrahepatic bile duct cancer.

Prognosis

Certain factors affect prognosis (chance of recovery) and treatment options. The prognosis and treatment options depend on the following:

- The stage of the cancer (whether it affects only the bile duct or has spread to other places in the body)

- Whether the tumor can be completely removed by surgery

- Whether the tumor is in the upper or lower part of the duct

- Whether the cancer has just been diagnosed or has recurred (come back)

Treatment options may also depend on the symptoms caused by the tumor. Extrahepatic bile duct cancer is usually found after it has spread and can rarely be removed completely by surgery. Palliative therapy may relieve symptoms and improve the patient's quality of life.

Stages of Extrahepatic Bile Duct Cancer

After extrahepatic bile duct cancer has been diagnosed, tests are done to find out if cancer cells have spread within the bile duct or to other parts of the body. The process used to find out if cancer has spread within the extrahepatic bile duct or to other parts of the body is called staging. The information gathered from the staging process determines the stage of the disease. It is important to know the stage in order to plan treatment.

Extrahepatic bile duct cancer is usually staged following a laparotomy. A surgical incision is made in the wall of the abdomen to check the inside of the abdomen for signs of disease and to remove tissue and fluid for examination under a microscope. The results of the diagnostic imaging tests, laparotomy, and biopsy are viewed together to determine the stage of the cancer. Sometimes, a laparoscopy will be done before the laparotomy to see if the cancer has spread. If the cancer has spread and cannot be removed by surgery, the surgeon may decide not to do a laparotomy.

Stage 0 (Carcinoma in Situ)

In stage 0, abnormal cells are found in the innermost layer of tissue lining the extrahepatic bile duct. These abnormal cells may become cancer and spread into nearby normal tissue. Stage 0 is also called carcinoma in situ.

Stage I

In stage I, cancer has formed. Stage I is divided into stage IA and stage IB.

Stage IA: Cancer is found in the bile duct only.

Stage IB: Cancer has spread through the wall of the bile duct.

Stage II

Stage II is divided into stage IIA and stage IIB.

Stage IIA: Cancer has spread to the liver, gallbladder, pancreas, and/or to either the right or left branch of the hepatic artery or to the right or left branch of the portal vein.

Stage IIB: Cancer has spread to nearby lymph nodes and:

- is found in the bile duct; or

- has spread through the wall of the bile duct; or

- has spread to the liver, gallbladder, pancreas, and/or the right or left branches of the hepatic artery or portal vein.

Stage III

In stage III, cancer has spread:

- to the main portal vein or to both right and left branches of the portal vein; or

- to the hepatic artery; or

- to other nearby organs or tissues, such as the colon, stomach, small intestine, or abdominal wall.

Cancer may have spread to nearby lymph nodes also.

Stage IV

In stage IV, cancer has spread to lymph nodes and/or organs far away from the extrahepatic bile duct.

Treatment Groups

Extrahepatic bile duct cancer can also be grouped according to how the cancer may be treated. There are two treatment groups:

Localized (and resectable): The cancer is in an area where it can be removed completely by surgery.

Unresectable: The cancer cannot be removed completely by surgery. The cancer may have spread to nearby blood vessels, the liver, the common bile duct, nearby lymph nodes, or other parts of the abdominal cavity.

Recurrent Extrahepatic Bile Duct Cancer

Recurrent extrahepatic bile duct cancer is cancer that has recurred (come back) after it has been treated. The cancer may come back in the bile duct or in other parts of the body.

Treatment Option Overview

Different types of treatment are available for patients with extra-hepatic bile duct cancer. Some treatments are standard (the currently used treatment), and some are being tested in clinical trials.

Surgery

The following types of surgery are used to treat extrahepatic bile duct cancer:

Removal of the bile duct: If the tumor is small and only in the bile duct, the entire bile duct may be removed. A new duct is made by connecting the duct openings in the liver to the intestine. Lymph nodes are removed and viewed under a microscope to see if they contain cancer.

Partial hepatectomy: Removal of the part of the liver where cancer is found. The part removed may be a wedge of tissue, an entire lobe, or a larger part of the liver, along with some normal tissue around it.

Whipple procedure: A surgical procedure in which the head of the pancreas, the gallbladder, part of the stomach, part of the small intestine, and the bile duct are removed. Enough of the pancreas is left to make digestive juices and insulin.

Surgical biliary bypass: If the tumor cannot be removed but is blocking the small intestine and causing bile to build up in the gallbladder, a biliary bypass may be done. During this operation, the gallbladder or bile duct will be cut and sewn to the small intestine to create a new pathway around the blocked area. This procedure helps to relieve jaundice caused by the build-up of bile.

Stent placement: If the tumor is blocking the bile duct, a stent (a thin tube) may be placed in the duct to drain bile that has built up in the area. The stent may drain to the outside of the body or it may go around the blocked area and drain the bile into the small intestine. The doctor may place the stent during surgery or PTC, or with an endoscope.

Radiation Therapy

Radiation therapy is a cancer treatment that uses high-energy x-rays or other types of radiation to kill cancer cells or keep them from growing. There are two types of radiation therapy. External radiation therapy uses a machine outside the body to send radiation toward the cancer. Internal radiation therapy uses a radioactive substance sealed in needles, seeds, wires, or catheters that are placed directly into or near the cancer. The way the radiation therapy is given depends on the type and stage of the cancer being treated.

Clinical Trials

A treatment clinical trial is a research study meant to help improve current treatments or obtain information on new treatments for patients with cancer. When clinical trials show that a new treatment is better than the standard treatment, the new treatment may become the standard treatment. Patients may want to think about taking part in a clinical trial. Some clinical trials are open only to patients who have not started treatment.

New types of treatment are being tested in clinical trials. This summary section describes treatments that are being studied in clinical trials. It may not mention every new treatment being studied.

Radiation Sensitizers

Clinical trials are studying ways to improve the effect of radiation therapy on tumor cells, including the following:

Hyperthermia therapy: A treatment in which body tissue is exposed to high temperatures to damage and kill cancer cells or to make cancer cells more sensitive to the effects of radiation therapy and certain anticancer drugs.

Radiosensitizers: Drugs that make tumor cells more sensitive to radiation therapy. Combining radiation therapy with radiosensitizers may kill more tumor cells.

Chemotherapy

Chemotherapy is a cancer treatment that uses drugs to stop the growth of cancer cells, either by killing the cells or by stopping them from dividing. When chemotherapy is taken by mouth or injected into a vein or muscle, the drugs enter the bloodstream and can reach cancer cells throughout the body (systemic chemotherapy). When chemotherapy is placed directly into the spinal column, an organ, or a body cavity such as the abdomen, the drugs mainly affect cancer cells in those areas (regional chemotherapy). The way the chemotherapy is given depends on the type and stage of the cancer being treated.

Biologic Therapy

Biologic therapy is a treatment that uses the patient's immune system to fight cancer. Substances made by the body or made in a laboratory are used to boost, direct, or restore the body's natural defenses against cancer. This type of cancer treatment is also called biotherapy or immunotherapy.

Follow-Up Tests

Some of the tests that were done to diagnose the cancer or to find out the stage of the cancer may be repeated. Some tests will be repeated in order to see how well the treatment is working. Decisions about whether to continue, change, or stop treatment may be based on the results of these tests. This is sometimes called re-staging.

Some of the tests will continue to be done from time to time after treatment has ended. The results of these tests can show if your condition has changed or if the cancer has recurred (come back). These tests are sometimes called follow-up tests or check-ups.

Chapter 32

Gastrointestinal Carcinoid Tumors

General Information about Gastrointestinal Carcinoid Tumors

A gastrointestinal carcinoid tumor is cancer that forms in the lining of the gastrointestinal tract. The gastrointestinal tract includes the stomach, small intestine, and large intestine. These organs are part of the digestive system, which processes nutrients (vitamins, minerals, carbohydrates, fats, proteins, and water) in foods that are eaten and helps pass waste material out of the body.

Gastrointestinal carcinoid tumors develop from a certain type of hormone-making cell in the lining of the gastrointestinal tract. These cells produce hormones that help regulate digestive juices and the muscles used in moving food through the stomach and intestines. A gastrointestinal carcinoid tumor may also produce hormones. Carcinoid tumors that start in the rectum (the last several inches of the large intestine) usually do not produce hormones.

Gastrointestinal carcinoid tumors grow slowly. Most of them occur in the appendix (an organ attached to the large intestine), small intestine, and rectum. It is common for more than one tumor to develop in the small intestine. Having a carcinoid tumor increases a person's chance of getting other cancers in the digestive system, either at the same time or later.

Excerpted from PDQ® Cancer Information Summary. National Cancer Institute; Bethesda, MD. "Gastrointestinal Carcinoid Tumors Treatment (PDQ) - Patient Version." Updated 06/2008. Available at: http://cancer.gov. Accessed January 20, 2010.

Risk Factors and Signs

Risk factors include having a family history of multiple endocrine neoplasia type 1 (MEN1) syndrome or having certain conditions that affect the stomach's ability to produce stomach acid, such as atrophic gastritis, pernicious anemia, or Zollinger-Ellison syndrome. Smoking tobacco is also a risk factor.

A gastrointestinal carcinoid tumor often has no signs in its early stages. Carcinoid syndrome may occur if the tumor spreads to the liver or other parts of the body.

The hormones produced by gastrointestinal carcinoid tumors are usually destroyed by blood and liver enzymes. If the tumor has spread to the liver, however, high amounts of these hormones may remain in the body and cause the following group of symptoms, called carcinoid syndrome:

- Redness or a feeling of warmth in the face and neck
- Diarrhea
- Shortness of breath, fast heartbeat, tiredness, or swelling of the feet and ankles
- Wheezing
- Pain or a feeling of fullness in the abdomen

These symptoms and others may be caused by gastrointestinal carcinoid tumors or by other conditions. A doctor should be consulted if any of these symptoms occur.

Detection and Diagnosis

The following tests and procedures may be used to detect (find) and diagnose gastrointestinal carcinoid tumors:

Complete blood count: A procedure in which a sample of blood is drawn and checked for the following:

- The number of red blood cells, white blood cells, and platelets
- The amount of hemoglobin (the protein that carries oxygen) in the red blood cells
- The portion of the sample made up of red blood cells

Physical exam and history: An exam of the body to check general signs of health, including checking for signs of disease, such as lumps or anything else that seems unusual. A history of the patient's health habits and past illnesses and treatments will also be taken.

Blood chemistry studies: A procedure in which a blood sample is checked to measure the amounts of certain substances, such as hormones, released into the blood by organs and tissues in the body. An unusual (higher or lower than normal) amount of a substance can be a sign of disease in the organ or tissue that produces it. The blood sample is checked to see if it contains a hormone produced by carcinoid tumors. This test is used to help diagnose carcinoid syndrome.

Twenty-four-hour urine test: A test in which a urine sample is checked to measure the amounts of certain substances, such as hormones. An unusual (higher or lower than normal) amount of a substance can be a sign of disease in the organ or tissue that produces it. The urine sample is checked to see if it contains a hormone produced by carcinoid tumors. This test is used to help diagnose carcinoid syndrome.

Prognosis

The prognosis (chance of recovery) and treatment options depend on the following:

- Whether the cancer can be completely removed by surgery
- Whether the cancer has spread from the stomach and intestines to other parts of the body, such as the liver or lymph nodes
- The size of the tumor
- Where the tumor is in the gastrointestinal tract
- Whether the cancer is newly diagnosed or has recurred

Treatment options also depend on whether the cancer is causing symptoms. Most gastrointestinal carcinoid tumors are slow-growing and can be treated and often cured. Even when not cured, many patients may live for a long time.

Stages of Gastrointestinal Carcinoid Tumors

After a gastrointestinal carcinoid tumor has been diagnosed, tests are done to find out if cancer cells have spread within the stomach and intestines or to other parts of the body.

Staging is the process used to find out how far the cancer has spread. The information gathered from the staging process determines the stage of the disease. There are no standard stages for gastrointestinal carcinoid tumors. In order to plan treatment, it is important to know the extent of the disease and whether the tumor can be removed by surgery. The following tests and procedures may be used:

Gastrointestinal endoscopy: A procedure to look inside the gastrointestinal tract for abnormal areas or cancer. An endoscope (a thin, lighted tube) is inserted through the mouth and esophagus into the stomach and first part of the small intestine. Also, a colonoscope (a thin, lighted tube) is inserted through the rectum into the colon (large intestine); this is called a colonoscopy.

CT scan (CAT scan): A procedure that makes a series of detailed pictures of areas inside the body, taken from different angles. The pictures are made by a computer linked to an x-ray machine. A dye may be injected into a vein or swallowed to help the organs or tissues show up more clearly. This procedure is also called computed tomography, computerized tomography, or computerized axial tomography.

Somatostatin receptor scintigraphy (SRS): A type of radionuclide scan used to find carcinoid tumors. In SRS, radioactive octreotide, a drug similar to somatostatin, is injected into a vein and travels through the bloodstream. The radioactive octreotide attaches to carcinoid tumor cells that have somatostatin receptors. A radiation-measuring device detects the radioactive material, showing where the carcinoid tumor cells are in the body. This procedure is also called an octreotide scan.

Biopsy: The removal of cells or tissues so they can be viewed under a microscope to check for signs of cancer. Tissue samples may be taken during endoscopy and colonoscopy.

Angiogram: A procedure to look at blood vessels and the flow of blood. A contrast dye is injected into the blood vessel. As the contrast dye moves through the blood vessel, x-rays are taken to see if there are any blockages.

PET scan (positron emission tomography scan): A procedure to find malignant tumor cells in the body. A small amount of radionuclide glucose (sugar) is injected into a vein. The PET scanner rotates around the body and makes a picture of where glucose is being used in the body. Malignant tumor cells show up brighter in the picture because they are more active and take up more glucose than normal cells.

X-ray of the abdomen: An x-ray of the organs and tissues inside the abdomen. An x-ray is a type of energy beam that can go through the body and onto film, making a picture of areas inside the body.

Treatment Groups

Gastrointestinal carcinoid tumors are grouped for treatment based on where they are in the body.

- **Localized:** Cancer is found in the appendix, colon, rectum, small intestine, and/or stomach only.

- **Regional:** Cancer has spread from the appendix, colon, rectum, stomach, and/or small intestine to nearby tissues or lymph nodes.

- **Metastatic:** Cancer has spread to other parts of the body.

Recurrent Gastrointestinal Carcinoid Tumors

A recurrent gastrointestinal carcinoid tumor is a tumor that has recurred (come back) after it has been treated. The tumor may come back in the stomach or intestines or in other parts of the body.

Treatment Option Overview

Different types of treatment are available for patients with gastrointestinal carcinoid tumors. Some treatments are standard (the currently used treatment), and some are being tested in clinical trials. Seven types of standard treatment are used:

Surgery

Treatment of gastrointestinal carcinoid tumors usually includes surgery. One of the following surgical procedures may be used:

- **Appendectomy:** Removal of the appendix.

- **Fulguration:** Use of an electric current to burn away the tumor using a special tool.

- **Cryosurgery:** A treatment that uses an instrument to freeze and destroy abnormal tissue, such as carcinoma in situ. This type of treatment is also called cryotherapy. The doctor may use ultrasound to guide the instrument.

- **Resection:** Surgery to remove part or all of the organ that contains cancer. Resection of the tumor and a small amount of normal tissue around it is called a local excision.

- **Bowel resection and anastomosis:** Removal of the bowel tumor and a small section of healthy bowel on each side. The healthy parts of the bowel are then sewn together (anastomosis). Lymph nodes are removed and checked by a pathologist to see if they contain cancer.

- **Radiofrequency ablation:** The use of a special probe with tiny electrodes that release high-energy radio waves (similar to microwaves) that kill cancer cells. The probe may be inserted through the skin or through an incision (cut) in the abdomen.

- **Hepatic resection:** Surgery to remove part or all of the liver.

- **Hepatic artery ligation or embolization:** A procedure to ligate (tie off) or embolize (block) the hepatic artery, the main blood vessel that brings blood into the liver. Blocking the flow of blood to the liver helps kill cancer cells growing there.

Radiation Therapy

Radiation therapy is a cancer treatment that uses high-energy x-rays or other types of radiation to kill cancer cells. There are two types of radiation therapy. External radiation therapy uses a machine outside the body to send radiation toward the cancer. Internal radiation therapy uses a radioactive substance sealed in needles, seeds, wires, or catheters that are placed directly into or near the cancer. The way the radiation therapy is given depends on the type and stage of the cancer being treated.

Chemotherapy

Chemotherapy is a cancer treatment that uses drugs to stop the growth of cancer cells, either by killing the cells or by stopping the cells from dividing. When chemotherapy is taken by mouth or injected into a vein or muscle, the drugs enter the bloodstream and can reach cancer cells throughout the body (systemic chemotherapy). When chemotherapy is placed directly into the spinal column, an organ, or a body cavity such as the abdomen, the drugs mainly affect cancer cells in those areas (regional chemotherapy).

Chemoembolization of the hepatic artery is a type of regional chemotherapy that may be used to treat a gastrointestinal carcinoid tumor that has spread to the liver. The anticancer drug is injected into the hepatic artery through a catheter (thin tube). The drug is mixed with a substance that embolizes (blocks) the artery, cutting off blood flow to the tumor. Most of the anticancer drug is trapped near the tumor and only a small amount of the drug reaches other parts of the body. The blockage may be temporary or permanent, depending on the substance used to block the artery. The tumor is prevented from getting the oxygen and nutrients it needs to grow. The liver continues to receive blood from the hepatic portal vein, which carries blood from the stomach and intestine.

The way the chemotherapy is given depends on the type and stage of the cancer being treated.

Percutaneous Ethanol Injection

Percutaneous ethanol injection is a cancer treatment in which a small needle is used to inject ethanol (alcohol) directly into a tumor to kill cancer cells. This procedure is also called intratumoral ethanol injection.

Biologic Therapy

Biologic therapy is a treatment that uses the patient's immune system to fight cancer. Substances made by the body or made in a laboratory are used to boost, direct, or restore the body's natural defenses against cancer. This type of cancer treatment is also called biotherapy or immunotherapy.

Hormone Therapy

Hormone therapy is a cancer treatment that removes hormones or blocks their action and stops cancer cells from growing. Hormones are substances produced by glands in the body and circulated in the bloodstream. The presence of some hormones can cause certain cancers to grow. If tests show that the cancer cells have places where hormones can attach (receptors), drugs, surgery, or radiation therapy are used to reduce the production of hormones or block them from working.

Other Drug Therapy

MIBG (metaiodobenzylguanidine) is sometimes used, with or without radioactive iodine (I131), to lessen the symptoms of gastrointestinal carcinoid tumors.

Clinical Trials

A treatment clinical trial is a research study meant to help improve current treatments or obtain information on new treatments for patients with cancer. When clinical trials show that a new treatment is better than the standard treatment, the new treatment may become the standard treatment. Patients may want to think about taking part in a clinical trial. Some clinical trials are open only to patients who have not started treatment.

Treatments being studied in clinical trials for gastrointestinal carcinoid tumors include new combinations of chemotherapy. Information about clinical trials is available from the National Cancer Institute website (www.cancer.gov).

Follow-Up Tests

Some of the tests that were done to diagnose the cancer or to find out the stage of the cancer may be repeated. Some tests will be repeated in order to see how well the treatment is working. Decisions about whether to continue, change, or stop treatment may be based on the results of these tests. This is sometimes called re-staging.

Some of the tests will continue to be done from time to time after treatment has ended. The results of these tests can show if your condition has changed or if the cancer has recurred (come back). These tests are sometimes called follow-up tests or check-ups.

Chapter 33

Small Intestine Cancer

General Information about Small Intestine Cancer

Small intestine cancer is a rare disease in which malignant (cancer) cells form in the tissues of the small intestine. The small intestine is part of the body's digestive system, which also includes the esophagus, stomach, and large intestine. The digestive system removes and processes nutrients (vitamins, minerals, carbohydrates, fats, proteins, and water) from foods and helps pass waste material out of the body. The small intestine is a long tube that connects the stomach to the large intestine. It folds many times to fit inside the abdomen.

There are five types of small intestine cancer. The types of cancer found in the small intestine are adenocarcinoma, sarcoma, carcinoid tumors, gastrointestinal stromal tumor, and lymphoma. This chapter discusses adenocarcinoma and leiomyosarcoma (a type of sarcoma). Other chapters discuss soft tissue sarcoma (chapter 53), non-Hodgkin lymphoma (chapter 45), and gastrointestinal carcinoid tumor (chapter 32).

Adenocarcinoma starts in glandular cells in the lining of the small intestine and is the most common type of small intestine cancer. Most of these tumors occur in the part of the small intestine near the stomach. They may grow and block the intestine.

Leiomyosarcoma starts in the smooth muscle cells of the small intestine. Most of these tumors occur in the part of the small intestine near the large intestine.

Excerpted from PDQ® Cancer Information Summary. National Cancer Institute; Bethesda, MD. "Small Intestine Cancer Treatment (PDQ) - Patient Version." Updated 08/2009. Available at: http://cancer.gov. Accessed January 20, 2010.

417

Risk Factors and Signs

Anything that increases your risk of getting a disease is called a risk factor. Having a risk factor does not mean that you will get cancer; not having risk factors doesn't mean that you will not get cancer. People who think they may be at risk should discuss this with their doctor. Risk factors for small intestine cancer include eating a high-fat diet, having Crohn disease, having celiac disease, and having familial adenomatous polyposis (FAP).

Possible signs of small intestine cancer include abdominal pain and unexplained weight loss. These and other symptoms may be caused by small intestine cancer or by other conditions. A doctor should be consulted if any of the following problems occur:

- Pain or cramps in the middle of the abdomen
- Weight loss with no known reason
- A lump in the abdomen
- Blood in the stool

Detection and Diagnosis

Procedures that create pictures of the small intestine and the area around it help diagnose small intestine cancer and show how far the cancer has spread. The process used to find out if cancer cells have spread within and around the small intestine is called staging.

In order to plan treatment, it is important to know the type of small intestine cancer and whether the tumor can be removed by surgery. Tests and procedures to detect, diagnose, and stage small intestine cancer are usually done at the same time. The following tests and procedures may be used:

Physical exam and history: An exam of the body to check general signs of health, including checking for signs of disease, such as lumps or anything else that seems unusual. A history of the patient's health habits and past illnesses and treatments will also be taken.

Blood chemistry studies: A procedure in which a blood sample is checked to measure the amounts of certain substances released into the blood by organs and tissues in the body. An unusual (higher or lower than normal) amount of a substance can be a sign of disease in the organ or tissue that produces it.

Liver function tests: A procedure in which a blood sample is checked to measure the amounts of certain substances released into the blood by the liver. A higher than normal amount of a substance can be a sign of liver disease that may be caused by small intestine cancer.

Abdominal x-ray: An x-ray of the organs in the abdomen. An x-ray is a type of energy beam that can go through the body onto film, making a picture of areas inside the body.

Barium enema: A series of x-rays of the lower gastrointestinal (GI) tract. A liquid that contains barium (a silver-white metallic compound) is put into the rectum. The barium coats the lower gastrointestinal tract and x-rays are taken. This procedure is also called a lower GI series.

Fecal occult blood test: A test to check stool (solid waste) for blood that can only be seen with a microscope. Small samples of stool are placed on special cards and returned to the doctor or laboratory for testing.

Upper endoscopy: A procedure to look at the inside of the esophagus, stomach, and duodenum (first part of the small intestine, near the stomach). An endoscope is inserted through the mouth and into the esophagus, stomach, and duodenum. An endoscope is a thin, tube-like instrument with a light and a lens for viewing. It may also have a tool to remove tissue samples, which are checked under a microscope for signs of cancer.

Upper GI series with small bowel follow-through: A series of x-rays of the esophagus, stomach, and small bowel. The patient drinks a liquid that contains barium (a silver-white metallic compound). The liquid coats the esophagus, stomach, and small bowel. X-rays are taken at different times as the barium travels through the upper GI tract and small bowel.

Biopsy: The removal of cells or tissues so they can be viewed under a microscope to check for signs of cancer. This may be done during the endoscopy. The sample is checked by a pathologist to see if it contains cancer cells.

CT scan (CAT scan): A procedure that makes a series of detailed pictures of areas inside the body, taken from different angles. The pictures are made by a computer linked to an x-ray machine. A dye may be injected into a vein or swallowed to help the organs or tissues show up more clearly. This procedure is also called computed tomography, computerized tomography, or computerized axial tomography.

Lymph node biopsy: The removal of all or part of a lymph node. A pathologist views the tissue under a microscope to look for cancer cells.

Laparotomy: A surgical procedure in which an incision (cut) is made in the wall of the abdomen to check the inside of the abdomen for signs of disease. The size of the incision depends on the reason the laparotomy is being done. Sometimes organs are removed or tissue samples are taken and checked under a microscope for signs of disease.

Prognosis

The prognosis (chance of recovery) and treatment options depend on the type of small intestine cancer, whether the cancer has spread to other places in the body, whether the cancer can be completely removed by surgery, and whether the cancer is newly diagnosed or has recurred.

Stages of Small Intestine Cancer

Tests and procedures to stage small intestine cancer are usually done at the same time as diagnosis. Staging is used to find out how far the cancer has spread, but treatment decisions are not based on stage. Treatment depends on whether the tumor can be removed by surgery and if the cancer is being treated as a primary tumor or is metastatic cancer.

Recurrent Small Intestine Cancer

Recurrent small intestine cancer is cancer that has recurred (come back) after it has been treated. The cancer may come back in the small intestine or in other parts of the body.

Treatment Option Overview

Different types of treatments are available for patients with small intestine cancer. Some treatments are standard (the currently used treatment), and some are being tested in clinical trials.

Three types of standard treatment are used: Surgery, radiation therapy, and chemotherapy.

Surgery

Surgery is the most common treatment of small intestine cancer. One of the following types of surgery may be done:

- **Resection:** Surgery to remove part or all of an organ that contains cancer. The resection may include the small intestine and nearby organs (if the cancer has spread). The doctor may remove the section of the small intestine that contains cancer and perform an anastomosis (joining the cut ends of the intestine together). The doctor will usually remove lymph nodes near the small intestine and examine them under a microscope to see whether they contain cancer.

- **Bypass:** Surgery to allow food in the small intestine to go around (bypass) a tumor that is blocking the intestine but cannot be removed.

Even if the doctor removes all the cancer that can be seen at the time of the surgery, some patients may be given radiation therapy after surgery to kill any cancer cells that are left. Treatment given after the surgery, to lower the risk that the cancer will come back, is called adjuvant therapy.

Radiation Therapy

Radiation therapy is a cancer treatment that uses high-energy x-rays or other types of radiation to kill cancer cells or keep them from growing. There are two types of radiation therapy. External radiation therapy uses a machine outside the body to send radiation toward the cancer. Internal radiation therapy uses a radioactive substance sealed in needles, seeds, wires, or catheters that are placed directly into or near the cancer. The way the radiation therapy is given depends on the type and stage of the cancer being treated.

Chemotherapy

Chemotherapy is a cancer treatment that uses drugs to stop the growth of cancer cells, either by killing the cells or by stopping them from dividing. When chemotherapy is taken by mouth or injected into a vein or muscle, the drugs enter the bloodstream and can reach cancer cells throughout the body (systemic chemotherapy). When chemotherapy is placed directly into the spinal column, an organ, or a body cavity such as the abdomen, the drugs mainly affect cancer cells in those areas (regional chemotherapy). The way the chemotherapy is given depends on the type and stage of the cancer being treated.

Clinical Trials

A treatment clinical trial is a research study meant to help improve current treatments or obtain information on new treatments for patients with cancer. When clinical trials show that a new treatment is better than the standard treatment, the new treatment may become the standard treatment. Patients may want to think about taking part in a clinical trial. Some clinical trials are open only to patients who have not started treatment.

New types of treatment are being tested in clinical trials. This summary describes treatments that are being studied in clinical trials. It may not mention every new treatment being studied. Information about clinical trials is available from the National Cancer Institute website (www.cancer.gov).

Biologic therapy: Biologic therapy is a treatment that uses the patient's immune system to fight cancer. Substances made by the body or made in a laboratory are used to boost, direct, or restore the body's natural defenses against cancer. This type of cancer treatment is also called biotherapy or immunotherapy.

Radiation therapy with radiosensitizers: Radiosensitizers are drugs that make tumor cells more sensitive to radiation therapy. Combining radiation therapy with radiosensitizers may kill more tumor cells.

Follow-Up Tests

Some of the tests that were done to diagnose the cancer or to find out the stage of the cancer may be repeated. Some tests will be repeated in order to see how well the treatment is working. Decisions about whether to continue, change, or stop treatment may be based on the results of these tests. This is sometimes called re-staging.

Some of the tests will continue to be done from time to time after treatment has ended. The results of these tests can show if your condition has changed or if the cancer has recurred (come back). These tests are sometimes called follow-up tests or check-ups.

Chapter 34

Colon Cancer

General Information about Colon Cancer

Colon cancer is a disease in which malignant (cancer) cells form in the tissues of the colon. The colon is part of the body's digestive system. The digestive system removes and processes nutrients (vitamins, minerals, carbohydrates, fats, proteins, and water) from foods and helps pass waste material out of the body. The digestive system is made up of the esophagus, stomach, and the small and large intestines. The first six feet of the large intestine are called the large bowel or colon. The last six inches are the rectum and the anal canal. The anal canal ends at the anus (the opening of the large intestine to the outside of the body).

Risk Factors and Signs

Anything that increases your chance of getting a disease is called a risk factor. Having a risk factor does not mean that you will get cancer; not having risk factors doesn't mean that you will not get cancer. People who think they may be at risk should discuss this with their doctor. Risk factors include the following:

- Age 50 or older

- A family history of cancer of the colon or rectum

Excerpted from PDQ® Cancer Information Summary. National Cancer Institute; Bethesda, MD. "Colon Cancer Treatment (PDQ) (PDQ) - Patient Version." Updated 9/2010. Available at: http://cancer.gov. Accessed September 28, 2010.

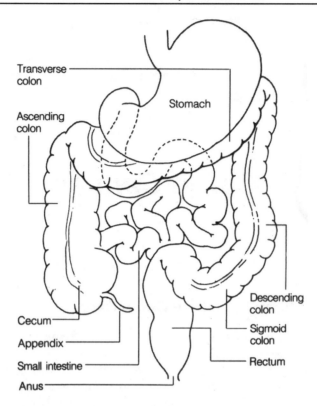

Figure 34.1. *The Colon and Nearby Organs (image by the National Cancer Institute, AV-0000-4096)*

- A personal history of cancer of the colon, rectum, ovary, endometrium, or breast

- A history of polyps (small pieces of bulging tissue) in the colon

- A history of ulcerative colitis (ulcers in the lining of the large intestine) or Crohn disease

- Certain hereditary conditions, such as familial adenomatous polyposis and hereditary nonpolyposis colon cancer (HNPCC; Lynch Syndrome)

Possible signs of colon cancer include a change in bowel habits or blood in the stool. These and other symptoms may be caused by colon cancer. Other conditions may cause the same symptoms. A doctor should be consulted if any of the following problems occur:

- A change in bowel habits
- Blood (either bright red or very dark) in the stool
- Diarrhea, constipation, or feeling that the bowel does not empty completely
- Stools that are narrower than usual
- Frequent gas pains, bloating, fullness, or cramps
- Weight loss for no known reason
- Feeling very tired
- Vomiting

Detection and Diagnosis

The following tests and procedures may be used:

Physical exam and history: An exam of the body to check general signs of health, including checking for signs of disease, such as lumps or anything else that seems unusual. A history of the patient's health habits and past illnesses and treatments will also be taken.

Digital rectal exam: An exam of the rectum. The doctor or nurse inserts a lubricated, gloved finger into the rectum to feel for lumps or anything else that seems unusual.

Fecal occult blood test: A test to check stool (solid waste) for blood that can only be seen with a microscope. Small samples of stool are placed on special cards and returned to the doctor or laboratory for testing.

Barium enema: A series of x-rays of the lower gastrointestinal tract. A liquid that contains barium (a silver-white metallic compound) is put into the rectum. The barium coats the lower gastrointestinal tract and x-rays are taken. This procedure is also called a lower GI series.

Sigmoidoscopy: A procedure to look inside the rectum and sigmoid (lower) colon for polyps (small pieces of bulging tissue), abnormal areas, or cancer. A sigmoidoscope is inserted through the rectum into the sigmoid colon. A sigmoidoscope is a thin, tube-like instrument with a light and a lens for viewing. It may also have a tool to remove polyps or tissue samples, which are checked under a microscope for signs of cancer.

Colonoscopy: A procedure to look inside the rectum and colon for polyps, abnormal areas, or cancer. A colonoscope is inserted through the rectum into the colon. A colonoscope is a thin, tube-like instrument with a light and a lens for viewing. It may also have a tool to remove polyps or tissue samples, which are checked under a microscope for signs of cancer.

Biopsy: The removal of cells or tissues so they can be viewed under a microscope by a pathologist to check for signs of cancer.

Virtual colonoscopy: A procedure that uses a series of x-rays called computed tomography to make a series of pictures of the colon. A computer puts the pictures together to create detailed images that may show polyps and anything else that seems unusual on the inside surface of the colon. This test is also called colonography or CT colonography.

Prognosis

The prognosis (chance of recovery) depends on the following:

- The stage of the cancer (whether the cancer is in the inner lining of the colon only, involves the whole colon, or has spread to other places in the body)
- Whether the cancer has blocked or created a hole in the colon
- Whether there are any cancer cells left after surgery
- The blood levels of carcinoembryonic antigen (CEA; a substance in the blood that may be increased when cancer is present) before treatment begins
- Whether the cancer has recurred
- The patient's general health

Treatment options depend on the stage of the cancer, whether the cancer has recurred, and the patient's general health.

Stages of Colon Cancer

After colon cancer has been diagnosed, tests are done to find out if cancer cells have spread within the colon or to other parts of the body. The process used to find out if cancer has spread within the colon or to other parts of the body is called staging. The information gathered from the staging process determines the stage of the disease. It is important to know the stage in order to plan treatment. The following tests and procedures may be used in the staging process:

CT scan (CAT scan): A procedure that makes a series of detailed pictures of areas inside the body, such as the abdomen, pelvis, or chest, taken from different angles. The pictures are made by a computer linked to an x-ray machine. A dye may be injected into a vein or swallowed to help the organs or tissues show up more clearly. This procedure is also called computed tomography, computerized tomography, or computerized axial tomography.

Lymph node biopsy: The removal of all or part of a lymph node. A pathologist views the tissue under a microscope to look for cancer cells.

Complete blood count (CBC): A procedure in which a sample of blood is drawn and checked for the following:

- The number of red blood cells, white blood cells, and platelets

- The amount of hemoglobin (the protein that carries oxygen) in the red blood cells

- The portion of the blood sample made up of red blood cells

Carcinoembryonic antigen (CEA) assay: A test that measures the level of CEA in the blood. CEA is released into the bloodstream from both cancer cells and normal cells. When found in higher than normal amounts, it can be a sign of colon cancer or other conditions.

MRI (magnetic resonance imaging): A procedure that uses a magnet, radio waves, and a computer to make a series of detailed pictures of areas inside the colon. A substance called gadolinium is injected into the patient through a vein. The gadolinium collects around the cancer cells so they show up brighter in the picture. This procedure is also called nuclear magnetic resonance imaging (NMRI).

Chest x-ray: An x-ray of the organs and bones inside the chest. An x-ray is a type of energy beam that can go through the body and onto film, making a picture of areas inside the body.

Surgery: A procedure to remove the tumor and see how far it has spread through the colon.

PET scan (positron emission tomography scan): A procedure to find malignant tumor cells in the body. A small amount of radioactive glucose (sugar) is injected into a vein. The PET scanner rotates around the body and makes a picture of where glucose is being used in the body. Malignant tumor cells show up brighter in the picture because they are more active and take up more glucose than normal cells do.

Stages of Colon Cancer

Stage 0 (Carcinoma in Situ)

In stage 0, abnormal cells are found in the mucosa (innermost layer) of the colon wall. These abnormal cells may become cancer and spread. Stage 0 is also called carcinoma in situ.

Stage I

In stage I, cancer has formed in the mucosa (innermost layer) of the colon wall and has spread to the submucosa (layer of tissue under the mucosa). Cancer may have spread to the muscle layer of the colon wall.

Stage II

Stage II colon cancer is divided into stage IIA, stage IIB, and stage IIC.

- **Stage IIA:** Cancer has spread through the muscle layer of the colon wall to the serosa (outermost layer) of the colon wall.

- **Stage IIB:** Cancer has spread through the serosa (outermost layer) of the colon wall but has not spread to nearby organs.

- **Stage IIC:** Cancer has spread through the serosa (outermost layer) of the colon wall to nearby organs.

Stage III

Stage III colon cancer is divided into stage IIIA, stage IIIB, and stage IIIC.

Stage IIIA: In stage IIIA:

- Cancer may have spread through the mucosa (innermost layer) of the colon wall to the submucosa (layer of tissue under the mucosa) and may have spread to the muscle layer of the colon wall. Cancer has spread to at least one but not more than three nearby lymph nodes or cancer cells have formed in tissues near the lymph nodes; or

- Cancer has spread through the mucosa (innermost layer) of the colon wall to the submucosa (layer of tissue under the mucosa). Cancer has spread to at least four but not more than six nearby lymph nodes.

428

Stage IIIB: In stage IIIB:

- Cancer has spread through the muscle layer of the colon wall to the serosa (outermost layer) of the colon wall or has spread through the serosa but not to nearby organs. Cancer has spread to at least one but not more than three nearby lymph nodes or cancer cells have formed in tissues near the lymph nodes; or

- Cancer has spread to the muscle layer of the colon wall or to the serosa (outermost layer) of the colon wall. Cancer has spread to at least four but not more than six nearby lymph nodes; or

- Cancer has spread through the mucosa (innermost layer) of the colon wall to the submucosa (layer of tissue under the mucosa) and may have spread to the muscle layer of the colon wall. Cancer has spread to seven or more nearby lymph nodes.

Stage IIIC: In stage IIIC:

- Cancer has spread through the serosa (outermost layer) of the colon wall but has not spread to nearby organs. Cancer has spread to at least four but not more than six nearby lymph nodes; or

- Cancer has spread through the muscle layer of the colon wall to the serosa (outermost layer) of the colon wall or has spread through the serosa but has not spread to nearby organs. Cancer has spread to seven or more nearby lymph nodes; or

- Cancer has spread through the serosa (outermost layer) of the colon wall and has spread to nearby organs. Cancer has spread to one or more nearby lymph nodes or cancer cells have formed in tissues near the lymph nodes.

Stage IV

Stage IV colon cancer is divided into stage IVA and stage IVB.

- **Stage IVA:** Cancer may have spread through the colon wall and may have spread to nearby organs or lymph nodes. Cancer has spread to one organ that is not near the colon, such as the liver, lung, or ovary, or to a distant lymph node.

- **Stage IVB:** Cancer may have spread through the colon wall and may have spread to nearby organs or lymph nodes. Cancer has spread to more than one organ that is not near the colon or into the lining of the abdominal wall.

Recurrent Colon Cancer

Recurrent colon cancer is cancer that has recurred (come back) after it has been treated. The cancer may come back in the colon or in other parts of the body, such as the liver, lungs, or both.

Treatment Option Overview

Different types of treatment are available for patients with colon cancer. Some treatments are standard (the currently used treatment), and some are being tested in clinical trials. Three types of standard treatment are used: Surgery, chemotherapy, and radiation therapy.

Surgery

Surgery (removing the cancer in an operation) is the most common treatment for all stages of colon cancer. A doctor may remove the cancer using one of the following types of surgery:

- **Local excision:** If the cancer is found at a very early stage, the doctor may remove it without cutting through the abdominal wall. Instead, the doctor may put a tube through the rectum into the colon and cut the cancer out. This is called a local excision. If the cancer is found in a polyp (a small bulging piece of tissue), the operation is called a polypectomy.

- **Resection:** If the cancer is larger, the doctor will perform a partial colectomy (removing the cancer and a small amount of healthy tissue around it). The doctor may then perform an anastomosis (sewing the healthy parts of the colon together). The doctor will also usually remove lymph nodes near the colon and examine them under a microscope to see whether they contain cancer.

- **Resection and colostomy:** If the doctor is not able to sew the two ends of the colon back together, a stoma (an opening) is made on the outside of the body for waste to pass through. This procedure is called a colostomy. A bag is placed around the stoma to collect the waste. Sometimes the colostomy is needed only until the lower colon has healed, and then it can be reversed. If the doctor needs to remove the entire lower colon, however, the colostomy may be permanent.

- **Radiofrequency ablation:** The use of a special probe with tiny electrodes that kill cancer cells. Sometimes the probe is inserted directly through the skin and only local anesthesia is needed. In other cases, the probe is inserted through an incision in the abdomen. This is done in the hospital with general anesthesia.

- **Cryosurgery:** A treatment that uses an instrument to freeze and destroy abnormal tissue, such as carcinoma in situ. This type of treatment is also called cryotherapy.

Even if the doctor removes all the cancer that can be seen at the time of the operation, some patients may be given chemotherapy or radiation therapy after surgery to kill any cancer cells that are left. Treatment given after the surgery, to lower the risk that the cancer will come back, is called adjuvant therapy.

Chemotherapy

Chemotherapy is a cancer treatment that uses drugs to stop the growth of cancer cells, either by killing the cells or by stopping them from dividing. When chemotherapy is taken by mouth or injected into a vein or muscle, the drugs enter the bloodstream and can reach cancer cells throughout the body (systemic chemotherapy). When chemotherapy is placed directly into the cerebrospinal fluid, an organ, or a body cavity such as the abdomen, the drugs mainly affect cancer cells in those areas (regional chemotherapy).

Chemoembolization of the hepatic artery may be used to treat cancer that has spread to the liver. This involves blocking the hepatic artery (the main artery that supplies blood to the liver) and injecting anticancer drugs between the blockage and the liver. The liver's arteries then deliver the drugs throughout the liver. Only a small amount of the drug reaches other parts of the body. The blockage may be temporary or permanent, depending on what is used to block the artery. The liver continues to receive some blood from the hepatic portal vein, which carries blood from the stomach and intestine.

The way the chemotherapy is given depends on the type and stage of the cancer being treated.

Radiation Therapy

Radiation therapy is a cancer treatment that uses high-energy x-rays or other types of radiation to kill cancer cells or keep them from growing. There are two types of radiation therapy. External radiation therapy uses a machine outside the body to send radiation toward the cancer. Internal radiation therapy uses a radioactive substance sealed in needles, seeds, wires, or catheters that are placed directly into or near the cancer. The way the radiation therapy is given depends on the type and stage of the cancer being treated.

Clinical Trials

A treatment clinical trial is a research study meant to help improve current treatments or obtain information on new treatments for patients with cancer. When clinical trials show that a new treatment is better than the standard treatment, the new treatment may become the standard treatment. Patients may want to think about taking part in a clinical trial. Some clinical trials are open only to patients who have not started treatment.

New types of treatment are being tested in clinical trials. This summary describes a type of treatment that is being studied in clinical trials. It may not mention every new treatment being studied. Information about clinical trials is available from the National Cancer website (www.cancer.gov).

Targeted therapy: Targeted therapy is a type of treatment that uses drugs or other substances to identify and attack specific cancer cells without harming normal cells. Monoclonal antibody therapy is a type of targeted therapy being studied in the treatment of colon cancer.

Monoclonal antibody therapy uses antibodies made in the laboratory from a single type of immune system cell. These antibodies can identify substances on cancer cells or normal substances that may help cancer cells grow. The antibodies attach to the substances and kill the cancer cells, block their growth, or keep them from spreading. Monoclonal antibodies are given by infusion. They may be used alone or to carry drugs, toxins, or radioactive material directly to cancer cells.

Follow-Up Tests

Some of the tests that were done to diagnose the cancer or to find out the stage of the cancer may be repeated. Some tests will be repeated in order to see how well the treatment is working. Decisions about whether to continue, change, or stop treatment may be based on the results of these tests. This is sometimes called re-staging.

Some of the tests will continue to be done from time to time after treatment has ended. The results of these tests can show if your condition has changed or if the cancer has recurred (come back). These tests are sometimes called follow-up tests or check-ups.

For colon cancer, a blood test to measure carcinoembryonic antigen (CEA; a substance in the blood that may be increased when colon cancer is present) may be done along with other tests to see if the cancer has come back.

Chapter 35

Rectal Cancer

General Information about Rectal Cancer

Rectal cancer is a disease in which malignant (cancer) cells form in the tissues of the rectum. The rectum is part of the body's digestive system. The digestive system removes and processes nutrients (vitamins, minerals, carbohydrates, fats, proteins, and water) from foods and helps pass waste material out of the body. The digestive system is made up of the esophagus, stomach, and the small and large intestines. The first six feet of the large intestine are called the large bowel or colon. The last six inches are the rectum and the anal canal. The anal canal ends at the anus (the opening of the large intestine to the outside of the body).

Risk Factors and Signs

Anything that increases your chance of getting a disease is called a risk factor. Having a risk factor does not mean that you will get cancer; not having risk factors doesn't mean that you will not get cancer. People who think they may be at risk should discuss this with their doctor. The following are possible risk factors for rectal cancer:

- Being aged 40 or older

Excerpted from PDQ® Cancer Information Summary. National Cancer Institute; Bethesda, MD. "Rectal Cancer Treatment (PDQ) - Patient Version." Updated 9/2010. Available at: http://cancer.gov. Accessed September 28, 2010.

- Having certain hereditary conditions, such as familial adenomatous polyposis (FAP) and hereditary nonpolyposis colon cancer (HNPCC or Lynch syndrome)

- Having a personal history of any of the following: colorectal cancer, polyps (small pieces of bulging tissue) in the colon or rectum, or cancer of the ovary, endometrium, or breast

- Having a parent, brother, sister, or child with a history of colorectal cancer or polyps.

Possible signs of rectal cancer include a change in bowel habits or blood in the stool. These and other symptoms may be caused by rectal cancer. Other conditions may cause the same symptoms. A doctor should be consulted if any of the following problems occur:

- A change in bowel habits: Diarrhea, constipation, feeling that the bowel does not empty completely, or stools that are narrower or have a different shape than usual

- Blood (either bright red or very dark) in the stool

- General abdominal discomfort (frequent gas pains, bloating, fullness, or cramps)

- Change in appetite

- Weight loss for no known reason

- Feeling very tired

Detection and Diagnosis

Tests used to diagnose rectal cancer include the following:

Physical exam and history: An exam of the body to check general signs of health, including checking for signs of disease, such as lumps or anything else that seems unusual. A history of the patient's health habits and past illnesses and treatments will also be taken.

Digital rectal exam (DRE): An exam of the rectum. The doctor or nurse inserts a lubricated, gloved finger into the lower part of the rectum to feel for lumps or anything else that seems unusual. In women, the vagina may also be examined.

Proctoscopy: An exam of the rectum using a proctoscope, inserted into the rectum. A proctoscope is a thin, tube-like instrument with a light and a lens for viewing. It may also have a tool to remove tissue to be checked under a microscope for signs of disease.

Colonoscopy: A procedure to look inside the rectum and colon for polyps (small pieces of bulging tissue), abnormal areas, or cancer. A colonoscope is a thin, tube-like instrument with a light and a lens for viewing. It may also have a tool to remove polyps or tissue samples, which are checked under a microscope for signs of cancer.

Biopsy: The removal of cells or tissues so they can be viewed under a microscope to check for signs of cancer. Tumor tissue that is removed during the biopsy may be checked to see if the patient is likely to have the gene mutation that causes HNPCC. This may help to plan treatment. The following tests may be used:

- **Reverse-transcription polymerase chain reaction (RT-PCR) test:** A laboratory test in which cells in a sample of tissue are studied using chemicals to look for certain changes in the structure or function of genes.

- **Immunohistochemistry study:** A laboratory test in which a substance such as an antibody, dye, or radioisotope is added to a sample of tissue to test for certain antigens. This type of study is used to tell the difference between different types of cancer.

Carcinoembryonic antigen (CEA) assay: A test that measures the level of CEA in the blood. CEA is released into the bloodstream from both cancer cells and normal cells. When found in higher than normal amounts, it can be a sign of rectal cancer or other conditions

Prognosis

The prognosis (chance of recovery) and treatment options depend on the following:

- The stage of the cancer (whether it affects the inner lining of the rectum only, involves the whole rectum, or has spread to lymph nodes, nearby organs, or other places in the body)

- Whether the tumor has spread into or through the bowel wall

- Where the cancer is found in the rectum

- Whether the bowel is blocked or has a hole in it

- Whether all of the tumor can be removed by surgery

- The patient's general health

- Whether the cancer has just been diagnosed or has recurred (come back)

Stages of Rectal Cancer

After rectal cancer has been diagnosed, tests are done to find out if cancer cells have spread within the rectum or to other parts of the body. The process used to find out whether cancer has spread within the rectum or to other parts of the body is called staging. The information gathered from the staging process determines the stage of the disease. It is important to know the stage in order to plan treatment. The following tests and procedures may be used in the staging process:

- **Chest x-ray:** An x-ray of the organs and bones inside the chest. An x-ray is a type of energy beam that can go through the body and onto film, making a picture of areas inside the body.

- **CT scan (CAT scan):** A procedure that makes a series of detailed pictures of areas inside the body, such as the abdomen, pelvis, or chest, taken from different angles. The pictures are made by a computer linked to an x-ray machine. A dye may be injected into a vein or swallowed to help the organs or tissues show up more clearly. This procedure is also called computed tomography, computerized tomography, or computerized axial tomography.

- **MRI (magnetic resonance imaging):** A procedure that uses a magnet, radio waves, and a computer to make a series of detailed pictures of areas inside the body. This procedure is also called nuclear magnetic resonance imaging (NMRI).

- **Endoscopic ultrasound (EUS):** A procedure in which an endoscope or rigid probe is inserted into the body through the rectum. The endoscope or probe has a light and a lens for viewing. A device at the end is used to bounce high-energy sound waves (ultrasound) off internal tissues or organs and make echoes. The echoes form a picture of body tissues called a sonogram. This procedure is also called endosonography.

- **PET scan (positron emission tomography scan):** A procedure to find malignant tumor cells in the body. A small amount of radioactive glucose (sugar) is injected into a vein. The PET scanner rotates around the body and makes a picture of where glucose is being used in the body. Malignant tumor cells show up brighter in the picture because they are more active and take up more glucose than normal cells do.

- **Carcinoembryonic antigen (CEA) assay:** A test that measures the level of CEA in the blood. CEA is released into the bloodstream from both cancer cells and normal cells. When found in higher than normal amounts, it can be a sign of rectal cancer or other conditions.

The following stages are used for rectal cancer:

Stage 0 (Carcinoma in Situ)

In stage 0, abnormal cells are found in the mucosa (innermost layer) of the rectal wall. These abnormal cells may become cancer and spread. Stage 0 is also called carcinoma in situ.

Stage I

In stage I, cancer has formed in the mucosa (innermost layer) of the rectal wall and has spread to the submucosa (layer of tissue under the mucosa). Cancer may have spread to the muscle layer of the rectal wall.

Stage II

Stage II rectal cancer is divided into stage IIA, stage IIB, and stage IIC.

- **Stage IIA:** Cancer has spread through the muscle layer of the rectal wall to the serosa (outermost layer) of the rectal wall.

- **Stage IIB:** Cancer has spread through the serosa (outermost layer) of the rectal wall but has not spread to nearby organs.

- **Stage IIC:** Cancer has spread through the serosa (outermost layer) of the rectal wall to nearby organs.

Stage III

Stage III rectal cancer is divided into stage IIIA, stage IIIB, and stage IIIC.

Stage IIIA: In stage IIIA:

- Cancer may have spread through the mucosa (innermost layer) of the rectal wall to the submucosa (layer of tissue under the mucosa) and may have spread to the muscle layer of the rectal wall. Cancer has spread to at least one but not more than three nearby lymph nodes or cancer cells have formed in tissues near the lymph nodes; or

- Cancer has spread through the mucosa (innermost layer) of the rectal wall to the submucosa (layer of tissue under the mucosa). Cancer has spread to at least four but not more than six nearby lymph nodes.

Stage IIIB: In stage IIIB:

- Cancer has spread through the muscle layer of the rectal wall to the serosa (outermost layer) of the rectal wall or has spread through the serosa but not to nearby organs. Cancer has spread to at least one but not more than three nearby lymph nodes or cancer cells have formed in tissues near the lymph nodes; or

- Cancer has spread to the muscle layer of the rectal wall or to the serosa (outermost layer) of the rectal wall. Cancer has spread to at least four but not more than six nearby lymph nodes; or

- Cancer has spread through the mucosa (innermost layer) of the rectal wall to the submucosa (layer of tissue under the mucosa) and may have spread to the muscle layer of the rectal wall. Cancer has spread to seven or more nearby lymph nodes.

Stage IIIC: In stage IIIC:

- Cancer has spread through the serosa (outermost layer) of the rectal wall but has not spread to nearby organs. Cancer has spread to at least four but not more than six nearby lymph nodes; or

- Cancer has spread through the muscle layer of the rectal wall to the serosa (outermost layer) of the rectal wall or has spread through the serosa but has not spread to nearby organs. Cancer has spread to seven or more nearby lymph nodes; or

- Cancer has spread through the serosa (outermost layer) of the rectal wall and has spread to nearby organs. Cancer has spread to one or more nearby lymph nodes or cancer cells have formed in tissues near the lymph nodes.

Stage IV

Stage IV rectal cancer is divided into stage IVA and stage IVB.

- **Stage IVA:** Cancer may have spread through the rectal wall and may have spread to nearby organs or lymph nodes. Cancer has spread to one organ that is not near the rectum, such as the liver, lung, or ovary, or to a distant lymph node.

- **Stage IVB:** Cancer may have spread through the rectal wall and may have spread to nearby organs or lymph nodes. Cancer has spread to more than one organ that is not near the rectum or into the lining of the abdominal wall.

Recurrent Rectal Cancer

Recurrent rectal cancer is cancer that has recurred (come back) after it has been treated. The cancer may come back in the rectum or in other parts of the body, such as the colon, pelvis, liver, or lungs.

Treatment Option Overview

Different types of treatment are available for patients with rectal cancer. Some treatments are standard (the currently used treatment), and some are being tested in clinical trials. Three types of standard treatment are used: Surgery, radiation therapy, and chemotherapy.

Surgery

Surgery is the most common treatment for all stages of rectal cancer. The cancer is removed using one of the following types of surgery:

- **Polypectomy:** If the cancer is found in a polyp (a small piece of bulging tissue), the polyp is often removed during a colonoscopy.

- **Local excision:** If the cancer is found on the inside surface of the rectum and has not spread into the wall of the rectum, the cancer and a small amount of surrounding healthy tissue is removed.

- **Resection:** If the cancer has spread into the wall of the rectum, the section of the rectum with cancer and nearby healthy tissue is removed. Sometimes the tissue between the rectum and the abdominal wall is also removed. The lymph nodes near the rectum are removed and checked under a microscope for signs of cancer.

- **Pelvic exenteration:** If the cancer has spread to other organs near the rectum, the lower colon, rectum, and bladder are removed. In women, the cervix, vagina, ovaries, and nearby lymph nodes may be removed. In men, the prostate may be removed. Artificial openings (stoma) are made for urine and stool to flow from the body to a collection bag.

After the cancer is removed, the surgeon will either do an anastomosis (sew the healthy parts of the rectum together, sew the remaining rectum to the colon, or sew the colon to the anus); or make a stoma (an opening) from the rectum to the outside of the body for waste to pass through. This procedure is done if the cancer is too close to the anus and is called a colostomy. A bag is placed around the stoma to collect the waste. Sometimes the colostomy is needed only until the rectum has healed, and then it can be reversed. If the entire rectum is removed, however, the colostomy may be permanent.

Radiation therapy or chemotherapy may be given before surgery to shrink the tumor, make it easier to remove the cancer, and lessen problems with bowel control after surgery. Treatment given before surgery is called neoadjuvant therapy. Even if all the cancer that can be seen at the time of the operation is removed, some patients may be given radiation therapy or chemotherapy after surgery to kill any cancer cells that are left. Treatment given after the surgery, to lower the risk that the cancer will come back, is called adjuvant therapy.

Radiation Therapy

Radiation therapy is a cancer treatment that uses high-energy x-rays or other types of radiation to kill cancer cells. There are two types of radiation therapy. External radiation therapy uses a machine outside the body to send radiation toward the cancer. Internal radiation therapy uses a radioactive substance sealed in needles, seeds, wires, or catheters that are placed directly into or near the cancer. The way the radiation therapy is given depends on the type and stage of the cancer being treated.

Chemotherapy

Chemotherapy is a cancer treatment that uses drugs to stop the growth of cancer cells, either by killing the cells or by stopping the cells from dividing. When chemotherapy is taken by mouth or injected into a vein or muscle, the drugs enter the bloodstream and can reach cancer cells throughout the body (systemic chemotherapy). When chemotherapy is placed directly in the cerebrospinal fluid, an organ, or a body cavity such as the abdomen, the drugs mainly affect cancer cells in those areas (regional chemotherapy). The way the chemotherapy is given depends on the type and stage of the cancer being treated.

Clinical Trials

A treatment clinical trial is a research study meant to help improve current treatments or obtain information on new treatments for patients with cancer. When clinical trials show that a new treatment is better than the standard treatment, the new treatment may become the standard treatment. Patients may want to think about taking part in a clinical trial. Some clinical trials are open only to patients who have not started treatment.

This summary describes a treatment that is being studied in clinical trials. It may not mention every treatment being studied. Information about clinical trials is available from the National Cancer Institute website (www.cancer.gov).

Targeted therapy: Targeted therapy is a type of treatment that uses drugs or other substances to identify and attack specific cancer cells without harming normal cells. Monoclonal antibody therapy is a type of targeted therapy being studied in the treatment of rectal cancer.

Monoclonal antibody therapy uses antibodies made in the laboratory from a single type of immune system cell. These antibodies can identify substances on cancer cells or normal substances that may help cancer cells grow. The antibodies attach to the substances and kill the cancer cells, block their growth, or keep them from spreading. Monoclonal antibodies are given by infusion. They may be used alone or to carry drugs, toxins, or radioactive material directly to cancer cells.

Follow-Up Tests

Some of the tests that were done to diagnose the cancer or to find out the stage of the cancer may be repeated. Some tests will be repeated in order to see how well the treatment is working. Decisions about whether to continue, change, or stop treatment may be based on the results of these tests. This is sometimes called re-staging.

Some of the tests will continue to be done from time to time after treatment has ended. The results of these tests can show if your condition has changed or if the cancer has recurred (come back). These tests are sometimes called follow-up tests or check-ups.

After treatment for rectal cancer, a blood test to measure amounts of carcinoembryonic antigen (a substance in the blood that may be increased when cancer is present) may be done to see if the cancer has come back.

Chapter 36

Anal Cancer

General Information about Anal Cancer

Anal cancer is a disease in which malignant (cancer) cells form in the tissues of the anus. The anus is the end of the large intestine, below the rectum, through which stool (solid waste) leaves the body. The anus is formed partly from the outer, skin layers of the body and partly from the intestine. Two ring-like muscles, called sphincter muscles, open and close the anal opening to let stool pass out of the body. The anal canal, the part of the anus between the rectum and the anal opening, is about 1½ inches long.

The skin around the outside of the anus is called the perianal area. Tumors in this area are skin tumors, not anal cancer.

Risk Factors and Signs

Risk factors include the following:

- Being over 50 years old

- Being infected with human papillomavirus (HPV)

- Having many sexual partners

- Having receptive anal intercourse (anal sex)

Excerpted from PDQ® Cancer Information Summary. National Cancer Institute; Bethesda, MD. Anal Cancer Treatment (PDQ) - Patient Version." Updated 06/2008. Available at: http://cancer.gov. Accessed January 20, 2010.

- Frequent anal redness, swelling, and soreness
- Having anal fistulas (abnormal openings)
- Smoking cigarettes

Possible signs of anal cancer include bleeding from the anus or rectum or a lump near the anus. These and other symptoms may be caused by anal cancer. Other conditions may cause the same symptoms. A doctor should be consulted if any of the following problems occur:

- Bleeding from the anus or rectum
- Pain or pressure in the area around the anus
- Itching or discharge from the anus
- A lump near the anus
- A change in bowel habits

Detection and Diagnosis

The following tests and procedures may be used:

Physical exam and history: An exam of the body to check general signs of health, including checking for signs of disease, such as lumps or anything else that seems unusual. A history of the patient's health habits and past illnesses and treatments will also be taken.

Digital rectal examination (DRE): An exam of the anus and rectum. The doctor or nurse inserts a lubricated, gloved finger into the lower part of the rectum to feel for lumps or anything else that seems unusual.

Anoscopy: An exam of the anus and lower rectum using a short, lighted tube called an anoscope.

Proctoscopy: An exam of the rectum using a short, lighted tube called a proctoscope.

Endo-anal or endorectal ultrasound: A procedure in which an ultrasound transducer (probe) is inserted into the anus or rectum and used to bounce high-energy sound waves (ultrasound) off internal tissues or organs and make echoes. The echoes form a picture of body tissues called a sonogram.

Biopsy: The removal of cells or tissues so they can be viewed under a microscope by a pathologist to check for signs of cancer. If an abnormal area is seen during the anoscopy, a biopsy may be done at that time.

Prognosis

The prognosis (chance of recovery) depends on the size of the tumor, where the tumor is in the anus, and whether the cancer has spread to the lymph nodes.

The treatment options depend on the stage of the cancer, where the tumor is in the anus, whether the patient has human immunodeficiency virus (HIV), and whether cancer remains after initial treatment or has recurred.

Stages of Anal Cancer

After anal cancer has been diagnosed, tests are done to find out if cancer cells have spread within the anus or to other parts of the body. The process used to find out if cancer has spread within the anus or to other parts of the body is called staging. The information gathered from the staging process determines the stage of the disease. It is important to know the stage in order to plan treatment. In addition to endo-anal or endorectal ultrasound, which may be used in diagnosis and is described above, the additional tests may be used in the staging process:

- **CT scan (CAT scan):** A procedure that makes a series of detailed pictures of areas inside the body, taken from different angles. The pictures are made by a computer linked to an x-ray machine. A dye may be injected into a vein or swallowed to help the organs or tissues show up more clearly. This procedure is also called computed tomography, computerized tomography, or computerized axial tomography. For anal cancer, a CT scan of the pelvis and abdomen may be done.

- **Chest x-ray:** An x-ray of the organs and bones inside the chest. An x-ray is a type of energy beam that can go through the body and onto film, making a picture of areas inside the body.

The following stages are used for anal cancer:

Stage 0 (Carcinoma in Situ)

In stage 0, abnormal cells are found in the innermost lining of the anus. These abnormal cells may become cancer and spread into nearby normal tissue. Stage 0 is also called carcinoma in situ.

Stage I

In stage I, cancer has formed and the tumor is two centimeters or smaller.

Stage II

In stage II, the tumor is larger than two centimeters.

Stage III

Stage IIIA: In stage IIIA, the tumor may be any size and has spread to either lymph nodes near the rectum; or nearby organs, such as the vagina, urethra, and bladder.

Stage IIIB: In stage IIIB, the tumor may be any size and has spread:

- to nearby organs and to lymph nodes near the rectum; or
- to lymph nodes on one side of the pelvis and/or groin, and may have spread to nearby organs; or
- to lymph nodes near the rectum and in the groin, and/or to lymph nodes on both sides of the pelvis and/or groin, and may have spread to nearby organs.

Stage IV

In stage IV, the tumor may be any size and cancer may have spread to lymph nodes or nearby organs and has spread to distant parts of the body.

Recurrent Anal Cancer

Recurrent anal cancer is cancer that has recurred (come back) after it has been treated. The cancer may come back in the anus or in other parts of the body.

Treatment Option Overview

Different types of treatments are available for patients with anal cancer. Some treatments are standard (the currently used treatment), and some are being tested in clinical trials.

Three types of standard treatment are used: Radiation therapy, chemotherapy, and surgery.

Radiation Therapy

Radiation therapy is a cancer treatment that uses high-energy x-rays or other types of radiation to kill cancer cells. There are two types of radiation therapy. External radiation therapy uses a machine outside the body to send radiation toward the cancer. Internal radiation therapy uses a radioactive substance sealed in needles, seeds, wires, or catheters that are placed directly into or near the cancer. The way the radiation therapy is given depends on the type and stage of the cancer being treated.

Chemotherapy

Chemotherapy is a cancer treatment that uses drugs to stop the growth of cancer cells, either by killing the cells or by stopping the cells from dividing. When chemotherapy is taken by mouth or injected into a vein or muscle, the drugs enter the bloodstream and can reach cancer cells throughout the body (systemic chemotherapy). When chemotherapy is placed directly into the spinal column, an organ, or a body cavity such as the abdomen, the drugs mainly affect cancer cells in those areas (regional chemotherapy). The way the chemotherapy is given depends on the type and stage of the cancer being treated.

Surgery

Local resection: A surgical procedure in which the tumor is cut from the anus along with some of the healthy tissue around it. Local resection may be used if the cancer is small and has not spread. This procedure may save the sphincter muscles so the patient can still control bowel movements. Tumors that develop in the lower part of the anus can often be removed with local resection.

Abdominoperineal resection: A surgical procedure in which the anus, the rectum, and part of the sigmoid colon are removed through an incision made in the abdomen. The doctor sews the end of the intestine to an opening, called a stoma, made in the surface of the abdomen so body waste can be collected in a disposable bag outside of the body. This is called a colostomy. Lymph nodes that contain cancer may also be removed during this operation.

HIV and Anal Cancer Treatment

Cancer therapy can further damage the already weakened immune systems of patients who have the human immunodeficiency virus (HIV). For this reason, patients who have anal cancer and HIV are usually treated with lower doses of anticancer drugs and radiation than patients who do not have HIV.

Clinical Trials

A treatment clinical trial is a research study meant to help improve current treatments or obtain information on new treatments for patients with cancer. When clinical trials show that a new treatment is better than the standard treatment, the new treatment may become the standard treatment. Patients may want to think about taking part in a clinical trial. Some clinical trials are open only to patients who have not started treatment.

New types of treatment are being tested in clinical trials. This summary describes a treatment that is being studied in clinical trials. It may not mention every new treatment being studied. Information about clinical trials is available from the National Cancer Institute website (www.cancer.gov).

Radiosensitizers: Radiosensitizers are drugs that make tumor cells more sensitive to radiation therapy. Combining radiation therapy with radiosensitizers may kill more tumor cells.

Follow-Up Tests

Some of the tests that were done to diagnose the cancer or to find out the stage of the cancer may be repeated. Some tests will be repeated in order to see how well the treatment is working. Decisions about whether to continue, change, or stop treatment may be based on the results of these tests. This is sometimes called re-staging.

Some of the tests will continue to be done from time to time after treatment has ended. The results of these tests can show if your condition has changed or if the cancer has recurred (come back). These tests are sometimes called follow-up tests or check-ups.

Chapter 37

Kidney Cancers

Chapter Contents

Section 37.1

Renal Cell Cancer

Excerpted from PDQ® Cancer Information Summary. National Cancer Institute; Bethesda, MD. "Renal Cell Cancer Treatment (PDQ) - Patient Version." Updated 09/2010. Available at: http://cancer.gov. Accessed September 28, 2010.

General Information about Renal Cell Cancer

Renal cell cancer is a disease in which malignant (cancer) cells form in tubules of the kidney. Renal cell cancer (also called kidney cancer or renal adenocarcinoma) is a disease in which malignant (cancer) cells are found in the lining of tubules (very small tubes) in the kidney. There are two kidneys, one on each side of the backbone, above the waist. The tiny tubules in the kidneys filter and clean the blood, taking out waste products and making urine. The urine passes from each kidney into the bladder through a long tube called a ureter. The bladder stores the urine until it is passed from the body.

Cancer that starts in the ureters or the renal pelvis (the part of the kidney that collects urine and drains it to the ureters) is different from renal cell cancer. It is discussed in chapter 38.

Risk Factors and Signs

Anything that increases your risk of getting a disease is called a risk factor. Having a risk factor does not mean that you will get cancer; not having risk factors doesn't mean that you will not get cancer. People who think they may be at risk should discuss this with their doctor. Risk factors for renal cell cancer include smoking, misusing certain pain medicines, including over-the-counter pain medicines, for a long time, and having certain genetic conditions, such as von Hippel-Lindau disease or hereditary papillary renal cell carcinoma.

Possible signs of renal cell cancer include blood in the urine and a lump in the abdomen. These and other symptoms may be caused by renal cell cancer. Other conditions may cause the same symptoms. There may be no symptoms in the early stages. Symptoms may appear as the tumor grows. A doctor should be consulted if any of the following problems occur:

- Blood in the urine
- A lump in the abdomen
- A pain in the side that doesn't go away.
- Loss of appetite
- Weight loss for no known reason
- Anemia

Detection and Diagnosis

The following tests and procedures may be used:

Physical exam and history: An exam of the body to check general signs of health, including checking for signs of disease, such as lumps or anything else that seems unusual. A history of the patient's health habits and past illnesses and treatments will also be taken.

Blood chemistry studies: A procedure in which a blood sample is checked to measure the amounts of certain substances released into the blood by organs and tissues in the body. An unusual (higher or lower than normal) amount of a substance can be a sign of disease in the organ or tissue that makes it.

Urinalysis: A test to check the color of urine and its contents, such as sugar, protein, red blood cells, and white blood cells.

Liver function test: A procedure in which a sample of blood is checked to measure the amounts of enzymes released into it by the liver. An abnormal amount of an enzyme can be a sign that cancer has spread to the liver. Certain conditions that are not cancer may also increase liver enzyme levels.

Intravenous pyelogram (IVP): A series of x-rays of the kidneys, ureters, and bladder to find out if cancer is present in these organs. A contrast dye is injected into a vein. As the contrast dye moves through the kidneys, ureters, and bladder, x-rays are taken to see if there are any blockages.

Ultrasound exam: A procedure in which high-energy sound waves (ultrasound) are bounced off internal tissues or organs and make echoes. The echoes form a picture of body tissues called a sonogram.

CT scan (CAT scan): A procedure that makes a series of detailed pictures of areas inside the body, taken from different angles. The pictures are made by a computer linked to an x-ray machine. A dye may be injected into a vein or swallowed to help the organs or tissues show up more clearly. This procedure is also called computed tomography, computerized tomography, or computerized axial tomography.

MRI (magnetic resonance imaging): A procedure that uses a magnet, radio waves, and a computer to make a series of detailed pictures of areas inside the body. This procedure is also called nuclear magnetic resonance imaging (NMRI).

Biopsy: The removal of cells or tissues so they can be viewed under a microscope by a pathologist to check for signs of cancer. To do a biopsy for renal cell cancer, a thin needle is inserted into the tumor and a sample of tissue is withdrawn.

Prognosis

The prognosis (chance of recovery) and treatment options depend on the stage of the disease and the patient's age and general health.

Stages of Renal Cell Cancer

After renal cell cancer has been diagnosed, tests are done to find out if cancer cells have spread within the kidney or to other parts of the body. The process used to find out if cancer has spread within the kidney or to other parts of the body is called staging. The information gathered from the staging process determines the stage of the disease. It is important to know the stage in order to plan treatment. Some of the tests used for diagnosis may also be used in staging, including CT scan and MRI. The following additional tests and procedures may be used in the staging process:

- **Chest x-ray:** An x-ray of the organs and bones inside the chest. An x-ray is a type of energy beam that can go through the body and onto film, making a picture of areas inside the body.

- **Bone scan:** A procedure to check if there are rapidly dividing cells, such as cancer cells, in the bone. A very small amount of radioactive material is injected into a vein and travels through the bloodstream. The radioactive material collects in the bones and is detected by a scanner.

The following stages are used for renal cell cancer:

Stage I

In stage I, the tumor is seven centimeters or smaller and is found only in the kidney.

Stage II

In stage II, the tumor is larger than seven centimeters and is found only in the kidney.

Stage III

- In stage III the tumor is any size and cancer is found only in the kidney and in one or more nearby lymph nodes; Or

- Cancer is found in the main blood vessels of the kidney or in the layer of fatty tissue around the kidney. Cancer may be found in one or more nearby lymph nodes.

Stage IV

- In stage IV, cancer has spread beyond the layer of fatty tissue around the kidney and may be found in the adrenal gland above the kidney with cancer, or in nearby lymph nodes; Or

- Cancer has spread to other organs, such as the lungs, liver, bones, or brain, and may have spread to lymph nodes.

Recurrent Renal Cell Cancer

Recurrent renal cell cancer is cancer that has recurred (come back) after it has been treated. The cancer may come back many years after initial treatment, in the kidney or in other parts of the body.

Treatment Option Overview

Different types of treatments are available for patients with renal cell cancer. Some treatments are standard (the currently used treatment), and some are being tested in clinical trials. Five types of standard treatment are used:

Surgery

Surgery to remove part or all of the kidney is often used to treat renal cell cancer. The following types of surgery may be used:

- **Partial nephrectomy:** A surgical procedure to remove the cancer within the kidney and some of the tissue around it. A partial nephrectomy may be done to prevent loss of kidney function when the other kidney is damaged or has already been removed.

- **Simple nephrectomy:** A surgical procedure to remove the kidney only.

- **Radical nephrectomy:** A surgical procedure to remove the kidney, the adrenal gland, surrounding tissue, and, usually, nearby lymph nodes.

A person can live with part of one working kidney, but if both kidneys are removed or not working, the person will need dialysis (a procedure to clean the blood using a machine outside of the body) or a kidney transplant (replacement with a healthy donated kidney). A kidney transplant may be done when the disease is in the kidney only and a donated kidney can be found. If the patient has to wait for a donated kidney, other treatment is given as needed.

When surgery to remove the cancer is not possible, a treatment called arterial embolization may be used to shrink the tumor. A small incision is made and a catheter (thin tube) is inserted into the main blood vessel that flows to the kidney. Small pieces of a special gelatin sponge are injected through the catheter into the blood vessel. The sponges block the blood flow to the kidney and prevent the cancer cells from getting oxygen and other substances they need to grow.

Even if the doctor removes all the cancer that can be seen at the time of the surgery, some patients may be given chemotherapy or radiation therapy after surgery to kill any cancer cells that are left. Treatment given after the surgery, to lower the risk that the cancer will come back, is called adjuvant therapy.

Radiation Therapy

Radiation therapy is a cancer treatment that uses high-energy x-rays or other types of radiation to kill cancer cells or keep them from growing. There are two types of radiation therapy. External radiation therapy uses a machine outside the body to send radiation toward the cancer. Internal radiation therapy uses a radioactive substance sealed in needles, seeds, wires, or catheters that are placed directly into or near the cancer. The way the radiation therapy is given depends on the type and stage of the cancer being treated.

Chemotherapy

Chemotherapy is a cancer treatment that uses drugs to stop the growth of cancer cells, either by killing the cells or by stopping them from dividing. When chemotherapy is taken by mouth or injected into a vein or muscle, the drugs enter the bloodstream and can reach cancer cells throughout the body (systemic chemotherapy). When chemotherapy is placed directly into the cerebrospinal fluid, an organ, or a body cavity such as the abdomen, the drugs mainly affect cancer cells in those areas (regional chemotherapy). The way the chemotherapy is given depends on the type and stage of the cancer being treated.

Biologic Therapy

Biologic therapy is a treatment that uses the patient's immune system to fight cancer. Substances made by the body or made in a laboratory are used to boost, direct, or restore the body's natural defenses against cancer. This type of cancer treatment is also called biotherapy or immunotherapy.

Targeted Therapy

Targeted therapy uses drugs or other substances that can find and attack specific cancer cells without harming normal cells. Antiangiogenic agents are a type of targeted therapy that may be used to treat advanced renal cell cancer. They keep blood vessels from forming in a tumor, causing the tumor to starve and stop growing or to shrink.

Clinical Trials

A treatment clinical trial is a research study meant to help improve current treatments or obtain information on new treatments for patients with cancer. When clinical trials show that a new treatment is better than the standard treatment, the new treatment may become the standard treatment. Patients may want to think about taking part in a clinical trial. Some clinical trials are open only to patients who have not started treatment.

This summary section describes a treatment that is being studied in clinical trials. It may not mention every new treatment being studied. Information about clinical trials is available from the National Cancer Institute website (www.cancer.gov).

Stem cell transplant: Stem cells (immature blood cells) are removed from the blood or bone marrow of a donor and given to the patient through an infusion. These reinfused stem cells grow into (and restore) the body's blood cells.

Follow-Up Tests

Some of the tests that were done to diagnose the cancer or to find out the stage of the cancer may be repeated. Some tests will be repeated in order to see how well the treatment is working. Decisions about whether to continue, change, or stop treatment may be based on the results of these tests. This is sometimes called re-staging.

Some of the tests will continue to be done from time to time after treatment has ended. The results of these tests can show if your condition has changed or if the cancer has recurred (come back). These tests are sometimes called follow-up tests or check-ups.

Section 37.2

Wilms Tumor and Other Childhood Kidney Tumors

Excerpted from PDQ® Cancer Information Summary. National Cancer Institute; Bethesda, MD. "Wilms Tumor and Other Childhood Kidney Tumors Treatment (PDQ) - Patient Version." Updated 06/2010. Available at: http://cancer.gov. Accessed September 29, 2010.

General Information about Wilms Tumor and Other Childhood Kidney Tumors

Wilms tumor and other childhood kidney tumors are diseases in which malignant (cancer) cells form in the tissues of the kidney.

Wilms tumor: In Wilms tumor, one or more tumors may be found in one or both kidneys. There are two kidneys, one on each side of the backbone, above the waist. Tiny tubules in the kidneys filter and clean the blood, taking out waste products and making urine. The urine passes from each kidney through a long tube called a ureter into the bladder. The bladder holds the urine until it is passed from the body. Wilms tumor may spread to the lungs, liver, or nearby lymph nodes.

Nephroblastomatosis: Nephroblastomatosis is a condition in which abnormal tissue grows on the outer part of one or both kidneys.

Children with this condition are at risk for developing a type of Wilms tumor that grows quickly. Frequent follow-up testing is important for at least seven years after the child is treated.

Other kidney tumors: Other childhood kidney tumors, which are diagnosed and treated in different ways:

- Clear cell sarcoma of the kidney is a type of kidney tumor that may spread to the lung, bone, brain, and soft tissue.

- Rhabdoid tumor of the kidney is a type of cancer that occurs mostly in infants and young children. It grows and spreads quickly, often to the lungs and brain.

- Neuroepithelial tumors of the kidney are rare and usually occur in young adults. They grow and spread quickly.

- Desmoplastic small round cell tumor of the kidney is a rare soft tissue sarcoma.

- Cystic partially differentiated nephroblastoma is a very rare type of Wilms tumor made up of cysts.

- Renal cell carcinoma is rare in children or in adolescents younger than 15 years of age. However, it is much more common in adolescents between 15 and 19 years of age. Renal cell carcinomas can spread to the lungs, bones, liver, and lymph nodes.

- Mesoblastic nephroma is a tumor of the kidney that is usually diagnosed within the first year of life and can usually be cured. One type of mesoblastic nephroma may appear on an ultrasound exam before birth or may occur within the first three months after the child is born. Mesoblastic nephroma occurs more often in males than females.

- Primary renal synovial sarcoma is a rare tumor of the kidney and is most common in young adults.

- Anaplastic sarcoma of the kidney is a rare tumor that is most commonly found in children or adolescents younger than 15 years of age. Anaplastic sarcoma of the kidney often spreads to the lungs, liver, or bones. There is no standard treatment for anaplastic sarcoma.

Risk Factors and Signs

Anything that increases the risk of getting a disease is called a risk factor. Having a risk factor does not mean that you will get cancer;

not having risk factors doesn't mean that you will not get cancer. Parents who think their child may be at risk should discuss this with the child's doctor.

Wilms tumor may be part of a genetic syndrome that affects growth or development. A genetic syndrome is a set of symptoms or conditions that occur together and is usually caused by abnormal genes. Certain birth defects can also increase a child's risk for developing Wilms tumor. The following genetic syndromes and birth defects have been linked to Wilms tumor:

- WAGR syndrome (Wilms tumor, aniridia, abnormal genitourinary system, and mental retardation)

- Beckwith-Wiedemann syndrome

- Hemihypertrophy (abnormally large growth of one side of the body or a body part)

- Denys-Drash syndrome

- Cryptorchidism

- Hypospadias

Children with these genetic syndromes and birth defects should be screened for Wilms tumor every three months until age eight. An ultrasound test may be used for screening.

Renal cell carcinoma may be related to the following conditions:

- Von Hippel-Lindau disease (an inherited condition that causes abnormal growth of blood vessels)

- Tuberous sclerosis (an inherited disease marked by noncancerous fatty cysts in the kidney)

- Neuroblastoma and/or sickle cell disease

Possible signs of Wilms tumor and other childhood kidney tumors include a lump in the abdomen and blood in the urine. These and other symptoms may be caused by kidney tumors. Other conditions may cause the same symptoms. A doctor should be consulted if any of the following problems occur in the child:

- A lump, swelling, or pain in the abdomen

- Blood in the urine

- Fever for no known reason

Detection

The following tests and procedures may be used:

Physical exam and history: An exam of the body to check general signs of health, including checking for signs of disease, such as lumps or anything else that seems unusual. A history of the patient's health habits and past illnesses and treatments will also be taken.

Complete blood count (CBC): A procedure in which a sample of blood is drawn and checked for the following:

- The number of red blood cells, white blood cells, and platelets

- The amount of hemoglobin (the protein that carries oxygen) in the red blood cells

- The portion of the blood sample made up of red blood cells

Blood chemistry studies: A procedure in which a blood sample is checked to measure the amounts of certain substances released into the blood by organs and tissues in the body. An unusual (higher or lower than normal) amount of a substance can be a sign of disease in the organ or tissue that makes it.

Liver function test: A procedure in which a blood sample is checked to measure the amounts of certain substances released into the blood by the liver. A higher than normal amount of a substance can be a sign that the liver is not working as it should.

Renal function test: A procedure in which blood or urine samples are checked to measure the amounts of certain substances released into the blood or urine by the kidneys. A higher or lower than normal amount of a substance can be a sign that the kidneys are not working as they should.

Urinalysis: A test to check the color of urine and its contents, such as sugar, protein, blood, and bacteria.

Ultrasound exam: A procedure in which high-energy sound waves (ultrasound) are bounced off internal tissues or organs and make echoes. The echoes form a picture of body tissues called a sonogram. An ultrasound of the abdomen is done to diagnose a kidney tumor.

CT scan (CAT scan): A procedure that makes a series of detailed pictures of areas inside the body, taken from different angles. The pictures are made by a computer linked to an x-ray machine. A dye may be injected into a vein or swallowed to help the organs or tissues show up more clearly. This procedure is also called computed tomography, computerized tomography, or computerized axial tomography.

Abdominal x-ray: An x-ray of the organs inside the abdomen. An x-ray is a type of energy beam that can go through the body and onto film, making a picture of areas inside the body.

Biopsy: The removal of cells or tissues so they can be viewed under a microscope by a pathologist to check for signs of cancer.

Diagnosis and Prognosis

Wilms tumor and other childhood kidney tumors are usually diagnosed and removed in surgery.

Once a kidney tumor is found, surgery is done to find out whether or not the tumor is cancer. If the tumor is only in the kidney, the surgeon will remove the whole kidney (nephrectomy). If there are tumors in both kidneys or if the tumor has spread outside the kidney, a piece of the tumor will be removed. In any case, a sample of tissue from the tumor is sent to a pathologist, who looks at it under a microscope to check for signs of cancer.

The prognosis (chance of recovery) and treatment options depend on the following:

- How different the tumor cells are from normal kidney cells
- The stage of the cancer
- The type and size of the tumor
- The age of the child
- Whether the tumor can be completely removed in surgery
- Whether the cancer has just been diagnosed or has recurred (come back)
- Whether there are any abnormal chromosomes or genes
- Whether the patient is treated by pediatric experts with experience in treating patients with Wilms tumor.

Stages of Wilms Tumor and Other Childhood Kidney Tumors

Wilms tumors and other childhood kidney tumors are staged during surgery and with imaging tests. The process used to find out if cancer has spread outside of the kidney to other parts of the body is called staging. The information gathered from the staging process determines the stage of the disease. It is important to know the stage in order to plan treatment.

For Wilms tumor, the stage is determined during the initial surgery and with the results from imaging tests. Some imaging tests, such as CT scan and ultrasound exam, are the same types of tests used in detecting Wilms tumor. Additional imaging tests that may be done to see if cancer has spread to other places in the body include the following:

- **X-ray of the chest and bones:** An x-ray is a type of energy beam that can go through the body and onto film, making a picture of areas inside the body.

- **MRI (magnetic resonance imaging):** A procedure that uses a magnet, radio waves, and a computer to make a series of detailed pictures of areas inside the body, such as the brain. This procedure is also called nuclear magnetic resonance imaging (NMRI).

- **Bone scan:** A procedure to check if there are rapidly dividing cells, such as cancer cells, in the bone. A very small amount of radioactive material is injected into a vein and travels through the bloodstream. The radioactive material collects in the bones and is detected by a scanner.

- **Cystoscopy:** A procedure to look inside the bladder and urethra to check for abnormal areas. A cystoscope is inserted through the urethra into the bladder. A cystoscope is a thin, tube-like instrument with a light and a lens for viewing. It may also have a tool to remove tissue samples, which are checked under a microscope for signs of cancer.

In addition to the stages, Wilms tumors are described by their histology. The histology (how the cells look under a microscope) of the tumor affects the prognosis and the treatment of Wilms tumor. The histology may be favorable or anaplastic (unfavorable). Tumors with a favorable histology have a better prognosis and respond better to chemotherapy than those with anaplastic histology. Tumor cells that are anaplastic divide rapidly and do not look like the type of cells they came from. Anaplastic tumors are harder to treat with chemotherapy than other Wilms tumors at the same stage.

The following stages are used for both favorable histology and anaplastic Wilms tumors:

Stage I

In stage I, the tumor was completely removed by surgery and all of the following are true:

- Cancer was found only in the kidney and did not spread to blood vessels of the kidney.
- The outer layer of the kidney did not break open.
- The tumor did not break open.
- A biopsy of the tumor was not done.
- No cancer cells were found at the edges of the area where the tumor was removed.

Stage II

In stage II, the tumor was completely removed by surgery and no cancer cells were found at the edges of the area where the cancer was removed. Before the tumor was removed, one of the following was true:

- Cancer had spread out of the kidney to nearby soft tissue.
- Cancer had spread to blood vessels of the kidney.

Stage III

In stage III, cancer remains in the abdomen after surgery and at least one of the following is true:

- Cancer spread to lymph nodes in the abdomen or pelvis (the part of the body between the hips).
- Cancer spread to or through the surface of the peritoneum (the layer of tissue that lines the abdominal cavity and covers most organs in the abdomen).
- Chemotherapy was given before surgery and a biopsy of the tumor was done during surgery to remove it.
- The tumor broke open before or during surgery to remove it.
- The tumor was removed in more than one piece.

Stage IV

In stage IV, cancer has spread through the blood to organs such as the lungs, liver, bone, or brain, or to lymph nodes outside of the abdomen and pelvis.

Stage V

In stage V, cancer cells are found in both kidneys when the disease is first diagnosed. Each kidney will be staged separately as I, II, III, or IV.

Recurrent Wilms Tumor and Other Childhood Kidney Tumors

Recurrent cancer is cancer that has recurred (come back) after it has been treated.

Treatment Option Overview

Different types of treatment are available for children with Wilms and other childhood kidney tumors. Some treatments are standard (the currently used treatment), and some are being tested in clinical trials. Because cancer in children is rare, taking part in a clinical trial should be considered. Some clinical trials are open only to patients who have not started treatment.

Children with Wilms tumor or other childhood kidney tumors should have their treatment planned by a team of health care providers who are experts in treating cancer in children. Your child's treatment will be overseen by a pediatric oncologist, a doctor who specializes in treating children with cancer. The pediatric oncologist works with other pediatric health care providers who are experts in treating children with Wilms tumor or other childhood kidney tumors and who specialize in certain areas of medicine. These may include the following specialists:

- Pediatric surgeon or urologist
- Radiation oncologist
- Rehabilitation specialist
- Pediatric nurse specialist
- Social worker

Side effects from cancer treatment that begin during or after treatment and continue for months or years are called late effects. Late effects of cancer treatment may include the following:

- Physical problems
- Changes in mood, feelings, thinking, learning, or memory
- Second cancers (new types of cancer)

Some late effects may be treated or controlled. It is important to talk with your child's doctors about the effects cancer treatment can have on your child. Clinical trials are ongoing to find out if lower doses of chemotherapy and radiation can be used.

Four types of standard treatment are used:

Surgery

Wilms tumor and other childhood kidney tumors are usually treated with nephrectomy (surgery to remove the whole kidney). Nearby lymph nodes may also be removed.

If cancer is found in both kidneys, surgery may include a partial nephrectomy (removal of the cancer in the kidney and a small amount of normal tissue around it). Partial nephrectomy is done to keep the kidney working.

Even if the doctor removes all the cancer that can be seen at the time of the surgery, some patients may be given chemotherapy or radiation therapy after surgery to kill any cancer cells that are left. Treatment given after the surgery, to lower the risk that the cancer will come back, is called adjuvant therapy. Sometimes, a second-look surgery is done to see if cancer remains after chemotherapy or radiation therapy.

Radiation Therapy

Radiation therapy is a cancer treatment that uses high-energy x-rays or other types of radiation to kill cancer cells or keep them from growing. There are two types of radiation therapy. External radiation therapy uses a machine outside the body to send radiation toward the cancer. Internal radiation therapy uses a radioactive substance sealed in needles, seeds, wires, or catheters that are placed directly into or near the cancer. The way the radiation therapy is given depends on the type and stage of the cancer being treated.

Chemotherapy

Chemotherapy is a cancer treatment that uses drugs to stop the growth of cancer cells, either by killing the cells or by stopping them from dividing. When chemotherapy is taken by mouth or injected into a vein or muscle, the drugs enter the bloodstream and can reach cancer cells throughout the body (systemic chemotherapy). When chemotherapy is placed directly into the cerebrospinal fluid, an organ, or a body cavity such as the abdomen, the drugs mainly affect cancer cells in those areas (regional chemotherapy). The way the chemotherapy is given depends on the type and stage of the cancer being treated.

Combination chemotherapy is treatment using two or more anti-cancer drugs.

Biologic Therapy

Biologic therapy is a treatment that uses the patient's immune system to fight cancer. Substances made by the body or made in a laboratory are used to boost, direct, or restore the body's natural defenses against cancer. This type of cancer treatment is also called biotherapy or immunotherapy.

Clinical Trials

A treatment clinical trial is a research study meant to help improve current treatments or obtain information on new treatments for patients with cancer. When clinical trials show that a new treatment is better than the standard treatment, the new treatment may become the standard treatment.

This summary describes a treatment that is being studied in clinical trials. It may not mention every new treatment being studied. Information about clinical trials is available from the National Cancer Institute website (www.cancer.gov).

High-dose chemotherapy with stem cell transplant: High-dose chemotherapy with stem cell transplant is a method of giving high doses of chemotherapy and replacing blood-forming cells destroyed by the cancer treatment. Stem cells (immature blood cells) are removed from the blood or bone marrow of the patient or a donor and are frozen and stored. After the chemotherapy is completed, the stored stem cells are thawed and given back to the patient through an infusion. These re-infused stem cells grow into (and restore) the body's blood cells.

Follow-Up Tests

Some of the tests that were done to diagnose the cancer or to find out the stage of the cancer may be repeated. Some tests will be repeated in order to see how well the treatment is working. Decisions about whether to continue, change, or stop treatment may be based on the results of these tests. This is sometimes called re-staging.

Some of the tests will continue to be done from time to time after treatment has ended. The results of these tests can show if your condition has changed or if the cancer has recurred (come back). These tests are sometimes called follow-up tests or check-ups.

Chapter 38

Transitional Cell Cancer of the Renal Pelvis and Ureter

General Information about Transitional Cell Cancer of the Renal Pelvis and Ureter

Transitional cell cancer of the renal pelvis and ureter is a disease in which malignant (cancer) cells form in the renal pelvis and ureter. The renal pelvis is part of the kidney and the ureter connects the kidney to the bladder. There are two kidneys, one on each side of the backbone, above the waist. The kidneys of an adult are about five inches long and three inches wide and are shaped like a kidney bean. The kidneys clean the blood and produce urine to rid the body of waste. The urine collects in the middle of each kidney in a large cavity called the renal pelvis. Urine drains from each kidney through a long tube called the ureter, into the bladder, where it is stored until it is passed from the body through the urethra.

The renal pelvis and ureters are lined with transitional cells. These cells can change shape and stretch without breaking apart. Transitional cell cancer starts in these cells. Transitional cell cancer can form in the renal pelvis or the ureter or both. Renal cell cancer is a more common type of kidney cancer; it is discussed in chapter 37.

Excerpted from PDQ® Cancer Information Summary. National Cancer Institute; Bethesda, MD. "Transitional Cell Cancer of the Renal Pelvis and Ureter Treatment (PDQ) - Patient Version." Updated 06/2010. Available at: http://cancer .gov. Accessed September 29, 2010.

Risk Factors and Signs

Risk factors include the following:

- Misusing certain pain medicines, including over-the-counter pain medicines, for a long time
- Being exposed to certain dyes and chemicals used in making leather goods, textiles, plastics, and rubber
- Smoking cigarettes

Possible signs of transitional cell cancer of the renal pelvis and ureter include blood in the urine and back pain. These and other symptoms may be caused by transitional cell cancer of the renal pelvis and ureter. Other conditions may cause the same symptoms. There may be no symptoms in the early stages. Symptoms may appear as the tumor grows. A doctor should be consulted if any of the following problems occur:

- Blood in the urine
- A pain in the back that doesn't go away
- Extreme tiredness
- Weight loss with no known reason
- Painful or frequent urination

Detection and Diagnosis

The following tests and procedures may be used:

Physical exam and history: An exam of the body to check general signs of health, including checking for signs of disease, such as lumps or anything else that seems unusual. A history of the patient's health habits and past illnesses and treatments will also be taken.

Urinalysis: A test to check the color of urine and its contents, such as sugar, protein, blood, and bacteria.

Ureteroscopy: A procedure to look inside the ureter and renal pelvis to check for abnormal areas. A ureteroscope (a thin, lighted tube) is inserted through the urethra into the bladder, ureter, and renal pelvis. Tissue samples may be taken for biopsy.

Urine cytology: Examination of urine under a microscope to check for abnormal cells. Cancer in the kidney, bladder, or ureter may shed cancer cells into the urine.

Intravenous pyelogram (IVP): A series of x-rays of the kidneys, ureters, and bladder to check for cancer. A contrast dye is injected into a vein. As the contrast dye moves through the kidneys, ureters, and bladder, x-rays are taken to see if there are any blockages.

CT scan (CAT scan): A procedure that makes a series of detailed pictures of areas inside the body, taken from different angles. The pictures are made by a computer linked to an x-ray machine. A dye may be injected into a vein or swallowed to help the organs or tissues show up more clearly. This procedure is also called computed tomography, computerized tomography, or computerized axial tomography.

Ultrasound: A procedure in which high-energy sound waves (ultrasound) are bounced off internal tissues or organs and make echoes. The echoes form a picture of body tissues called a sonogram. An ultrasound of the abdomen may be done to help diagnose cancer of the renal pelvis and ureter.

Prognosis

The prognosis (chance of recovery) depends on the stage and grade of the tumor. The treatment options depend the stage and grade of the tumor, where the tumor is, whether the patient's other kidney is healthy, and whether the cancer has recurred. Most transitional cell cancer of the renal pelvis and ureter can be cured if found early.

Stages of Transitional Cell Cancer of the Renal Pelvis and Ureter

After transitional cell cancer of the renal pelvis and ureter has been diagnosed, tests are done to find out if cancer cells have spread within the renal pelvis and ureter or to other parts of the body. The process used to find out if cancer has spread within the renal pelvis and ureter or to other parts of the body is called staging. The information gathered from the staging process determines the stage of the disease. It is important to know the stage in order to plan treatment. Intravenous pyelogram (IVP), CT scan, ultrasound, and ureteroscopy may be used in the staging process along with surgical procedures to remove tissues that will be examined by a pathologist.

The following stages are used for transitional cell cancer of the renal pelvis and/or ureter:

Stage 0 (Papillary Carcinoma and Carcinoma in Situ)

In stage 0, abnormal cells are found in tissue lining the inside of the renal pelvis or ureter. These abnormal cells may become cancer and spread into nearby normal tissue. Stage 0 is divided into stage 0a and stage 0is, depending on the type of tumor:

- Stage 0a may look like tiny mushrooms growing from the lining. Stage 0a is also called noninvasive papillary carcinoma.

- Stage 0is is a flat tumor on the tissue lining the inside of the renal pelvis or ureter. Stage 0is is also called carcinoma in situ.

Stage I

In stage I, cancer has formed and spread through the lining of the renal pelvis and/or ureter, into the layer of connective tissue.

Stage II

In stage II, cancer has spread through the layer of connective tissue to the muscle layer of the renal pelvis and/or ureter.

Stage III

In stage III, cancer has spread to the layer of fat outside the renal pelvis and/or ureter; or into the wall of the kidney.

Stage IV

In stage IV, cancer has spread to at least one of the following:

- A nearby organ
- The layer of fat surrounding the kidney
- One or more lymph nodes
- Other parts of the body

Other Descriptions

Transitional cell cancer of the renal pelvis and ureter is also described as localized, regional, or metastatic:

- **Localized:** The cancer is found only in the kidney.
- **Regional:** The cancer has spread to tissues around the kidney and to nearby lymph nodes and blood vessels in the pelvis.
- **Metastatic:** The cancer has spread to other parts of the body.

Recurrent Transitional Cell Cancer of the Renal Pelvis and Ureter

Recurrent transitional cell cancer of the renal pelvis and ureter is cancer that has recurred (come back) after it has been treated. The cancer may come back in the renal pelvis, ureter, or other parts of the body.

Treatment Option Overview

Different types of treatments are available for patients with transitional cell cancer of the renal pelvis and ureter. Some treatments are standard (the currently used treatment), and some are being tested in clinical trials. One type of standard treatment is used:

Surgery

One of the following surgical procedures may be used to treat transitional cell cancer of the renal pelvis and ureter:

- **Nephroureterectomy:** Surgery to remove the entire kidney, the ureter, and the bladder cuff (tissue that connects the ureter to the bladder)

- **Segmental resection of the ureter:** A surgical procedure to remove the part of the ureter that contains cancer and some of the healthy tissue around it. The ends of the ureter are then re-attached. This treatment is used when the cancer is superficial and in the lower third of the ureter only, near the bladder.

Clinical Trials

A treatment clinical trial is a research study meant to help improve current treatments or obtain information on new treatments for patients with cancer. When clinical trials show that a new treatment is better than the standard treatment, the new treatment may become the standard treatment. Patients may want to think about taking part in a clinical trial. Some clinical trials are open only to patients who have not started treatment.

This summary describes treatments that are being studied in clinical trials. It may not mention every new treatment being studied. Information about clinical trials is available from the National Cancer Institute website (www.cancer.gov).

Fulguration: Fulguration is a surgical procedure that destroys tissue using an electric current. A tool with a small wire loop on the end is used to remove the cancer or to burn away the tumor with electricity.

Segmental resection of the renal pelvis: This is a surgical procedure to remove localized cancer from the renal pelvis without removing the entire kidney. Segmental resection may be done to save kidney function when the other kidney is damaged or has already been removed.

Laser surgery: A laser beam (narrow beam of intense light) is used as a knife to remove the cancer. A laser beam can also be used to kill the cancer cells. This procedure may be called laser therapy or laser fulguration.

Regional chemotherapy and regional biologic therapy: Chemotherapy is a cancer treatment that uses drugs to stop the growth of cancer cells, either by killing the cells or by stopping the cells from dividing. Biologic therapy is a treatment that uses the patient's immune system to fight cancer; substances made by the body or made in a laboratory are used to boost, direct, or restore the body's natural defenses against cancer. Regional treatment means the anticancer drugs or biologic substances are placed directly into an organ or a body cavity such as the abdomen, so the drugs will affect cancer cells in that area. Clinical trials are studying the effectiveness of chemotherapy or biologic therapy using drugs placed directly into the renal pelvis or the ureter.

Follow-Up Tests

Some of the tests that were done to diagnose the cancer or to find out the stage of the cancer may be repeated. Some tests will be repeated in order to see how well the treatment is working. Decisions about whether to continue, change, or stop treatment may be based on the results of these tests. This is sometimes called re-staging.

Some of the tests will continue to be done from time to time after treatment has ended. The results of these tests can show if your condition has changed or if the cancer has recurred (come back). These tests are sometimes called follow-up tests or check-ups.

Chapter 39

Urethral Cancer

General Information about Urethral Cancer

Urethral cancer is a disease in which malignant (cancer) cells form in the tissues of the urethra. The urethra is the tube that carries urine from the bladder to outside the body. In women, the urethra is about 1½ inches long and is just above the vagina. In men, the urethra is about 8 inches long, and goes through the prostate gland and the penis to the outside of the body. In men, the urethra also carries semen.

Urethral cancer is a rare cancer that occurs more often in women than in men. There are different types of urethral cancer that begin in cells that line the urethra. These cancers are named for the types of cells that become malignant (cancerous):

- Squamous cell carcinoma is the most common type of urethral cancer. It forms in cells in the part of the urethra near the bladder in women, and in the lining of the urethra in the penis in men.

- Transitional cell carcinoma forms in the area near the urethral opening in women, and in the part of the urethra that goes through the prostate gland in men.

- Adenocarcinoma forms in glands near the urethra in both men and women.

Excerpted from PDQ® Cancer Information Summary. National Cancer Institute; Bethesda, MD. "Urethral Cancer Treatment (PDQ) - Patient Version." Updated 05/2010. Available at: http://cancer.gov. Accessed September 29, 2010.

Urethral cancer can metastasize (spread) quickly to tissues around the urethra and is often found in nearby lymph nodes by the time it is diagnosed.

Risk Factors and Signs

Risk factors include the following:

- Having a history of bladder cancer
- Having conditions that cause chronic inflammation in the urethra, including sexually transmitted diseases (STDs) and frequent urinary tract infections (UTIs)
- Being 60 or older
- Being a white female

Possible signs of urethral cancer include bleeding or trouble with urination. These and other symptoms may be caused by urethral cancer. Other conditions may cause the same symptoms. Sometimes early cancer of the urethra does not cause any symptoms at all. A doctor should be consulted if any of the following problems occur:

- Bleeding from the urethra or blood in the urine
- Weak or interrupted ("stop-and-go") flow of urine
- Frequent urination
- A lump or thickness in the perineum or penis
- Discharge from the urethra
- Enlarged lymph nodes in the groin area

Detection and Diagnosis

The following tests and procedures may be used:

Physical exam and history: An exam of the body to check general signs of health, including checking for signs of disease, such as lumps or anything else that seems unusual. A history of the patient's health habits and past illnesses and treatments will also be taken.

Laboratory tests: Medical procedures that test samples of tissue, blood, urine, or other substances in the body. These tests help to diagnose disease, plan and check treatment, or monitor the disease over time.

Urine cytology: Examination of urine under a microscope to check for abnormal cells.

Urinalysis: A test to check the color of urine and its contents, such as sugar, protein, blood, and white blood cells. If white blood cells (a sign of infection) are found, a urine culture is usually done to find out what type of infection it is.

Digital rectal exam: An exam of the rectum. The doctor or nurse inserts a lubricated, gloved finger into the lower part of the rectum to feel for lumps or anything else that seems unusual. This procedure may be done while the patient is under anesthesia.

Pelvic exam: An exam of the vagina, cervix, uterus, fallopian tubes, ovaries, and rectum. The doctor or nurse inserts one or two lubricated, gloved fingers of one hand into the vagina and places the other hand over the lower abdomen to feel the size, shape, and position of the uterus and ovaries. A speculum is also inserted into the vagina and the doctor or nurse looks at the vagina and cervix for signs of disease. This may be done while the patient is under anesthesia.

Cystoscopy: A procedure to look inside the urethra and bladder to check for abnormal areas. A cystoscope (a thin, lighted tube) is inserted through the urethra into the bladder. Tissue samples may be taken for biopsy.

Biopsy: The removal of cells or tissues from the urethra, bladder, and, sometimes, the prostate gland, so they can be viewed under a microscope by a pathologist to check for signs of cancer.

Prognosis

The prognosis (chance of recovery) depends on the stage and size of the cancer (whether it is in only one area or has spread to other areas), where in the urethra the cancer first formed, the patient's general health, and whether the cancer has just been diagnosed or has recurred (come back).

Treatment options depend on the stage of the cancer and where it is in the urethra, the patient's sex and general health, and whether the cancer has just been diagnosed or has recurred.

Stages of Urethral Cancer

After urethral cancer has been diagnosed, tests are done to find out if cancer cells have spread within the urethra or to other parts of the body. The process used to find out if cancer has spread within the urethra or to other parts of the body is called staging. The information gathered from the staging process determines the stage of the disease. It is important to know the stage in order to plan treatment. The following procedures may be used in the staging process:

Chest x-ray: An x-ray of the organs and bones inside the chest. An x-ray is a type of energy beam that can go through the body and onto film, making a picture of areas inside the body.

CT scan (CAT scan) of the pelvis and abdomen: A procedure that makes a series of detailed pictures of the pelvis and abdomen, taken from different angles. The pictures are made by a computer linked to an x-ray machine. A dye may be injected into a vein or swallowed to help the organs or tissues show up more clearly. This procedure is also called computed tomography, computerized tomography, or computerized axial tomography.

MRI (magnetic resonance imaging): A procedure that uses a magnet, radio waves, and a computer to make a series of detailed pictures of the urethra, nearby lymph nodes, and other soft tissue and bones in the pelvis. A substance called gadolinium is injected into the patient through a vein. The gadolinium collects around the cancer cells so they show up brighter in the picture. This procedure is also called nuclear magnetic resonance imaging (NMRI).

Blood chemistry studies: A procedure in which a blood sample is checked to measure the amounts of certain substances released into the blood by organs and tissues in the body. An unusual (higher or lower than normal) amount of a substance can be a sign of disease in the organ or tissue that produces it.

Complete blood count (CBC): A procedure in which a sample of blood is drawn and checked for the following:

- The number of red blood cells, white blood cells, and platelets

- The amount of hemoglobin (the protein that carries oxygen) in the red blood cells

- The portion of the blood sample made up of red blood cells

Urethral cancer is staged and treated based on the part of the urethra that is affected and how deeply the tumor has spread into tissue around the urethra. Urethral cancer can be described as anterior or posterior.

- **Anterior urethral cancer:** In anterior urethral cancer, the tumors are not deep and they affect the part of the urethra that is closest to the outside of the body.

- **Posterior urethral cancer:** In posterior urethral cancer, the tumors are deep and affect the part of the urethra closest to the bladder. In women, the entire urethra may be affected. In men, the prostate gland may be affected.

The following stages are also used to describe urethral cancer:

Stage 0 (Carcinoma in Situ)

In stage 0, abnormal cells are found in the inside lining of the urethra. These abnormal cells may become cancer and spread into nearby normal tissue. Stage 0 is also called carcinoma in situ.

Stage A

In stage A, cancer has formed and spread into the layer of tissue beneath the lining of the urethra.

Stage B

In stage B, cancer is found in the muscle around the urethra. In men, the penile tissue surrounding the urethra may be affected.

Stage C

In stage C, cancer has spread beyond the tissue surrounding the urethra, and in women, may be found in the vagina, vaginal lips, or nearby muscle; in men, may be found in the penis or in nearby muscle.

Stage D

Stage D is divided into stage D1 and stage D2, based on where the cancer has spread.

- In stage D1, cancer has spread to nearby lymph nodes in the pelvis and groin.
- In stage D2, cancer has spread to distant lymph nodes or to other organs in the body, such as the lungs, liver, and bone.

Associated with Invasive Bladder Cancer

A small number of patients who have bladder cancer are also diagnosed with cancer of the urethra, or will develop it in the future.

Recurrent Urethral Cancer

Recurrent urethral cancer is cancer that has recurred (come back) after it has been treated. The cancer may come back in the urethra or in other parts of the body.

Treatment Option Overview

Different types of treatments are available for patients with urethral cancer. Some treatments are standard (the currently used treatment), and some are being tested in clinical trials.

Three types of standard treatment are used: Surgery, radiation therapy, and watchful waiting.

Surgery

Surgery is the most common treatment for cancer of the urethra. One of the following types of surgery may be done:

- **Open excision:** Removal of the cancer by surgery.

- **Electro-resection with fulguration:** Surgery to remove the cancer by electric current. A lighted tool with a small wire loop on the end is used to remove the cancer or to burn the tumor away with high-energy electricity.

- **Laser surgery:** A surgical procedure that uses a laser beam (a narrow beam of intense light) as a knife to make bloodless cuts in tissue or to remove or destroy tissue.

- **Lymph node dissection:** Lymph nodes in the pelvis and groin may be removed.

- **Cystourethrectomy:** Surgery to remove the bladder and the urethra.

- **Cystoprostatectomy:** Surgery to remove the bladder and the prostate.

- **Anterior exenteration:** Surgery to remove the urethra, the bladder, and the vagina. Plastic surgery may be done to rebuild the vagina.

- **Partial penectomy:** Surgery to remove the part of the penis surrounding the urethra where cancer has spread. Plastic surgery may be done to rebuild the penis.

- **Radical penectomy:** Surgery to remove the entire penis. Plastic surgery may be done to rebuild the penis.

If the urethra is removed, the surgeon will make a new way for the urine to pass from the body. This is called urinary diversion. If the bladder is removed, the surgeon will make a new way for urine to be stored and passed from the body. The surgeon may use part of the small intestine to make a tube that passes urine through an opening (stoma). This is called an ostomy or urostomy. If a patient has an ostomy, a disposable bag to collect urine is worn under clothing. The surgeon may also use part of the small intestine to make a new storage pouch (continent reservoir) inside the body where the urine can collect. A tube (catheter) is then used to drain the urine through a stoma.

Even if the doctor removes all the cancer that can be seen at the time of the surgery, some patients may be given chemotherapy or radiation therapy after surgery to kill any cancer cells that are left. Treatment given after the surgery, to lower the risk that the cancer will come back, is called adjuvant therapy.

Radiation Therapy

Radiation therapy is a cancer treatment that uses high-energy x-rays or other types of radiation to kill cancer cells. There are two types of radiation therapy. External radiation therapy uses a machine outside the body to send radiation toward the cancer. Internal radiation therapy uses a radioactive substance sealed in needles, seeds, wires, or catheters that are placed directly into or near the cancer. The way the radiation therapy is given depends on the type and stage of the cancer being treated.

Watchful Waiting

Watchful waiting is closely monitoring a patient's condition without giving any treatment until symptoms appear or change.

Clinical Trials

A treatment clinical trial is a research study meant to help improve current treatments or obtain information on new treatments for patients with cancer. When clinical trials show that a new treatment is better than the standard treatment, the new treatment may become the standard treatment. Patients may want to think about taking part in a clinical trial. Some clinical trials are open only to patients who have not started treatment.

This summary describes a treatment that is being studied in clinical trials. It may not mention every new treatment being studied.

Information about clinical trials is available from the National Cancer Institute website (www.cancer.gov).

Chemotherapy: Chemotherapy is a cancer treatment that uses drugs to stop the growth of cancer cells, either by killing the cells or by stopping the cells from dividing. When chemotherapy is taken by mouth or injected into a vein or muscle, the drugs enter the bloodstream and can reach cancer cells throughout the body (systemic chemotherapy). When chemotherapy is placed directly into the spinal column, an organ, or a body cavity such as the abdomen, the drugs mainly affect cancer cells in those areas (regional chemotherapy). The way the chemotherapy is given depends on the type and stage of the cancer being treated.

Follow-Up Tests

Some of the tests that were done to diagnose the cancer or to find out the stage of the cancer may be repeated. Some tests will be repeated in order to see how well the treatment is working. Decisions about whether to continue, change, or stop treatment may be based on the results of these tests. This is sometimes called re-staging.

Some of the tests will continue to be done from time to time after treatment has ended. The results of these tests can show if your condition has changed or if the cancer has recurred (come back). These tests are sometimes called follow-up tests or check-ups.

Chapter 40

Bladder Cancer

General Information about Bladder Cancer

Bladder cancer is a disease in which malignant (cancer) cells form in the tissues of the bladder. The bladder is a hollow organ in the lower part of the abdomen. It is shaped like a small balloon and has a muscular wall that allows it to get larger or smaller. The bladder stores urine until it is passed out of the body. Urine is the liquid waste that is made by the kidneys when they clean the blood. The urine passes from the two kidneys into the bladder through two tubes called ureters. When the bladder is emptied during urination, the urine goes from the bladder to the outside of the body through another tube called the urethra.

There are three types of bladder cancer that begin in cells in the lining of the bladder. These cancers are named for the type of cells that become malignant (cancerous):

- **Transitional cell carcinoma:** Cancer that begins in cells in the innermost tissue layer of the bladder. These cells are able to stretch when the bladder is full and shrink when it is emptied. Most bladder cancers begin in the transitional cells.

- **Squamous cell carcinoma:** Cancer that begins in squamous cells, which are thin, flat cells that may form in the bladder after long-term infection or irritation.

Excerpted from PDQ® Cancer Information Summary. National Cancer Institute; Bethesda, MD. "Bladder Cancer Treatment (PDQ) - Patient Version." Updated 08/2010. Available at: http://cancer.gov. Accessed September 29, 2010.

- **Adenocarcinoma:** Cancer that begins in glandular (secretory) cells that may form in the bladder after long-term irritation and inflammation.

Cancer that is confined to the lining of the bladder is called superficial bladder cancer. Cancer that begins in the transitional cells may spread through the lining of the bladder and invade the muscle wall of the bladder or spread to nearby organs and lymph nodes; this is called invasive bladder cancer.

Risk Factors and Signs

Anything that increases your chance of getting a disease is called a risk factor. Risk factors for bladder cancer include the following:

- Smoking
- Being exposed to certain substances at work, such as rubber, certain dyes and textiles, paint, and hairdressing supplies
- A diet high in fried meats and fat
- Being older, male, or white
- Having an infection caused by a certain parasite

Possible signs of bladder cancer include blood in the urine or pain during urination. These and other symptoms may be caused by bladder cancer. Other conditions may cause the same symptoms. A doctor should be consulted if any of the following problems occur:

- Blood in the urine (slightly rusty to bright red in color)
- Frequent urination, or feeling the need to urinate without being able to do so
- Pain during urination
- Lower back pain

Detection and Diagnosis

Tests that examine the urine, vagina, or rectum are used to help detect (find) and diagnose bladder cancer. The following tests and procedures may be used:

CT scan (CAT scan): A procedure that makes a series of detailed pictures of areas inside the body, taken from different angles. The pictures are made by a computer linked to an x-ray machine. A dye may be injected into a vein or swallowed to help the organs or tissues show up more clearly. This procedure is also called computed tomography, computerized tomography, or computerized axial tomography.

Urinalysis: A test to check the color of urine and its contents, such as sugar, protein, red blood cells, and white blood cells.

Internal exam: An exam of the vagina and/or rectum. The doctor inserts gloved fingers into the vagina and/or rectum to feel for lumps.

Intravenous pyelogram (IVP): A series of x-rays of the kidneys, ureters, and bladder to find out if cancer is present in these organs. A contrast dye is injected into a vein. As the contrast dye moves through the kidneys, ureters, and bladder, x-rays are taken to see if there are any blockages.

Cystoscopy: A procedure to look inside the bladder and urethra to check for abnormal areas. A cystoscope is inserted through the urethra into the bladder. A cystoscope is a thin, tube-like instrument with a light and a lens for viewing. It may also have a tool to remove tissue samples, which are checked under a microscope for signs of cancer.

Biopsy: The removal of cells or tissues so they can be viewed under a microscope by a pathologist to check for signs of cancer. A biopsy for bladder cancer is usually done during cystoscopy. It may be possible to remove the entire tumor during biopsy.

Urine cytology: Examination of urine under a microscope to check for abnormal cells.

Prognosis

The prognosis (chance of recovery) depends on the following:

- The stage of the cancer (whether it is superficial or invasive bladder cancer, and whether it has spread to other places in the body). Bladder cancer in the early stages can often be cured.

- The type of bladder cancer cells and how they look under a microscope

- The patient's age and general health

Treatment options depend on the stage of bladder cancer.

Stages of Bladder Cancer

After bladder cancer has been diagnosed, tests are done to find out if cancer cells have spread within the bladder or to other parts of the body. The process used to find out if cancer has spread within the bladder lining and muscle or to other parts of the body is called staging. The information gathered from the staging process determines the stage of the disease. It is important to know the stage in order to plan treatment. Cystoscopy and CT scan, which are described above, may be used in the staging process. The following additional tests and procedures may also be used:

- **MRI (magnetic resonance imaging):** A procedure that uses a magnet, radio waves, and a computer to make a series of detailed pictures of areas inside the body. This procedure is also called nuclear magnetic resonance imaging (NMRI).

- **Physical exam and history:** An exam of the body to check general signs of health, including checking for signs of disease, such as lumps or anything else that seems unusual. A history of the patient's health habits and past illnesses and treatments will also be taken.

- **Chest x-ray:** An x-ray of the organs and bones inside the chest. An x-ray is a type of energy beam that can go through the body and onto film, making a picture of areas inside the body.

- **Bone scan:** A procedure to check if there are rapidly dividing cells, such as cancer cells, in the bone. A very small amount of radioactive material is injected into a vein and travels through the bloodstream. The radioactive material collects in the bones and is detected by a scanner.

The following stages are used for bladder cancer:

Stage 0 (Papillary Carcinoma and Carcinoma in Situ)

In stage 0, abnormal cells are found in tissue lining the inside of the bladder. These abnormal cells may become cancer and spread into nearby normal tissue. Stage 0 is divided into stage 0a and stage 0is, depending on the type of the tumor:

- Stage 0a is also called papillary carcinoma, which may look like tiny mushrooms growing from the lining of the bladder

- Stage 0is is also called carcinoma in situ, which is a flat tumor on the tissue lining the inside of the bladder.

Stage I

In stage I, cancer has formed and spread to the layer of tissue under the inner lining of the bladder.

Stage II

In stage II, cancer has spread to either the inner half or outer half of the muscle wall of the bladder.

Stage III

In stage III, cancer has spread from the bladder to the fatty layer of tissue surrounding it and may have spread to the reproductive organs (prostate, seminal vesicles, uterus, or vagina).

Stage IV

In stage IV, cancer has spread from the bladder to the wall of the abdomen or pelvis. Cancer may have spread to one or more lymph nodes or to other parts of the body.

Recurrent Bladder Cancer

Recurrent bladder cancer is cancer that has recurred (come back) after it has been treated. The cancer may come back in the bladder or in other parts of the body.

Treatment Option Overview

Different types of treatment are available for patients with bladder cancer. Some treatments are standard (the currently used treatment), and some are being tested in clinical trials. Four types of standard treatment are used:

Surgery

One of the following types of surgery may be done:

- **Transurethral resection (TUR) with fulguration:** Surgery in which a cystoscope (a thin lighted tube) is inserted into the bladder through the urethra. A tool with a small wire loop on the end is then used to remove the cancer or to burn the tumor away with high-energy electricity. This is known as fulguration.

- **Radical cystectomy:** Surgery to remove the bladder and any lymph nodes and nearby organs that contain cancer. This surgery may be done when the bladder cancer invades the muscle wall, or when superficial cancer involves a large part of the bladder. In men, the nearby organs that are removed are the prostate and the seminal vesicles. In women, the uterus, the ovaries, and part of the vagina are removed. Sometimes, when the cancer has spread outside the bladder and cannot be completely removed, surgery to remove only the bladder may be done to reduce urinary symptoms caused by the cancer. When the bladder must be removed, the surgeon creates another way for urine to leave the body.

- **Segmental cystectomy:** Surgery to remove part of the bladder. This surgery may be done for patients who have a low-grade tumor that has invaded the wall of the bladder but is limited to one area of the bladder. Because only a part of the bladder is removed, patients are able to urinate normally after recovering from this surgery.

- **Urinary diversion:** Surgery to make a new way for the body to store and pass urine.

Even if the doctor removes all the cancer that can be seen at the time of the surgery, some patients may be given chemotherapy after surgery to kill any cancer cells that are left. Treatment given after surgery, to lower the risk that the cancer will come back, is called adjuvant therapy.

Radiation Therapy

Radiation therapy is a cancer treatment that uses high-energy x-rays or other types of radiation to kill cancer cells or keep them from growing. There are two types of radiation therapy. External radiation therapy uses a machine outside the body to send radiation toward the cancer. Internal radiation therapy uses a radioactive substance sealed in needles, seeds, wires, or catheters that are placed directly into or near the cancer. The way the radiation therapy is given depends on the type and stage of the cancer being treated.

Chemotherapy

Chemotherapy is a cancer treatment that uses drugs to stop the growth of cancer cells, either by killing the cells or by stopping them from dividing. When chemotherapy is taken by mouth or injected into a vein or muscle, the drugs enter the bloodstream and can reach cancer cells throughout the body (systemic chemotherapy). When chemotherapy is placed directly into the cerebrospinal fluid, an organ, or a body cavity such as the abdomen, the drugs mainly affect cancer cells in those areas (regional chemotherapy). Bladder cancer may be treated with intravesical (into the bladder through a tube inserted into the urethra) chemotherapy. The way the chemotherapy is given depends on the type and stage of the cancer being treated.

Biologic Therapy

Biologic therapy is a treatment that uses the patient's immune system to fight cancer. Substances made by the body or made in a laboratory are used to boost, direct, or restore the body's natural defenses against cancer. This type of cancer treatment is also called biotherapy or immunotherapy.

Clinical Trials

A treatment clinical trial is a research study meant to help improve current treatments or obtain information on new treatments for patients with cancer. When clinical trials show that a new treatment is better than the standard treatment, the new treatment may become the standard treatment. Patients may want to think about taking part in a clinical trial. Some clinical trials are open only to patients who have not started treatment.

This summary describes treatments that are being studied in clinical trials. It may not mention every new treatment being studied. Information about clinical trials is available from the National Cancer Institute website (www.cancer.gov).

Chemoprevention: Chemoprevention is the use of drugs, vitamins, or other substances to reduce the risk of developing cancer or to reduce the risk that cancer will recur (come back).

Photodynamic therapy: Photodynamic therapy (PDT) is a cancer treatment that uses a drug and a certain type of laser light to kill cancer cells. A drug that is not active until it is exposed to light is injected into a vein. The drug collects more in cancer cells than in normal cells. Fiberoptic tubes are then used to carry the laser light to the cancer cells, where the drug becomes active and kills the cells. Photodynamic therapy causes little damage to healthy tissue.

Follow-Up Tests

Some of the tests that were done to diagnose the cancer or to find out the stage of the cancer may be repeated. Some tests will be repeated in order to see how well the treatment is working. Decisions about whether to continue, change, or stop treatment may be based on the results of these tests. This is sometimes called re-staging.

Some of the tests will continue to be done from time to time after treatment has ended. The results of these tests can show if your condition has changed or if the cancer has recurred (come back). These tests are sometimes called follow-up tests or check-ups.

Chapter 41

Breast Cancer

General Information about Breast Cancer

Inside a woman's breast are 15 to 20 sections called lobes. Each lobe is made of many smaller sections called lobules. Lobules have groups of tiny glands that can make milk. After a baby is born, a woman's breast milk flows from the lobules through thin tubes called ducts to the nipple. Fat and fibrous tissue fill the spaces between the lobules and ducts.

The breasts also contain lymph vessels. These vessels are connected to small, round masses of tissue called lymph nodes. Groups of lymph nodes are near the breast in the underarm (axilla), above the collarbone, and in the chest behind the breastbone.

Cancer begins in cells, the building blocks that make up tissues. Tissues make up the breasts and other parts of the body.

Risk Factors

When you're told that you have breast cancer, it's natural to wonder what may have caused the disease. But no one knows the exact causes of breast cancer. Doctors seldom know why one woman develops breast cancer and another doesn't.

Doctors do know that bumping, bruising, or touching the breast does not cause cancer. And breast cancer is not contagious. You can't catch it from another person.

Excerpted from "What You Need to Know about Breast Cancer," National Cancer Institute (www.cancer.gov), October 15, 2009.

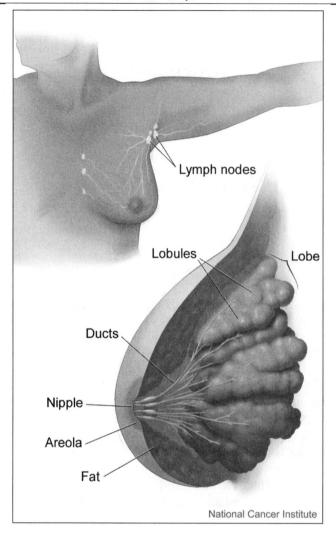

Figure 41.1. *The Breast and Adjacent Lymph Nodes (image by Don Bliss, National Cancer Institute)*

Doctors also know that women with certain risk factors are more likely than others to develop breast cancer. A risk factor is something that may increase the chance of getting a disease. Some risk factors (such as drinking alcohol) can be avoided. But most risk factors (such as having a family history of breast cancer) can't be avoided. Studies have found the following risk factors for breast cancer:

- **Age:** The chance of getting breast cancer increases as you get older. Most women are over 60 years old when they are diagnosed.

- **Personal health history:** Having breast cancer in one breast increases your risk of getting cancer in your other breast. Also, having certain types of abnormal breast cells (atypical hyperplasia, lobular carcinoma in situ [LCIS], or ductal carcinoma in situ [DCIS]) increases the risk of invasive breast cancer. These conditions are found with a breast biopsy.

- **Family health history:** Your risk of breast cancer is higher if your mother, father, sister, or daughter had breast cancer. The risk is even higher if your family member had breast cancer before age 50. Having other relatives (in either your mother's or father's family) with breast cancer or ovarian cancer may also increase your risk.

- **Certain genome changes:** Changes in certain genes, such as BRCA1 or BRCA2, substantially increase the risk of breast cancer. Tests can sometimes show the presence of these rare, specific gene changes in families with many women who have had breast cancer, and health care providers may suggest ways to try to reduce the risk of breast cancer or to improve the detection of this disease in women who have these genetic changes. Also, researchers have found specific regions on certain chromosomes that are linked to the risk of breast cancer. If a woman has a genetic change in one or more of these regions, the risk of breast cancer may be slightly increased. The risk increases with the number of genetic changes that are found. Although these genetic changes are more common among women than BRCA1 or BRCA2, the risk of breast cancer is far lower.

- **Radiation therapy to the chest:** Women who had radiation therapy to the chest (including the breasts) before age 30 are at an increased risk of breast cancer. This includes women treated with radiation for Hodgkin lymphoma. Studies show that the younger a woman was when she received radiation treatment, the higher her risk of breast cancer later in life.

- **Reproductive and menstrual history:** The older a woman is when she has her first child, the greater her chance of breast cancer. Women who never had children are at an increased risk of breast cancer. Women who had their first menstrual period before age 12 are at an increased risk of breast cancer. Women who went through menopause after age 55 are at an increased risk of breast cancer. Women who take menopausal hormone therapy for many years have an increased risk of breast cancer.

- **Race:** In the United States, breast cancer is diagnosed more often in white women than in African American/black, Hispanic/Latina, Asian/Pacific Islander, or American Indian/Alaska Native women.

- **Breast density:** Breasts appear on a mammogram (breast x-ray) as having areas of dense and fatty (not dense) tissue. Women whose mammograms show a larger area of dense tissue than the mammograms of women of the same age are at increased risk of breast cancer.

- **History of taking DES:** DES was given to some pregnant women in the United States between about 1940 and 1971. (It is no longer given to pregnant women.) Women who took DES during pregnancy may have a slightly increased risk of breast cancer. The possible effects on their daughters are under study.

- **Being overweight or obese after menopause:** The chance of getting breast cancer after menopause is higher in women who are overweight or obese.

- **Lack of physical activity:** Women who are physically inactive throughout life may have an increased risk of breast cancer.

- **Drinking alcohol:** Studies suggest that the more alcohol a woman drinks, the greater her risk of breast cancer.

Having a risk factor does not mean that a woman will get breast cancer. Most women who have risk factors never develop breast cancer.

Many other possible risk factors have been studied. For example, researchers are studying whether women who have a diet high in fat or who are exposed to certain substances in the environment have an increased risk of breast cancer. Researchers continue to study these and other possible risk factors.

Symptoms

Early breast cancer usually doesn't cause symptoms. But as the tumor grows, it can change how the breast looks or feels. The common changes include the following:

- A lump or thickening in or near the breast or in the underarm area
- A change in the size or shape of the breast
- Dimpling or puckering in the skin of the breast
- A nipple turned inward into the breast
- Discharge (fluid) from the nipple, especially if it's bloody
- Scaly, red, or swollen skin on the breast, nipple, or areola (the dark area of skin at the center of the breast). The skin may have ridges or pitting so that it looks like the skin of an orange.

You should see your health care provider about any symptom that does not go away. Most often, these symptoms are not due to cancer. Another health problem could cause them. If you have any of these symptoms, you should tell your health care provider so that the problems can be diagnosed and treated.

Breast Cancer Detection and Diagnosis

Your doctor can check for breast cancer before you have any symptoms. During an office visit, your doctor will ask about your personal and family medical history. You'll have a physical exam. Your doctor may order one or more imaging tests, such as a mammogram.

Doctors recommend that women have regular clinical breast exams and mammograms to find breast cancer early. Treatment is more likely to work well when breast cancer is detected early.

Clinical Breast Exam

During a clinical breast exam, your health care provider checks your breasts. You may be asked to raise your arms over your head, let them hang by your sides, or press your hands against your hips. Your health care provider looks for differences in size or shape between your breasts. The skin of your breasts is checked for a rash, dimpling, or other abnormal signs. Your nipples may be squeezed to check for fluid.

Using the pads of the fingers to feel for lumps, your health care provider checks your entire breast, underarm, and collarbone area. A lump is generally the size of a pea before anyone can feel it. The exam is done on one side and then the other. Your health care provider checks the lymph nodes near the breast to see if they are enlarged.

If you have a lump, your health care provider will feel its size, shape, and texture. Your health care provider will also check to see if the lump moves easily. Benign lumps often feel different from cancerous ones. Lumps that are soft, smooth, round, and movable are likely to be benign. A hard, oddly shaped lump that feels firmly attached within the breast is more likely to be cancer, but further tests are needed to diagnose the problem.

Mammogram

A mammogram is an x-ray picture of tissues inside the breast. Mammograms can often show a breast lump before it can be felt. They also can show a cluster of tiny specks of calcium. These specks are called microcalcifications. Lumps or specks can be from cancer, precancerous cells, or other conditions. Further tests are needed to find out if abnormal cells are present.

Before they have symptoms, women should get regular screening mammograms to detect breast cancer early:

- Women in their 40s and older should have mammograms every one or two years.

- Women who are younger than 40 and have risk factors for breast cancer should ask their health care provider whether to have mammograms and how often to have them.

If the mammogram shows an abnormal area of the breast, your doctor may order clearer, more detailed images of that area. Doctors use diagnostic mammograms to learn more about unusual breast changes, such as a lump, pain, thickening, nipple discharge, or change in breast size or shape. Diagnostic mammograms may focus on a specific area of the breast. They may involve special techniques and more views than screening mammograms.

Other Imaging Tests

If an abnormal area is found during a clinical breast exam or with a mammogram, the doctor may order other imaging tests:

- **Ultrasound:** A woman with a lump or other breast change may have an ultrasound test. An ultrasound device sends out sound waves that people can't hear. The sound waves bounce off breast tissues. A computer uses the echoes to create a picture. The picture may show whether a lump is solid, filled with fluid (a cyst), or a mixture of both. Cysts usually are not cancer. But a solid lump may be cancer.

- **MRI:** MRI uses a powerful magnet linked to a computer. It makes detailed pictures of breast tissue. These pictures can show the difference between normal and diseased tissue.

Biopsy

A biopsy is the removal of tissue to look for cancer cells. A biopsy is the only way to tell for sure if cancer is present.

You may need to have a biopsy if an abnormal area is found. An abnormal area may be felt during a clinical breast exam but not seen on a mammogram. Or an abnormal area could be seen on a mammogram but not be felt during a clinical breast exam. In this case, doctors can use imaging procedures (such as a mammogram, an ultrasound, or MRI) to help see the area and remove tissue.

Your doctor may refer you to a surgeon or breast disease specialist for a biopsy. The surgeon or doctor will remove fluid or tissue from your breast in one of several ways:

- **Fine-needle aspiration biopsy:** Your doctor uses a thin needle to remove cells or fluid from a breast lump.

- **Core biopsy:** Your doctor uses a wide needle to remove a sample of breast tissue.

- **Skin biopsy:** If there are skin changes on your breast, your doctor may take a small sample of skin.

- **Surgical biopsy:** Your surgeon removes a sample of tissue. An incisional biopsy takes a part of the lump or abnormal area. An excisional biopsy takes the entire lump or abnormal area.

A pathologist will check the tissue or fluid removed from your breast for cancer cells. If cancer cells are found, the pathologist can tell what kind of cancer it is. The most common type of breast cancer is ductal carcinoma. It begins in the cells that line the breast ducts. Lobular carcinoma is another type. It begins in the lobules of the breast.

Lab Tests with Breast Tissue

If you are diagnosed with breast cancer, your doctor may order special lab tests on the breast tissue that was removed:

- **Hormone receptor tests:** Some breast tumors need hormones to grow. These tumors have receptors for the hormones estrogen, progesterone, or both. If the hormone receptor tests show that the breast tumor has these receptors, then hormone therapy is most often recommended as a treatment option.

- **HER2/neu test:** HER2/neu protein is found on some types of cancer cells. This test shows whether the tissue either has too much HER2/neu protein or too many copies of its gene. If the breast tumor has too much HER2/neu, then targeted therapy may be a treatment option.

It may take several weeks to get the results of these tests. The test results help your doctor decide which cancer treatments may be options for you.

Staging

If the biopsy shows that you have breast cancer, your doctor needs to learn the extent (stage) of the disease to help you choose the best treatment. The stage is based on the size of the cancer, whether the cancer has invaded nearby tissues, and whether the cancer has spread to other parts of the body.

Staging may involve blood tests and other tests:

- **Bone scan:** The doctor injects a small amount of a radioactive substance into a blood vessel. It travels through the bloodstream and collects in the bones. A machine called a scanner detects and measures the radiation. The scanner makes pictures of the bones. The pictures may show cancer that has spread to the bones.

- **CT scan:** Doctors sometimes use CT scans to look for breast cancer that has spread to the liver or lungs. An x-ray machine linked to a computer takes a series of detailed pictures of your chest or abdomen. You may receive contrast material by injection into a blood vessel in your arm or hand. The contrast material makes abnormal areas easier to see.

- **Lymph node biopsy:** The stage often is not known until after surgery to remove the tumor in your breast and one or more lymph nodes under your arm. Surgeons use a method called sentinel lymph node biopsy to remove the lymph node most likely to have breast cancer cells. The surgeon injects a blue dye, a radioactive substance, or both near the breast tumor. Or the surgeon may inject a radioactive substance under the nipple. The surgeon then uses a scanner to find the sentinel lymph node containing the radioactive substance or looks for the lymph node stained with dye. The sentinel node is removed and checked for cancer cells. Cancer cells may appear first in the sentinel node before spreading to other lymph nodes and other places in the body.

These tests can show whether the cancer has spread and, if so, to what parts of your body. When breast cancer spreads, cancer cells are often found in lymph nodes under the arm (axillary lymph nodes). Also, breast cancer can spread to almost any other part of the body, such as the bones, liver, lungs, and brain.

When breast cancer spreads from its original place to another part of the body, the new tumor has the same kind of abnormal cells and the same name as the primary (original) tumor. For example, if breast cancer spreads to the bones, the cancer cells in the bones are actually breast cancer cells. The disease is metastatic breast cancer, not bone cancer. For that reason, it is treated as breast cancer, not bone cancer. Doctors call the new tumor "distant" or metastatic disease.

These are the stages of breast cancer:

Stage 0

Stage 0 is sometimes used to describe abnormal cells that are not invasive cancer. For example, Stage 0 is used for ductal carcinoma in situ (DCIS). DCIS is diagnosed when abnormal cells are in the lining of a breast duct, but the abnormal cells have not invaded nearby breast tissue or spread outside the duct. Although many doctors don't consider DCIS to be cancer, DCIS sometimes becomes invasive breast cancer if not treated.

Stage I

Stage I is an early stage of invasive breast cancer. Cancer cells have invaded breast tissue beyond where the cancer started, but the cells have not spread beyond the breast. The tumor is no more than two centimeters (three-quarters of an inch) across.

Stage II

Stage II is one of the following:

- The tumor is no more than two centimeters (three-quarters of an inch) across. The cancer has spread to the lymph nodes under the arm.

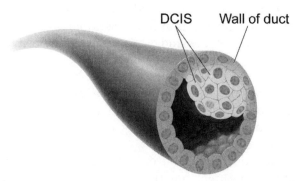

DCIS   Wall of duct

Figure 41.2. Ductal Carcinoma in Situ (image by Don Bliss, National Cancer Institute)

- The tumor is between two and five centimeters (three-quarters of an inch to two inches). The cancer has not spread to the lymph nodes under the arm.

- The tumor is between two and five centimeters (three-quarters of an inch to two inches). The cancer has spread to the lymph nodes under the arm.

- The tumor is larger than five centimeters (two inches). The cancer has not spread to the lymph nodes under the arm.

Stage III

Stage III is locally advanced cancer. It is divided into Stage IIIA, IIIB, and IIIC.

Stage IIIA is one of the following:

- The tumor is no more than five centimeters (two inches) across. The cancer has spread to underarm lymph nodes that are attached to each other or to other structures. Or the cancer may have spread to lymph nodes behind the breastbone.

- The tumor is more than five centimeters across. The cancer has spread to underarm lymph nodes that are either alone or attached to each other or to other structures. Or the cancer may have spread to lymph nodes behind the breastbone.

Stage IIIB is a tumor of any size that has grown into the chest wall or the skin of the breast. It may be associated with swelling of the breast or with nodules (lumps) in the breast skin:

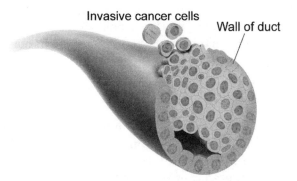

Figure 41.3. *Invasive Breast Cancer (image by Don Bliss, National Cancer Institute)*

- The cancer may have spread to lymph nodes under the arm.

- The cancer may have spread to underarm lymph nodes that are attached to each other or other structures. Or the cancer may have spread to lymph nodes behind the breastbone.

- Inflammatory breast cancer is a rare type of breast cancer. The breast looks red and swollen because cancer cells block the lymph vessels in the skin of the breast. When a doctor diagnoses inflammatory breast cancer, it is at least Stage IIIB, but it could be more advanced.

Stage IIIC is a tumor of any size. It has spread in one of the following ways:

- The cancer has spread to the lymph nodes behind the breastbone and under the arm.

- The cancer has spread to the lymph nodes above or below the collarbone.

Stage IV

Stage IV is distant metastatic cancer. The cancer has spread to other parts of the body, such as the bones or liver.

Recurrent Cancer

Recurrent cancer is cancer that has come back after a period of time when it could not be detected. Even when the cancer seems to be completely destroyed, the disease sometimes returns because undetected cancer cells remained somewhere in your body after treatment. It may return in the breast or chest wall. Or it may return in any other part of the body, such as the bones, liver, lungs, or brain.

Breast Cancer Treatment

Women with breast cancer have many treatment options. The treatment that's best for one woman may not be best for another.

The options are surgery, radiation therapy, hormone therapy, chemotherapy, and targeted therapy. Surgery and radiation therapy are types of local therapy. They remove or destroy cancer in the breast. Hormone therapy, chemotherapy, and targeted therapy are types of systemic therapy. The drug enters the bloodstream and destroys or controls cancer throughout the body.

You may receive more than one type of treatment. The treatment that's right for you depends mainly on the stage of the cancer, the results of the hormone receptor tests, the result of the HER2/neu test, and your general health.

You may want to talk with your doctor about taking part in a clinical trial, a research study of new treatment methods. Clinical trials are an important option for women at any stage of breast cancer.

Your doctor can describe your treatment choices, the expected results, and the possible side effects. Because cancer therapy often damages healthy cells and tissues, side effects are common. Before treatment starts, ask your health care team about possible side effects, how to prevent or reduce these effects, and how treatment may change your normal activities.

You may want to know how you will look during and after treatment. You and your health care team can work together to develop a treatment plan that meets your medical and personal needs.

Your doctor may refer you to a specialist, or you may ask for a referral. Specialists who treat breast cancer include surgeons, medical oncologists, and radiation oncologists. You also may be referred to a plastic surgeon or reconstructive surgeon. Your health care team may also include an oncology nurse and a registered dietitian.

At any stage of disease, supportive care is available to control pain and other symptoms, to relieve the side effects of treatment, and to ease emotional concerns.

You may want to ask your doctor these questions before you begin treatment:

- What did the hormone receptor tests show? What did other lab tests show? Would genetic testing be helpful to me or my family?

- Do any lymph nodes show signs of cancer?

- What is the stage of the disease? Has the cancer spread?

- What are my treatment choices? Which do you recommend for me? Why?

- What are the expected benefits of each kind of treatment?

- What can I do to prepare for treatment?

- Will I need to stay in the hospital? If so, for how long?

- What are the risks and possible side effects of each treatment? How can side effects be managed?

- What is the treatment likely to cost? Will my insurance cover it?

- How will treatment affect my normal activities?

- Would a research study (clinical trial) be appropriate for me?

- Can you recommend other doctors who could give me a second opinion about my treatment options?

- How often should I have checkups?

Surgery

Surgery is the most common treatment for breast cancer. Your doctor can explain each type, discuss and compare the benefits and risks, and describe how each will change the way you look:

- **Breast-sparing surgery:** This is an operation to remove the cancer but not the breast. It's also called breast-conserving surgery. It can be a lumpectomy or a segmental mastectomy (also called a partial mastectomy). Sometimes an excisional biopsy is the only surgery a woman needs because the surgeon removed the whole lump.

- **Mastectomy:** This is an operation to remove the entire breast (or as much of the breast tissue as possible). In some cases, a skin-sparing mastectomy may be an option. For this approach, the surgeon removes as little skin as possible.

The surgeon usually removes one or more lymph nodes from under the arm to check for cancer cells. If cancer cells are found in the lymph nodes, other cancer treatments will be needed.

You may choose to have breast reconstruction. This is plastic surgery to rebuild the shape of the breast. It may be done at the same time as the cancer surgery or later. If you're considering breast reconstruction, you may wish to talk with a plastic surgeon before having cancer surgery.

The time it takes to heal after surgery is different for each woman. Surgery causes pain and tenderness. Medicine can help control the pain. Before surgery, you should discuss the plan for pain relief with your doctor or nurse. After surgery, your doctor can adjust the plan if you need more relief.

Any kind of surgery also carries a risk of infection, bleeding, or other problems. You should tell your health care team right away if you develop any problems.

You may feel off balance if you've had one or both breasts removed. You may feel more off balance if you have large breasts. This imbalance can cause discomfort in your neck and back.

Also, the skin where your breast was removed may feel tight. Your arm and shoulder muscles may feel stiff and weak. These problems usually go away. The doctor, nurse, or physical therapist can suggest exercises to help you regain movement and strength in your arm and shoulder. Exercise can also reduce stiffness and pain. You may be able to begin gentle exercise within days of surgery.

Because nerves may be injured or cut during surgery, you may have numbness and tingling in your chest, underarm, shoulder, and upper arm. These feelings usually go away within a few weeks or months. But for some women, numbness does not go away.

Removing the lymph nodes under the arm slows the flow of lymph fluid. The fluid may build up in your arm and hand and cause swelling. This swelling is called lymphedema. It can develop soon after surgery or months or even years later. You'll always need to protect the arm and hand on the treated side of your body from cuts, burns, or other injuries. Information about preventing and treating lymphedema is available on the National Cancer Institute's website (www.cancer.gov) or from the NCI's Information Specialists at 800-4-CANCER (800-422-6237) or LiveHelp (http://www.cancer.gov/help).

Radiation Therapy

Radiation therapy (also called radiotherapy) uses high-energy rays to kill cancer cells. It affects cells only in the part of the body that is treated. Radiation therapy may be used after surgery to destroy breast cancer cells that remain in the area.

Doctors use two types of radiation therapy to treat breast cancer. Some women receive both types:

- **External radiation therapy:** The radiation comes from a large machine outside the body. You will go to a hospital or clinic for treatment. Treatments are usually five days a week for four to six weeks. External radiation is the most common type used for breast cancer.

- **Internal radiation therapy (implant radiation therapy or brachytherapy):** The doctor places one or more thin tubes inside the breast through a tiny incision. A radioactive substance is loaded into the tube. The treatment session may last for a few minutes, and the substance is removed. When it's removed, no radioactivity remains in your body. Internal radiation therapy may be repeated every day for a week.

Side effects depend mainly on the dose and type of radiation. It's common for the skin in the treated area to become red, dry, tender, and itchy. Your breast may feel heavy and tight. Internal radiation therapy may make your breast look red or bruised. These problems usually go away over time.

Bras and tight clothes may rub your skin and cause soreness. You may want to wear loose-fitting cotton clothes during this time.

Gentle skin care also is important. You should check with your doctor before using any deodorants, lotions, or creams on the treated area. Toward the end of treatment, your skin may become moist and "weepy." Exposing this area to air as much as possible can help the skin heal. After treatment is over, the skin will slowly heal. However, there may be a lasting change in the color of your skin.

You're likely to become very tired during radiation therapy, especially in the later weeks of treatment. Resting is important, but doctors usually advise patients to try to stay active, unless it leads to pain or other problems.

You may wish to discuss with your doctor the possible long-term effects of radiation therapy. For example, radiation therapy to the chest may harm the lung or heart. Also, it can change the size of your breast and the way it looks. If any of these problems occur, your health care team can tell you how to manage them.

Hormone Therapy

Hormone therapy may also be called anti-hormone treatment. If lab tests show that the tumor in your breast has hormone receptors, then hormone therapy may be an option. Hormone therapy keeps cancer cells from getting or using the natural hormones (estrogen and progesterone) they need to grow.

If you have not gone through menopause, the options for hormone therapy include the following:

- **Tamoxifen:** This drug can prevent the original breast cancer from returning and also helps prevent the development of new cancers in the other breast. As treatment for metastatic breast cancer, tamoxifen slows or stops the growth of cancer cells that are in the body. It's a pill that you take every day for five years. In general, the side effects of tamoxifen are similar to some of the symptoms of menopause. The most common are hot flashes and vaginal discharge. Others are irregular menstrual periods, thinning bones, headaches, fatigue, nausea, vomiting, vaginal dryness or itching, irritation of the skin around the vagina, and skin rash. Serious side effects are rare, but they include blood clots, strokes, uterine cancer, and cataracts.

- **LH-RH agonist:** This type of drug can prevent the ovaries from making estrogen. The estrogen level falls slowly. Examples are leuprolide and goserelin. This type of drug may be given by injection under the skin in the stomach area. Side effects include hot flashes, headaches, weight gain, thinning bones, and bone pain.

- **Surgery to remove your ovaries:** Until you go through menopause, your ovaries are your body's main source of estrogen. When the surgeon removes your ovaries, this source of estrogen is also removed. (A woman who has gone through menopause wouldn't benefit from this kind of surgery because her ovaries produce much less estrogen.) When the ovaries are removed, menopause occurs right away. The side effects are often more severe than those caused by natural menopause. Your health care team can suggest ways to cope with these side effects.

The following options are for hormone therapy are available for women who have gone through menopause:

Aromatase inhibitor: This type of drug prevents the body from making a form of estrogen (estradiol). Examples are anastrazole, exemestane, and letrozole. Common side effects include hot flashes, nausea, vomiting, and painful bones or joints. Serious side effects include thinning bones and an increase in cholesterol.

Tamoxifen: Hormone therapy is given for at least five years. Women who have gone through menopause receive tamoxifen for two to five years. If tamoxifen is given for less than five years, then an aromatase inhibitor often is given to complete the five years. Some women have hormone therapy for more than five years.

Chemotherapy

Chemotherapy uses drugs to kill cancer cells. The drugs that treat breast cancer are usually given through a vein (intravenous) or as a pill. You'll probably receive a combination of drugs.

You may receive chemotherapy in an outpatient part of the hospital, at the doctor's office, or at home. Some women need to stay in the hospital during treatment.

The side effects depend mainly on which drugs are given and how much. Chemotherapy kills fast-growing cancer cells, but the drugs can also harm normal cells that divide rapidly:

- **Blood cells:** When drugs lower the levels of healthy blood cells, you're more likely to get infections, bruise or bleed easily, and feel very weak and tired. Your health care team will check for low levels of blood cells. If your levels are low, your health care team may stop the chemotherapy for a while or reduce the dose of the drug. There are also medicines that can help your body make new blood cells.

- **Cells in hair roots:** Chemotherapy may cause hair loss. If you lose your hair, it will grow back after treatment, but the color and texture may be changed.

- **Cells that line the digestive tract:** Chemotherapy can cause a poor appetite, nausea and vomiting, diarrhea, or mouth and lip sores. Your health care team can give you medicines and suggest other ways to help with these problems.

Some drugs used for breast cancer can cause tingling or numbness in the hands or feet. This problem often goes away after treatment is over.

Other problems may not go away. For example, some of the drugs used for breast cancer may weaken the heart. Your doctor may check your heart before, during, and after treatment. A rare side effect of chemotherapy is that years after treatment, a few women have developed leukemia (cancer of the blood cells).

Some anticancer drugs can damage the ovaries. If you have not gone through menopause yet, you may have hot flashes and vaginal dryness.

Your menstrual periods may no longer be regular or may stop. You may become infertile (unable to become pregnant). For women over the age of 35, this damage to the ovaries is likely to be permanent.

On the other hand, you may remain able to become pregnant during chemotherapy. Before treatment begins, you should talk with your doctor about birth control because many drugs given during the first trimester are known to cause birth defects.

Targeted Therapy

Some women with breast cancer may receive drugs called targeted therapy. Targeted therapy uses drugs that block the growth of breast cancer cells. For example, targeted therapy may block the action of an abnormal protein (such as HER2) that stimulates the growth of breast cancer cells.

Trastuzumab (Herceptin®) or lapatinib (TYKERB®) may be given to a woman whose lab tests show that her breast tumor has too much HER2:

- **Trastuzumab:** This drug is given through a vein. It may be given alone or with chemotherapy. Side effects that most commonly occur during the first treatment include fever and chills. Other possible side effects include weakness, nausea, vomiting, diarrhea, headaches, difficulty breathing, and rashes. These side effects generally become less severe after the first treatment. Trastuzumab also may cause heart damage, heart failure, and serious breathing problems. Before and during treatment, your doctor will check your heart and lungs.

- **Lapatinib:** The tablet is taken by mouth. Lapatinib is given with chemotherapy. Side effects include nausea, vomiting, diarrhea, tiredness, mouth sores, and rashes. It can also cause red, painful hands and feet. Before treatment, your doctor will check your heart and liver. During treatment, your doctor will watch for signs of heart, lung, or liver problems.

Second Opinion

Before starting treatment, you might want a second opinion from another doctor about your diagnosis and treatment plan. Some women worry that their doctor will be offended if they ask for a second opinion. Usually the opposite is true. Most doctors welcome a second opinion. And many health insurance companies will pay for a second opinion if you or your doctor requests it. Some companies require a second opinion.

If you get a second opinion, the doctor may agree with your first doctor's diagnosis and treatment plan. Or the second doctor may suggest another approach. Either way, you'll have more information and perhaps a greater sense of control. You may also feel more confident about the decisions you make, knowing that you've looked carefully at your options.

It may take some time and effort to gather your medical records and see another doctor. Usually it's not a problem if it takes you several weeks to get a second opinion. In most cases, the delay in starting treatment will not make treatment less effective. To make sure, you should discuss this possible delay with your doctor. Some women with breast cancer need treatment right away.

There are many ways to find a doctor for a second opinion. You can ask your doctor, a local or state medical society, a nearby hospital, or a medical school for names of specialists.

The NCI Cancer Information Service at 800-4-CANCER (800-422-6237) or at LiveHelp (http://www.cancer.gov/help) can tell you about nearby treatment centers.

Breast Reconstruction

Some women who plan to have a mastectomy decide to have breast reconstruction. Other women prefer to wear a breast form (prosthesis) inside their bra. Others decide to do nothing after surgery. All of these options have pros and cons. What is right for one woman may not be right for another. What is important is that nearly every woman treated for breast cancer has choices.

Breast reconstruction may be done at the same time as the mastectomy or later on. If radiation therapy is part of the treatment plan, some doctors suggest waiting until after radiation therapy is complete.

If you are thinking about breast reconstruction, you should talk to a plastic surgeon before the mastectomy, even if you plan to have your reconstruction later on.

There are many ways for a surgeon to reconstruct the breast. Some women choose to have breast implants, which are filled with saline or silicone gel.

You also may have breast reconstruction with tissue that the plastic surgeon removes from another part of your body. Skin, muscle, and fat can come from your lower abdomen, back, or buttocks. The surgeon uses this tissue to create a breast shape.

The type of reconstruction that is best for you depends on your age, body type, and the type of cancer surgery that you had. The plastic surgeon can explain the risks and benefits of each type of reconstruction.

You may want to ask your doctor these questions about breast reconstruction:

- Which type of surgery would give me the best results? How will I look afterward?

- When can my reconstruction begin?

- How many surgeries will I need?

- What are the risks at the time of surgery? Later?

- Will I have scars? Where? What will they look like?

- If tissue from another part of my body is used, will there be any permanent changes where the tissue was removed?

- What activities should I avoid? When can I return to my normal activities?

- Will I need follow-up care?

- How much will reconstruction cost? Will my health insurance pay for it?

Nutrition and Physical Activity

It's important for you to take very good care of yourself before, during, and after cancer treatment. Taking care of yourself includes eating well and staying as active as you can.

You need the right amount of calories to maintain a good weight. You also need enough protein to keep up your strength. Eating well may help you feel better and have more energy.

Sometimes, especially during or soon after treatment, you may not feel like eating. You may be uncomfortable or tired. You may find that foods don't taste as good as they used to. In addition, the side effects of treatment (such as poor appetite, nausea, vomiting, or mouth blisters) can make it hard to eat well. On the other hand, some women treated for breast cancer may have a problem with weight gain. Your doctor, a registered dietitian, or another health care provider can suggest ways to help you meet your nutrition needs.

Many women find that they feel better when they stay active. Walking, yoga, swimming, and other activities can keep you strong and increase your energy. Exercise may reduce nausea and pain and make treatment easier to handle. It also can help relieve stress. Whatever physical activity you choose, be sure to talk to your doctor before you start. Also, if your activity causes you pain or other problems, be sure to let your doctor or nurse know.

Follow-Up Care

You'll need regular checkups after treatment for breast cancer. Checkups help ensure that any changes in your health are noted and treated if needed. If you have any health problems between checkups, you should contact your doctor.

Your doctor will check for return of the cancer. Also, checkups help detect health problems that can result from cancer treatment.

You should report any changes in the treated area or in your other breast to the doctor right away. Tell your doctor about any health problems, such as pain, loss of appetite or weight, changes in menstrual cycles, unusual vaginal bleeding, or blurred vision. Also talk to your doctor about headaches, dizziness, shortness of breath, coughing or hoarseness, backaches, or digestive problems that seem unusual or that don't go away. Such problems may arise months or years after treatment. They may suggest that the cancer has returned, but they can also be symptoms of other health problems. It's important to share your concerns with your doctor so that problems can be diagnosed and treated as soon as possible.

Checkups usually include an exam of the neck, underarm, chest, and breast areas. Since a new breast cancer may develop, you should have regular mammograms. You probably won't need a mammogram of a reconstructed breast or if you had a mastectomy without reconstruction. Your doctor may order other imaging procedures or lab tests.

Chapter 42

Gynecological Cancers

Chapter Contents

Section 42.1

Cervical Cancer

Excerpted from "What You Need to Know about Cancer of the Cervix,"
National Cancer Institute (www.cancer.gov), November 20, 2008.

General Information about Cancer of the Cervix

The cervix is part of a woman's reproductive system. It is in the pelvis. The cervix is the lower, narrow part of the uterus (womb). The cervix is a passageway. It connects the uterus to the vagina, and during a menstrual period, blood flows from the uterus through the cervix into the vagina. The vagina leads to the outside of the body.

The cervix makes mucus. During sex, mucus helps sperm move from the vagina through the cervix into the uterus.

During pregnancy, the cervix is tightly closed to help keep the baby inside the uterus. During childbirth, the cervix opens to allow the baby to pass through the vagina.

Growths on the cervix can be benign or malignant. Benign growths are not cancer. They are not as harmful as malignant growths (cancer). Cervical cancer begins in cells on the surface of the cervix. Over time, the cervical cancer can invade more deeply into the cervix and nearby tissues.

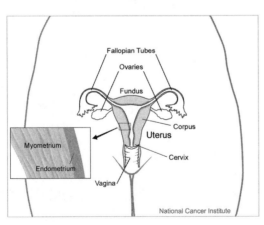

Figure 42.1. *Organs in the Female Reproductive Tract (image by NIH Medical Arts, National Cancer Institute)*

Risk Factors for Cervical Cancer

Doctors cannot always explain why one woman develops cervical cancer and another does not. However, we do know that a woman with certain risk factors may be more likely than others to develop cervical cancer.

Studies have found a number of factors that may increase the risk of cervical cancer. For example, infection with HPV (human papillomavirus) is the main cause of cervical cancer. HPV infection and other risk factors may act together to increase the risk even more. Having an HPV infection or other risk factors does not mean that a woman will develop cervical cancer. Most women who have risk factors for cervical cancer never develop it.

HPV infection: HPV is a group of viruses that can infect the cervix. An HPV infection that doesn't go away can cause cervical cancer in some women. HPV is the cause of nearly all cervical cancers.

HPV infections are very common. These viruses are passed from person to person through sexual contact. Most adults have been infected with HPV at some time in their lives, but most infections clear up on their own.

Some types of HPV can cause changes to cells in the cervix. If these changes are found early, cervical cancer can be prevented by removing or killing the changed cells before they can become cancer cells. A vaccine for females ages 9 to 26 protects against two types of HPV infection that cause cervical cancer.

Lack of regular Pap tests: Cervical cancer is more common among women who don't have regular Pap tests. The Pap test helps doctors find abnormal cells. Removing or killing the abnormal cells usually prevents cervical cancer.

Smoking: Among women who are infected with HPV, smoking cigarettes slightly increases the risk of cervical cancer.

Weakened immune system (the body's natural defense system): Infection with HIV (the virus that causes AIDS) or taking drugs that suppress the immune system increases the risk of cervical cancer.

Sexual history: Women who have had many sexual partners have a higher risk of developing cervical cancer. Also, a woman who has had sex with a man who has had many sexual partners may be at higher risk of developing cervical cancer. In both cases, the risk of developing cervical cancer is higher because these women have a higher risk of HPV infection.

Using birth control pills for a long time: Using birth control pills for a long time (five or more years) may slightly increase the risk of cervical cancer among women with HPV infection. However, the risk decreases quickly when women stop using birth control pills.

Having many children: Studies suggest that giving birth to many children (five or more) may slightly increase the risk of cervical cancer among women with HPV infection.

DES (diethylstilbestrol): DES may increase the risk of a rare form of cervical cancer in daughters exposed to this drug before birth. DES was given to some pregnant women in the United States between about 1940 and 1971. (It is no longer given to pregnant women.)

Symptoms

Early cervical cancers usually don't cause symptoms. When the cancer grows larger, women may notice one or more of these symptoms:

- Abnormal vaginal bleeding
- Bleeding that occurs between regular menstrual periods
- Bleeding after sexual intercourse, douching, or a pelvic exam
- Menstrual periods that last longer and are heavier than before
- Bleeding after going through menopause
- Increased vaginal discharge
- Pelvic pain
- Pain during sex

Infections or other health problems may also cause these symptoms. Only a doctor can tell for sure. A woman with any of these symptoms should tell her doctor so that problems can be diagnosed and treated as early as possible.

Detection and Diagnosis

Doctors recommend that women help reduce their risk of cervical cancer by having regular Pap tests. A Pap test (sometimes called Pap smear or cervical smear) is a simple test used to look at cervical cells. Pap tests can find cervical cancer or abnormal cells that can lead to cervical cancer.

Finding and treating abnormal cells can prevent most cervical cancer. Also, the Pap test can help find cancer early, when treatment is more likely to be effective.

For most women, the Pap test is not painful. It's done in a doctor's office or clinic during a pelvic exam. The doctor or nurse scrapes a sample of cells from the cervix. A lab checks the cells under a microscope for cell changes. Most often, abnormal cells found by a Pap test are not cancerous. The same sample of cells may be tested for HPV infection.

If you have abnormal Pap or HPV test results, your doctor will suggest other tests, such as colposcopy or biopsy, to make a diagnosis. Colposcopy is a test in which the doctor uses a colposcope to look at the cervix. The colposcope combines a bright light with a magnifying lens to make tissue easier to see. It is not inserted into the vagina. A colposcopy is usually done in the doctor's office or clinic.

A biopsy involves removing tissue for examination. Most women have tissue removed in the doctor's office with local anesthesia. A pathologist checks the tissue under a microscope for abnormal cells. There are several types of biopsy used to diagnose cervical cancer:

- **Punch biopsy:** The doctor uses a sharp tool to pinch off small samples of cervical tissue.

- **LEEP:** The doctor uses an electric wire loop to slice off a thin, round piece of cervical tissue.

- **Endocervical curettage:** The doctor uses a curette (a small, spoon-shaped instrument) to scrape a small sample of tissue from the cervix. Some doctors may use a thin, soft brush instead of a curette.

- **Conization:** The doctor removes a cone-shaped sample of tissue. A conization, or cone biopsy, lets the pathologist see if abnormal cells are in the tissue beneath the surface of the cervix. The doctor may do this test in the hospital under general anesthesia.

Removing tissue from the cervix may cause some bleeding or other discharge. The area usually heals quickly. Some women also feel some pain similar to menstrual cramps. Your doctor can suggest medicine that will help relieve your pain.

Staging

The stage is based on where cancer is found. These are the stages of invasive cervical cancer:

Stage I: The tumor has invaded the cervix beneath the top layer of cells. Cancer cells are found only in the cervix.

Stage II: The tumor extends to the upper part of the vagina. It may extend beyond the cervix into nearby tissues toward the pelvic wall (the lining of the part of the body between the hips). The tumor does not invade the lower third of the vagina or the pelvic wall.

Stage III: The tumor extends to the lower part of the vagina. It may also have invaded the pelvic wall. If the tumor blocks the flow of urine, one or both kidneys may not be working well.

Stage IV: The tumor invades the bladder or rectum. Or the cancer has spread to other parts of the body. When cervical cancer spreads, it most often spreads to nearby tissues in the pelvis, lymph nodes, or the lungs. It may also spread to the liver or bones.

Recurrent cancer: The cancer was treated, but has returned after a period of time during which it could not be detected. The cancer may show up again in the cervix or in other parts of the body.

Treatment Options for Cervical Cancer

Women with cervical cancer have many treatment options. The options are surgery, radiation therapy, chemotherapy, or a combination of methods.

Surgery is an option for women with Stage I or II cervical cancer. The surgeon removes tissue that may contain cancer cells.

Radiation therapy (also called radiotherapy) is an option for women with any stage of cervical cancer. Women with early stage cervical cancer may choose radiation therapy instead of surgery. It also may be used after surgery to destroy any cancer cells that remain in the area. Women with cancer that extends beyond the cervix may have radiation therapy and chemotherapy.

For the treatment of cervical cancer, chemotherapy is usually combined with radiation therapy. For cancer that has spread to distant organs, chemotherapy alone may be used.

Additional information about these types of treatments can be found in Section 42.7.

Section 42.2

Endometrial Cancer

Excerpted from PDQ® Cancer Information Summary. National Cancer Institute; Bethesda, MD. "Endometrial Cancer Treatment (PDQ) - Patient Version." Updated 10/2009. Available at: http://cancer.gov. Accessed January 20, 2010.

General Information about Endometrial Cancer

Endometrial cancer is a disease in which malignant (cancer) cells form in the tissues of the endometrium. The endometrium is the lining of the uterus, a hollow, muscular organ in a woman's pelvis. The uterus is where a fetus grows. In most nonpregnant women, the uterus is about three inches long. The lower, narrow end of the uterus is the cervix, which leads to the vagina.

Cancer of the endometrium is different from cancer of the muscle of the uterus, which is called sarcoma of the uterus. Sarcoma of the uterus is discussed in Section 42.5.

Risk Factors and Signs

Endometrial cancer may develop in breast cancer patients who have been treated with tamoxifen. A patient taking this drug should have a pelvic exam every year and report any vaginal bleeding (other than menstrual bleeding) as soon as possible. Women taking estrogen (a hormone that can affect the growth of some cancers) alone have an increased risk of developing endometrial cancer. Taking estrogen in combination with progesterone (another hormone) does not increase a woman's risk of this cancer.

Possible signs of endometrial cancer include unusual vaginal discharge or pain in the pelvis. These and other symptoms may be caused by endometrial cancer. Other conditions may cause the same symptoms. A doctor should be consulted if any of the following problems occur:

- Bleeding or discharge not related to menstruation (periods).
- Difficult or painful urination.
- Pain during sexual intercourse.
- Pain in the pelvic area.

Detection, Diagnosis, and Prognosis

Because endometrial cancer begins inside the uterus, it does not usually show up in the results of a Pap test. For this reason, a sample of endometrial tissue must be removed and examined under a microscope to look for cancer cells. One of the following procedures may be used: endometrial biopsy or dilatation and curettage (D&C). Additional information about these procedures can be found in Section 42.7.

The prognosis (chance of recovery) and treatment options depend on the stage of the cancer (whether it is in the endometrium only, involves the whole uterus, or has spread to other places in the body), how the cancer cells look under a microscope, and whether the cancer cells are affected by progesterone. Endometrial cancer is highly curable.

Stages of Endometrial Cancer

After endometrial cancer has been diagnosed, tests are done to find out if cancer cells have spread within the uterus or to other parts of the body. This process is called staging. The information gathered from the staging process determines the stage of the disease. It is important to know the stage in order to plan treatment. Certain tests and procedures are used in the staging process. A hysterectomy (an operation in which the uterus is removed) will usually be done to help find out how far the cancer has spread. The following stages are used for endometrial cancer:

Stage I

In stage I, cancer is found in the uterus only. Stage I is divided into stages IA, IB, and IC, based on how far the cancer has spread.

- **Stage IA:** Cancer is in the endometrium only.

- **Stage IB:** Cancer has spread into the inner half of the myometrium (muscle layer of the uterus).

- **Stage IC:** Cancer has spread into the outer half of the myometrium.

Stage II

In stage II, cancer has spread from the uterus to the cervix, but has not spread outside the uterus. Stage II is divided into stages IIA and IIB, based on how far the cancer has spread into the cervix.

- **Stage IIA:** Cancer has spread to the glands where the cervix and uterus meet.

- **Stage IIB:** Cancer has spread into the connective tissue of the cervix.

Stage III

In stage III, cancer has spread beyond the uterus and cervix, but has not spread beyond the pelvis. Stage III is divided into stages IIIA, IIIB, and IIIC, based on how far the cancer has spread within the pelvis.

- **Stage IIIA:** Cancer has spread to one or more of the following: the outermost layer of the uterus; or tissue just beyond the uterus; or the peritoneum.

- **Stage IIIB:** Cancer has spread beyond the uterus and cervix, into the vagina.

- **Stage IIIC:** Cancer has spread to lymph nodes near the uterus.

Stage IV

In stage IV, cancer has spread beyond the pelvis. Stage IV is divided into stages IVA and IVB, based on how far the cancer has spread.

- **Stage IVA:** Cancer has spread to the bladder and/or bowel wall.

- **Stage IVB:** Cancer has spread to other parts of the body beyond the pelvis, including lymph nodes in the abdomen and/or groin.

Recurrent Endometrial Cancer

Recurrent endometrial cancer is cancer that has recurred (come back) after it has been treated. The cancer may come back in the pelvis, in lymph nodes in the abdomen, or in other parts of the body.

Treatment Option Overview

Different types of treatment are available for patients with endometrial cancer. Some treatments are standard (the currently used treatment), and some are being tested in clinical trials. Three types of standard treatment are used: Surgery, radiation therapy, and hormone therapy. Details about treatments can be found in Section 42.7. In addition, chemotherapy for endometrial cancer is being tested in clinical trials.

Section 42.3

Gestational Trophoblastic Tumors

Excerpted from PDQ® Cancer Information Summary. National Cancer Institute; Bethesda, MD. "Gestational Trophoblastic Tumors Treatment (PDQ) - Patient Version." Updated 06/2008. Available at: http://cancer.gov. Accessed January 20, 2010.

General Information about Gestational Trophoblastic Tumors

Gestational trophoblastic tumor, a rare cancer in women, is a disease in which cancer (malignant) cells grow in the tissues that are formed following conception (the joining of sperm and egg). Gestational trophoblastic tumors start inside the uterus, the hollow, muscular, pear-shaped organ where a baby grows. This type of cancer occurs in women during the years when they are able to have children. There are two types of gestational trophoblastic tumors: hydatidiform mole and choriocarcinoma.

If a patient has a hydatidiform mole (also called a molar pregnancy), the sperm and egg cells have joined without the development of a baby in the uterus. Instead, the tissue that is formed resembles grape-like cysts. Hydatidiform mole does not spread outside of the uterus to other parts of the body.

If a patient has a choriocarcinoma, the tumor may have started from a hydatidiform mole or from tissue that remains in the uterus following an abortion or delivery of a baby. Choriocarcinoma can spread from the uterus to other parts of the body. A very rare type of gestational trophoblastic tumor starts in the uterus where the placenta was attached. This type of cancer is called placental-site trophoblastic disease.

Gestational trophoblastic tumor is not always easy to find. In its early stages, it may look like a normal pregnancy. A doctor should be seen if the there is vaginal bleeding (not menstrual bleeding) and if a woman is pregnant and the baby hasn't moved at the expected time.

If there are symptoms, a doctor may use several tests to see if the patient has a gestational trophoblastic tumor. An internal (pelvic) examination is usually the first of these tests. The doctor will feel for any lumps or strange feeling in the shape or size of the uterus. The doctor may then do an ultrasound, a test that uses sound waves to find tumors. A blood test will also be done to look for high levels of a hormone called beta-HCG (beta human chorionic gonadotropin) which is present during normal pregnancy. If a woman is not pregnant and HCG is in the blood, it can be a sign of gestational trophoblastic tumor.

The chance of recovery (prognosis) and choice of treatment depend on the type of gestational trophoblastic tumor, whether it has spread to other places, and the patient's general state of health.

Stage Explanation

Once gestational trophoblastic tumor has been found, more tests will be done to find out if the cancer has spread from inside the uterus to other parts of the body (staging). Treatment of gestational trophoblastic tumor depends on the stage of the disease and the patient's age and general health. The following stages are used for gestational trophoblastic tumor:

Hydatidiform mole: Cancer is found only in the space inside the uterus. If the cancer is found in the muscle of the uterus, it is called an invasive mole (choriocarcinoma destruens).

Placental-site gestational trophoblastic tumors: Cancer is found in the place where the placenta was attached and in the muscle of the uterus.

Nonmetastatic: Cancer cells have grown inside the uterus from tissue remaining following treatment of a hydatidiform mole or following an abortion or delivery of a baby. Cancer has not spread outside the uterus.

Metastatic: Cancer cells have grown inside the uterus from tissue remaining following treatment of a hydatidiform mole or following an abortion or delivery of a baby. The cancer has spread from the uterus to other parts of the body. Metastatic gestational trophoblastic tumors are considered good prognosis or poor prognosis.

Metastatic gestational trophoblastic tumor is considered good prognosis if all of the following are true:

- The last pregnancy was less than four months ago.
- The level of beta-HCG in the blood is low.
- Cancer has not spread to the liver or brain.
- The patient has not received chemotherapy earlier.

Metastatic gestational trophoblastic tumor is considered poor prognosis if any the following are true:

- The last pregnancy was more than four months ago.

- The level of beta-HCG in the blood is high.

- Cancer has spread to the liver or brain.

- The patient received chemotherapy earlier and the cancer did not go away.

- The tumor began after the completion of a normal pregnancy.

Recurrent: Recurrent disease means that the cancer has come back (recurred) after it has been treated. It may come back in the uterus or in another part of the body.

Treatment Option Overview

Different types of treatment are available for patients with gestational trophoblastic tumor. Some treatments are standard (the currently used treatment), and some are being tested in clinical trials.

Two kinds of standard treatment are used: surgery (taking out the cancer) and chemotherapy (using drugs to kill cancer cells). Radiation therapy (using high-energy x-rays to kill cancer cells) may be used in certain cases to treat cancer that has spread to other parts of the body.

Dilation and curettage (D & C) with suction evacuation is stretching the opening of the uterus (the cervix) and removing the material inside the uterus with a small vacuum-like device. The walls of the uterus are then scraped gently to remove any material that may remain in the uterus. This is used only for molar pregnancies.

Hysterectomy is an operation to take out the uterus. The ovaries usually are not removed in the treatment of this disease.

For more information about these and other treatments, see Section 42.7.

Section 42.4

Ovarian Epithelial Cancer

PDQ® Cancer Information Summary. National Cancer Institute; Bethesda, MD. "Ovarian Epithelial Cancer Treatment (PDQ) - Patient Version." Updated 01/2010. Available at: http://cancer.gov. Accessed October 1, 2010.

General Information about Ovarian Epithelial Cancer

Ovarian epithelial cancer is a disease in which malignant (cancer) cells form in the tissue covering the ovary. The ovaries are a pair of organs in the female reproductive system. They are located in the pelvis, one on each side of the uterus (the hollow, pear-shaped organ where a fetus grows). Each ovary is about the size and shape of an almond. The ovaries produce eggs and female hormones (chemicals that control the way certain cells or organs function).

Ovarian epithelial cancer is one type of cancer that affects the ovary. Others are ovarian germ cell tumors and ovarian low malignant potential tumors.

Risk Factors

Women who have one first-degree relative (mother, daughter, or sister) with ovarian cancer are at an increased risk of developing ovarian cancer. This risk is higher in women who have one first-degree relative and one second-degree relative (grandmother or aunt) with ovarian cancer. This risk is even higher in women who have two or more first-degree relatives with ovarian cancer.

Inherited gene mutations: The genes in cells carry the hereditary information that is received from a person's parents. Hereditary ovarian cancer makes up approximately 5% to 10% of all cases of ovarian cancer. Three hereditary patterns have been identified: ovarian cancer alone, ovarian and breast cancers, and ovarian and colon cancers.

Tests that can detect mutated genes have been developed. These genetic tests are sometimes done for members of families with a high risk of cancer.

Prophylactic surgery: Some women who have an increased risk of ovarian cancer may choose to have a prophylactic oophorectomy (the removal of healthy ovaries so that cancer cannot grow in them). In high-risk women, this procedure has been shown to greatly decrease the risk of developing ovarian cancer.

Signs and Symptoms

Early ovarian cancer may not cause any symptoms. When symptoms do appear, ovarian cancer is often advanced. Symptoms of ovarian cancer may include the following:

- Pain or swelling in the abdomen
- Pain in the pelvis
- Gastrointestinal problems, such as gas, bloating, or constipation

These symptoms may be caused by other conditions and not by ovarian cancer. If the symptoms get worse or do not go away on their own, a doctor should be consulted so that any problem can be diagnosed and treated as early as possible. When found in its early stages, ovarian epithelial cancer can often be cured.

Detection, Diagnosis, and Prognosis

Tests that examine the ovaries, pelvic area, blood, and ovarian tissue are used to detect (find) and diagnose ovarian cancer. The following tests and procedures may be used: pelvic exam, abdominal ultrasound, CA 125 assay, barium enema, intravenous pyelogram, CT scan, and biopsy. For more information about these tests, see Section 42.7.

The prognosis (chance of recovery) and treatment options depend on the following:

- The stage of the cancer
- The type and size of the tumor
- The patient's age and general health
- Whether the cancer has just been diagnosed or has recurred (come back)

Stages of Ovarian Epithelial Cancer

The process used to find out if cancer has spread within the ovary or to other parts of the body is called staging. The information gathered from the staging process determines the stage of the disease. It is important to know the stage in order to plan treatment.

An operation called a laparotomy is usually done to find out the stage of the disease. A doctor must cut into the abdomen and carefully look at all the organs to see if they contain cancer. The doctor will also perform a biopsy (cut out small pieces of tissue so they can be looked at under a microscope to see whether they contain cancer). Usually the doctor will remove the cancer and organs that contain cancer during the laparotomy.

The following stages are used for ovarian epithelial cancer:

Stage I

In stage I, cancer is found in one or both of the ovaries. Stage I is divided into stage IA, stage IB, and stage IC.

- **Stage IA:** Cancer is found in a single ovary.
- **Stage IB:** Cancer is found in both ovaries.
- **Stage IC:** Cancer is found in one or both ovaries and one of the following is true: cancer is found on the outside surface of one or both ovaries; or the capsule (outer covering) of the tumor has ruptured (broken open); or cancer cells are found in the fluid of the peritoneal cavity (the body cavity that contains most of the organs in the abdomen) or in washings of the peritoneum (tissue lining the peritoneal cavity).

Stage II

In stage II, cancer is found in one or both ovaries and has spread into other areas of the pelvis. Stage II is divided into stage IIA, stage IIB, and stage IIC.

- **Stage IIA:** Cancer has spread to the uterus and/or the fallopian tubes (the long slender tubes through which eggs pass from the ovaries to the uterus).
- **Stage IIB:** Cancer has spread to other tissue within the pelvis.
- **Stage IIC:** Cancer has spread to the uterus and/or fallopian tubes and/or other tissue within the pelvis and cancer cells are found in the fluid of the peritoneal cavity (the body cavity that contains most of the organs in the abdomen) or in washings of the peritoneum (tissue lining the peritoneal cavity).

Stage III

In stage III, cancer is found in one or both ovaries and has spread to other parts of the abdomen. Stage III is divided into stage IIIA, stage IIIB, and stage IIIC.

- **Stage IIIA:** The tumor is found in the pelvis only, but cancer cells have spread to the surface of the peritoneum (tissue that lines the abdominal wall and covers most of the organs in the abdomen).

- **Stage IIIB:** Cancer has spread to the peritoneum but is two centimeters or smaller in diameter.

- **Stage IIIC:** Cancer has spread to the peritoneum and is larger than two centimeters in diameter and/or has spread to lymph nodes in the abdomen.

Cancer that has spread to the surface of the liver is also considered stage III disease.

Stage IV

In stage IV, cancer is found in one or both ovaries and has metastasized (spread) beyond the abdomen to other parts of the body, such as the lungs, liver, lymph nodes, or bones. Cancer that has spread to tissues in the liver is also considered stage IV disease.

Recurrent or Persistent Ovarian Epithelial Cancer

Recurrent ovarian epithelial cancer is cancer that has recurred (come back) after it has been treated. Persistent cancer is cancer that does not go away with treatment.

Treatment Option Overview

Different types of treatment are available for patients with ovarian epithelial cancer. Some treatments are standard, and some are being tested in clinical trials.

Three kinds of standard treatment are used. One is surgery. Most patients have surgery to remove as much of the tumor as possible. The others are radiation therapy and chemotherapy. A type of regional chemotherapy used to treat ovarian cancer is intraperitoneal (IP) chemotherapy. In IP chemotherapy, the anticancer drugs are carried directly into the peritoneal cavity (the space that contains the abdominal organs) through a thin tube.

New types of treatment for ovarian epithelial cancer being tested in clinical trials include biologic therapy and targeted therapy.

For more information about these and other treatments, see Section 42.7.

Section 42.5

Uterine Sarcoma

PDQ® Cancer Information Summary. National Cancer Institute; Bethesda, MD. "Uterine Sarcoma Treatment (PDQ) - Patient Version." Updated 08/2009. Available at: http://cancer.gov. Accessed January 20, 2010.

General Information about Uterine Sarcoma

Uterine sarcoma is a disease in which malignant (cancer) cells form in the muscles of the uterus or other tissues that support the uterus. The uterus is part of the female reproductive system. The uterus is the hollow, pear-shaped organ in the pelvis, where a fetus grows. The cervix is at the lower, narrow end of the uterus, and leads to the vagina.

Uterine sarcoma is different from cancer of the endometrium, a disease in which cancer cells start growing inside the lining of the uterus. For information about endometrial cancer, see Section 42.2.

Risk Factors

Risk factors for uterine sarcoma include past treatment with radiation therapy to the pelvis, and treatment with tamoxifen for breast cancer. A patient taking this drug should have a pelvic exam every year and report any vaginal bleeding (other than menstrual bleeding) as soon as possible.

Signs, Symptoms, and Diagnosis

Abnormal bleeding from the vagina and other symptoms may be caused by uterine sarcoma. Other conditions may cause the same symptoms. A doctor should be consulted if any of the following problems occur:

- Bleeding that is not part of menstrual periods.
- Bleeding after menopause.
- A mass in the vagina.
- Pain or a feeling of fullness in the abdomen.
- Frequent urination.

The following tests and procedures may be used: physical exam and history, pelvic exam, Pap test, dilatation and curettage, and endometrial biopsy. Additional information about these and other procedures can be found in Section 42.7.

The prognosis (chance of recovery) and treatment options depend on the stage of the cancer, the type and size of the tumor, the patient's general health, and whether the cancer has just been diagnosed or has recurred (come back).

Stages of Uterine Sarcoma

After uterine sarcoma has been diagnosed, tests are done to find out if cancer cells have spread within the uterus or to other parts of the body.

The process used to find out if cancer has spread within the uterus or to other parts of the body is called staging. The information gathered from the staging process determines the stage of the disease. It is important to know the stage in order to plan treatment. The following procedures may be used in the staging process:

- Barium enema
- Blood chemistry studies
- CA 125 assay
- Chest x-ray
- CT scan (CAT scan)
- Cystoscopy
- Sigmoidoscopy
- Transvaginal ultrasound exam

Surgery is also used to diagnose, stage, and treat uterine sarcoma. During this surgery, the doctor removes as much of the cancer as possible. The following procedures may be used to diagnose, stage, and treat uterine sarcoma: laparotomy, abdominal and pelvic washings, total abdominal hysterectomy, bilateral salpingo-oophorectomy, and lymphadenectomy.

For more information about the tests and procedures used for diagnosing and staging uterine sarcoma, see Section 42.7.

The following stages are used for uterine sarcoma:

Stage I

In stage I, cancer is found in the uterus only. Stage I is divided into stage IA, stage IB, and stage IC, based on how far the cancer has spread.

- **Stage IA:** Cancer is in the endometrium only.
- **Stage IB:** Cancer has spread into the inner half of the myometrium (muscle layer of the uterus).
- **Stage IC:** Cancer has spread into the outer half of the myometrium.

Stage II

In stage II, cancer has spread from the uterus to the cervix. Stage II is divided into stage IIA and stage IIB, based on how far the cancer has spread.

- **Stage IIA:** Cancer has spread to the glands where the cervix and uterus meet.
- **Stage IIB:** Cancer has spread into the connective tissue of the cervix.

Stage III

In stage III, cancer has spread beyond the uterus and cervix, but has not spread beyond the pelvis. Stage III is divided into stage IIIA and stage IIIB, based on how far the cancer has spread within the pelvis.

- **Stage IIIA:** Cancer has spread to one or more of the following: the outermost layer of the uterus; and/or tissues just beyond the uterus; and/or the peritoneum.
- **Stage IIIB:** Cancer has spread to lymph nodes in the pelvis and/or near the uterus.

Stage IV

In stage IV, cancer has spread beyond the pelvis. Stage IV is divided into stage IVA and stage IVB, based on how far the cancer has spread.

- **Stage IVA:** Cancer has spread to the lining of the bladder and/or bowel.
- **Stage IVB:** Cancer has spread to other parts of the body beyond the pelvis, including lymph nodes in the abdomen and/or groin.

Recurrent Uterine Sarcoma

Recurrent uterine sarcoma is cancer that has recurred (come back) after it has been treated. The cancer may come back in the uterus or in other parts of the body.

Treatment Option Overview

Different types of treatments are available for patients with uterine sarcoma. Some treatments are standard (the currently used treatment), and some are being tested in clinical trials. Four types of standard treatment are used: Surgery is the most common treatment for uterine sarcoma. Other standard treatments are radiation therapy, chemotherapy, and hormone therapy. For more information about these treatments, see Section 42.7.

Section 42.6

Vaginal and Vulvar Cancers

Excerpted from PDQ® Cancer Information Summary. National Cancer Institute; Bethesda, MD. "Vaginal Cancer Treatment (PDQ) - Patient Version." Updated 07/2010. Available at: http://cancer.gov. Accessed October 1, 2010, And, PDQ® Cancer Information Summary. National Cancer Institute; Bethesda, MD. "Vulvar Cancer Treatment (PDQ) - Patient Version." Updated 08/2009. Available at: http://cancer.gov. Accessed January 20, 2010.

General Information about Vaginal Cancer

Vaginal cancer is a disease in which malignant (cancer) cells form in the vagina. The vagina is the canal leading from the cervix (the opening of uterus) to the outside of the body. At birth, a baby passes out of the body through the vagina (also called the birth canal).

Vaginal cancer is not common. When found in early stages, it can often be cured. There are two main types of vaginal cancer:

Squamous cell carcinoma: Cancer that forms in squamous cells, the thin, flat cells lining the vagina. Squamous cell vaginal cancer spreads slowly and usually stays near the vagina, but may spread to the lungs and liver. This is the most common type of vaginal cancer. It is found most often in women aged 60 or older.

Adenocarcinoma: Cancer that begins in glandular (secretory) cells. Glandular cells in the lining of the vagina make and release fluids such as mucus. Adenocarcinoma is more likely than squamous cell cancer to spread to the lungs and lymph nodes. It is found most often in women aged 30 or younger.

Risk Factors for Vaginal Cancer

Risk factors for vaginal cancer include the following:

- Being aged 60 or older.

- Being exposed to DES while in the mother's womb. In the 1950s, the drug DES was given to some pregnant women to prevent miscarriage (premature birth of a fetus that cannot survive). Women who were exposed to DES before birth have an increased risk of developing vaginal cancer. Some of these women develop a rare form of cancer called clear cell adenocarcinoma.

- Having human papilloma virus (HPV) infection.

- Having a history of abnormal cells in the cervix or cervical cancer.

Vaginal Cancer Symptoms, Diagnosis, and Prognosis

Vaginal cancer often does not cause early symptoms and may be found during a routine Pap test. When symptoms occur they may be caused by vaginal cancer or by other conditions. A doctor should be consulted if any of the following problems occur:

- Bleeding or discharge not related to menstrual periods

- Pain during sexual intercourse

- Pain in the pelvic area

- A lump in the vagina

Tests that examine the vagina and other organs in the pelvis are used to detect (find) and diagnose vaginal cancer. The following tests and procedures may be used: Physical exam and history, pelvic exam, Pap smear, biopsy, and colposcopy. Additional information about these and other tests can be found in Section 42.7.

The prognosis (chance of recovery) depends on the following:

- The stage of the cancer (whether it is in the vagina only or has spread to other areas)

- The size of the tumor

- The grade of tumor cells (how different they are from normal cells)

- Where the cancer is within the vagina
- Whether there are symptoms
- The patient's age and general health
- Whether the cancer has just been diagnosed or has recurred (come back)

Treatment options depend on the stage, size, and location of the cancer, whether the tumor cells are squamous cell or adenocarcinoma, whether the patient has a uterus or has had a hysterectomy, and whether the patient has had past radiation treatment to the pelvis.

Stages of Vaginal Cancer

The process used to find out if cancer has spread within the vagina or to other parts of the body is called staging. The information gathered from the staging process determines the stage of the disease. It is important to know the stage in order to plan treatment. The following procedures may be used in the staging process:

- Biopsy
- Chest x-ray
- Cystoscopy
- Ureteroscopy
- Proctoscopy
- CT scan (CAT scan)
- MRI (magnetic resonance imaging)
- Lymphangiogram

These and other procedures used for staging cancer are discussed in Section 42.7.

The following stages are used for vaginal cancer:

Stage 0 (carcinoma in situ): In stage 0, abnormal cells are found in tissue lining the inside of the vagina. These abnormal cells may become cancer and spread into nearby normal tissue. Stage 0 is also called carcinoma in situ.

Stage I: In stage I, cancer has formed and is found in the vagina only.

Stage II: In stage II, cancer has spread from the vagina to the tissue around the vagina.

Stage III: In stage III, cancer has spread from the vagina to the lymph nodes in the pelvis or groin, or to the pelvis, or both.

Stage IV: Stage IV is divided into stage IVA and stage IVB:

- **Stage IVA:** Cancer may have spread to lymph nodes in the pelvis or groin and has spread to one or both of the following areas: The lining of the bladder or rectum; and/or beyond the pelvis.

- **Stage IVB:** Cancer has spread to parts of the body that are not near the vagina, such as the lungs. Cancer may also have spread to the lymph nodes.

Recurrent vaginal cancer: Recurrent vaginal cancer is cancer that has recurred (come back) after it has been treated. The cancer may come back in the vagina or in other parts of the body.

Treatment Option Overview

Different types of treatments are available for patients with vaginal cancer. Some treatments are standard (the currently used treatment), and some are being tested in clinical trials.

Surgery, one of three types of standard treatment used, is the most common treatment of vaginal cancer. The following surgical procedures may be used: Laser surgery, wide local excision, vaginectomy, total hysterectomy, lymph node dissection, and pelvic exenteration.

Skin grafting may follow surgery, to repair or reconstruct the vagina. Skin grafting is a surgical procedure in which skin is moved from one part of the body to another. A piece of healthy skin is taken from a part of the body that is usually hidden, such as the buttock or thigh, and used to repair or rebuild the area treated with surgery.

Other standard treatments are radiation therapy and chemotherapy. Topical chemotherapy for squamous cell vaginal cancer may be applied to the vagina in a cream or lotion.

For more information about these treatments, see Section 42.7.

In addition to standard treatments, radiosensitizers are being tested in clinical trials. Radiosensitizers are drugs that make tumor cells more sensitive to radiation therapy. Combining radiation therapy with radiosensitizers may kill more tumor cells. For more information about clinical trials, visit www.clinicaltrials.gov.

General Information about Vulvar Cancer

Vulvar cancer is a rare disease in which malignant (cancer) cells form in the tissues of the vulva. Vulvar cancer forms in a woman's external genitalia. The vulva includes the inner and outer lips of the vagina, the clitoris (sensitive tissue between the lips), and the opening of the vagina and its glands.

Vulvar cancer most often affects the outer vaginal lips. Less often, cancer affects the inner vaginal lips or the clitoris.

Vulvar cancer usually develops slowly over a period of years. Abnormal cells can grow on the surface of the vulvar skin for a long time. This precancerous condition is called vulvar intraepithelial neoplasia (VIN) or dysplasia. Because it is possible for VIN or dysplasia to develop into vulvar cancer, treatment of this condition is very important.

Vulvar Cancer Risk Factors, Symptoms, Diagnosis, and Prognosis

Risk factors include the following having human papillomavirus (HPV) infection and older age.

Vulvar cancer often does not cause early symptoms. When symptoms occur, they may be caused by vulvar cancer or by other conditions. A doctor should be consulted if any of the following problems occur:

- A lump in the vulva

- Itching that does not go away in the vulvar area

- Bleeding not related to menstruation (periods)

- Tenderness in the vulvar area

The following tests and procedures may be used to detect and diagnose vulvar cancer: Physical exam and history; and biopsy. These procedures are discussed in Section 42.7.

The prognosis (chance of recovery) and treatment options depend on the stage of the cancer, the patient's age and general health, and whether the cancer has just been diagnosed or has recurred (come back).

Stages of Vulvar Cancer

The process used to find out if cancer has spread within the vulva or to other parts of the body is called staging. The information gathered from the staging process determines the stage of the disease. It is important to know the stage in order to plan treatment. The following tests and procedures may be used in the staging process: pelvic exam, cystoscopy, proctoscopy, x-rays, intravenous pyelogram (IVP), CT scan (CAT scan), and MRI (magnetic resonance imaging). Information about these procedures can be found in Section 42.7

The following stages are used for vulvar cancer:

Stage 0 (carcinoma in situ): In stage 0, abnormal cells are found on the surface of the vulvar skin. These abnormal cells may become cancer and spread into nearby normal tissue. Stage 0 is also called carcinoma in situ.

Stage I: In stage I, cancer has formed and is found in the vulva only or in the vulva and perineum (area between the rectum and the vagina). The tumor is two centimeters or smaller and has spread to tissue under the skin. Stage I vulvar cancer is further divided into stage IA and stage IB.

- **Stage IA:** The tumor has spread one millimeter or less into the tissue of the vulva.

- **Stage IB:** The tumor has spread more than one millimeter into the tissue of the vulva.

Stage II: In stage II, cancer is found in the vulva or the vulva and perineum (space between the rectum and the vagina), and the tumor is larger than two centimeters.

Stage III: In stage III vulvar cancer, the cancer is of any size and either is found only in the vulva or the vulva and perineum and has spread to tissue under the skin and to nearby lymph nodes on one side of the groin; or has spread to nearby tissues such as the lower part of the urethra and/or vagina or anus, and may have spread to nearby lymph nodes on one side of the groin.

Stage IV: Stage IV is divided into stage IVA and stage IVB, based on where the cancer has spread.

- **Stage IVA:** Cancer has spread to nearby lymph nodes on both sides of the groin, or has spread beyond nearby tissues to the upper part of the urethra, bladder, or rectum, or has attached to the pelvic bone and may have spread to lymph nodes.

- **Stage IVB:** Cancer has spread to distant parts of the body.

Recurrent vulvar cancer: Recurrent vulvar cancer is cancer that has recurred (come back) after it has been treated. The cancer may come back in the vulva or in other parts of the body.

Treatment Option Overview

Different types of treatments are available for patients with vulvar cancer. Some treatments are standard (the currently used treatment), and some are being tested in clinical trials.

Four types of standard treatment are used. The most common is surgery. The goal of surgery is to remove all the cancer without any loss of the woman's sexual function. One of the following types of surgery may be done: Wide local excision, radical local excision, vulvectomy, skinning vulvectomy, simple vulvectomy, modified radical vulvectomy, radical vulvectomy, and pelvic exenteration.

The other three types of standard treatment that are used for vulvar cancer are laser therapy, radiation therapy, and chemotherapy. Topical chemotherapy for vulvar cancer may be applied to the skin in a cream or lotion.

For more information about these treatment procedures, see Section 42.7.

Section 42.7

Common Procedures for Cancers of the Female Reproductive Organs

Excerpted from "What You Need to Know about Cancer of the Cervix," National Cancer Institute (www.cancer.gov), November 20, 2008; PDQ® Cancer Information Summary. National Cancer Institute; Bethesda, MD. "Endometrial Cancer Treatment (PDQ) - Patient Version." Updated 10/2009. Available at: http://cancer.gov. Accessed January 20, 2010; PDQ® Cancer Information Summary. National Cancer Institute; Bethesda, MD. "Gestational Trophoblastic Tumors Treatment (PDQ) - Patient Version." Updated 06/2008. Available at: http://cancer.gov. Accessed January 20, 2010; PDQ® Cancer Information Summary. National Cancer Institute; Bethesda, MD. "Ovarian Epithelial Cancer Treatment (PDQ) - Patient Version." Updated 01/2010. Available at: http://cancer.gov. Accessed October 1, 2010; PDQ® Cancer Information Summary. National Cancer Institute; Bethesda, MD. "Uterine Sarcoma Treatment (PDQ) - Patient Version." Updated 08/2009. Available at: http://cancer.gov. Accessed January 20, 2010; Excerpted from PDQ® Cancer Information Summary. National Cancer Institute; Bethesda, MD. "Vaginal Cancer Treatment (PDQ) - Patient Version." Updated 07/2010. Available at: http://cancer.gov. Accessed October 1, 2010; And, PDQ® Cancer Information Summary. National Cancer Institute; Bethesda, MD. "Vulvar Cancer Treatment (PDQ) - Patient Version." Updated 08/2009. Available at: http://cancer.gov. Accessed January 20, 2010.

Cancer Cells: What You Should Know

Cancer begins in cells, the building blocks that make up tissues. Tissues make up the organs of the body. Normal cells grow and divide to form new cells as the body needs them. When normal cells grow old or get damaged, they die, and new cells take their place.

Sometimes, this process goes wrong. New cells form when the body does not need them, and old or damaged cells do not die as they should. The buildup of extra cells often forms a mass of tissue called a growth or tumor.

Benign growths (polyps, cysts, or genital warts) are rarely a threat to life, and they don't invade the tissues around them. Malignant growths may sometimes be a threat to life. They can invade nearby tissues and organs, and they can spread to other parts of the body.

The cancer cells can spread by breaking away from the original (primary) tumor. There are three ways that cancer spreads in the body:

- **Through tissue:** Cancer invades the surrounding normal tissue.

- **Through the lymph system:** Cancer invades the lymph system and travels through the lymph vessels to other places in the body.

- **Through the blood:** Cancer invades the veins and capillaries and travels through the blood to other places in the body.

The spread of cancer is called metastasis. When cancer spreads from its original place to another part of the body, the new tumor has the same kind of cancer cells and the same name as the original tumor. For example, if cervical cancer spreads to the lungs, the cancer cells in the lungs are actually cervical cancer cells. The disease is metastatic cervical cancer, not lung cancer. For that reason, it's treated as cervical cancer, not lung cancer. Doctors call the new tumor "distant" or metastatic disease.

Diagnostic and Staging Procedures

To diagnose cancer of the female reproductive organs or to determine whether or not the cancer has spread, your doctor may order some of the following tests:

Abdominal and pelvic washings: A procedure in which a saline solution is placed into the abdominal and pelvic body cavities. After a short time, the fluid is removed and viewed under a microscope to check for cancer cells.

Barium enema: A series of x-rays of the lower gastrointestinal tract. A liquid that contains barium (a silver-white metallic compound) is put into the rectum. The barium coats the lower gastrointestinal tract and x-rays are taken. This procedure is also called a lower GI series.

Biopsy: The removal of cells or tissues so they can be viewed under a microscope by a pathologist to check for signs of cancer. A biopsy that removes only a small amount of tissue is usually done in the doctor's office. A woman may need to go to a hospital for a cone biopsy (removal of a larger, cone-shaped piece of tissue from the cervix and cervical canal). You may want to ask the doctor these questions before having a biopsy:

- Which biopsy method do you recommend?

- How will tissue be removed?

- Will I have to go to the hospital?

- How long will it take? Will I be awake? Will it hurt?

- Are there any risks? What are the chances of infection or bleeding after the test?

- For how many days afterward should I avoid using tampons, douching, or having sex?

- Can the test affect my ability to get pregnant and have children?

- How soon will I know the results? Who will explain them to me?

- If I do have cancer, who will talk to me about the next steps? When?

Blood chemistry studies: A procedure in which a blood sample is checked to measure the amounts of certain substances released into the blood by organs and tissues in the body. An unusual (higher or lower than normal) amount of a substance can be a sign of disease in the organ or tissue that makes it.

CA 125 assay: A test that measures the level of CA 125 in the blood. CA 125 is a substance released by cells into the bloodstream. An increased CA 125 level is sometimes a sign of cancer or other condition.

Chest x-ray: An x-ray of the organs and bones inside the chest. An x-ray is a type of energy beam that can go through the body and onto film, making a picture of areas inside the body. X-rays often can show whether cancer has spread to the lungs.

Colposcopy: A procedure in which a colposcope (a lighted, magnifying instrument) is used to check the vagina and cervix for abnormal areas. Tissue samples may be taken using a curette (spoon-shaped instrument) and checked under a microscope for signs of disease.

CT scan (CAT scan): A procedure that makes a series of detailed pictures of areas inside the body, taken from different angles. The pictures are made by a computer linked to an x-ray machine. A dye may be injected into a vein or swallowed to help the organs or tissues show up more clearly. This procedure is also called computed tomography, computerized tomography, or computerized axial tomography.

Cystoscopy: A procedure to look inside the bladder and urethra to check for abnormal areas. A cystoscope is inserted through the urethra into the bladder. A cystoscope is a thin, tube-like instrument with a light and a lens for viewing. It may also have a tool to remove tissue samples, which are checked under a microscope for signs of cancer.

Dilatation and curettage: Surgery to remove samples of tissue or the inner lining of the uterus. The cervix is dilated and a curette (spoon-shaped instrument) is inserted into the uterus to remove tissue. Tissue samples may be taken and checked under a microscope for signs of disease. This procedure is also called a D&C.

Endometrial biopsy: The removal of tissue from the endometrium (inner lining of the uterus) by inserting a thin, flexible tube through the cervix and into the uterus. The tube is used to gently scrape a small amount of tissue from the endometrium and then remove the tissue samples. A pathologist views the tissue under a microscope to look for cancer cells.

Intravenous pyelogram (IVP): A series of x-rays of the kidneys, ureters, and bladder to find out if cancer has spread to these organs. A contrast dye is injected into a vein. As the contrast dye moves through the kidneys, ureters, and bladder, x-rays are taken to see if there are any blockages. This procedure is also called intravenous urography.

Lymphangiogram: A procedure used to x-ray the lymph system. A dye is injected into the lymph vessels in the feet. The dye travels upward through the lymph nodes and lymph vessels and x-rays are taken to see if there are any blockages. This test helps find out whether cancer has spread to the lymph nodes.

MRI (magnetic resonance imaging): A procedure that uses a magnet, radio waves, and a computer to make a series of detailed pictures of areas inside the body. The doctor can view these pictures on a monitor and can print them on film. An MRI can show whether cancer has spread. Sometimes contrast material makes abnormal areas show up more clearly on the picture. This procedure is also called nuclear magnetic resonance imaging (NMRI).

Pap test: A procedure to collect cells from the surface of the cervix and vagina. A piece of cotton, a brush, or a small wooden stick is used to gently scrape cells from the cervix and vagina. The cells are viewed under a microscope to find out if they are abnormal. This procedure is also called a Pap smear.

Pelvic exam: An exam of the vagina, cervix, uterus, fallopian tubes, ovaries, and rectum. The doctor or nurse inserts one or two lubricated, gloved fingers of one hand into the vagina and the other hand is placed over the lower abdomen to feel the size, shape, and position of the uterus and ovaries. A speculum is also inserted into the vagina and the doctor or nurse looks at the vagina and cervix for signs of disease. A Pap test or Pap smear of the cervix is usually done. The doctor or nurse also inserts a lubricated, gloved finger into the rectum to feel for lumps or abnormal areas.

PET scan: During a positron emission tomography scan, you receive an injection of a small amount of radioactive sugar. A machine makes computerized pictures of the sugar being used by cells in your body. Cancer cells use sugar faster than normal cells, and areas with cancer look brighter on the pictures.

Physical exam and history: An exam of the body to check general signs of health, including checking for signs of disease, such as lumps or anything else that seems unusual. A history of the patient's health habits and past illnesses and treatments will also be taken.

Proctoscopy: A procedure to look inside the rectum to check for abnormal areas. A proctoscope is inserted through the rectum. A proctoscope is a thin, tube-like instrument with a light and a lens for viewing. It may also have a tool to remove tissue to be checked under a microscope for signs of disease.

Sigmoidoscopy: A procedure to look inside the rectum and sigmoid (lower) colon for polyps, abnormal areas, or cancer. A sigmoidoscope is inserted through the rectum into the sigmoid colon. A sigmoidoscope is a thin, tube-like instrument with a light and a lens for viewing. It may also have a tool to remove polyps or tissue samples, which are checked under a microscope for signs of cancer.

Ultrasound exam: A procedure in which high-energy sound waves (ultrasound) are bounced off internal tissues or organs and make echoes. The echoes form a picture of body tissues called a sonogram. The picture can be printed to be looked at later. An abdominal ultrasound or a transvaginal ultrasound may be done. In a transvaginal ultrasound, the ultrasound transducer (probe) is inserted into the vagina.

Ureteroscopy: A procedure to look inside the ureters to check for abnormal areas. A ureteroscope is inserted through the bladder and into the ureters. A ureteroscope is a thin, tube-like instrument with a light and a lens for viewing. It may also have a tool to remove tissue to be checked under a microscope for signs of disease. A ureteroscopy and cystoscopy may be done during the same procedure.

X-rays: An x-ray is a type of energy beam that can go through the body and onto film, making a picture of areas inside the body.

Treatment Options

The choice of treatment depends mainly on the size of the tumor and whether the cancer has spread. The treatment choice may also depend on whether you would like to become pregnant someday.

Your doctor can describe your treatment choices, the expected results of each, and the possible side effects. You and your doctor can work together to develop a treatment plan that meets your medical and personal needs.

Your doctor may refer you to a specialist, or you may ask for a referral. You may want to see a gynecologic oncologist, a surgeon who specializes in treating female cancers. Other specialists who treat gynecological cancer include gynecologists, medical oncologists, and radiation oncologists. Your health care team may also include an oncology nurse and a registered dietitian.

Before treatment starts, ask your health care team about possible side effects and how treatment may change your normal activities. Because cancer treatments often damage healthy cells and tissues, side effects are common. Side effects may not be the same for each person, and they may change from one treatment session to the next.

Questions to Ask before Treatment Begins

You may want to ask the doctor these questions before treatment begins:

- What is the stage of my disease? Has the cancer spread? If so, where?

- May I have a copy of the report from the pathologist?

- What are my treatment choices? Which do you recommend for me? Will I have more than one kind of treatment?

- What are the expected benefits of each kind of treatment?

- What are the risks and possible side effects of each treatment?

What can we do to control the side effects?

- What can I do to prepare for treatment?

- Will I have to stay in the hospital? If so, for how long?

- What is the treatment likely to cost? Will my insurance cover the cost?

- How will treatment affect my normal activities?

- What can I do to take care of myself during treatment?

- What is my chance of a full recovery?

- How often will I need checkups after treatment?

- Would a clinical trial (research study) be right for me?

Types of Surgical Treatments

If your treatment includes a surgical procedure, the type of procedure will depend on the type of cancer, its stage, and other factors. The following definitions explain some of the most commonly used procedures:

- **Hysterectomy:** In a *total hysterectomy*, surgery is performed to remove the uterus, including the cervix. If the uterus and cervix are taken out through the vagina, the operation is called a vaginal hysterectomy. If the uterus and cervix are taken out through a large incision (cut) in the abdomen, the operation is called a total abdominal hysterectomy. If the uterus and cervix are taken out through a small incision (cut) in the abdomen using a laparoscope, the operation is called a total laparoscopic hysterectomy. In a *radical hysterectomy*, surgery is performed to remove the uterus, cervix, and part of the vagina. The ovaries, fallopian tubes, or nearby lymph nodes may also be removed.

- **Laparotomy:** A surgical procedure in which an incision (cut) is made in the wall of the abdomen to check the inside of the abdomen for signs of disease. The size of the incision depends on the reason the laparotomy is being done. Sometimes organs are removed or tissue samples are taken and checked under a microscope for signs of disease.

- **Laser surgery:** A surgical procedure that uses a laser beam (a narrow beam of intense light) as a knife to make bloodless cuts in tissue or to remove a surface lesion such as a tumor.

- **Lymph node biopsy:** The removal of all or part of a lymph node. A pathologist views the tissue under a microscope to look for cancer cells.

- **Lymphadenectomy:** A surgical procedure in which lymph nodes are removed and checked under a microscope for signs of cancer. For a regional lymphadenectomy, some of the lymph nodes in the tumor area are removed. For a radical lymphadenectomy, most or all of the lymph nodes in the tumor area are removed. This procedure is also called lymph node dissection.

- **Omentectomy:** A surgical procedure to remove the omentum (a piece of the tissue lining the abdominal wall).

- **Pelvic exenteration:** Surgery to remove the lower colon, rectum, and bladder. In women, the cervix, vagina, ovaries, and nearby lymph nodes are also removed. Artificial openings (stoma) are made for urine and stool to flow from the body into a collection bag.

- **Radical local excision:** A surgical procedure to remove the cancer and a large amount of normal tissue around it. Nearby lymph nodes in the groin may also be removed.

- **Radical trachelectomy:** The surgeon removes the cervix, part of the vagina, and the lymph nodes in the pelvis. This option is for a small number of women with small tumors who want to try to get pregnant later on. After a radical trachelectomy, some women have bladder problems for a few days. The hospital stay usually is about two to five days.

- **Salpingo-oophorectomy:** In a *bilateral salpingo-oophorectomy*, surgery is performed to remove both ovaries and both fallopian tubes. When the ovaries are removed, menopause occurs at once. Hot flashes and other symptoms of menopause caused by surgery may be more severe than those caused by natural menopause. You may wish to discuss this with your doctor before surgery. Some drugs have been shown to help with these symptoms, and they may be more effective if started before surgery. A *unilateral salpingo-oophorectomy* is a surgical procedure to remove one ovary and one fallopian tube.

- **Vaginectomy:** Surgery to remove all or part of the vagina.

- **Vulvectomy:** A surgical procedure to remove part or all of the vulva. In a *skinning vulvectomy* the top layer of vulvar skin where the cancer is found is removed. Skin grafts from other parts of the body may be needed to cover the area. In a *simple vulvectomy* the entire vulva is removed. In a *modified radical vulvectomy* the part of the vulva that contains cancer and some of the normal tissue around it are removed. In a *radical vulvectomy* the entire vulva, including the clitoris, and nearby tissue are removed. Nearby lymph nodes may also be removed.

- **Wide local excision:** A surgical procedure that takes out the cancer and some of the healthy tissue around it.

Even if the doctor removes all the cancer that can be seen at the time of the surgery, some patients may have chemotherapy or radiation therapy after surgery to kill any cancer cells that are left. Treatment given after the surgery, to lower the risk that the cancer will come back, is called adjuvant therapy

The time it takes to heal after surgery is different for each woman. You may have pain or discomfort for the first few days. Medicine can help control your pain. Before surgery, you should discuss the plan for pain relief with your doctor or nurse. After surgery, your doctor can adjust the plan if you need more pain control.

After a hysterectomy, the length of the hospital stay may vary from several days to a week. It is common to feel tired or weak for a while. You may have problems with nausea and vomiting, and you may have bladder and bowel problems. The doctor may restrict your diet to liquids at first, with a gradual return to solid food. Most women return to their normal activities within four to eight weeks after surgery.

After a hysterectomy, women no longer have menstrual periods. They cannot become pregnant.

For some women, a hysterectomy can affect sexual intimacy. You may have feelings of loss that make intimacy difficult. Sharing these feelings with your partner may be helpful. Sometimes couples talk with a counselor to help them express their concerns.

You may want to ask the doctor these questions before having surgery:

- Do you recommend surgery for me? If so, which kind? Will my ovaries be removed? Do I need to have lymph nodes removed?

- What is the goal of surgery?

- What are the risks of surgery?

- How will I feel after surgery? If I have pain, how will it be controlled?

- How long will I have to be in the hospital?

- Will I have any lasting side effects? If I don't have a hysterectomy, will I be able to get pregnant and have children? If I get pregnant later on, is there a bigger chance that I could have a miscarriage?

- When will I be able to resume normal activities?

- How will the surgery affect my sex life?

Radiation Therapy

Radiation therapy uses high-energy rays to kill cancer cells. It affects cells only in the treated area. Doctors use two types of radiation therapy. Some women receive both types:

- **External radiation therapy:** A large machine directs radiation at your pelvis or other tissues where the cancer has spread. The treatment usually is given in a hospital or clinic. You may receive external radiation five days a week for several weeks. Each treatment takes only a few minutes.

- **Internal radiation therapy:** A thin tube is placed inside the vagina. A radioactive substance is loaded into the tube. You may need to stay in the hospital while the radioactive source is in place (up to three days). Or the treatment session may last a few minutes, and you can go home afterward. Once the radioactive substance is removed, no radioactivity is left in your body. Internal radiation may be repeated two or more times over several weeks.

Side effects depend mainly on how much radiation is given and which part of your body is treated. Radiation to the abdomen and pelvis may cause nausea, vomiting, diarrhea, or urinary problems. You may lose hair in your genital area. Also, your skin in the treated area may become red, dry, and tender.

You may have dryness, itching, or burning in your vagina. Your doctor may advise you to wait to have sex until a few weeks after radiation treatment ends.

You are likely to become tired during radiation therapy, especially in the later weeks of treatment. Resting is important, but doctors usually advise patients to try to stay as active as they can.

Although the side effects of radiation therapy can be upsetting, they can usually be treated or controlled. Talk with your doctor or nurse about ways to relieve discomfort.

It may also help to know that most side effects go away when treatment ends. However, you may wish to discuss with your doctor the possible long-term effects of radiation therapy. For example, the radiation may make the vagina narrower. A narrow vagina can make sex or follow-up exams difficult. There are ways to prevent this problem. If it does occur, however, your health care team can tell you about ways to expand the vagina.

Another long-term effect is that radiation aimed at the pelvic area can harm the ovaries. Menstrual periods usually stop, and women may have hot flashes and vaginal dryness. Menstrual periods are more likely to return for younger women. Women who may want to get pregnant after radiation therapy should ask their health care team about ways to preserve their eggs before treatment starts.

You may want to ask the doctor these questions before having radiation therapy:

- What is the goal of this treatment?

- How will the radiation be given?

- Will I need to stay in the hospital? If so, for how long?

- When will the treatments begin? How often will I have them? When will they end?

- How will I feel during treatment? Are there side effects?

- How will we know if the radiation therapy is working?

- Will I be able to continue my normal activities during treatment?

- How will radiation therapy affect my sex life?

- Are there lasting side effects?

- Will I be able to get pregnant and have children after my treatment is over?

Chemotherapy

Chemotherapy is a cancer treatment that uses drugs to stop the growth of cancer cells, either by killing the cells or by stopping the cells from dividing. When chemotherapy is taken by mouth or injected into a vein or muscle, the drugs enter the bloodstream and can reach cancer cells throughout the body (systemic chemotherapy). When chemotherapy is placed directly into the spinal column, an organ, or a body cavity such as the abdomen, the drugs mainly affect cancer cells in those areas (regional chemotherapy). The way the chemotherapy is given depends on the type and stage of the cancer being treated. You may receive chemotherapy in a clinic, at the doctor's office, or at home. Some women need to stay in the hospital during treatment.

The side effects depend mainly on which drugs are given and how much. Chemotherapy kills fast-growing cancer cells, but the drugs can also harm normal cells that divide rapidly:

- **Blood cells:** When chemotherapy lowers the levels of healthy blood cells, you're more likely to get infections, bruise or bleed easily, and feel very weak and tired. Your health care team will check for low levels of blood cells. If your levels are low, your health care team may stop the chemotherapy for a while or reduce the dose of drug. There are also medicines that can help your body make new blood cells.

- **Cells in hair roots:** Chemotherapy may cause hair loss. If you lose your hair, it will grow back, but it may change in color and texture.

- **Cells that line the digestive tract:** Chemotherapy can cause a poor appetite, nausea and vomiting, diarrhea, or mouth and lip sores. Your health care team can give you medicines and suggest other ways to help with these problems.

Other side effects include skin rash, tingling or numbness in your hands and feet, hearing problems, loss of balance, joint pain, or swollen legs and feet. Your health care team can suggest ways to control many of these problems. Most go away when treatment ends.

You may want to ask the doctor these questions before having chemotherapy:

- Why do I need this treatment?
- Which drug or drugs will I have?
- How do the drugs work?
- What are the expected benefits of the treatment?
- What are the risks and possible side effects of treatment? What can we do about them?
- When will treatment start? When will it end?
- How will treatment affect my normal activities?

Hormone Therapy

Hormone therapy is a cancer treatment that removes hormones or blocks their action and stops cancer cells from growing. Hormones are substances made by glands in the body and circulated in the blood-stream. Some hormones can cause certain cancers to grow. If tests show that the cancer cells have places where hormones can attach (receptors), drugs, surgery, or radiation therapy are used to reduce the production of hormones or block them from working.

Biologic Therapy

Biologic therapy is a treatment that uses the patient's immune system to fight cancer. Substances made by the body or made in a laboratory are used to boost, direct, or restore the body's natural defenses against cancer. This type of cancer treatment is also called biotherapy or immunotherapy.

Targeted Therapy

Targeted therapy is a type of treatment that uses drugs or other substances to identify and attack specific cancer cells without harming normal cells.

Laser Therapy

Laser therapy is a cancer treatment that uses a laser beam (a narrow beam of intense light) to kill cancer cells.

Clinical Trials

New types of treatment are being tested in clinical trials. For some patients, taking part in a clinical trial may be the best treatment choice. Clinical trials are part of the cancer research process. Clinical trials are done to find out if new cancer treatments are safe and effective or better than the standard treatment.

Many of today's standard treatments for cancer are based on earlier clinical trials. Patients who take part in a clinical trial may receive the standard treatment or be among the first to receive a new treatment.

Patients who take part in clinical trials also help improve the way cancer will be treated in the future. Even when clinical trials do not lead to effective new treatments, they often answer important questions and help move research forward.

Patients can enter clinical trials before, during, or after starting their cancer treatment. Some clinical trials only include patients who have not yet received treatment. Other trials test treatments for patients whose cancer has not gotten better. There are also clinical trials that test new ways to stop cancer from recurring (coming back) or reduce the side effects of cancer treatment.

Clinical trials are taking place in many parts of the country. For more information, visit the website at www.clinicaltrials.gov, a service of the National Institutes of Health.

Getting a Second Opinion

Before starting treatment, you might want a second opinion about your diagnosis and treatment plan. Some people worry that the doctor will be offended if they ask for a second opinion. Usually the opposite is true. Most doctors welcome a second opinion. And many health insurance companies will pay for a second opinion if you or your doctor requests it.

If you get a second opinion, the doctor may agree with your first doctor's diagnosis and treatment plan. Or the second doctor may suggest another approach. Either way, you have more information and perhaps a greater sense of control. You can feel more confident about the decisions you make, knowing that you've looked at your options.

It may take some time and effort to gather your medical records and see another doctor. In most cases, it's not a problem to take several weeks to get a second opinion. The delay in starting treatment usually will not make treatment less effective. To make sure, you should discuss this delay with your doctor.

There are many ways to find a doctor for a second opinion. You can ask your doctor, a local or state medical society, a nearby hospital, or a medical school for names of specialists. The National Cancer Institute's Cancer Information Service at 800-4-CANCER can tell you about nearby treatment centers.

Follow-Up Care

You'll need regular checkups after treatment for cancers of the reproductive organs. Checkups help ensure that any changes in your health are noted and treated if needed. If you have any health problems between checkups, you should contact your doctor.

Your doctor will check for the return of cancer. Even when the cancer seems to have been completely removed or destroyed, the disease sometimes returns because undetected cancer cells remained somewhere in the body after treatment. Checkups may include a physical exam, Pap tests, and chest x-rays.

You may want to ask your doctor these questions after you have finished treatment:

- How often will I need checkups?

- How often will I need a Pap test?

- What other follow-up tests do you suggest for me?

- Between checkups, what health problems or symptoms should I tell you about?

Chapter 43

Andrological Cancers

Chapter Contents

Section 43.1

Penile Cancer

Excerpted from PDQ® Cancer Information Summary. National Cancer Institute; Bethesda, MD. "Penile Cancer Treatment (PDQ) - Patient Version." Updated 10/2010. Available at: http://cancer.gov. Accessed October 19, 2010.

General Information about Penile Cancer

Penile cancer is a disease in which malignant (cancer) cells form in the tissues of the penis. The penis is a rod-shaped male reproductive organ that passes sperm and urine from the body. It contains two types of erectile tissue (spongy tissue with blood vessels that fill with blood to make an erection):

- **Corpora cavernosa:** The two columns of erectile tissue that form most of the penis.

- **Corpus spongiosum:** The single column of erectile tissue that forms a small portion of the penis. The corpus spongiosum surrounds the urethra (the tube through which urine and sperm pass from the body).

The erectile tissue is wrapped in connective tissue and covered with skin. The glans (head of the penis) is covered with loose skin called the foreskin.

Risk Factors

Anything that increases your chance of getting a disease is called a risk factor. Having a risk factor does not mean that you will get cancer; not having risk factors doesn't mean that you will not get cancer. People who think they may be at risk should discuss this with their doctor.

Human papillomavirus infection may increase the risk of developing penile cancer. Circumcision may help prevent infection with the human papillomavirus (HPV). A circumcision is an operation in which the doctor removes part or all of the foreskin from the penis. Many boys are circumcised shortly after birth. Men who were not circumcised at birth may have a higher risk of developing penile cancer.

Other risk factors for penile cancer include the following:

- Being age 60 or older
- Having phimosis (a condition in which the foreskin of the penis cannot be pulled back over the glans)
- Having poor personal hygiene
- Having many sexual partners
- Using tobacco products

Detection, Diagnosis, and Prognosis

Possible signs of penile cancer include sores, discharge, and bleeding. These and other symptoms may be caused by penile cancer. Other conditions may cause the same symptoms. A doctor should be consulted if any of the following problems occur:

- Redness, irritation, or a sore on the penis
- A lump on the penis

The following tests and procedures may be used:

- **Physical exam and history:** An exam of the body to check general signs of health, including checking the penis for signs of disease, such as lumps or anything else that seems unusual. A history of the patient's health habits and past illnesses and treatments will also be taken.
- **Biopsy:** The removal of cells or tissues so they can be viewed under a microscope by a pathologist to check for signs of cancer.

The prognosis (chance of recovery) and treatment options depend on the stage of the cancer, the location and size of the tumor, and whether the cancer has just been diagnosed or has recurred (come back).

Stages of Penile Cancer

After penile cancer has been diagnosed, tests are done to find out if cancer cells have spread within the penis or to other parts of the body. The process used to find out if cancer has spread within the penis or to other parts of the body is called staging. The information gathered from the staging process determines the stage of the disease. It is important to know the stage in order to plan treatment. The following tests and procedures may be used in the staging process:

- **CT scan (CAT scan):** A procedure that makes a series of detailed pictures of areas inside the body, taken from different angles. The pictures are made by a computer linked to an x-ray machine. A dye may be injected into a vein or swallowed to help the organs or tissues show up more clearly. This procedure is also called computed tomography, computerized tomography, or computerized axial tomography.

- **MRI (magnetic resonance imaging):** A procedure that uses a magnet, radio waves, and a computer to make a series of detailed pictures of areas inside the body. A substance called gadolinium is injected into a vein. The gadolinium collects around the cancer cells so they show up brighter in the picture. This procedure is also called nuclear magnetic resonance imaging (NMRI).

- **Ultrasound exam:** A procedure in which high-energy sound waves (ultrasound) are bounced off internal tissues or organs and make echoes. The echoes form a picture of body tissues called a sonogram.

- **Chest x-ray:** An x-ray of the organs and bones inside the chest. An x-ray is a type of energy beam that can go through the body and onto film, making a picture of areas inside the body.
  The following stages are used for penile cancer:

Stage 0 (Carcinoma in Situ)

In stage 0, abnormal cells or growths that look like warts are found on the surface of the skin of the penis. These abnormal cells or growths may become cancer and spread into nearby normal tissue. Stage 0 is also called carcinoma in situ.

Stage I

In stage I, cancer has formed and spread to connective tissue just under the skin of the penis. Cancer has not spread to lymph vessels or blood vessels. The tumor cells look a lot like normal cells under a microscope.

Stage II

In stage II, cancer has spread to one of the following areas:

- Connective tissue just under the skin of the penis. Also, cancer has spread to lymph vessels or blood vessels or the tumor cells may look very different from normal cells under a microscope

- Through connective tissue to erectile tissue (spongy tissue that fills with blood to make an erection)

- Beyond erectile tissue to the urethra

Stage III

Stage III is divided into stage IIIa and stage IIIb. In stage IIIa, cancer has spread to one lymph node in the groin. In stage IIIb, cancer has spread to more than one lymph node on one side of the groin or to lymph nodes on both sides of the groin. In both stage IIIa and IIIb cancer has also spread to one of the areas identified in stage II.

Stage IV

In stage IV, cancer has spread to one of the following areas:

- To tissues near the penis such as the prostate, and may have spread to lymph nodes in the groin or pelvis

- To one or more lymph nodes in the pelvis, or cancer has spread from the lymph nodes to the tissues around the lymph nodes

- To distant parts of the body

Recurrent Penile Cancer

Recurrent penile cancer is cancer that has recurred (come back) after it has been treated. The cancer may come back in the penis or in other parts of the body.

Treatment Option Overview

Different types of treatments are available for patients with penile cancer. Some treatments are standard (the currently used treatment), and some are being tested in clinical trials. Three types of standard treatment are used: surgery, radiation therapy, and chemotherapy.

Surgery

Surgery is the most common treatment for all stages of penile cancer. A doctor may remove the cancer using one of the following operations:

- **Mohs microsurgery:** A procedure in which the tumor is cut from the skin in thin layers. During the surgery, the edges of the tumor and each layer of tumor removed are viewed through a microscope to check for cancer cells. Layers continue to be removed until no more cancer cells are seen. This type of surgery removes as little normal tissue as possible and is often used to remove cancer on the skin. It is also called Mohs surgery.

- **Laser surgery:** A surgical procedure that uses a laser beam (a narrow beam of intense light) as a knife to make bloodless cuts in tissue or to remove a surface lesion such as a tumor.

- **Cryosurgery:** A treatment that uses an instrument to freeze and destroy abnormal tissue. This type of treatment is also called cryotherapy.

- **Circumcision:** Surgery to remove part or all of the foreskin of the penis.

- **Wide local excision:** Surgery to remove only the cancer and some normal tissue around it.

- **Amputation of the penis:** Surgery to remove part or all of the penis. If part of the penis is removed, it is a partial penectomy. If all of the penis is removed, it is a total penectomy.

Lymph nodes in the groin may be taken out during surgery.

Even if the doctor removes all the cancer that can be seen at the time of the surgery, some patients may be given chemotherapy or radiation therapy after surgery to kill any cancer cells that are left. Treatment given after the surgery, to lower the risk that the cancer will come back, is called adjuvant therapy.

Radiation Therapy

Radiation therapy is a cancer treatment that uses high-energy x-rays or other types of radiation to kill cancer cells or keep them from growing. There are two types of radiation therapy. External radiation therapy uses a machine outside the body to send radiation toward the cancer. Internal radiation therapy uses a radioactive substance sealed in needles, seeds, wires, or catheters that are placed directly into or near the cancer. The way the radiation therapy is given depends on the type and stage of the cancer being treated.

Chemotherapy

Chemotherapy is a cancer treatment that uses drugs to stop the growth of cancer cells, either by killing the cells or by stopping them from dividing. When chemotherapy is taken by mouth or injected into a vein or muscle, the drugs enter the bloodstream and can reach cancer cells throughout the body (systemic chemotherapy). When chemotherapy is placed directly onto the skin (topical chemotherapy) or into the cerebrospinal fluid, an organ, or a body cavity such as the abdomen, the drugs mainly affect cancer cells in those areas (regional chemotherapy). The way the chemotherapy is given depends on the type and stage of the cancer being treated. Topical chemotherapy may be used to treat stage 0 penile cancer.

Clinical Trials

A treatment clinical trial is a research study meant to help improve current treatments or obtain information on new treatments for patients with cancer. When clinical trials show that a new treatment is better than the standard treatment, the new treatment may become the standard treatment. Patients may want to think about taking part in a clinical trial. Some clinical trials are open only to patients who have not started treatment.

This summary section describes treatments that are being studied in clinical trials. It may not mention every new treatment being studied. Information about clinical trials is available from the National Cancer Institute website (www.cancer.gov).

Biologic Therapy

Biologic therapy is a treatment that uses the patient's immune system to fight cancer. Substances made by the body or made in a laboratory are used to boost, direct, or restore the body's natural defenses against cancer. This type of cancer treatment is also called biotherapy or immunotherapy. Topical biologic therapy may be used to treat stage 0 penile cancer.

Radiosensitizers

Radiosensitizers are drugs that make tumor cells more sensitive to radiation therapy. Combining radiation therapy with radiosensitizers helps kill more tumor cells.

Sentinel Lymph Node Biopsy Followed by Surgery

Sentinel lymph node biopsy is the removal of the sentinel lymph node during surgery. The sentinel lymph node is the first lymph node to receive lymphatic drainage from a tumor. It is the first lymph node the cancer is likely to spread to from the tumor. A radioactive substance and/or blue dye is injected near the tumor. The substance or dye flows through the lymph ducts to the lymph nodes. The first lymph node to receive the substance or dye is removed. A pathologist views the tissue under a microscope to look for cancer cells. If cancer cells are not found, it may not be necessary to remove more lymph nodes. After the sentinel lymph node biopsy, the surgeon removes the cancer.

Follow-Up Tests

Some of the tests that were done to diagnose the cancer or to find out the stage of the cancer may be repeated. Some tests will be repeated in order to see how well the treatment is working. Decisions about whether to continue, change, or stop treatment may be based on the results of these tests. This is sometimes called re-staging.

Some of the tests will continue to be done from time to time after treatment has ended. The results of these tests can show if your condition has changed or if the cancer has recurred (come back). These tests are sometimes called follow-up tests or check-ups.

Section 43.2

Prostate Cancer

Excerpted from "What You Need to Know About Prostate Cancer,"
National Cancer Institute (www.cancer.gov), November 20, 2008.

The Prostate

The prostate is part of a man's reproductive system. It's an organ located in front of the rectum and under the bladder. The prostate surrounds the urethra, the tube through which urine flows.

A healthy prostate is about the size of a walnut. If the prostate grows too large, it squeezes the urethra. This may slow or stop the flow of urine from the bladder to the penis.

The prostate is a gland. It makes part of the seminal fluid. During ejaculation, the seminal fluid helps carry sperm out of the man's body as part of semen.

Male hormones (androgens) make the prostate grow. The testicles are the main source of male hormones, including testosterone. The adrenal gland also makes testosterone, but in small amounts.

Benign Prostatic Hyperplasia

Benign prostatic hyperplasia (BPH) is a benign growth of prostate cells. It is not cancer. The prostate grows larger and squeezes the urethra. This prevents the normal flow of urine. BPH is a very common problem. In the United States, most men over the age of 50 have symptoms of BPH. For some men, the symptoms may be severe enough to need treatment.

Prostate Cancer Risk Factors

Doctors seldom know why one man develops prostate cancer and another doesn't. However, research has shown that men with certain risk factors are more likely than others to develop prostate cancer. A risk factor is something that may increase the chance of getting a disease. Having a risk factor doesn't mean that a man will develop prostate cancer. Most men who have risk factors never develop the disease.

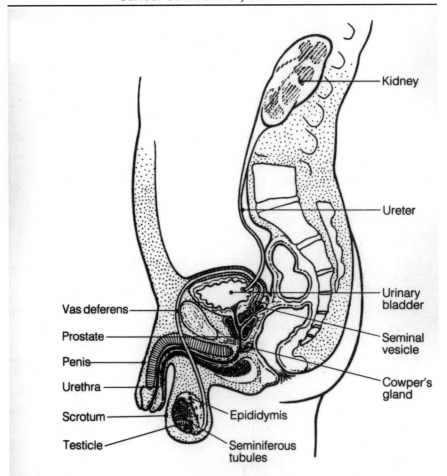

Figure 43.1. *Organs in the Male Reproductive Tract (image by the National Cancer Institute, AV-0000-4110)*

Studies have found the following risk factors for prostate cancer:

- **Age over 65:** Age is the main risk factor for prostate cancer. The chance of getting prostate cancer increases as you get older. In the United States, most men with prostate cancer are over 65. This disease is rare in men under 45.

- **Family history:** Your risk is higher if your father, brother, or son had prostate cancer.

- **Race:** Prostate cancer is more common among black men than white or Hispanic/Latino men. It's less common among Asian/Pacific Islander and American Indian/Alaska Native men.

- **Certain prostate changes:** Men with cells called high-grade prostatic intraepithelial neoplasia (PIN) may be at increased risk of prostate cancer. These prostate cells look abnormal under a microscope.

- **Certain genome changes:** Researchers have found specific regions on certain chromosomes that are linked to the risk of prostate cancer. According to recent studies, if a man has a genetic change in one or more of these regions, the risk of prostate cancer may be increased. The risk increases with the number of genetic changes that are found. Also, other studies have shown an elevated risk of prostate cancer among men with changes in certain genes, such as BRCA1 and BRCA2.

Many other possible risk factors are under study. For example, researchers have studied whether vasectomy (surgery to cut or tie off the tubes that carry sperm out of the testicles) may pose a risk, but most studies have found no increased risk. Also, most studies have shown that the chance of getting prostate cancer is not increased by tobacco or alcohol use, BPH, a sexually transmitted disease, obesity, a lack of exercise, or a diet high in animal fat or meat. Researchers continue to study these and other possible risk factors.

Researchers are also studying how prostate cancer may be prevented. For example, they are studying the possible benefits of certain drugs, vitamin E, selenium, green tea extract, and other substances. These studies are with men who have not yet developed prostate cancer.

Symptoms, Detection, and Diagnosis

A man with prostate cancer may not have any symptoms. For men who do have symptoms, the common symptoms include the following:

- Urinary problems
- Not being able to pass urine
- Having a hard time starting or stopping the urine flow
- Needing to urinate often, especially at night
- Weak flow of urine
- Urine flow that starts and stops
- Pain or burning during urination
- Difficulty having an erection
- Blood in the urine or semen

- Frequent pain in the lower back, hips, or upper thighs

Most often, these symptoms are not due to cancer. BPH, an infection, or another health problem may cause them. If you have any of these symptoms, you should tell your doctor so that problems can be diagnosed and treated.

Your doctor can check for prostate cancer before you have any symptoms. During an office visit, your doctor will ask about your personal and family medical history. You'll have a physical exam. You may also have one or both of the following tests:

- **Digital rectal exam:** Your doctor inserts a lubricated, gloved finger into the rectum and feels your prostate through the rectal wall. Your prostate is checked for hard or lumpy areas.

- **Blood test for prostate-specific antigen (PSA):** A lab checks the level of PSA in your blood sample. The prostate makes PSA. A high PSA level is commonly caused by BPH or prostatitis (inflammation of the prostate). Prostate cancer may also cause a high PSA level.

The digital rectal exam and PSA test can detect a problem in the prostate. However, they can't show whether the problem is cancer or a less serious condition. If you have abnormal test results, your doctor may suggest other tests to make a diagnosis. For example, your visit may include other lab tests, such as a urine test to check for blood or infection. Your doctor may order other procedures:

Transrectal ultrasound: The doctor inserts a probe into the rectum to check your prostate for abnormal areas. The probe sends out sound waves that people cannot hear (ultrasound). The waves bounce off the prostate. A computer uses the echoes to create a picture called a sonogram.

Transrectal biopsy: A biopsy is the removal of tissue to look for cancer cells. It's the only sure way to diagnose prostate cancer. The doctor inserts needles through the rectum into the prostate. The doctor removes small tissue samples (called cores) from many areas of the prostate. Transrectal ultrasound is usually used to guide the insertion of the needles. A pathologist checks the tissue samples for cancer cells.

If Cancer Is Found

If cancer cells are found, the pathologist studies tissue samples from the prostate under a microscope to report the grade of the tumor. The grade tells how much the tumor tissue differs from normal prostate tissue. It suggests how fast the tumor is likely to grow.

Tumors with higher grades tend to grow faster than those with lower grades. They are also more likely to spread. Doctors use tumor grade along with your age and other factors to suggest treatment options.

One system of grading is with the Gleason score. Gleason scores range from 2 to 10. To come up with the Gleason score, the pathologist uses a microscope to look at the patterns of cells in the prostate tissue. The most common pattern is given a grade of 1 (most like normal cells) to 5 (most abnormal). If there is a second most common pattern, the pathologist gives it a grade of 1 to 5, and adds the two most common grades together to make the Gleason score. If only one pattern is seen, the pathologist counts it twice. For example, 5 + 5 = 10. A high Gleason score (such as 10) means a high-grade prostate tumor. High-grade tumors are more likely than low-grade tumors to grow quickly and spread.

Another system of grading prostate cancer uses grades 1 through 4 (G1 to G4). G4 is more likely than G1, G2, or G3 to grow quickly and spread.

Staging

If the biopsy shows that you have cancer, your doctor needs to learn the extent (stage) of the disease to help you choose the best treatment. Staging is a careful attempt to find out whether the tumor has invaded nearby tissues, whether the cancer has spread and, if so, to what parts of the body.

Some men may need tests that make pictures of the body:

- **Bone scan:** The doctor injects a small amount of a radioactive substance into a blood vessel. It travels through the bloodstream and collects in the bones. A machine called a scanner detects and measures the radiation. The scanner makes pictures of the bones on a computer screen or on film. The pictures may show cancer that has spread to the bones.

- **CT scan:** An x-ray machine linked to a computer takes a series of detailed pictures of your pelvis or other parts of the body. Doctors use CT scans to look for prostate cancer that has spread to lymph nodes and other areas. You may receive contrast material by injection into a blood vessel in your arm or hand, or by enema. The contrast material makes abnormal areas easier to see.

- **MRI:** A strong magnet linked to a computer is used to make detailed pictures of areas inside your body. The doctor can view these pictures on a monitor and can print them on film. An MRI can show whether cancer has spread to lymph nodes or other areas. Sometimes contrast material makes abnormal areas show up more clearly on the picture.

When prostate cancer spreads, it's often found in nearby lymph nodes. If cancer has reached these nodes, it also may have spread to other lymph nodes, the bones, or other organs.

When cancer spreads from its original place to another part of the body, the new tumor has the same kind of abnormal cells and the same name as the primary tumor. For example, if prostate cancer spreads to bones, the cancer cells in the bones are actually prostate cancer cells. The disease is metastatic prostate cancer, not bone cancer. For that reason, it's treated as prostate cancer, not bone cancer. Doctors call the new tumor "distant" or metastatic disease.

These are the stages of prostate cancer:

- **Stage I:** The cancer can't be felt during a digital rectal exam, and it can't be seen on a sonogram. It's found by chance when surgery is done for another reason, usually for BPH. The cancer is only in the prostate. The grade is G1, or the Gleason score is no higher than 4.

- **Stage II:** The tumor is more advanced or a higher grade than Stage I, but the tumor doesn't extend beyond the prostate. It may be felt during a digital rectal exam, or it may be seen on a sonogram.

- **Stage III:** The tumor extends beyond the prostate. The tumor may have invaded the seminal vesicles, but cancer cells haven't spread to the lymph nodes.

- **Stage IV:** The tumor may have invaded the bladder, rectum, or nearby structures (beyond the seminal vesicles). It may have spread to the lymph nodes, bones, or to other parts of the body.

Treatment

Men with prostate cancer have many treatment options. The treatment that's best for one man may not be best for another. The options include active surveillance (also called watchful waiting), surgery, radiation therapy, hormone therapy, and chemotherapy. You may have a combination of treatments.

The treatment that's right for you depends mainly on your age, the grade of the tumor (the Gleason score), the number of biopsy tissue samples that contain cancer cells, the stage of the cancer, your symptoms, and your general health. Your doctor can describe your treatment choices, the expected results of each, and the possible side effects. You and your doctor can work together to develop a treatment plan that meets your medical and personal needs.

Your doctor may refer you to a specialist, or you may ask for a referral. You may want to see a urologist, a surgeon who specializes in treating problems in the urinary or male sex organs. Other specialists who treat prostate cancer include urologic oncologists, medical oncologists, and radiation oncologists. Your health care team may also include an oncology nurse and a registered dietitian.

Active Surveillance

You may choose active surveillance if the risks and possible side effects of treatment outweigh the possible benefits. Your doctor may suggest active surveillance if you're diagnosed with early stage prostate cancer that seems to be slowly growing. Your doctor may also offer this option if you are older or have other serious health problems.

Choosing active surveillance doesn't mean you're giving up. It means you're putting off the side effects of surgery or radiation therapy. Having surgery or radiation therapy is no guarantee that a man will live longer than a man who chooses to put off treatment.

If you and your doctor agree that active surveillance is a good idea, your doctor will check you regularly (such as every three to six months, at first). After about one year, your doctor may order another biopsy to check the Gleason score. You may begin treatment if your Gleason score rises, your PSA level starts to rise, or you develop symptoms. You'll receive surgery, radiation therapy, or another approach.

Active surveillance avoids or delays the side effects of surgery and radiation therapy, but this choice has risks. For some men, it may reduce the chance to control cancer before it spreads. Also, it may be harder to cope with surgery or radiation therapy when you're older.

If you choose active surveillance but grow concerned later, you should discuss your feelings with your doctor. Another approach is an option for most men.

Surgery

Surgery is an option for men with early (Stage I or II) prostate cancer. It's sometimes an option for men with Stage III or IV prostate cancer. The surgeon may remove the whole prostate or only part of it.

Before the surgeon removes the prostate, the lymph nodes in the pelvis may be removed. If prostate cancer cells are found in the lymph nodes, the disease may have spread to other parts of the body. If cancer has spread to the lymph nodes, the surgeon does not always remove the prostate and may suggest other types of treatment.

There are several types of surgery for prostate cancer. Each type has benefits and risks. You and your doctor can talk about the types of surgery and which may be right for you:

- **Open surgery:** The surgeon makes a large incision (cut) into your body to remove the tumor. There are two approaches. One is through the abdomen. The surgeon removes the entire prostate through a cut in the abdomen. This is called a radical retropubic prostatectomy. The other is between the scrotum and anus. The surgeon removes the entire prostate through a cut between the scrotum and the anus. This is called a radical perineal prostatectomy.

- **Laparoscopic prostatectomy:** The surgeon removes the entire prostate through small cuts, rather than a single long cut in the abdomen. A thin, lighted tube (a laparoscope) helps the surgeon remove the prostate.

- **Robotic laparoscopic surgery:** The surgeon removes the entire prostate through small cuts. A laparoscope and a robot are used to help remove the prostate. The surgeon uses handles below a computer display to control the robot's arms.

- **Cryosurgery:** For some men, cryosurgery is an option. The surgeon inserts a tool through a small cut between the scrotum and anus. The tool freezes and kills prostate tissue. Cryosurgery is under study.

- **TURP:** A man with advanced prostate cancer may choose TURP (transurethral resection of the prostate) to relieve symptoms. The surgeon inserts a long, thin scope through the urethra. A cutting tool at the end of the scope removes tissue from the inside of the prostate. TURP may not remove all of the cancer, but it can remove tissue that blocks the flow of urine.

You may be uncomfortable for the first few days or weeks after surgery. However, medicine can help control the pain. Before surgery, you should discuss the plan for pain relief with your doctor or nurse. After surgery, your doctor can adjust the plan if you need more pain relief.

The time it takes to heal after surgery is different for each man and depends on the type of surgery. You may be in the hospital for one to three days.

After surgery, the urethra needs time to heal. You'll have a catheter. A catheter is a tube put through the urethra into the bladder to drain urine. You'll have the catheter for five days to three weeks. Your nurse or doctor will show you how to care for it.

After surgery, some men may lose control of the flow of urine (urinary incontinence). Most men regain at least some bladder control after a few weeks.

Surgery can damage the nerves around the prostate. Damaging these nerves can make a man impotent (unable to have an erection). In some cases, your surgeon can protect the nerves that control erection. But if you have a large tumor or a tumor that's very close to the nerves, surgery may cause impotence. Impotence can be permanent. You can talk with your doctor about medicine and other ways to help manage the sexual side effects of cancer treatment.

If your prostate is removed, you will no longer produce semen. You'll have dry orgasms. If you wish to father children, you may consider sperm banking or a sperm retrieval procedure before surgery.

Radiation Therapy

Radiation therapy is an option for men with any stage of prostate cancer. Men with early stage prostate cancer may choose radiation therapy instead of surgery. It also may be used after surgery to destroy any cancer cells that remain in the area. In later stages of prostate cancer, radiation treatment may be used to help relieve pain.

Radiation therapy (also called radiotherapy) uses high-energy rays to kill cancer cells. It affects cells only in the treated area. Doctors use two types of radiation therapy to treat prostate cancer. Some men receive both types:

- **External radiation:** The radiation comes from a large machine outside the body. You will go to a hospital or clinic for treatment. Treatments are usually five days a week for several weeks. Many men receive 3-dimensional conformal radiation therapy or intensity-modulated radiation therapy. These types of treatment use computers to more closely target the cancer to lessen the damage to healthy tissue near the prostate.

- **Internal radiation (implant radiation or brachytherapy):**
  The radiation comes from radioactive material usually contained in very small implants called seeds. Dozens of seeds are placed inside needles, and the needles are inserted into the prostate. The needles are removed, leaving the seeds behind. The seeds give off radiation for months. They don't need to be removed once the radiation is gone.

Side effects depend mainly on the dose and type of radiation. You're likely to be very tired during radiation therapy, especially in the later weeks of treatment. Resting is important, but doctors usually advise patients to try to stay active, unless it leads to pain or other problems.

If you have external radiation, you may have diarrhea or frequent and uncomfortable urination. Some men have lasting bowel or urinary problems. Your skin in the treated area may become red, dry, and tender. You may lose hair in the treated area. The hair may not grow back.

Internal radiation therapy may cause incontinence. This side effect usually goes away.

Both internal and external radiation can cause impotence. You can talk with your doctor about ways to help cope with this side effect.

Hormone Therapy

A man with prostate cancer may have hormone therapy before, during, or after radiation therapy. Hormone therapy is also used alone for prostate cancer that has returned after treatment.

Male hormones (androgens) can cause prostate cancer to grow. Hormone therapy keeps prostate cancer cells from getting the male hormones they need to grow. The testicles are the body's main source of the male hormone testosterone. The adrenal gland makes other male hormones and a small amount of testosterone.

Hormone therapy uses drugs or surgery:

Drugs: Your doctor may suggest a drug that can block natural hormones:

- **Luteinizing hormone-releasing hormone (LH-RH) agonists:** These drugs can prevent the testicles from making testosterone. Examples are leuprolide, goserelin, and triptorelin. The testosterone level falls slowly. Without testosterone, the tumor shrinks, or its growth slows. These drugs are also called gonadotropin-releasing hormone (GnRH) agonists.

- **Antiandrogens:** These drugs can block the action of male hormones. Examples are flutamide, bicalutamide, and nilutamide.

- **Other drugs:** Some drugs can prevent the adrenal gland from making testosterone. Examples are ketoconazole and aminoglutethimide.

Surgery: Surgery to remove the testicles is called orchiectomy. After orchiectomy or treatment with an LH-RH agonist, your body no longer gets testosterone from the testicles, the major source of male hormones. Because the adrenal gland makes small amounts of male hormones, you may receive an antiandrogen to block the action of the male hormones that remain. This combination of treatments is known as total androgen blockade (also called combined androgen blockade). However, studies have shown that total androgen blockade is no more effective than surgery or an LH-RH agonist alone.

Side effects: Hormone therapy causes side effects such as impotence, hot flashes, and loss of sexual desire. Also, any treatment that lowers hormone levels can weaken your bones. Your doctor can suggest medicines that may reduce your risk of bone fractures.

An LH-RH agonist may make your symptoms worse for a short time at first. This temporary problem is called "flare." To prevent flare, your doctor may give you an antiandrogen for a few weeks along with the LH-RH agonist.

An LH-RH agonist such as leuprolide can increase body fat, especially around the waist. The levels of sugar and cholesterol in your blood may increase too. Because these changes increase the risk of diabetes and heart disease, your health care team will monitor you for these side effects.

Antiandrogens (such as nilutamide) can cause nausea, diarrhea, or breast growth or tenderness. Rarely, they may cause liver problems (pain in the abdomen, yellow eyes, or dark urine). Some men who use nilutamide may have shortness of breath or develop heart failure. Some may have trouble adjusting to sudden changes in light.

If you receive total androgen blockade, you may have more side effects than if you have just one type of hormone treatment.

If used for a long time, ketoconazole may cause liver problems, and aminoglutethimide can cause skin rashes.

When hormone therapy response diminishes: Doctors usually treat prostate cancer that has spread to other parts of the body with hormone therapy. For some men, the cancer will be controlled for two or three years, but others will have a much shorter response to hormone therapy. In time, most prostate cancers can grow with very little or no male hormones, and hormone therapy alone is no longer helpful. At that time, your doctor may suggest chemotherapy or other forms of treatment that are under study. In many cases, the doctor may suggest continuing with hormone therapy because it may still be effective against some of the cancer cells.

Chemotherapy

Chemotherapy may be used for prostate cancer that has spread and no longer responds to hormone therapy. Chemotherapy uses drugs to kill cancer cells. The drugs for prostate cancer are usually given through a vein (intravenous). You may receive chemotherapy in a clinic, at the doctor's office, or at home. Some men need to stay in the hospital during treatment.

The side effects depend mainly on which drugs are given and how much. Chemotherapy kills fast-growing cancer cells, but the drugs can also harm normal cells that divide rapidly:

- **Blood cells:** When chemotherapy lowers the levels of healthy blood cells, you're more likely to get infections, bruise or bleed easily, and feel very weak and tired. Your health care team will check for low levels of blood cells. If your levels are low, your health care team may stop the chemotherapy for a while or reduce the dose of drug. There are also medicines that can help your body make new blood cells.

- **Cells in hair roots:** Chemotherapy may cause hair loss. If you lose your hair, it will grow back, but it may change in color and texture.

- **Cells that line the digestive tract:** Chemotherapy can cause a poor appetite, nausea and vomiting, or diarrhea. Your health care team can give you medicines and suggest other ways to help with these problems.

Other side effects include shortness of breath and a problem with your body holding extra water. Your health care team can give you medicine to protect against too much water building up in the body. Also, chemotherapy may cause a skin rash, tingling or numbness in your hands and feet, and watery eyes. Your health care team can suggest ways to control many of these problems. Most go away when treatment ends.

Second Opinion

Before starting treatment, you might want a second opinion about your diagnosis and treatment plan. You may even want to talk to several different doctors about all of the treatment options, their side effects, and the expected results. For example, you may want to talk to a urologist, radiation oncologist, and medical oncologist.

Some people worry that the doctor will be offended if they ask for a second opinion. Usually the opposite is true. Most doctors welcome a second opinion. And many health insurance companies will pay for a second opinion if you or your doctor requests it.

If you get a second opinion, the doctor may agree with your first doctor's diagnosis and treatment plan. Or, the second doctor may suggest another approach. Either way, you have more information and perhaps a greater sense of control. You can feel more confident about the decisions you make, knowing that you've looked at your options.

It may take some time and effort to gather your medical records and see another doctor. In most cases, it's not a problem to take several weeks to get a second opinion. The delay in starting treatment usually will not make treatment less effective. To make sure, you should discuss this delay with your doctor.

There are many ways to find a doctor for a second opinion. You can ask your doctor, a local or state medical society, a nearby hospital, or a medical school for names of specialists. The National Cancer Institute's Cancer Information Service at 800-4-CANCER can tell you about nearby treatment centers.

Follow-Up Care

You'll need regular checkups after treatment for prostate cancer. Checkups help ensure that any changes in your health are noted and treated if needed. If you have any health problems between checkups, you should contact your doctor.

Your doctor will check for return of cancer. Even when the cancer seems to have been completely removed or destroyed, the disease sometimes returns because undetected cancer cells remained somewhere in the body after treatment.

Checkups may include a digital rectal exam and a PSA test. A rise in PSA level can mean that cancer has returned after treatment. Your doctor may also order a biopsy, a bone scan, CT scans, an MRI, or other tests.

Section 43.3

Testicular Cancer

Excerpted from PDQ® Cancer Information Summary. National Cancer Institute; Bethesda, MD. "Testicular Cancer Treatment (PDQ) - Patient Version." Updated 10/2010. Available at: http://cancer.gov. Accessed October 19, 2010.

General Information about Testicular Cancer

Testicular cancer is the most common cancer in men 20 to 35 years old. Testicular cancer is a disease in which malignant (cancer) cells form in the tissues of one or both testicles. The testicles are two egg-shaped glands located inside the scrotum (a sac of loose skin that lies directly below the penis). The testicles are held within the scrotum by the spermatic cord, which also contains the vas deferens and vessels and nerves of the testicles.

The testicles are the male sex glands and produce testosterone and sperm. Germ cells within the testicles produce immature sperm that travel through a network of tubules (tiny tubes) and larger tubes into the epididymis (a long coiled tube next to the testicles) where the sperm mature and are stored.

Almost all testicular cancers start in the germ cells. The two main types of testicular germ cell tumors are seminomas and nonseminomas. These two types grow and spread differently and are treated differently. Nonseminomas tend to grow and spread more quickly than seminomas. Seminomas are more sensitive to radiation. A testicular tumor that contains both seminoma and nonseminoma cells is treated as a nonseminoma.

Risk Factors and Symptoms

Anything that increases the chance of getting a disease is called a risk factor. Having a risk factor does not mean that you will get cancer; not having risk factors doesn't mean that you will not get cancer. People who think they may be at risk should discuss this with their doctor. Risk factors for testicular cancer include:

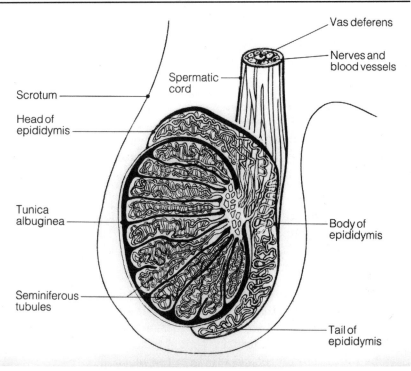

Figure 43.2. Cross Section of Testicle (image by the National Cancer Institute, AV-0000-4097)

- Having had an undescended testicle
- Having had abnormal development of the testicles
- Having a personal or family history of testicular cancer
- Being white

Possible signs of testicular cancer include swelling or discomfort in the scrotum. These and other symptoms may be caused by testicular cancer. Other conditions may cause the same symptoms. A doctor should be consulted if any of the following problems occur:

- A painless lump or swelling in either testicle
- A change in how the testicle feels
- A dull ache in the lower abdomen or the groin
- A sudden build-up of fluid in the scrotum
- Pain or discomfort in a testicle or in the scrotum

Detection, Diagnosis, and Prognosis

Tests that examine the testicles and blood are used to detect (find) and diagnose testicular cancer. The following tests and procedures may be used:

- **Physical exam and history:** An exam of the body to check general signs of health, including checking for signs of disease, such as lumps or anything else that seems unusual. The testicles will be examined to check for lumps, swelling, or pain. A history of the patient's health habits and past illnesses and treatments will also be taken.

- **Ultrasound exam:** A procedure in which high-energy sound waves (ultrasound) are bounced off internal tissues or organs and make echoes. The echoes form a picture of body tissues called a sonogram.

- **Serum tumor marker test:** A procedure in which a sample of blood is examined to measure the amounts of certain substances released into the blood by organs, tissues, or tumor cells in the body. Certain substances are linked to specific types of cancer when found in increased levels in the blood. These are called tumor markers. The following three tumor markers are used to detect testicular cancer: alpha-fetoprotein (AFP); beta-human chorionic gonadotropin (beta-hCG); and lactate dehydrogenase (LDH). Tumor marker levels are measured before radical inguinal orchiectomy and biopsy, to help diagnose testicular cancer.

- **Radical inguinal orchiectomy and biopsy:** A procedure to remove the entire testicle through an incision in the groin. A tissue sample from the testicle is then viewed under a microscope to check for cancer cells. (The surgeon does not cut through the scrotum into the testicle to remove a sample of tissue for biopsy, because if cancer is present, this procedure could cause it to spread into the scrotum and lymph nodes.) If cancer is found, the cell type (seminoma or nonseminoma) is determined in order to help plan treatment.

The prognosis (chance of recovery) and treatment options depend on the stage of the cancer (whether it is in or near the testicle or has spread to other places in the body, and blood levels of AFP, beta-hCG, and LDH), type of cancer, size of the tumor, and number and size of retroperitoneal lymph nodes. Testicular cancer is often curable.

Certain treatments for testicular cancer can cause infertility that may be permanent. Patients who may wish to have children should consider sperm banking before having treatment. Sperm banking is the process of freezing sperm and storing it for later use.

Stages of Testicular Cancer

After testicular cancer has been diagnosed, tests are done to find out if cancer cells have spread within the testicles or to other parts of the body. The process used to find out if cancer has spread within the testicles or to other parts of the body is called staging. The information gathered from the staging process determines the stage of the disease. It is important to know the stage in order to plan treatment. In addition to serum marker tests and radical inguinal orchiectomy and biopsy, which are described above, the following tests and procedures may be used in the staging process:

- **Chest x-ray:** An x-ray of the organs and bones inside the chest. An x-ray is a type of energy beam that can go through the body and onto film, making a picture of areas inside the body.

- **CT scan (CAT scan):** A procedure that makes a series of detailed pictures of areas inside the body, taken from different angles. The pictures are made by a computer linked to an x-ray machine. A dye may be injected into a vein or swallowed to help the organs or tissues show up more clearly. This procedure is also called computed tomography, computerized tomography, or computerized axial tomography.

- **Lymphangiography:** A procedure used to x-ray the lymph system. A dye is injected into the lymph vessels in the feet. The dye travels upward through the lymph nodes and lymph vessels, and x-rays are taken to see if there are any blockages. This test helps find out whether cancer has spread to the lymph nodes.

- **Abdominal lymph node dissection:** A surgical procedure in which lymph nodes in the abdomen are removed and a sample of tissue is checked under a microscope for signs of cancer. This procedure is also called lymphadenectomy. For patients with nonseminoma, removing the lymph nodes may help stop the spread of disease. Cancer cells in the lymph nodes of seminoma patients can be treated with radiation therapy.

The following stages are used for testicular cancer:

Stage 0 (Carcinoma in Situ)

In stage 0, abnormal cells are found in the tiny tubules where the sperm cells begin to develop. These abnormal cells may become cancer and spread into nearby normal tissue. All tumor marker levels are normal. Stage 0 is also called carcinoma in situ.

Stage I

In stage I, cancer has formed. Stage I is divided into stage IA, stage IB, and stage IS and is determined after a radical inguinal orchiectomy is done.

- In stage IA, cancer is in the testicle and epididymis and may have spread to the inner layer of the membrane surrounding the testicle. All tumor marker levels are normal.

- In stage IB, all tumor marker levels are normal and cancer is in the testicle and the epididymis and has spread to the blood vessels or lymph vessels in the testicle; or has spread to the outer layer of the membrane surrounding the testicle; or is in the spermatic cord or the scrotum and may be in the blood vessels or lymph vessels of the testicle.

- In stage IS, cancer is found anywhere within the testicle, spermatic cord, or the scrotum and either all tumor marker levels are slightly above normal or one or more tumor marker levels are moderately above normal or high.

Stage II

Stage II is divided into stage IIA, stage IIB, and stage IIC and is determined after a radical inguinal orchiectomy is done.

In stage IIA, all tumor marker levels are normal or slightly above normal and cancer is anywhere within the testicle, spermatic cord, or scrotum and has spread to up to five lymph nodes in the abdomen, none larger than two centimeters.

In stage IIB, all tumor marker levels are normal or slightly above normal, and cancer is anywhere within the testicle, spermatic cord, or scrotum; and either has spread to up to five lymph nodes in the abdomen and at least one of the lymph nodes is larger than two centimeters, but none are larger than five centimeters; or has spread to more than five lymph nodes and the lymph nodes are not larger than five centimeters.

In stage IIC, all tumor marker levels are normal or slightly above normal and cancer is anywhere within the testicle, spermatic cord, or scrotum and has spread to a lymph node in the abdomen that is larger than five centimeters.

Stage III

Stage III is divided into stage IIIA, stage IIIB, and stage IIIC and is determined after a radical inguinal orchiectomy is done.

In stage IIIA, tumor marker levels may range from normal to slightly above normal, and cancer is anywhere within the testicle, spermatic cord, or scrotum and may have spread to one or more lymph nodes in the abdomen and has spread to distant lymph nodes or to the lungs.

In stage IIIB, the level of one or more tumor markers is moderately above normal, and cancer is anywhere within the testicle, spermatic cord, or scrotum and may have spread to one or more lymph nodes in the abdomen, to distant lymph nodes, or to the lungs.

In stage IIIC, the level of one or more tumor markers is high, and cancer is anywhere within the testicle, spermatic cord, or scrotum and may have spread to one or more lymph nodes in the abdomen, to distant lymph nodes, or to the lungs. Or, tumor marker levels may range from normal to high, and cancer is anywhere within the testicle, spermatic cord, or scrotum; and may have spread to one or more lymph nodes in the abdomen; and has not spread to distant lymph nodes or the lung but has spread to other parts of the body.

Recurrent Testicular Cancer

Recurrent testicular cancer is cancer that has recurred (come back) after it has been treated. The cancer may come back many years after the initial cancer, in the other testicle or in other parts of the body.

Treatment Option Overview

Different types of treatments are available for patients with testicular cancer. Some treatments are standard (the currently used treatment), and some are being tested in clinical trials. Three types of standard treatment are used: surgery, radiation therapy, and chemotherapy.

Testicular tumors are divided into three groups, based on how well the tumors are expected to respond to treatment.

Good Prognosis

For nonseminoma, all of the following must be true:

- The tumor is found only in the testicle or in the retroperitoneum (area outside or behind the abdominal wall); and

- The tumor has not spread to organs other than the lungs; and

- The levels of all the tumor markers are slightly above normal.

For seminoma, all of the following must be true:

- The tumor has not spread to organs other than the lungs; and

- The level of alpha-fetoprotein (AFP) is normal. Beta-human chorionic gonadotropin (beta-hCG) and lactate dehydrogenase (LDH) may be at any level.

Intermediate Prognosis

For nonseminoma, all of the following must be true:

- The tumor is found in one testicle only or in the retroperitoneum (area outside or behind the abdominal wall); and

- The tumor has not spread to organs other than the lungs; and

- The level of any one of the tumor markers is more than slightly above normal.

For seminoma, all of the following must be true:

- The tumor has spread to organs other than the lungs; and

- The level of AFP is normal. Beta-hCG and LDH may be at any level.

Poor Prognosis

For nonseminoma, at least one of the following must be true:

- The tumor is in the center of the chest between the lungs; or

- The tumor has spread to organs other than the lungs; or

- The level of any one of the tumor markers is high.

There is no poor prognosis grouping for seminoma testicular tumors.

Surgery

Surgery to remove the testicle (radical inguinal orchiectomy) and some of the lymph nodes may be done at diagnosis and staging. Tumors that have spread to other places in the body may be partly or entirely removed by surgery.

Even if the doctor removes all the cancer that can be seen at the time of the surgery, some patients may be given chemotherapy or radiation therapy after surgery to kill any cancer cells that are left. Treatment given after the surgery, to lower the risk that the cancer will come back, is called adjuvant therapy.

Radiation Therapy

Radiation therapy is a cancer treatment that uses high-energy x-rays or other types of radiation to kill cancer cells. There are two types of radiation therapy. External radiation therapy uses a machine outside the body to send radiation toward the cancer. Internal radiation therapy uses a radioactive substance sealed in needles, seeds, wires, or catheters that are placed directly into or near the cancer. The way the radiation therapy is given depends on the type and stage of the cancer being treated.

Chemotherapy

Chemotherapy is a cancer treatment that uses drugs to stop the growth of cancer cells, either by killing the cells or by stopping the cells from dividing. When chemotherapy is taken by mouth or injected into a vein or muscle, the drugs enter the bloodstream and can reach cancer cells throughout the body (systemic chemotherapy). When chemotherapy is placed directly into the cerebrospinal fluid, an organ, or a body cavity such as the abdomen, the drugs mainly affect cancer cells in those areas (regional chemotherapy). The way the chemotherapy is given depends on the type and stage of the cancer being treated.

Clinical Trials

A treatment clinical trial is a research study meant to help improve current treatments or obtain information on new treatments for patients with cancer. When clinical trials show that a new treatment is better than the standard treatment, the new treatment may become the standard treatment. Patients may want to think about taking part in a clinical trial. Some clinical trials are open only to patients who have not started treatment.

High-dose chemotherapy with stem cell transplant is being studied in clinical trials. High-dose chemotherapy with stem cell transplant is a method of giving high doses of chemotherapy and replacing blood-forming cells destroyed by the cancer treatment. Stem cells (immature blood cells) are removed from the blood or bone marrow of the patient or a donor and are frozen and stored. After the chemotherapy is completed, the stored stem cells are thawed and given back to the patient through an infusion. These reinfused stem cells grow into (and restore) the body's blood cells.

Other new treatment may also be being studied. Information about clinical trials is available from the National Cancer Institute website (www.cancer.gov).

Follow-Up Tests

Some of the tests that were done to diagnose the cancer or to find out the stage of the cancer may be repeated. Some tests will be repeated in order to see how well the treatment is working. Decisions about whether to continue, change, or stop treatment may be based on the results of these tests. This is sometimes called re-staging.

Some of the tests will continue to be done from time to time after treatment has ended. The results of these tests can show if your condition has changed or if the cancer has recurred (come back). These tests are sometimes called follow-up tests or check-ups.

Men who have had testicular cancer have an increased risk of developing cancer in the other testicle. A patient is advised to regularly check the other testicle and report any unusual symptoms to a doctor right away.

Lifelong clinical exams are very important. The patient will probably have check-ups once per month during the first year after surgery, every other month during the next year, and less often after that.

Chapter 44

Leukemia

Basic Information about Leukemia

Leukemia is cancer that starts in the tissue that forms blood. To understand cancer, it helps to know how normal blood cells form.

Normal Blood Cells

Most blood cells develop from cells in the bone marrow called stem cells. Bone marrow is the soft material in the center of most bones. Stem cells mature into different kinds of blood cells. Each kind has a special job:

- White blood cells help fight infection. There are several types of white blood cells.

- Red blood cells carry oxygen to tissues throughout the body.

- Platelets help form blood clots that control bleeding.

White blood cells, red blood cells, and platelets are made from stem cells as the body needs them. When cells grow old or get damaged, they die, and new cells take their place.

First, a stem cell matures into either a myeloid stem cell or a lymphoid stem cell:

Excerpted from "What You Need to Know about Leukemia," National Cancer Institute (www.cancer.gov), November 25, 2008.

- A myeloid stem cell matures into a myeloid blast. The blast can form a red blood cell, platelets, or one of several types of white blood cells.

- A lymphoid stem cell matures into a lymphoid blast. The blast can form one of several types of white blood cells, such as B cells or T cells.

The white blood cells that form from myeloid blasts are different from the white blood cells that form from lymphoid blasts.

Most blood cells mature in the bone marrow and then move into the blood vessels. Blood flowing through the blood vessels and heart is called the peripheral blood.

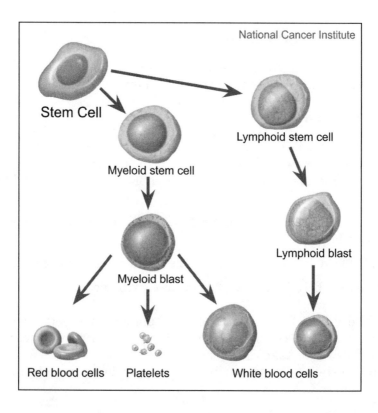

Figure 44.1. Blood Cells Maturing from Stem Cells (image by Alan Hoofring, National Cancer Institute)

Leukemia Cells

In a person with leukemia, the bone marrow makes abnormal white blood cells. The abnormal cells are leukemia cells. Unlike normal blood cells, leukemia cells don't die when they should. They may crowd out normal white blood cells, red blood cells, and platelets. This makes it hard for normal blood cells to do their work.

Types of Leukemia

The types of leukemia can be grouped based on how quickly the disease develops and gets worse. Leukemia is either chronic (which usually gets worse slowly) or acute (which usually gets worse quickly):

- **Chronic leukemia:** Early in the disease, the leukemia cells can still do some of the work of normal white blood cells. People may not have any symptoms at first. Doctors often find chronic leukemia during a routine checkup—before there are any symptoms. Slowly, chronic leukemia gets worse. As the number of leukemia cells in the blood increases, people get symptoms, such as swollen lymph nodes or infections. When symptoms do appear, they are usually mild at first and get worse gradually.

- **Acute leukemia:** The leukemia cells can't do any of the work of normal white blood cells. The number of leukemia cells increases rapidly. Acute leukemia usually worsens quickly.

The types of leukemia also can be grouped based on the type of white blood cell that is affected. Leukemia can start in lymphoid cells or myeloid cells. Leukemia that affects lymphoid cells is called lymphoid, lymphocytic, or lymphoblastic leukemia. Leukemia that affects myeloid cells is called myeloid, myelogenous, or myeloblastic leukemia. There are four common types of leukemia:

- **Chronic lymphocytic leukemia (CLL):** CLL affects lymphoid cells and usually grows slowly. It accounts for more than 15,000 new cases of leukemia each year. Most often, people diagnosed with the disease are over age 55. It almost never affects children.

- **Chronic myeloid leukemia (CML):** CML affects myeloid cells and usually grows slowly at first. It accounts for nearly 5,000 new cases of leukemia each year. It mainly affects adults.

- **Acute lymphocytic (lymphoblastic) leukemia (ALL):** ALL affects lymphoid cells and grows quickly. It accounts for more

587

than 5,000 new cases of leukemia each year. ALL is the most common type of leukemia in young children. It also affects adults.

- **Acute myeloid leukemia (AML):** AML affects myeloid cells and grows quickly. It accounts for more than 13,000 new cases of leukemia each year. It occurs in both adults and children.

Hairy cell leukemia is a rare type of chronic leukemia. This chapter is not about hairy cell leukemia or other rare types of leukemia. Together, these rare leukemias account for fewer than 6,000 new cases of leukemia each year. The National Cancer Institute's Cancer Information Service (800-4-CANCER) can provide information about rare types of leukemia.

Leukemia Risk Factors

When you're told that you have cancer, it's natural to wonder what may have caused the disease. No one knows the exact causes of leukemia. Doctors seldom know why one person gets leukemia and another doesn't. However, research shows that certain risk factors increase the chance that a person will get this disease, and the risk factors may be different for the different types of leukemia:

- **Radiation:** People exposed to very high levels of radiation are much more likely than others to get acute myeloid leukemia, chronic myeloid leukemia, or acute lymphocytic leukemia.

  - **Atomic bomb explosions:** Very high levels of radiation have been caused by atomic bomb explosions (such as those in Japan during World War II). People, especially children, who survive atomic bomb explosions are at increased risk of leukemia.

  - **Radiation therapy:** Another source of exposure to high levels of radiation is medical treatment for cancer and other conditions. Radiation therapy can increase the risk of leukemia.

  - **Diagnostic x-rays:** Dental x-rays and other diagnostic x-rays (such as CT scans) expose people to much lower levels of radiation. It's not known yet whether this low level of radiation to children or adults is linked to leukemia. Researchers are studying whether having many x-rays may increase the risk of leukemia. They are also studying whether CT scans during childhood are linked with increased risk of developing leukemia.

- **Smoking:** Smoking cigarettes increases the risk of acute myeloid leukemia.

- **Benzene:** Exposure to benzene in the workplace can cause acute myeloid leukemia. It may also cause chronic myeloid leukemia or acute lymphocytic leukemia. Benzene is used widely in the chemical industry. It's also found in cigarette smoke and gasoline.

- **Chemotherapy:** Cancer patients treated with certain types of cancer-fighting drugs sometimes later get acute myeloid leukemia or acute lymphocytic leukemia. For example, being treated with drugs known as alkylating agents or topoisomerase inhibitors is linked with a small chance of later developing acute leukemia.

- **Down syndrome and certain other inherited diseases:** Down syndrome and certain other inherited diseases increase the risk of developing acute leukemia.

- **Myelodysplastic syndrome and certain other blood disorders:** People with certain blood disorders are at increased risk of acute myeloid leukemia.

- **Human T-cell leukemia virus type I (HTLV-I):** People with HTLV-I infection are at increased risk of a rare type of leukemia known as adult T-cell leukemia. Although the HTLV-I virus may cause this rare disease, adult T-cell leukemia and other types of leukemia are not contagious.

- **Family history of leukemia:** It's rare for more than one person in a family to have leukemia. When it does happen, it's most likely to involve chronic lymphocytic leukemia. However, only a few people with chronic lymphocytic leukemia have a father, mother, brother, sister, or child who also has the disease.

Having one or more risk factors does not mean that a person will get leukemia. Most people who have risk factors never develop the disease.

Symptoms

Like all blood cells, leukemia cells travel through the body. The symptoms of leukemia depend on the number of leukemia cells and where these cells collect in the body.

People with chronic leukemia may not have symptoms. The doctor may find the disease during a routine blood test.

People with acute leukemia usually go to their doctor because they feel sick. If the brain is affected, they may have headaches, vomiting, confusion, loss of muscle control, or seizures. Leukemia also can affect other parts of the body such as the digestive tract, kidneys, lungs, heart, or testes.

Common symptoms of chronic or acute leukemia may include:

- Swollen lymph nodes that usually don't hurt (especially lymph nodes in the neck or armpit)
- Fevers or night sweats
- Frequent infections
- Feeling weak or tired
- Bleeding and bruising easily (bleeding gums, purplish patches in the skin, or tiny red spots under the skin)
- Swelling or discomfort in the abdomen (from a swollen spleen or liver)
- Weight loss for no known reason
- Pain in the bones or joints

Most often, these symptoms are not due to cancer. An infection or other health problems may also cause these symptoms. Only a doctor can tell for sure. Anyone with these symptoms should tell the doctor so that problems can be diagnosed and treated as early as possible.

Diagnosis

Doctors sometimes find leukemia after a routine blood test. If you have symptoms that suggest leukemia, your doctor will try to find out what's causing the problems. Your doctor may ask about your personal and family medical history. You may have one or more of the following tests:

- **Physical exam:** Your doctor checks for swollen lymph nodes, spleen, or liver.
- **Blood tests:** The lab does a complete blood count to check the number of white blood cells, red blood cells, and platelets. Leukemia causes a very high level of white blood cells. It may also cause low levels of platelets and hemoglobin, which is found inside red blood cells.

- **Biopsy:** Your doctor removes tissue to look for cancer cells. A biopsy is the only sure way to know whether leukemia cells are in your bone marrow. Before the sample is taken, local anesthesia is used to numb the area. This helps reduce the pain. Your doctor removes some bone marrow from your hipbone or another large bone. A pathologist uses a microscope to check the tissue for leukemia cells.

There are two ways your doctor can obtain bone marrow. Some people will have both procedures during the same visit:

- **Bone marrow aspiration:** The doctor uses a thick, hollow needle to remove samples of bone marrow.

- **Bone marrow biopsy:** The doctor uses a very thick, hollow needle to remove a small piece of bone and bone marrow.

The tests that your doctor orders for you depend on your symptoms and type of leukemia. You may have other tests:

- **Cytogenetics:** The lab looks at the chromosomes of cells from samples of blood, bone marrow, or lymph nodes. If abnormal chromosomes are found, the test can show what type of leukemia you have. For example, people with CML have an abnormal chromosome called the Philadelphia chromosome.

- **Spinal tap:** Your doctor may remove some of the cerebrospinal fluid (the fluid that fills the spaces in and around the brain and spinal cord). The doctor uses a long, thin needle to remove fluid from the lower spine. The procedure takes about 30 minutes and is performed with local anesthesia. You must lie flat for several hours afterward to keep from getting a headache. The lab checks the fluid for leukemia cells or other signs of problems.

- **Chest x-ray:** An x-ray can show swollen lymph nodes or other signs of disease in your chest.

Treatment Options

People with leukemia have many treatment options. The options are watchful waiting, chemotherapy, targeted therapy, biological therapy, radiation therapy, and stem cell transplant. If your spleen is enlarged, your doctor may suggest surgery to remove it. Sometimes a combination of these treatments is used. The choice of treatment depends mainly on the type of leukemia (acute or chronic), your age, and whether leukemia cells were found in your cerebrospinal fluid. It also may depend on certain features of the leukemia cells. Your doctor also considers your symptoms and general health.

People with acute leukemia need to be treated right away. The goal of treatment is to destroy signs of leukemia in the body and make symptoms go away. This is called a remission. After people go into remission, more therapy may be given to prevent a relapse. This type of therapy is called consolidation therapy or maintenance therapy. Many people with acute leukemia can be cured.

If you have chronic leukemia without symptoms, you may not need cancer treatment right away. Your doctor will watch your health closely so that treatment can start when you begin to have symptoms. Not getting cancer treatment right away is called watchful waiting.

When treatment for chronic leukemia is needed, it can often control the disease and its symptoms. People may receive maintenance therapy to help keep the cancer in remission, but chronic leukemia can seldom be cured with chemotherapy. However, stem cell transplants offer some people with chronic leukemia the chance for cure.

Your doctor can describe your treatment choices, the expected results, and the possible side effects. You and your doctor can work together to develop a treatment plan that meets your medical and personal needs. You may want to talk with your doctor about taking part in a clinical trial, a research study of new treatment methods.

Your doctor may refer you to a specialist, or you may ask for a referral. Specialists who treat leukemia include hematologists, medical oncologists, and radiation oncologists. Pediatric oncologists and hematologists treat childhood leukemia. Your health care team may also include an oncology nurse and a registered dietitian.

Whenever possible, people should be treated at a medical center that has doctors experienced in treating leukemia. If this isn't possible, your doctor may discuss the treatment plan with a specialist at such a center.

Before treatment starts, ask your health care team to explain possible side effects and how treatment may change your normal activities. Because cancer treatments often damage healthy cells and tissues, side effects are common. Side effects may not be the same for each person, and they may change from one treatment session to the next.

Watchful Waiting

People with chronic lymphocytic leukemia who do not have symptoms may be able to put off having cancer treatment. By delaying treatment, they can avoid the side effects of treatment until they have symptoms.

If you and your doctor agree that watchful waiting is a good idea, you'll have regular checkups (such as every three months). You can start treatment if symptoms occur.

Although watchful waiting avoids or delays the side effects of cancer treatment, this choice has risks. It may reduce the chance to control leukemia before it gets worse.

You may decide against watchful waiting if you don't want to live with an untreated leukemia. Some people choose to treat the cancer right away.

If you choose watchful waiting but grow concerned later, you should discuss your feelings with your doctor. A different approach is nearly always available.

Chemotherapy

Many people with leukemia are treated with chemotherapy. Chemotherapy uses drugs to destroy leukemia cells. Depending on the type of leukemia, you may receive a single drug or a combination of two or more drugs. You may receive chemotherapy in several different ways:

- **By mouth:** Some drugs are pills that you can swallow.

- **Into a vein (IV):** The drug is given through a needle or tube inserted into a vein.

- **Through a catheter (a thin, flexible tube):** The tube is placed in a large vein, often in the upper chest. A tube that stays in place is useful for patients who need many IV treatments. The health care professional injects drugs into the catheter, rather than directly into a vein. This method avoids the need for many injections, which can cause discomfort and injure the veins and skin.

- **Into the cerebrospinal fluid:** If the pathologist finds leukemia cells in the fluid that fills the spaces in and around the brain and spinal cord, the doctor may order intrathecal chemotherapy. The doctor injects drugs directly into the cerebrospinal fluid. Intrathecal chemotherapy is given in two ways: Into the spinal fluid—the doctor injects the drugs into the spinal fluid; and, under the scalp—children and some adult patients receive chemotherapy through a special catheter called an Ommaya reservoir. The doctor places the catheter under the scalp. The doctor injects the drugs into the catheter. This method avoids the pain of injections into the spinal fluid. Intrathecal chemotherapy is used because many drugs given by IV or taken by mouth can't pass through the tightly packed blood vessel walls found in the brain and spinal cord. This network of blood vessels is known as the blood-brain barrier.

Chemotherapy is usually given in cycles. Each cycle has a treatment period followed by a rest period. You may have your treatment in a clinic, at the doctor's office, or at home. Some people may need to stay in the hospital for treatment.

The side effects depend mainly on which drugs are given and how much. Chemotherapy kills fast-growing leukemia cells, but the drug can also harm normal cells that divide rapidly:

- **Blood cells:** When chemotherapy lowers the levels of healthy blood cells, you're more likely to get infections, bruise or bleed easily, and feel very weak and tired. You'll get blood tests to check for low levels of blood cells. If your levels are low, your health care team may stop the chemotherapy for a while or reduce the dose of drug. There also are medicines that can help your body make new blood cells. Or, you may need a blood transfusion.

- **Cells in hair roots:** Chemotherapy may cause hair loss. If you lose your hair, it will grow back, but it may be somewhat different in color and texture.

- **Cells that line the digestive tract:** Chemotherapy can cause poor appetite, nausea and vomiting, diarrhea, or mouth and lip sores. Ask your health care team about medicines and other ways to help you cope with these problems.

- **Sperm or egg cells:** Some types of chemotherapy can cause infertility. Most children treated for leukemia appear to have normal fertility when they grow up. However, depending on the drugs and doses used and the age of the patient, some boys and girls may be infertile as adults. Among adult men, chemotherapy may damage sperm cells. Men may stop making sperm. Because these changes to sperm may be permanent, some men have their sperm frozen and stored before treatment (sperm banking). Among adult women, chemotherapy may damage the ovaries. Women may have irregular menstrual periods or periods may stop altogether. Women may have symptoms of menopause, such as hot flashes and vaginal dryness. Women who may want to get pregnant in the future should ask their health care team about ways to preserve their eggs before treatment starts.

Targeted Therapy

People with chronic myeloid leukemia and some with acute lymphoblastic leukemia may receive drugs called targeted therapy. Imatinib (Gleevec) tablets were the first targeted therapy approved for chronic myeloid leukemia. Other targeted therapy drugs are now used too.

Targeted therapies use drugs that block the growth of leukemia cells. For example, a targeted therapy may block the action of an abnormal protein that stimulates the growth of leukemia cells.

Side effects include swelling, bloating, and sudden weight gain. Targeted therapy can also cause anemia, nausea, vomiting, diarrhea, muscle cramps, or a rash. Your health care team will monitor you for signs of problems.

Biological Therapy

Some people with leukemia receive drugs called biological therapy. Biological therapy for leukemia is treatment that improves the body's natural defenses against the disease.

One type of biological therapy is a substance called a monoclonal antibody. It's given by IV infusion. This substance binds to the leukemia cells. One kind of monoclonal antibody carries a toxin that kills the leukemia cells. Another kind helps the immune system destroy leukemia cells.

For some people with chronic myeloid leukemia, the biological therapy is a drug called interferon. It is injected under the skin or into a muscle. It can slow the growth of leukemia cells.

You may have your treatment in a clinic, at the doctor's office, or in the hospital. Other drugs may be given at the same time to prevent side effects.

The side effects of biological therapy differ with the types of substances used, and from person to person. Biological therapies commonly cause a rash or swelling where the drug is injected. They also may cause a headache, muscle aches, a fever, or weakness. Your health care team may check your blood for signs of anemia and other problems.

Radiation Therapy

Radiation therapy (also called radiotherapy) uses high-energy rays to kill leukemia cells. People receive radiation therapy at a hospital or clinic.

Some people receive radiation from a large machine that is aimed at the spleen, the brain, or other parts of the body where leukemia cells have collected. This type of therapy takes place five days a week for several weeks. Others may receive radiation that is directed to the whole body. The radiation treatments are given once or twice a day for a few days, usually before a stem cell transplant.

The side effects of radiation therapy depend mainly on the dose of radiation and the part of the body that is treated. For example, radiation to your abdomen can cause nausea, vomiting, and diarrhea. In addition, your skin in the area being treated may become red, dry, and tender. You also may lose your hair in the treated area.

You are likely to be very tired during radiation therapy, especially after several weeks of treatment. Resting is important, but doctors usually advise patients to try to stay as active as they can.

Although the side effects of radiation therapy can be distressing, they can usually be treated or controlled. You can talk with your doctor about ways to ease these problems.

It may also help to know that, in most cases, the side effects are not permanent. However, you may want to discuss with your doctor the possible long-term effects of radiation treatment.

Stem Cell Transplant

Some people with leukemia receive a stem cell transplant. A stem cell transplant allows you to be treated with high doses of drugs, radiation, or both. The high doses destroy both leukemia cells and normal blood cells in the bone marrow. After you receive high-dose chemotherapy, radiation therapy, or both, you receive healthy stem cells through a large vein. (It's like getting a blood transfusion.) New blood cells develop from the transplanted stem cells. The new blood cells replace the ones that were destroyed by treatment.

Stem cell transplants take place in the hospital. Stem cells may come from you or from someone who donates their stem cells to you:

- **From you:** An autologous stem cell transplant uses your own stem cells. Before you get the high-dose chemotherapy or radiation therapy, your stem cells are removed. The cells may be treated to kill any leukemia cells present. Your stem cells are frozen and stored. After you receive high-dose chemotherapy or radiation therapy, the stored stem cells are thawed and returned to you.

- **From a family member or other donor:** An allogeneic stem cell transplant uses healthy stem cells from a donor. Your brother, sister, or parent may be the donor. Sometimes the stem cells come from a donor who isn't related. Doctors use blood tests to learn how closely a donor's cells match your cells.

- **From your identical twin:** If you have an identical twin, a syngeneic stem cell transplant uses stem cells from your healthy twin.

Stem cells come from a few sources. The stem cells usually come from the blood (peripheral stem cell transplant). Or they can come from the bone marrow (bone marrow transplant). Another source of stem cells is umbilical cord blood. Cord blood is taken from a newborn baby and stored in a freezer. When a person gets cord blood, it's called an umbilical cord blood transplant.

After a stem cell transplant, you may stay in the hospital for several weeks or months. You'll be at risk for infections and bleeding because of the large doses of chemotherapy or radiation you received. In time, the transplanted stem cells will begin to produce healthy blood cells.

Another problem is that graft-versus-host disease (GVHD) may occur in people who receive donated stem cells. In GVHD, the donated white blood cells in the stem cell graft react against the patient's normal tissues. Most often, the liver, skin, or digestive tract is affected. GVHD can be mild or very severe. It can occur any time after the transplant, even years later. Steroids or other drugs may help.

Second Opinion

Before starting treatment, you might want a second opinion about your diagnosis and treatment plan. Some people worry that the doctor will be offended if they ask for a second opinion. Usually the opposite is true. Most doctors welcome a second opinion. And many health insurance companies will pay for a second opinion if you or your doctor requests it.

If you get a second opinion, the doctor may agree with your first doctor's diagnosis and treatment plan. Or the second doctor may suggest another approach. Either way, you have more information and perhaps a greater sense of control. You can feel more confident about the decisions you make, knowing that you've looked at your options.

It may take some time and effort to gather your medical records and see another doctor. In most cases, it's not a problem to take several weeks to get a second opinion. The delay in starting treatment usually won't make treatment less effective. To make sure, you should discuss this delay with your doctor. Some people with leukemia need treatment right away.

There are many ways to find a doctor for a second opinion. You can ask your doctor, a local or state medical society, a nearby hospital, or a medical school for names of specialists. The National Cancer Institute's Cancer Information Service at 800-4-CANCER can tell you about nearby treatment centers.

Nonprofit groups with an interest in leukemia may be of help. Many such groups are listed in end section of this book.

Supportive Care

Leukemia and its treatment can lead to other health problems. You can have supportive care before, during, or after cancer treatment.

Supportive care is treatment to prevent or fight infections, to control pain and other symptoms, to relieve the side effects of therapy, and to help you cope with the feelings that a diagnosis of cancer can bring. You may receive supportive care to prevent or control these problems and to improve your comfort and quality of life during treatment.

- **Infections:** Because people with leukemia get infections very easily, you may receive antibiotics and other drugs. Some people receive vaccines against the flu and pneumonia. The health care team may advise you to stay away from crowds and from people with colds and other contagious diseases. If an infection develops, it can be serious and should be treated promptly. You may need to stay in the hospital for treatment.

- **Anemia and bleeding:** Anemia and bleeding are other problems that often require supportive care. You may need a transfusion of red blood cells or platelets. Transfusions help treat anemia and reduce the risk of serious bleeding.

- **Dental problems:** Leukemia and chemotherapy can make the mouth sensitive, easily infected, and likely to bleed. Doctors often advise patients to have a complete dental exam and, if possible, undergo needed dental care before chemotherapy begins. Dentists show patients how to keep their mouth clean and healthy during treatment.

Follow-Up Care

You'll need regular checkups after treatment for leukemia. Checkups help ensure that any changes in your health are noted and treated if needed. If you have any health problems between checkups, you should contact your doctor.

Your doctor will check for return of the cancer. Even when the cancer seems to be completely destroyed, the disease sometimes returns because undetected leukemia cells remained somewhere in your body after treatment. Also, checkups help detect health problems that can result from cancer treatment.

Checkups may include a careful physical exam, blood tests, cytogenetics, x-rays, bone marrow aspiration, or spinal tap.

Chapter 45

Lymphoma

Chapter Contents

Section 45.1

Hodgkin Lymphoma

Excerpted from "What You Need to Know about Hodgkin Lymphoma,"
National Cancer Institute (www.cancer.gov), February 5, 2008.

Basic Facts about Hodgkin Lymphoma

Hodgkin lymphoma is a cancer that begins in cells of the immune system. The immune system fights infections and other diseases. The lymphatic system is part of the immune system. The lymphatic system includes the following:

- **Lymph vessels:** The lymphatic system has a network of lymph vessels. Lymph vessels branch into all the tissues of the body.

- **Lymph:** The lymph vessels carry clear fluid called lymph. Lymph contains white blood cells, especially lymphocytes such as B cells and T cells.

- **Lymph nodes:** Lymph vessels are connected to small, round masses of tissue called lymph nodes. Groups of lymph nodes are found in the neck, underarms, chest, abdomen, and groin. Lymph nodes store white blood cells. They trap and remove bacteria or other harmful substances that may be in the lymph.

- **Other parts of the lymphatic system:** Other parts of the lymphatic system include the tonsils, thymus, and spleen. Lymphatic tissue is also found in other parts of the body including the stomach, skin, and small intestine.

Because lymphatic tissue is in many parts of the body, Hodgkin lymphoma can start almost anywhere. Usually, it's first found in a lymph node above the diaphragm, the thin muscle that separates the chest from the abdomen. But Hodgkin lymphoma also may be found in a group of lymph nodes. Sometimes it starts in other parts of the lymphatic system.

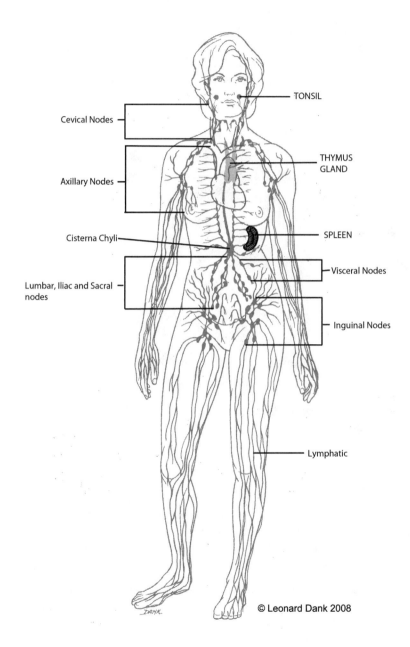

Figure 45.1. *Components of the Lymphatic System (image by Leonard Dank)*

Hodgkin Lymphoma Cells

Hodgkin lymphoma begins when a lymphocyte (usually a B cell) becomes abnormal. The abnormal cell is called a Reed-Sternberg cell. Reed-Sternberg cells are much larger than normal cells and they divide to make copies of themselves. The new cells divide again and again, making more and more abnormal cells. The abnormal cells don't die when they should. They don't protect the body from infections or other diseases. The buildup of extra cells often forms a mass of tissue called a growth or tumor.

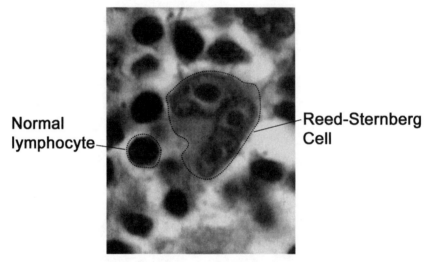

Figure 45.2. Reed-Sternberg Cell (National Cancer Institute, AV No. CDR576466)

Risk Factors

Doctors seldom know why one person develops Hodgkin lymphoma and another does not. But research shows that certain risk factors increase the chance that a person will develop this disease. The risk factors for Hodgkin lymphoma include the following:

- **Certain viruses:** Having an infection with the Epstein-Barr virus (EBV) or the human immunodeficiency virus (HIV) may increase the risk of developing Hodgkin lymphoma. However, lymphoma is not contagious. You can't catch lymphoma from another person.

- **Weakened immune system:** The risk of developing Hodgkin lymphoma may be increased by having a weakened immune system (such as from an inherited condition or certain drugs used after an organ transplant).

- **Age:** Hodgkin lymphoma is most common among teens and adults aged 15 to 35 years and adults aged 55 years and older.

- **Family history:** Family members, especially brothers and sisters, of a person with Hodgkin lymphoma or other lymphomas may have an increased chance of developing this disease.

Having one or more risk factors does not mean that a person will develop Hodgkin lymphoma. Most people who have risk factors never develop cancer.

Symptoms

Hodgkin lymphoma can cause many symptoms:

- Swollen lymph nodes (that do not hurt) in the neck, underarms, or groin
- Becoming more sensitive to the effects of alcohol or having painful lymph nodes after drinking alcohol
- Weight loss for no known reason
- Fever that does not go away
- Soaking night sweats
- Itchy skin
- Coughing, trouble breathing, or chest pain
- Weakness and tiredness that don't go away

Most often, these symptoms are not due to cancer. Infections or other health problems may also cause these symptoms. Anyone with symptoms that last more than two weeks should see a doctor so that problems can be diagnosed and treated.

Diagnosis

If you have swollen lymph nodes or another symptom that suggests Hodgkin lymphoma, your doctor will try to find out what's causing the problem. Your doctor may ask about your personal and family medical history. You may have some of the following exams and tests:

- **Physical exam:** Your doctor checks for swollen lymph nodes in your neck, underarms, and groin. Your doctor also checks for a swollen spleen or liver.

- **Blood tests:** The lab does a complete blood count to check the number of white blood cells and other cells and substances.

- **Chest x-rays:** X-ray pictures may show swollen lymph nodes or other signs of disease in your chest.

- **Biopsy:** A biopsy is the only sure way to diagnose Hodgkin lymphoma. Your doctor may remove an entire lymph node (excisional biopsy) or only part of a lymph node (incisional biopsy). A thin needle (fine needle aspiration) usually cannot remove a large enough sample for the pathologist to diagnose Hodgkin lymphoma. Removing an entire lymph node is best. The pathologist uses a microscope to check the tissue for Hodgkin lymphoma cells. A person with Hodgkin lymphoma usually has large, abnormal cells known as Reed-Sternberg cells. They are not found in people with non-Hodgkin lymphoma.

Types of Hodgkin Lymphoma

When Hodgkin lymphoma is found, the pathologist reports the type. There are two major types of Hodgkin lymphoma:

- **Classical Hodgkin lymphoma:** Most people with Hodgkin lymphoma have the classical type.

- **Nodular lymphocyte-predominant Hodgkin lymphoma:** This is a rare type of Hodgkin lymphoma. The abnormal cell is called a popcorn cell. It may be treated differently from the classical type.

Staging Hodgkin Lymphoma

Your doctor needs to know the extent (stage) of Hodgkin lymphoma to plan the best treatment. Staging is a careful attempt to find out what parts of the body are affected by the disease.

Hodgkin lymphoma tends to spread from one group of lymph nodes to the next group. For example, Hodgkin lymphoma that starts in the lymph nodes in the neck may spread first to the lymph nodes above the collarbones, and then to the lymph nodes under the arms and within the chest.

In time, the Hodgkin lymphoma cells can invade blood vessels and spread to almost any other part of the body. For example, it can spread to the liver, lungs, bone, and bone marrow.

Staging may involve one or more of the following tests:

- **CT scan:** An x-ray machine linked to a computer takes a series of detailed pictures of your chest, abdomen, and pelvis. You may receive an injection of contrast material. Also, you may be asked to drink another type of contrast material. The contrast material makes it easier for the doctor to see swollen lymph nodes and other abnormal areas on the x-ray.

- **MRI:** A powerful magnet linked to a computer is used to make detailed pictures of your bones, brain, or other tissues. Your doctor can view these pictures on a monitor and can print them on film.

- **PET scan:** You receive an injection of a small amount of radioactive sugar. A machine makes computerized pictures of the sugar being used by cells in your body. Lymphoma cells use sugar faster than normal cells, and areas with lymphoma look brighter on the pictures.

- **Bone marrow biopsy:** The doctor uses a thick needle to remove a small sample of bone and bone marrow from your hipbone or another large bone. Local anesthesia can help control pain. A pathologist looks for Hodgkin lymphoma cells in the sample.

Other staging procedures may include biopsies of other lymph nodes, the liver, or other tissue.

The doctor considers the following to determine the stage of Hodgkin lymphoma:

- The number of lymph nodes that have Hodgkin lymphoma cells

- Whether these lymph nodes are on one or both sides of the diaphragm

- Whether the disease has spread to the bone marrow, spleen, liver, or lung.

The stages of Hodgkin lymphoma are as follows:

- **Stage I:** The lymphoma cells are in one lymph node group (such as in the neck or underarm). Or, if the lymphoma cells are not in the lymph nodes, they are in only one part of a tissue or an organ (such as the lung).

- **Stage II:** The lymphoma cells are in at least two lymph node groups on the same side of (either above or below) the diaphragm. Or, the lymphoma cells are in one part of a tissue or an organ and the lymph nodes near that organ (on the same side of the diaphragm). There may be lymphoma cells in other lymph node groups on the same side of the diaphragm.

- **Stage III:** The lymphoma cells are in lymph nodes above and below the diaphragm. Lymphoma also may be found in one part of a tissue or an organ (such as the liver, lung, or bone) near these lymph node groups. It may also be found in the spleen.

- **Stage IV:** Lymphoma cells are found in several parts of one or more organs or tissues. Or, the lymphoma is in an organ (such as the liver, lung, or bone) and in distant lymph nodes.

- **Recurrent:** The disease returns after treatment.

In addition to these stage numbers, your doctor may also describe the stage as A or B:

- **A:** You have not had weight loss, drenching night sweats, or fevers.
- **B:** You have had weight loss, drenching night sweats, or fevers.

Treatment Options

Your doctor can describe your treatment choices and the expected results. You and your doctor can work together to develop a treatment plan that meets your needs.

Your doctor may refer you to a specialist, or you may ask for a referral. Specialists who treat Hodgkin lymphoma include hematologists, medical oncologists, and radiation oncologists. Your doctor may suggest that you choose an oncologist who specializes in the treatment of Hodgkin lymphoma. Often, such doctors are associated with major academic centers. Your health care team may also include an oncology nurse and a registered dietitian.

The choice of treatment depends mainly on the following the type of your Hodgkin lymphoma (most people have classical Hodgkin lymphoma), its stage (where the lymphoma is found), whether you have a tumor that is more than four inches (10 centimeters) wide, your age, and whether you've had weight loss, drenching night sweats, or fevers. People with Hodgkin lymphoma may be treated with chemotherapy, radiation therapy, or both.

If Hodgkin lymphoma comes back after treatment, doctors call this a relapse or recurrence. People with Hodgkin lymphoma that comes back after treatment may receive high doses of chemotherapy, radiation therapy, or both, followed by stem cell transplantation.

You may want to know about side effects and how treatment may change your normal activities. Because chemotherapy and radiation therapy often damage healthy cells and tissues, side effects are common. Side effects may not be the same for each person, and they may change from one treatment session to the next. Before treatment starts, your health care team will explain possible side effects and suggest ways to help you manage them. The younger a person is, the easier it may be to cope with treatment and its side effects.

At any stage of the disease, you can have supportive care. Supportive care is treatment to prevent or fight infections, to control pain and other symptoms, to relieve the side effects of therapy, and to help you cope with the feelings that a diagnosis of cancer can bring. You may want to talk to your doctor about taking part in a clinical trial, a research study of new treatment methods.

Chemotherapy

Chemotherapy for Hodgkin lymphoma uses drugs to kill lymphoma cells. It is called systemic therapy because the drugs travel through the bloodstream. The drugs can reach lymphoma cells in almost all parts of the body.

Usually, more than one drug is given. Most drugs for Hodgkin lymphoma are given through a vein (intravenous), but some are taken by mouth.

Chemotherapy is given in cycles. You have a treatment period followed by a rest period. The length of the rest period and the number of treatment cycles depend on the stage of your disease and on the anticancer drugs used.

You may have your treatment in a clinic, at the doctor's office, or at home. Some people may need to stay in the hospital for treatment.

The side effects depend mainly on which drugs are given and how much. The drugs can harm normal cells that divide rapidly:

Blood cells: When chemotherapy lowers the levels of healthy blood cells, you are more likely to get infections, bruise or bleed easily, and feel very weak and tired. Your health care team gives you blood tests to check for low levels of blood cells. If levels are low, there are medicines that can help your body make new blood cells.

- **Cells in hair roots:** Chemotherapy may cause hair loss. If you lose your hair, it will grow back, but it may be somewhat different in color and texture.

- **Cells that line the digestive tract:** Chemotherapy can cause poor appetite, nausea and vomiting, diarrhea, or mouth and lip sores. Ask your health care team about medicines and other ways to help you cope with these problems.

- **Some types of chemotherapy can cause infertility:** In men, chemotherapy may damage sperm cells. Because these changes to sperm may be permanent, some men have their sperm frozen and stored before treatment (sperm banking). In women, chemotherapy may damage the ovaries. Women who may want to get pregnant in the future should ask their health care team about ways to preserve their eggs before treatment starts.

Some of the drugs used for Hodgkin lymphoma may cause heart disease or cancer later on.

Radiation Therapy

Radiation therapy (also called radiotherapy) for Hodgkin lymphoma uses high-energy rays to kill lymphoma cells. It can shrink tumors and help control pain.

A large machine aims the rays at the lymph node areas affected by lymphoma. This is local therapy because it affects cells in the treated area only. Most people go to a hospital or clinic for treatment five days a week for several weeks.

The side effects of radiation therapy depend mainly on the dose of radiation and the part of the body that is treated. For example, radiation to your abdomen can cause nausea, vomiting, and diarrhea. When your chest and neck are treated, you may have a dry, sore throat and some trouble swallowing.

In addition, your skin in the area being treated may become red, dry, and tender. You also may lose your hair in the treated area.

Many people become very tired during radiation therapy, especially in the later weeks of treatment. Resting is important, but doctors usually advise people to try to stay as active as they can.

Although the side effects of radiation therapy can be distressing, they can usually be treated or controlled. You can talk with your doctor about ways to ease these problems.

It may also help to know that, in most cases, the side effects are not permanent. However, you may want to discuss with your doctor the possible long-term effects of radiation treatment. After treatment is over, you may have an increased chance of developing a second cancer. Also, radiation therapy aimed at the chest may cause heart disease or lung damage.

Radiation therapy aimed at the pelvis can cause infertility. Loss of fertility may be temporary or permanent, depending on your age. In men, if radiation therapy is aimed at the pelvic area, the testes may be harmed. Sperm banking before treatment may be a choice. In women radiation aimed at the pelvic area can harm the ovaries. Menstrual periods may stop, and women may have hot flashes and vaginal dryness. Menstrual periods are more likely to return for younger women. Women who may want to get pregnant after radiation therapy should ask their health care team about ways to preserve their eggs before treatment starts.

Stem Cell Transplantation

If Hodgkin lymphoma returns after treatment, you may receive stem cell transplantation. A transplant of your own blood-forming stem cells (autologous stem cell transplantation) allows you to receive high doses of chemotherapy, radiation therapy, or both. The high doses destroy both Hodgkin lymphoma cells and healthy blood cells in the bone marrow.

Stem cell transplants take place in the hospital. Before you receive high-dose treatment, your stem cells are removed and may be treated to kill lymphoma cells that may be present. Your stem cells are frozen and stored. After you receive high-dose treatment to kill Hodgkin lymphoma cells, your stored stem cells are thawed and given back to you through a flexible tube placed in a large vein in your neck or chest area. New blood cells develop from the transplanted stem cells.

Second Opinion

Before starting treatment, you might want a second opinion about your diagnosis and your treatment plan. Many insurance companies cover a second opinion if you or your doctor requests it.

It may take some time and effort to gather your medical records and see another doctor. In most cases, a brief delay in starting treatment will not make treatment less effective. To make sure, you should discuss this delay with your doctor. Sometimes people with Hodgkin lymphoma need treatment right away.

There are many ways to find a doctor for a second opinion. You can ask your doctor, a local or state medical society, a nearby hospital, or a medical school for names of specialists. Nonprofit groups with an interest in lymphoma may be of help. Some such groups are listed in the resources at the end of this book.

Follow-Up Care

You'll need regular checkups after treatment for Hodgkin lymphoma. Even when there are no longer any signs of cancer, the disease sometimes returns because undetected lymphoma cells may remain somewhere in your body after treatment.

Also, checkups help detect health problems that can result from cancer treatment. People treated for Hodgkin lymphoma have an increased chance of developing heart disease; leukemia; melanoma; non-Hodgkin lymphoma; and cancers of the bone, breast, lung, stomach, and thyroid. Checkups help ensure that any changes in your health are noted and treated if needed. Checkups may include a physical exam, blood tests, chest x-rays, CT scans, and other tests.

After treatment, people with Hodgkin lymphoma may receive the flu vaccine and other vaccines. You may want to talk with your health care team about when to get certain vaccines.

If you have any health problems between checkups, you should contact your doctor.

Section 45.2

Non-Hodgkin Lymphoma

Excerpted from "What You Need to Know about Non-Hodgkin Lympho-ma," National Cancer Institute (www.cancer.gov), February 12, 2008.

Basic Facts about Non-Hodgkin Lymphoma

Non-Hodgkin lymphoma is cancer that begins in cells of the immune system. The immune system fights infections and other diseases. The lymphatic system is part of the immune system. For more information about the lymphatic system, see Section 45.1.

Non-Hodgkin Lymphoma Cells

Non-Hodgkin lymphoma begins when a lymphocyte (usually a B cell) becomes abnormal. The abnormal cell divides to make copies of itself. The new cells divide again and again, making more and more abnormal cells. The abnormal cells don't die when they should. They don't protect the body from infections or other diseases. The buildup of extra cells often forms a mass of tissue called a growth or tumor.

Risk Factors

Doctors seldom know why one person develops non-Hodgkin lym-phoma and another does not. But research shows that certain risk factors increase the chance that a person will develop this disease. In general, the risk factors for non-Hodgkin lymphoma include the following:

Weakened immune system: The risk of developing lymphoma may be increased by having a weakened immune system (such as from an inherited condition or certain drugs used after an organ transplant).

Certain infections: Having certain types of infections increases the risk of developing lymphoma. However, lymphoma is not contagious. You cannot catch lymphoma from another person. The following are the main types of infection that can increase the risk of lymphoma:

- **Human immunodeficiency virus (HIV):** HIV is the virus that causes AIDS. People who have HIV infection are at much greater risk of some types of non-Hodgkin lymphoma.

- **Epstein-Barr virus (EBV):** Infection with EBV has been linked to an increased risk of lymphoma. In Africa, EBV infection is linked to Burkitt lymphoma.

- *Helicobacter pylori: H. pylori* are bacteria that can cause stomach ulcers. They also increase a person's risk of lymphoma in the stomach lining.

- **Human T-cell leukemia/lymphoma virus type 1 (HTLV-1):** Infection with HTLV-1 increases a person's risk of lymphoma and leukemia.

- **Hepatitis C virus:** Some studies have found an increased risk of lymphoma in people with hepatitis C virus. More research is needed to understand the role of hepatitis C virus.

Age: Although non-Hodgkin lymphoma can occur in young people, the chance of developing this disease goes up with age. Most people with non-Hodgkin lymphoma are older than 60.

Other Risks: Researchers are studying obesity and other possible risk factors for non-Hodgkin lymphoma. People who work with herbicides or certain other chemicals may be at increased risk of this disease. Researchers are also looking at a possible link between using hair dyes before 1980 and non-Hodgkin lymphoma.

Having one or more risk factors does not mean that a person will develop non-Hodgkin lymphoma. Most people who have risk factors never develop cancer.

Symptoms

Non-Hodgkin lymphoma can cause many symptoms:

- Swollen, painless lymph nodes in the neck, armpits, or groin
- Unexplained weight loss
- Fever
- Soaking night sweats
- Coughing, trouble breathing, or chest pain
- Weakness and tiredness that don't go away
- Pain, swelling, or a feeling of fullness in the abdomen

Most often, these symptoms are not due to cancer. Infections or other health problems may also cause these symptoms. Anyone with symptoms that do not go away within two weeks should see a doctor so that problems can be diagnosed and treated.

Diagnosis

If you have swollen lymph nodes or another symptom that suggests non-Hodgkin lymphoma, your doctor will try to find out what's causing the problem. Your doctor may ask about your personal and family medical history. You may have some of the following exams and tests:

- **Physical exam:** Your doctor checks for swollen lymph nodes in your neck, underarms, and groin. Your doctor also checks for a swollen spleen or liver.

- **Blood tests:** The lab does a complete blood count to check the number of white blood cells. The lab also checks for other cells and substances, such as lactate dehydrogenase (LDH). Lymphoma may cause a high level of LDH.

- **Chest x-rays:** You may have x-rays to check for swollen lymph nodes or other signs of disease in your chest.

- **Biopsy:** A biopsy is the only sure way to diagnose lymphoma. Your doctor may remove an entire lymph node (excisional biopsy) or only part of a lymph node (incisional biopsy). A thin needle (fine needle aspiration) usually cannot remove a large enough sample for the pathologist to diagnose lymphoma. Removing an entire lymph node is best. The pathologist uses a microscope to check the tissue for lymphoma cells.

Types of Non-Hodgkin Lymphoma

When lymphoma is found, the pathologist reports the type. There are many types of lymphoma. The most common types are diffuse large B-cell lymphoma and follicular lymphoma. Lymphomas may be grouped by how quickly they are likely to grow:

- **Indolent** (also called low-grade) lymphomas grow slowly. They tend to cause few symptoms.

- **Aggressive** (also called intermediate-grade and high-grade) lymphomas grow and spread more quickly. They tend to cause severe symptoms. Over time, many indolent lymphomas become aggressive lymphomas.

It's a good idea to get a second opinion about the type of lymphoma that you have. The treatment plan varies by the type of lymphoma. A pathologist at a major referral center can review your biopsy.

Staging Lymphoma

Your doctor needs to know the extent (stage) of non-Hodgkin lymphoma to plan the best treatment. Staging is a careful attempt to find out what parts of the body are affected by the disease. Lymphoma usually starts in a lymph node. It can spread to nearly any other part of the body. For example, it can spread to the liver, lungs, bone, and bone marrow. Some of the staging tests for non-Hodgkin lymphoma are the same as those for Hodgkin lymphoma (see Section 45.1). Additional staging procedures for non-Hodgkin lymphoma may also involve one or more of the following tests:

- **Ultrasound:** An ultrasound device sends out sound waves that you cannot hear. A small hand-held device is held against your body. The waves bounce off nearby tissues, and a computer uses the echoes to create a picture. Tumors may produce echoes that are different from the echoes made by healthy tissues. The picture can show possible tumors.

- **Spinal tap:** The doctor uses a long, thin needle to remove fluid from the spinal column. Local anesthesia can help control pain. You must lie flat for a few hours afterward so that you don't get a headache. The lab checks the fluid for lymphoma cells or other problems.

The stage is based on where lymphoma cells are found (in the lymph nodes or in other organs or tissues). The stage also depends on how many areas are affected. The stages of non-Hodgkin lymphoma are as follows:

- **Stage I:** The lymphoma cells are in one lymph node group (such as in the neck or underarm). Or, if the abnormal cells are not in the lymph nodes, they are in only one part of a tissue or organ (such as the lung, but not the liver or bone marrow).

- **Stage II:** The lymphoma cells are in at least two lymph node groups on the same side of (either above or below) the diaphragm. Or, the lymphoma cells are in one part of an organ and the lymph nodes near that organ (on the same side of the diaphragm). There may be lymphoma cells in other lymph node groups on the same side of the diaphragm.

- **Stage III:** The lymphoma is in lymph nodes above and below the diaphragm. It also may be found in one part of a tissue or an organ near these lymph node groups.

- **Stage IV:** Lymphoma cells are found in several parts of one or more organs or tissues (in addition to the lymph nodes). Or, it is in the liver, blood, or bone marrow.

- **Recurrent:** The disease returns after treatment.

In addition to these stage numbers, your doctor may also describe the stage as A or B:

- **A:** You have not had weight loss, drenching night sweats, or fevers.

- **B:** You have had weight loss, drenching night sweats, or fevers.

Treatment Options

Your doctor can describe your treatment choices and the expected results. You and your doctor can work together to develop a treatment plan that meets your needs.

Your doctor may refer you to a specialist, or you may ask for a referral. Specialists who treat non-Hodgkin lymphoma include hematologists, medical oncologists, and radiation oncologists. Your doctor may suggest that you choose an oncologist who specializes in the treatment of lymphoma. Often, such doctors are associated with major academic centers. Your health care team may also include an oncology nurse and a registered dietitian.

The choice of treatment depends mainly on the following the type of non-Hodgkin lymphoma (for example, follicular lymphoma), its stage (where the lymphoma is found), how quickly the cancer is growing (whether it is indolent or aggressive lymphoma), your age, and whether you have other health problems.

If you have indolent non-Hodgkin lymphoma without symptoms, you may not need treatment for the cancer right away. The doctor watches your health closely so that treatment can start when you begin to have symptoms. Not getting cancer treatment right away is called watchful waiting.

If you have indolent lymphoma with symptoms, you will probably receive chemotherapy and biological therapy. Radiation therapy may be used for people with Stage I or Stage II lymphoma.

If you have aggressive lymphoma, the treatment is usually chemotherapy and biological therapy. Radiation therapy also may be used.

If non-Hodgkin lymphoma comes back after treatment, doctors call this a relapse or recurrence. People with lymphoma that comes back after treatment may receive high doses of chemotherapy, radiation therapy, or both, followed by stem cell transplantation.

You may want to know about side effects and how treatment may change your normal activities. Because chemotherapy and radiation therapy often damage healthy cells and tissues, side effects are common. Side effects may not be the same for each person, and they may change from one treatment session to the next. Before treatment starts, your health care team will explain possible side effects and suggest ways to help you manage them.

At any stage of the disease, you can have supportive care. Supportive care is treatment to control pain and other symptoms, to relieve the side effects of therapy, and to help you cope with the feelings that a diagnosis of cancer can bring.

Watchful Waiting

People who choose watchful waiting put off having cancer treatment until they have symptoms. Doctors sometimes suggest watchful waiting for people with indolent lymphoma. People with indolent lymphoma may not have problems that require cancer treatment for a long time. Sometimes the tumor may even shrink for a while without therapy. By putting off treatment, they can avoid the side effects of chemotherapy or radiation therapy.

If you and your doctor agree that watchful waiting is a good idea, the doctor will check you regularly (every three months). You will receive treatment if symptoms occur or get worse.

Some people do not choose watchful waiting because they don't want to worry about having cancer that is not treated. Those who choose watchful waiting but later become worried should discuss their feelings with the doctor.

Chemotherapy

Chemotherapy for lymphoma uses drugs to kill lymphoma cells. It is called systemic therapy because the drugs travel through the bloodstream. The drugs can reach lymphoma cells in almost all parts of the body.

You may receive chemotherapy by mouth, through a vein, or in the space around the spinal cord. Treatment is usually in an outpatient part of the hospital, at the doctor's office, or at home. Some people need to stay in the hospital during treatment.

Chemotherapy is given in cycles. You have a treatment period followed by a rest period. The length of the rest period and the number of treatment cycles depend on the stage of your disease and on the anticancer drugs used.

If you have lymphoma in the stomach caused by *H. pylori* infection, your doctor may treat this lymphoma with antibiotics. After the drug cures the infection, the lymphoma also may go away.

The side effects depend mainly on which drugs are given and how much. The drugs can harm normal cells that divide rapidly, such as blood cells, cells in hair roots, and cells that line the digestive track. For more information about these side effects, see Section 45.1.

The drugs used for non-Hodgkin lymphoma also may cause skin rashes or blisters, and headaches or other aches. Your skin may become darker. Your nails may develop ridges or dark bands. Your doctor can suggest ways to control many of these side effects.

Biological Therapy

People with certain types of non-Hodgkin lymphoma may have biological therapy. This type of treatment helps the immune system fight cancer.

Monoclonal antibodies are the type of biological therapy used for lymphoma. They are proteins made in the lab that can bind to cancer cells. They help the immune system kill lymphoma cells. People receive this treatment through a vein at the doctor's office, clinic, or hospital.

Flu-like symptoms such as fever, chills, headache, weakness, and nausea may occur. Most side effects are easy to treat. Rarely, a person may have more serious side effects, such as breathing problems, low blood pressure, or severe skin rashes. Your doctor or nurse can tell you about the side effects that you can expect and how to manage them.

Radiation Therapy

Radiation therapy (also called radiotherapy) uses high-energy rays to kill lymphoma cells. It can shrink tumors and help control pain. Two types of radiation therapy are used for people with lymphoma:

- **External radiation:** A large machine aims the rays at the part of the body where lymphoma cells have collected. This is local therapy because it affects cells in the treated area only. Most people go to a hospital or clinic for treatment five days a week for several weeks.

- **Systemic radiation:** Some people with lymphoma receive an injection of radioactive material that travels throughout the body. The radioactive material is bound to monoclonal antibodies that seek out lymphoma cells. The radiation destroys the lymphoma cells.

The side effects of radiation therapy depend mainly on the type of radiation therapy, the dose of radiation, and the part of the body that is treated. For example, external radiation to your abdomen can cause nausea, vomiting, and diarrhea. When your chest and neck are treated, you may have a dry, sore throat and some trouble swallowing. In addition, your skin in the treated area may become red, dry, and tender. You also may lose your hair in the treated area.

You are likely to become very tired during external radiation therapy, especially in the later weeks of treatment. Resting is important, but doctors usually advise people to try to stay as active as they can.

People who get systemic radiation also may feel very tired. They may be more likely to get infections.

If you have radiation therapy and chemotherapy at the same time, your side effects may be worse. The side effects can be distressing. You can talk with your doctor about ways to relieve them.

Stem Cell Transplantation

If lymphoma returns after treatment, you may receive stem cell transplantation. A transplant of your own blood-forming stem cells allows you to receive high doses of chemotherapy, radiation therapy, or both. The high doses destroy both lymphoma cells and healthy blood cells in the bone marrow.

Stem cell transplants take place in the hospital. After you receive high-dose treatment, healthy blood-forming stem cells are given to you through a flexible tube placed in a large vein in your neck or chest area. New blood cells develop from the transplanted stem cells.

The stem cells may come from your own body or from a donor:

- **Autologous stem cell transplantation:** This type of transplant uses your own stem cells. Your stem cells are removed before high-dose treatment. The cells may be treated to kill lymphoma cells that may be present. The stem cells are frozen and stored. After you receive high-dose treatment, the stored stem cells are thawed and returned to you.

- **Allogeneic stem cell transplantation:** Sometimes healthy stem cells from a donor are available. Your brother, sister, or parent may be the donor. Or the stem cells may come from an unrelated donor. Doctors use blood tests to be sure the donor's cells match your cells.

- **Syngeneic stem cell transplantation:** This type of transplant uses stem cells from a patient's healthy identical twin.

Second Opinion

Before starting treatment, you might want a second opinion about your diagnosis and your treatment plan. Many insurance companies cover a second opinion if you or your doctor requests it.

It may take some time and effort to gather your medical records and see another doctor. In most cases, a brief delay in starting treatment will not make treatment less effective. To make sure, you should discuss this delay with your doctor. Sometimes people with non-Hodgkin lymphoma need treatment right away.

There are many ways to find a doctor for a second opinion. You can ask your doctor, a local or state medical society, a nearby hospital, or a medical school for names of specialists. Nonprofit groups with an interest in lymphoma may be of help. Some such groups are listed in resources at the end of this book.

Supportive Care

Non-Hodgkin lymphoma and its treatment can lead to other health problems. You may receive supportive care to prevent or control these problems and to improve your comfort and quality of life during treatment.

You may receive antibiotics and other drugs to help protect you from infections. Your health care team may advise you to stay away from crowds and from people with colds and other contagious diseases. If an infection develops, it can be serious, and you will need treatment right away.

Non-Hodgkin lymphoma and its treatment also can lead to anemia, which may make you feel very tired. Drugs or blood transfusions can help with this problem.

Follow-Up Care

You'll need regular checkups after treatment for non-Hodgkin lymphoma. Your doctor will watch your recovery closely and check for recurrence of the lymphoma. Checkups help make sure that any changes in your health are noted and treated as needed. Checkups may include a physical exam, lab tests, chest x-rays, and other procedures. Between scheduled visits, you should contact the doctor right away if you have any health problems.

Chapter 46

Multiple Myeloma

Basic Facts about Multiple Myeloma

Multiple myeloma is a type of cancer. Cancer is a group of many related diseases. Myeloma is a cancer that starts in plasma cells, a type of white blood cell. It's the most common type of plasma cell cancer.

Normal Blood Cells

Most blood cells develop from cells in the bone marrow called stem cells. Bone marrow is the soft material in the center of most bones.

Stem cells mature into different types of blood cells. Each type has a special job. White blood cells help fight infection. There are several types of white blood cells. Red blood cells carry oxygen to tissues throughout the body. Platelets help form blood clots that control bleeding.

Plasma cells are white blood cells that make antibodies. Antibodies are part of the immune system. They work with other parts of the immune system to help protect the body from germs and other harmful substances. Each type of plasma cell makes a different antibody. Normal plasma cells help protect the body from germs and other harmful substances.

Myeloma Cells

Myeloma, like other cancers, begins in cells. In cancer, new cells form when the body doesn't need them, and old or damaged cells don't

Excerpted from "What You Need to Know about Multiple Myeloma," National Cancer Institute (www.cancer.gov), November 20, 2008.

die when they should. These extra cells can form a mass of tissue called a growth or tumor.

Myeloma begins when a plasma cell becomes abnormal. The abnormal cell divides to make copies of itself. The new cells divide again and again, making more and more abnormal cells. These abnormal plasma cells are called myeloma cells.

In time, myeloma cells collect in the bone marrow. They may damage the solid part of the bone. When myeloma cells collect in several of your bones, the disease is called "multiple myeloma." This disease may also harm other tissues and organs, such as the kidneys.

Myeloma cells make antibodies called M proteins and other proteins. These proteins can collect in the blood, urine, and organs.

Risk Factors

No one knows the exact causes of multiple myeloma. Doctors seldom know why one person develops this disease and another doesn't. However, we do know that multiple myeloma isn't contagious. You cannot catch it from another person.

Research has shown that certain risk factors increase the chance that a person will develop this disease. Studies have found the following risk factors for multiple myeloma:

- **Age over 65:** Growing older increases the chance of developing multiple myeloma. Most people with myeloma are diagnosed after age 65. This disease is rare in people younger than 35.

- **Race:** The risk of multiple myeloma is highest among African Americans and lowest among Asian Americans. The reason for the difference between racial groups is not known.

- **Being a man:** Each year in the United States, about 11,200 men and 8,700 women are diagnosed with multiple myeloma. It is not known why more men are diagnosed with the disease.

- **Personal history of monoclonal gammopathy of undetermined significance (MGUS):** MGUS is a benign condition in which abnormal plasma cells make M proteins. Usually, there are no symptoms, and the abnormal level of M protein is found with a blood test. Sometimes, people with MGUS develop certain cancers, such as multiple myeloma. There is no treatment, but people with MGUS get regular lab tests (every one or two years) to check for a further increase in the level of M protein. They also get regular exams to check for the development of symptoms.

- **Family history of multiple myeloma:** Studies have found that a person's risk of multiple myeloma may be higher if a close relative had the disease.

Many other suspected risk factors are under study. Researchers have studied whether being exposed to certain chemicals or germs (especially viruses), having alterations in certain genes, eating certain foods, or being obese increases the risk of developing multiple myeloma. Researchers continue to study these and other possible risk factors.

Having one or more risk factors does not mean that a person will develop myeloma. Most people who have risk factors never develop cancer.

Symptoms

Common symptoms of multiple myeloma include the following:

- Bone pain, usually in the back and ribs
- Broken bones, usually in the spine
- Feeling weak and very tired
- Feeling very thirsty
- Frequent infections and fevers
- Weight loss
- Nausea or constipation
- Frequent urination

Most often, these symptoms are not due to cancer. Other health problems may also cause these symptoms. Only a doctor can tell for sure. Anyone with these symptoms should tell the doctor so that problems can be diagnosed and treated as early as possible.

Diagnosis

Doctors sometimes find multiple myeloma after a routine blood test. More often, doctors suspect multiple myeloma after an x-ray for a broken bone. Usually though, patients go to the doctor because they are having other symptoms.

To find out whether such problems are from multiple myeloma or some other condition, your doctor may ask about your personal and family medical history and do a physical exam. Your doctor also may order some of the following tests:

- **Blood tests:** The lab does several blood tests: Multiple myeloma causes high levels of proteins in the blood. The lab checks the levels of many different proteins, including M protein and other immunoglobulins (antibodies), albumin, and beta-2-microglobulin. Myeloma may also cause anemia and low levels of white blood cells and platelets. The lab does a complete blood count to check the number of white blood cells, red blood cells, and platelets. The lab also checks for high levels of calcium, and to see how well the kidneys are working, the lab tests for creatinine.

- **Urine tests:** The lab checks for Bence Jones protein, a type of M protein, in urine. The lab measures the amount of Bence Jones protein in urine collected over a 24-hour period. If the lab finds a high level of Bence Jones protein in your urine sample, doctors will monitor your kidneys. Bence Jones protein can clog the kidneys and damage them.

- **X-rays:** You may have x-rays to check for broken or thinning bones. An x-ray of your whole body can be done to see how many bones could be damaged by the myeloma.

- **Biopsy:** Your doctor removes tissue to look for cancer cells. A biopsy is the only sure way to know whether myeloma cells are in your bone marrow. Before the sample is taken, local anesthesia is used to numb the area. This helps reduce the pain. Your doctor removes some bone marrow from your hip bone or another large bone. A pathologist uses a microscope to check the tissue for myeloma cells.

There are two ways your doctor can obtain bone marrow. Some people will have both procedures during the same visit:

- **Bone marrow aspiration:** The doctor uses a thick, hollow needle to remove samples of bone marrow.

- **Bone marrow biopsy:** The doctor uses a very thick, hollow needle to remove a small piece of bone and bone marrow.

Staging Multiple Myeloma

If the biopsy shows that you have multiple myeloma, your doctor needs to learn the extent (stage) of the disease to plan the best treatment. Staging may involve having more tests:

- **Blood tests:** For staging, the doctor considers the results of blood tests, including albumin and beta-2-microglobulin.

- **CT scan**: An x-ray machine linked to a computer takes a series of detailed pictures of your bones.

- **MRI:** A powerful magnet linked to a computer is used to make detailed pictures of your bones.

Doctors may describe multiple myeloma as smoldering, Stage I, Stage II, or Stage III. The stage takes into account whether the cancer is causing problems with your bones or kidneys. Smoldering multiple myeloma is early disease without any symptoms. For example, there is no bone damage. Early disease with symptoms (such as bone damage) is Stage I. Stage II or III is more advanced, and more myeloma cells are found in the body.

Treatment Options

People with multiple myeloma have many treatment options. The options are watchful waiting, induction therapy, and stem cell transplant. Sometimes a combination of methods is used.

Radiation therapy is used sometimes to treat painful bone disease. It may be used alone or along with other therapies.

The choice of treatment depends mainly on how advanced the disease is and whether you have symptoms. If you have multiple myeloma without symptoms (smoldering myeloma), you may not need cancer treatment right away. The doctor monitors your health closely (watchful waiting) so that treatment can start when you begin to have symptoms.

If you have symptoms, you will likely get induction therapy. Sometimes a stem cell transplant is part of the treatment plan.

When treatment for myeloma is needed, it can often control the disease and its symptoms. People may receive therapy to help keep the cancer in remission, but myeloma can seldom be cured. Because standard treatment may not control myeloma, you may want to talk to your doctor about taking part in a clinical trial. Clinical trials are research studies of new treatment methods.

Your doctor can describe your treatment choices, the expected results, and the possible side effects. You and your doctor can work together to develop a treatment plan that meets your needs.

Your doctor may refer you to a specialist, or you may ask for a referral. Specialists who treat multiple myeloma include hematologists and medical oncologists. Your health care team may also include an oncology nurse and a registered dietitian.

Before treatment starts, ask your health care team to explain possible side effects and how treatment may change your normal activities. Because cancer treatments often damage healthy cells and tissues, side effects are common. Side effects may not be the same for each person, and they may change from one treatment session to the next.

Watchful Waiting

People with smoldering myeloma or Stage I myeloma may be able to put off having cancer treatment. By delaying treatment, you can avoid the side effects of treatment until you have symptoms.

If you and your doctor agree that watchful waiting is a good idea, you will have regular checkups (such as every three months). You will receive treatment if symptoms occur.

Although watchful waiting avoids or delays the side effects of cancer treatment, this choice has risks. In some cases, it may reduce the chance to control myeloma before it gets worse.

You may decide against watchful waiting if you don't want to live with untreated myeloma. If you choose watchful waiting but grow concerned later, you should discuss your feelings with your doctor. Another approach is an option in most cases.

Induction Therapy

Many different types of drugs are used to treat myeloma. People often receive a combination of drugs, and many different combinations are used to treat myeloma. Each type of drug kills cancer cells in a different way:

- **Chemotherapy:** Chemotherapy kills fast-growing myeloma cells, but the drug can also harm normal cells that divide rapidly.

- **Targeted therapy:** Targeted therapies use drugs that block the growth of myeloma cells. The targeted therapy blocks the action of an abnormal protein that stimulates the growth of myeloma cells.

- **Steroids:** Some steroids have antitumor effects. It is thought that steroids can trigger the death of myeloma cells. A steroid may be used alone or with other drugs to treat myeloma.

You may receive the drugs by mouth or through a vein (IV). The treatment usually takes place in an outpatient part of the hospital, at your doctor's office, or at home. Some people may need to stay in the hospital for treatment.

The side effects depend mainly on which drugs are given and how much:

- **Blood cells:** When a drug used for myeloma treatment lowers the levels of healthy blood cells, you're more likely to get infections, bruise or bleed easily, and feel very weak and tired. Your health care team will check for low levels of blood cells. If your levels are low, your health care team may stop therapy for a while or reduce the dose of drug. There are also medicines that can help your body make new blood cells.

- **Cells in hair roots:** Chemotherapy may cause hair loss. If you lose your hair, it will grow back, but it may be somewhat different in color and texture.

- **Cells that line the digestive tract:** Chemotherapy and targeted therapy can cause poor appetite, nausea and vomiting, diarrhea, constipation, or mouth and lip sores. Ask your health care team about medicines and other ways to help you cope with these problems.

The drugs used for myeloma may also cause dizziness, drowsiness, numbness or tingling in hands or feet, and low blood pressure. Most of these problems go away when treatment ends.

Stem Cell Transplant

Many people with multiple myeloma may get a stem cell transplant. A stem cell transplant allows you to be treated with high doses of drugs. The high doses destroy both myeloma cells and normal blood cells in the bone marrow. After you receive high-dose treatment, you receive healthy stem cells through a vein. (It's like getting a blood transfusion.) New blood cells develop from the transplanted stem cells. The new blood cells replace the ones that were destroyed by treatment.

Stem cell transplants take place in the hospital. Some people with myeloma have two or more transplants.

Stem cells may come from you or from someone who donates their stem cells to you:

- **From you:** An autologous stem cell transplant uses your own stem cells. Before you get the high-dose chemotherapy, your stem cells are removed. The cells may be treated to kill any myeloma cells present. Your stem cells are frozen and stored. After you receive high-dose chemotherapy, the stored stem cells are thawed and returned to you.

- **From a family member or other donor:** An allogeneic stem cell transplant uses healthy stem cells from a donor. Your brother, sister, or parent may be the donor. Sometimes the stem cells come from a donor who isn't related. Doctors use blood tests to be sure the donor's cells match your cells. Allogeneic stem cell transplants are under study for the treatment of multiple myeloma.

- **From your identical twin:** If you have an identical twin, a syngeneic stem cell transplant uses stem cells from your healthy twin.

There are two ways to get stem cells for people with myeloma. They usually come from the blood (peripheral blood stem cell transplant). Or they can come from the bone marrow (bone marrow transplant).

After a stem cell transplant, you may stay in the hospital for several weeks or months. You'll be at risk for infections because of the large doses of chemotherapy you received. In time, the transplanted stem cells will begin to produce healthy blood cells.

Second Opinion

Before starting treatment, you might want a second opinion about your diagnosis and treatment plan. Some people worry that the doctor will be offended if they ask for a second opinion. Usually the opposite is true. Most doctors welcome a second opinion. And many health insurance companies will pay for a second opinion if you or your doctor requests it.

If you get a second opinion, the doctor may agree with your first doctor's diagnosis and treatment plan. Or the second doctor may suggest another approach. Either way, you have more information and perhaps a greater sense of control. You can feel more confident about the decisions you make, knowing that you've looked at your options.

It may take some time and effort to gather your medical records and see another doctor. In most cases, it's not a problem to take several weeks to get a second opinion. The delay in starting treatment usually won't make treatment less effective. To make sure, you should discuss this delay with your doctor. Some people with multiple myeloma need treatment right away.

There are many ways to find a doctor for a second opinion. You can ask your doctor, a local or state medical society, a nearby hospital, or a medical school for names of specialists. The National Cancer Institute's Cancer Information Service at 800-4-CANCER can tell you about nearby treatment centers. Nonprofit groups with an interest in multiple myeloma may be of help. Some such groups are listed in the resources section of this book.

Supportive Care

Multiple myeloma and its treatment can lead to other health problems. At any stage of the disease, you can have supportive care.

Supportive care is treatment to prevent or fight infections, to control pain and other symptoms, to relieve the side effects of therapy, and to help you cope with the feelings that a diagnosis of cancer can bring. You may receive supportive care to prevent or control these problems and to improve your comfort and quality of life during treatment.

Infections: Because people with multiple myeloma get infections very easily, you may receive antibiotics and other drugs.

Some people receive vaccines against the flu and pneumonia. You may want to talk with your health care team about when to get certain vaccines.

The health care team may advise you to stay away from crowds and from people with colds and other contagious diseases. If an infection develops, it can be serious and should be treated promptly. You may need to stay in the hospital for treatment.

Anemia: Myeloma and its treatment can lead to anemia, which may make you feel very tired. Drugs or a blood transfusion can help with this problem.

Pain: Multiple myeloma often causes bone pain. Your health care provider can suggest ways to relieve or reduce pain, such as a brace that relieves pain in the neck or back, drugs that fight pain anywhere in the body, radiation therapy from a large machine aimed at the bone, or surgery to fix a compressed (squeezed) spinal cord.

Some people get pain relief from massage or acupuncture when used along with other approaches. Also, you may learn relaxation techniques such as listening to slow music or breathing slowly and comfortably.

Thinning bones: Myeloma cells keep new bone cells from forming, and bones become thin wherever there are myeloma cells. Your doctor may give you drugs to prevent bone thinning and help reduce the risk of fractures. Physical activity, such as walking, also helps keep bones strong.

Too much calcium in the blood: Multiple myeloma may cause calcium to leave the bones and enter the bloodstream. If you have a very high level of calcium in your blood, you may lose your appetite. You also may feel nauseated, restless, or confused. A high calcium level can also make you very tired, weak, dehydrated, and thirsty. Drinking a lot of fluids and taking drugs that lower the calcium in the blood can be helpful.

Kidney problems: Some people with multiple myeloma have kidney problems. If the problems are severe, a person may need dialysis. Dialysis removes wastes from the blood. A person with serious kidney problems may need a kidney transplant.

Amyloidosis: Some people with myeloma develop amyloidosis. This problem is caused by abnormal proteins collecting in tissues of the body. The buildup of proteins can cause many problems, some of them severe. For example, proteins can build up in the heart, causing chest pain and swollen feet. There are drugs to treat amyloidosis.

Follow-Up Care

You'll need regular checkups after treatment for multiple myeloma. Checkups help ensure that any changes in your health are noted and treated if needed. If you have any health problems between checkups, you should contact your doctor.

Your doctor will check for return of cancer. Even when the cancer seems to have been completely destroyed, the disease sometimes returns because undetected myeloma cells remained somewhere in the body after treatment. Also, checkups help detect health problems that can result from cancer treatment.

Checkups may include a careful physical exam, blood tests, x-rays, or bone marrow biopsy.

Chapter 47

Myelodysplastic and Myeloproliferative Diseases

General Information about Myelodysplastic/ Myeloproliferative Neoplasms

Myelodysplastic/myeloproliferative neoplasms are diseases of the blood and bone marrow. Normally, the bone marrow makes blood stem cells (immature cells) that become mature blood cells over time. A blood stem cell may become a myeloid stem cell or a lymphoid stem cell. The lymphoid stem cell develops into a white blood cell. The myeloid stem cell develops into one of three types of mature blood cells:

- Red blood cells that carry oxygen and other materials to all tissues of the body

- White blood cells that fight infection and disease

- Platelets that help prevent bleeding by causing blood clots to form

A blood stem cell goes through several steps to become a red blood cell, platelet, or white blood cell.

Myelodysplastic/myeloproliferative neoplasms have features of both myelodysplastic syndromes and myeloproliferative disorders.

Excerpted from PDQ® Cancer Information Summary. National Cancer Institute; Bethesda, MD. "Myelodysplastic/Myeloproliferative Neoplasms Treatment (PDQ) - Patient Version." Updated 03/2010. Available at: http://cancer.gov. Accessed October 23, 2010.

In myelodysplastic diseases, the blood stem cells do not mature into healthy red blood cells, white blood cells, or platelets. The immature blood cells, called blasts, do not work the way they should and die in the bone marrow or soon after they enter the blood. As a result, there are fewer healthy red blood cells, white blood cells, and platelets.

In myeloproliferative diseases, a greater than normal number of blood stem cells develop into one or more types of blood cells and the total number of blood cells slowly increases.

The three main types of myelodysplastic/myeloproliferative neoplasms are chronic myelomonocytic leukemia (CMML), juvenile myelomonocytic leukemia (JMML), and atypical chronic myelogenous leukemia (aCML). When a myelodysplastic/myeloproliferative neoplasm does not match any of these types, it is called myelodysplastic/myeloproliferative neoplasm, unclassifiable (MDS/MPN-UC).

Myelodysplastic/myeloproliferative neoplasms may progress to acute leukemia.

Detection and Diagnosis

The following tests and procedures may be used:

- **Physical exam and history:** An exam of the body to check general signs of health, including checking for signs of disease such as an enlarged spleen and liver. A history of the patient's health habits and past illnesses and treatments will also be taken.

- **Complete blood count (CBC) with differential:** A procedure in which a sample of blood is drawn and checked for the number of red blood cells and platelets, the number and type of white blood cells, the amount of hemoglobin (the protein that carries oxygen) in the red blood cells, and the portion of the sample made up of red blood cells.

- **Blood chemistry studies:** A procedure in which a blood sample is checked to measure the amounts of certain substances released into the blood by organs and tissues in the body. An unusual (higher or lower than normal) amount of a substance can be a sign of disease in the organ or tissue that produces it.

- **Peripheral blood smear:** A procedure in which a sample of blood is checked for the presence of blast cells, number and kinds of white blood cells, the number of platelets, and changes in the shape of blood cells.

- **Cytogenetic analysis:** A test in which cells in a sample of blood or bone marrow are viewed under a microscope to look for certain changes in the chromosomes. The cancer cells in myelodysplastic/myeloproliferative neoplasms do not contain the Philadelphia chromosome that is present in chronic myelogenous leukemia.

- **Bone marrow aspiration and biopsy:** The removal of a small piece of bone and bone marrow by inserting a needle into the hipbone or breastbone. A pathologist views both the bone and bone marrow samples under a microscope to look for abnormal cells.

Chronic Myelomonocytic Leukemia

Chronic myelomonocytic leukemia (CMML) is a disease in which too many myelocytes and monocytes (immature white blood cells) are made in the bone marrow.

In CMML, the body tells too many blood stem cells to develop into two types of white blood cells called myelocytes and monocytes. Some of these blood stem cells never become mature white blood cells. These immature white blood cells are called blasts. Over time, the myelocytes, monocytes, and blasts crowd out the red blood cells and platelets in the bone marrow. When this happens, infection, anemia, or easy bleeding may occur.

CMML Risk Factors, Symptoms, and Prognosis

Anything that increases your chance of getting a disease is called a risk factor. Possible risk factors for CMML include the following:

- Older age

- Being male

- Being exposed to certain substances at work or in the environment

- Being exposed to radiation

- Past treatment with certain anticancer drugs

Possible signs of chronic myelomonocytic leukemia include fever, feeling very tired, and weight loss. These and other symptoms may be caused by CMML. Other conditions may cause the same symptoms. A doctor should be consulted if any of the following problems occur:

- Fever for no known reason
- Infection
- Feeling very tired
- Weight loss for no known reason
- Easy bruising or bleeding
- Pain or a feeling of fullness below the ribs

The prognosis (chance of recovery) and treatment options for CMML depend on the number of white blood cells or platelets in the blood or bone marrow, whether the patient is anemic, the amount of blasts in the blood or bone marrow, the amount of hemoglobin in red blood cells, and whether there are certain changes in the chromosomes.

Juvenile Myelomonocytic Leukemia

Juvenile myelomonocytic leukemia (JMML) is a rare childhood cancer that occurs more often in children younger than two years. Children who have neurofibromatosis type 1 and males have an increased risk of developing juvenile myelomonocytic leukemia.

In JMML, the body tells too many blood stem cells to develop into two types of white blood cells called myelocytes and monocytes. Some of these blood stem cells never become mature white blood cells. These immature white blood cells are called blasts. Over time, the myelocytes, monocytes, and blasts crowd out the red blood cells and platelets in the bone marrow. When this happens, infection, anemia, or easy bleeding may occur.

JMML Symptoms and Prognosis

Possible signs of juvenile myelomonocytic leukemia include fever, feeling very tired, and weight loss. These and other symptoms may be caused by JMML. Other conditions may cause the same symptoms. A doctor should be consulted if any of the following problems occur:

- Fever for no known reason
- Having infections, such as bronchitis or tonsillitis
- Feeling very tired
- Easy bruising or bleeding
- Skin rash

- Painless swelling of the lymph nodes in the neck, underarm, stomach, or groin

- Pain or a feeling of fullness below the ribs

The prognosis (chance of recovery) and treatment options for JMML depend on the age of the child at diagnosis, the number of platelets in the blood, and the amount of a certain type of hemoglobin in red blood cells.

Atypical Chronic Myelogenous Leukemia

In atypical chronic myelogenous leukemia (aCML), the body tells too many blood stem cells to develop into a type of white blood cell called granulocytes. Some of these blood stem cells never become mature white blood cells. These immature white blood cells are called blasts. Over time, the granulocytes and blasts crowd out the red blood cells and platelets in the bone marrow.

The leukemia cells in aCML and chronic myelogenous leukemia (CML) look alike under a microscope. However, in aCML a certain chromosome change, called the "Philadelphia chromosome" is not present.

Symptoms and Prognosis

Possible signs of atypical chronic myelogenous leukemia include easy bruising or bleeding and feeling tired and weak. These and other symptoms may be caused by aCML. Other conditions may cause the same symptoms. A doctor should be consulted if any of the following problems occur:

- Shortness of breath

- Pale skin

- Feeling very tired and weak

- Easy bruising or bleeding

- Petechiae (flat, pinpoint spots under the skin caused by bleeding)

- Pain or a feeling of fullness below the ribs on the left side

The prognosis (chance of recovery) for aCML depends on the number of red blood cells and platelets in the blood.

Myelodysplastic/Myeloproliferative Neoplasm, Unclassifiable

Myelodysplastic/myeloproliferative neoplasm, unclassifiable, is a disease that has features of both myelodysplastic and myeloproliferative diseases but is not chronic myelomonocytic leukemia, juvenile myelomonocytic leukemia, or atypical chronic myelogenous leukemia.

In myelodysplastic /myeloproliferative neoplasm, unclassifiable (MDS/MPD-UC), the body tells too many blood stem cells to develop into red blood cells, white blood cells, or platelets. Some of these blood stem cells never become mature blood cells. These immature blood cells are called blasts. Over time, the abnormal blood cells and blasts in the bone marrow crowd out the healthy red blood cells, white blood cells, and platelets.

MDS/MPN-UC is a very rare disease. Because it is so rare, the factors that affect risk and prognosis are not known.

Symptoms

Possible signs of myelodysplastic/myeloproliferative neoplasm, unclassifiable, include fever, feeling very tired, and weight loss. These and other symptoms may be caused by MDS/MPN-UC. Other conditions may cause the same symptoms. A doctor should be consulted if any of the following problems occur:

- Fever or frequent infections
- Shortness of breath
- Feeling very tired and weak
- Pale skin
- Easy bruising or bleeding
- Petechiae (flat, pinpoint spots under the skin caused by bleeding)
- Pain or a feeling of fullness below the ribs

Stages of Myelodysplastic/Myeloproliferative Neoplasms

Staging is the process used to find out how far the cancer has spread. There is no standard staging system for myelodysplastic /myeloproliferative neoplasms. Treatment is based on the type of myelodysplastic/myeloproliferative neoplasm the patient has. It is important to know the type in order to plan treatment.

When cancer cells spread outside the blood, a solid tumor may form. This process is called metastasis. The new (metastatic) tumor is the same type of cancer as the primary cancer. For example, if leukemia cells spread to the brain, the cancer cells in the brain are actually leukemia cells. The disease is metastatic leukemia, not brain cancer.

Treatment Option Overview

Different types of treatments are available for patients with myelodysplastic /myeloproliferative neoplasms. Some treatments are standard (the currently used treatment), and some are being tested in clinical trials. Four types of standard treatment are used:

Chemotherapy

Chemotherapy is a cancer treatment that uses drugs to stop the growth of cancer cells, either by killing the cells or by stopping them from dividing. When chemotherapy is taken by mouth or injected into a vein or muscle, the drugs enter the bloodstream and can reach cancer cells throughout the body (systemic chemotherapy). When chemotherapy is placed directly into the spinal column, an organ, or a body cavity such as the abdomen, the drugs mainly affect cancer cells in those areas (regional chemotherapy). The way the chemotherapy is given depends on the type and stage of the cancer being treated. Combination chemotherapy is treatment using more than one anticancer drug.

Other drug therapy: 13-cis retinoic acid is a vitamin-like drug that slows the cancer's ability to make more cancer cells and changes the way these cells look and act.

Stem Cell Transplant

Stem cell transplant is a method of replacing blood-forming cells that are destroyed by chemotherapy. Stem cells (immature blood cells) are removed from the blood or bone marrow of the patient or a donor and are frozen and stored. After the chemotherapy is completed, the stored stem cells are thawed and given back to the patient through an infusion. These reinfused stem cells grow into (and restore) the body's blood cells.

Supportive Care

Supportive care is given to lessen the problems caused by the disease or its treatment. Supportive care may include transfusion therapy or drug therapy, such as antibiotics to fight infection.

Clinical Trials

New types of treatment are being tested in clinical trials. A treatment clinical trial is a research study meant to help improve current treatments or obtain information on new treatments for patients with cancer. When clinical trials show that a new treatment is better than the standard treatment, the new treatment may become the standard treatment. Patients may want to think about taking part in a clinical trial. Some clinical trials are open only to patients who have not started treatment.

One treatment that is currently being studied is targeted therapy. Targeted therapy is a cancer treatment that uses drugs or other substances to attack cancer cells without harming normal cells. Farnesyltransferase inhibitors are one type of targeted therapy that is being studied in the treatment of JMML.

For more information about clinical trials, visit the National Cancer Center's clinical trials website at www.cancer.gov/clinicaltrials.

Follow-Up Tests

Some of the tests that were done to diagnose the cancer or to find out the stage of the cancer may be repeated. Some tests will be repeated in order to see how well the treatment is working. Decisions about whether to continue, change, or stop treatment may be based on the results of these tests. This is sometimes called re-staging.

Some of the tests will continue to be done from time to time after treatment has ended. The results of these tests can show if your condition has changed or if the cancer has recurred (come back). These tests are sometimes called follow-up tests or check-ups.

Chapter 48

Thymoma and Thymic Carcinoma

General Information about Thymoma and Thymic Carcinoma

Thymoma and thymic carcinoma are diseases in which malignant (cancer) cells form on the outside surface of the thymus. The thymus, a small organ that lies in the upper chest under the breastbone, is part of the lymph system. It makes white blood cells, called lymphocytes, that protect the body against infections.

There are different types of tumors of the thymus. Thymomas and thymic carcinomas are rare tumors of the cells that are on the outside surface of the thymus. The tumor cells in a thymoma look similar to the normal cells of the thymus, grow slowly, and rarely spread beyond the thymus. On the other hand, the tumor cells in a thymic carcinoma look very different from the normal cells of the thymus, grow more quickly, and have usually spread to other parts of the body when the cancer is found. Thymic carcinoma is more difficult to treat than thymoma.

People with thymoma often have autoimmune diseases as well. These diseases cause the immune system to attack healthy tissue and organs. They include the following:

- Myasthenia gravis

Excerpted from PDQ® Cancer Information Summary. National Cancer Institute; Bethesda, MD. "Thymoma and Thymic Carcinoma Treatment (PDQ) - Patient Version." Updated 04/2010. Available at: http://cancer.gov. Accessed October 23, 2010.

- Autoimmune pure red cell aplasia
- Hypogammaglobulinemia
- Polymyositis
- Lupus erythematosus
- Rheumatoid arthritis
- Thyroiditis
- Sjögren syndrome

Signs and Symptoms

Possible signs of thymoma and thymic carcinoma include a cough and chest pain. Sometimes thymoma and thymic carcinoma do not cause symptoms. The cancer may be found during a routine chest x-ray. The following symptoms may be caused by thymoma, thymic carcinoma, or other conditions. A doctor should be consulted if any of the following problems occur: a cough that doesn't go away; chest pain; trouble breathing.

Detection and Diagnosis

Tests that examine the thymus are used to detect thymoma or thymic carcinoma. The following tests and procedures may be used:

Physical exam and history: An exam of the body to check general signs of health, including checking for signs of disease, such as lumps or anything else that seems unusual. A history of the patient's health habits and past illnesses and treatments will also be taken.

Chest x-ray: An x-ray of the organs and bones inside the chest. An x-ray is a type of energy beam that can go through the body and onto film, making a picture of areas inside the body.

CT scan (CAT scan): A procedure that makes a series of detailed pictures of areas inside the body, such as the chest, taken from different angles. The pictures are made by a computer linked to an x-ray machine. A dye may be injected into a vein or swallowed to help the organs or tissues show up more clearly. This procedure is also called computed tomography, computerized tomography, or computerized axial tomography.

MRI (magnetic resonance imaging): A procedure that uses a magnet, radio waves, and a computer to make a series of detailed pictures of areas inside the body, such as the chest. This procedure is also called nuclear magnetic resonance imaging (NMRI).

PET scan (positron emission tomography scan): A procedure to find malignant tumor cells in the body. A small amount of radioactive glucose (sugar) is injected into a vein. The PET scanner rotates around the body and makes a picture of where glucose is being used in the body. Malignant tumor cells show up brighter in the picture because they are more active and take up more glucose than normal cells do.

Biopsy: Thymoma and thymic carcinoma are usually diagnosed, staged, and treated during surgery. A biopsy of the tumor is done to diagnose the disease. The biopsy may be done before or during surgery, using a thin needle to remove a sample of cells. This is called a fine-needle aspiration (FNA) biopsy. A pathologist will view the sample under a microscope to check for cancer. If thymoma or thymic carcinoma is diagnosed, the pathologist will determine the type of cancer cell in the tumor. There may be more than one type of cancer cell in a thymoma. The surgeon will decide if all or part of the tumor can be removed by surgery. In some cases, lymph nodes and other tissues may be removed as well.

Prognosis

Certain factors affect prognosis (chance of recovery) and treatment options. The prognosis and treatment options depend on the following:

- The stage of the cancer
- The type of cancer cell
- Whether the tumor can be removed completely by surgery
- The patient's general health
- Whether the cancer has just been diagnosed or has recurred (come back)

Stages of Thymoma and Thymic Carcinoma

Staging is the process used to find out if cancer has spread from the thymus to other parts of the body. The findings made during surgery and the results of tests and procedures are used to determine the stage of the disease. It is important to know the stage in order to plan treatment. The following stages are used for thymoma.

Stage I

In stage I, cancer is found only within the thymus. All cancer cells are inside the capsule (sac) that surrounds the thymus.

Stage II

In stage II, cancer has spread through the capsule and into the fat around the thymus or into the lining of the chest cavity.

Stage III

In stage III, cancer has spread to nearby organs in the chest, including the lung, the sac around the heart, or large blood vessels that carry blood to the heart.

Stage IV

Stage IV is divided into stage IVA and stage IVB, depending on where the cancer has spread.

- In stage IVA, cancer has spread widely around the lungs and heart.
- In stage IVB, cancer has spread to the blood or lymph system.

Thymic carcinomas have usually spread to other parts of the body when diagnosed. The staging system used for thymomas is sometimes used for thymic carcinomas.

Recurrent Thymoma and Thymic Carcinoma

Recurrent thymoma and thymic carcinoma is cancer that has recurred (come back) after it has been treated. The cancer may come back in the thymus or in other parts of the body. Thymic carcinomas commonly recur. Thymomas may recur after a long time. There is also an increased risk of having another type of cancer after having a thymoma. For these reasons, lifelong follow-up is needed.

Treatment Option Overview

Different types of treatments are available for patients with thymoma and thymic carcinoma. Some treatments are standard (the currently used treatment), and some are being tested in clinical trials. A treatment clinical trial is a research study meant to help improve current treatments or obtain information on new treatments for patients with cancer. When clinical trials show that a new treatment is better than the standard treatment, the new treatment may become the standard treatment. Patients may want to think about taking part in a clinical trial. Some clinical trials are open only to patients who have not started treatment. Four types of standard treatment are used.

Surgery

Surgery to remove the tumor is the most common treatment of thymoma. Even if the doctor removes all the cancer that can be seen at the time of the surgery, some patients may be given radiation therapy after surgery to kill any cancer cells that are left. Treatment given after the surgery, to lower the risk that the cancer will come back, is called adjuvant therapy.

Radiation Therapy

Radiation therapy is a cancer treatment that uses high-energy x-rays or other types of radiation to kill cancer cells or keep them from growing. There are two types of radiation therapy. External radiation therapy uses a machine outside the body to send radiation toward the cancer. Internal radiation therapy uses a radioactive substance sealed in needles, seeds, wires, or catheters that are placed directly into or near the cancer. The way the radiation therapy is given depends on the type and stage of the cancer being treated.

Chemotherapy

Chemotherapy is a cancer treatment that uses drugs to stop the growth of cancer cells, either by killing the cells or by stopping them from dividing. When chemotherapy is taken by mouth or injected into a vein or muscle, the drugs enter the bloodstream and can reach cancer cells throughout the body (systemic chemotherapy). When chemotherapy is placed directly into the spinal column, an organ, or a body cavity such as the abdomen, the drugs mainly affect cancer cells in those areas (regional chemotherapy). The way the chemotherapy is given depends on the type and stage of the cancer being treated.

Chemotherapy may be used to shrink the tumor before surgery or radiation therapy. This is called neoadjuvant chemotherapy.

Hormone Therapy

Hormone therapy is a cancer treatment that removes hormones or blocks their action and stops cancer cells from growing. Hormones are substances produced by glands in the body and circulated in the bloodstream. Some hormones can cause certain cancers to grow. If tests show that the cancer cells have places where hormones can attach (receptors), drugs, surgery, or radiation therapy is used to reduce the production of hormones or block them from working.

Hormone therapy with drugs called corticosteroids may be used to treat thymoma or thymic carcinoma.

Clinical Trials

Patients may want to think about taking part in a clinical trial. For some patients, taking part in a clinical trial may be the best treatment choice. Clinical trials are part of the cancer research process. Clinical trials are done to find out if new cancer treatments are safe and effective or better than the standard treatment.

Many of today's standard treatments for cancer are based on earlier clinical trials. Patients who take part in a clinical trial may receive the standard treatment or be among the first to receive a new treatment.

Patients who take part in clinical trials also help improve the way cancer will be treated in the future. Even when clinical trials do not lead to effective new treatments, they often answer important questions and help move research forward.

Patients can enter clinical trials before, during, or after starting their cancer treatment.

Some clinical trials only include patients who have not yet received treatment. Other trials test treatments for patients whose cancer has not gotten better. There are also clinical trials that test new ways to stop cancer from recurring (coming back) or reduce the side effects of cancer treatment.

For more information about current clinical trials, visit the National Cancer Institute's clinical trials website at www.cancer.gov/clinicaltrials.gov.

Follow-Up Tests

Some of the tests that were done to diagnose the cancer or to find out the stage of the cancer may be repeated. Some tests will be repeated in order to see how well the treatment is working. Decisions

646

about whether to continue, change, or stop treatment may be based on the results of these tests. This is sometimes called re-staging.

Some of the tests will continue to be done from time to time after treatment has ended. The results of these tests can show if your condition has changed or if the cancer has recurred (come back). These tests are sometimes called follow-up tests or check-ups.

Chapter 49

Melanoma

General Information about Melanoma

The skin is the body's largest organ. It protects against heat, sunlight, injury, and infection. The skin has two main layers: the epidermis (upper or outer layer) and the dermis (lower or inner layer).

Melanoma is a disease in which malignant (cancer) cells form in the skin cells called melanocytes (cells that color the skin). Melanocytes are in the layer of basal cells at the deepest part of the epidermis. They make melanin, the pigment that gives skin its natural color. When skin is exposed to the sun, melanocytes make more pigment, causing the skin to tan, or darken.

When melanoma starts in the skin, the disease is called cutaneous melanoma. This chapter is about cutaneous (skin) melanoma. Melanoma may also occur in the eye and is called intraocular or ocular melanoma.

There are three types of skin cancer: melanoma, basal cell skin cancer, and squamous cell skin cancer. Melanoma is more aggressive than basal cell skin cancer or squamous cell skin cancer. Melanoma can occur anywhere on the body.

In men, melanoma is often found on the trunk (the area from the shoulders to the hips) or the head and neck. In women, melanoma often develops on the arms and legs. Melanoma usually occurs in adults, but it is sometimes found in children and adolescents.

Excerpted from PDQ® Cancer Information Summary. National Cancer Institute; Bethesda, MD. "Melanoma Treatment (PDQ) - Patient Version." Updated 07/2010. Available at: http://cancer.gov. Accessed October 23, 2010.

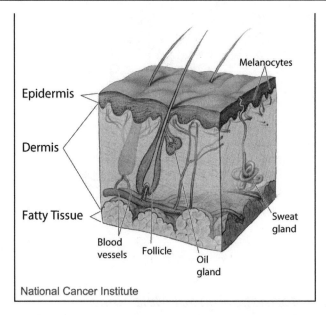

National Cancer Institute

Figure 49.1. *The Skin and Its Layers (image by Don Bliss, National Cancer Institute)*

Risk Factors

Anything that increases your risk of getting a disease is called a risk factor. Having a risk factor does not mean that you will get cancer; not having risk factors doesn't mean that you will not get cancer. People who think they may be at risk should discuss this with their doctor. Risk factors for melanoma include the following:

- Having a fair complexion, which includes the following:
  - Fair skin that freckles and burns easily, does not tan, or tans poorly
  - Blue or green or other light-colored eyes
  - Red or blond hair
- Being exposed to natural sunlight or artificial sunlight (such as from tanning beds) over long periods of time
- Having a history of many blistering sunburns as a child
- Having several large or many small moles
- Having a family history of unusual moles (atypical nevus syndrome)

- Having a family or personal history of melanoma
- Being white and male

Signs and Symptoms

Possible signs of melanoma include a change in the appearance of a mole or pigmented area. These and other symptoms may be caused by melanoma. Other conditions may cause the same symptoms. A doctor should be consulted if any of the following problems occur:

- A mole that:
  - changes in size, shape, or color
  - has irregular edges or borders
  - is more than one color
  - is asymmetrical (if the mole is divided in half, the two halves are different in size or shape)
  - itches
  - oozes, bleeds, or is ulcerated (a hole forms in the skin when the top layer of cells breaks down and the tissue below shows through)
  - Change in pigmented (colored) skin
- Satellite moles (new moles that grow near an existing mole).

Detection

Tests that examine the skin are used to detect and diagnose melanoma. If a mole or pigmented area of the skin changes or looks abnormal, the following tests and procedures can help detect and diagnose melanoma:

Skin examination: A doctor or nurse checks the skin for moles, birthmarks, or other pigmented areas that look abnormal in color, size, shape, or texture.

Biopsy: A local excision is done to remove as much of the suspicious mole or lesion as possible. A pathologist then looks at the tissue under a microscope to check for cancer cells. Because melanoma can be hard to diagnose, patients should consider having their biopsy sample checked by a second pathologist.

Suspicious areas of the skin should be biopsied and not be shaved off or cauterized (destroyed with a hot instrument, an electrical current, or a caustic substance).

Prognosis

Certain factors affect prognosis (chance of recovery) and treatment options. The prognosis and treatment options depend on the following:

- The thickness of the tumor and where it is in the body

- How quickly the cancer cells are dividing

- Whether there was bleeding or ulceration at the primary site

- Whether cancer has spread to the lymph nodes or to other places in the body

- The number of places cancer has spread to in the body and the level of lactate dehydrogenase (LDH) in the blood

- The patient's general health

Although many people are successfully treated, melanoma can recur (come back).

Stages of Melanoma

After melanoma has been diagnosed, tests are done to find out if cancer cells have spread within the skin or to other parts of the body.

The process used to find out whether cancer has spread within the skin or to other parts of the body is called staging. The information gathered from the staging process determines the stage of the disease. It is important to know the stage in order to plan treatment. Talk with your doctor about what the stage of your cancer is. The following tests and procedures may be used in the staging process, and the results of these tests are viewed together with the results of the tumor biopsy to determine the melanoma stage.

Wide local excision: A surgical procedure to remove some of the normal tissue surrounding the area where melanoma was found, to check for cancer cells.

Lymph node mapping and sentinel lymph node biopsy: Procedures in which a radioactive substance and/or blue dye is injected near the tumor. The substance or dye flows through lymph ducts to the sentinel node or nodes (the first lymph node or nodes where cancer cells are likely to have spread). The surgeon removes only the nodes with the radioactive substance or dye. A pathologist then checks the sentinel lymph nodes for cancer cells. If no cancer cells are detected, it may not be necessary to remove additional nodes.

Chest x-ray: An x-ray of the organs and bones inside the chest. An x-ray is a type of energy beam that can go through the body and onto film, making a picture of areas inside the body.

CT scan (CAT scan): A procedure that makes a series of detailed pictures of areas inside the body, taken from different angles. The pictures are made by a computer linked to an x-ray machine. A dye may be injected into a vein or swallowed to help the organs or tissues show up more clearly. This procedure is also called computed tomography, computerized tomography, or computerized axial tomography. For melanoma, pictures may be taken of the chest, abdomen, and pelvis.

MRI (magnetic resonance imaging): A procedure that uses a magnet, radio waves, and a computer to make a series of detailed pictures of areas inside the body. This procedure is also called nuclear magnetic resonance imaging (NMRI).

PET scan (positron emission tomography scan): A procedure to find malignant tumor cells in the body. A small amount of radioactive glucose (sugar) is injected into a vein. The PET scanner rotates around the body and makes a picture of where glucose is being used in the body. Malignant tumor cells show up brighter in the picture because they are more active and take up more glucose than normal cells do.

Laboratory tests: Medical procedures that test samples of tissue, blood, urine, or other substances in the body. These tests help to diagnose disease, plan and check treatment, or monitor the disease over time.

Blood chemistry studies: A procedure in which a blood sample is checked to measure the amounts of certain substances released into the blood by organs and tissues in the body. For melanoma, the blood is checked for an enzyme called lactate dehydrogenase (LDH).

Clark Levels

The Clark levels are used for thin tumors to describe how deeply the cancer has spread into the different layers of the skin:

Level I: The cancer is in the epidermis only.

Level II: The cancer has begun to spread into the papillary dermis (upper layer of the dermis).

Level III: The cancer has spread through the papillary dermis (upper layer of the dermis) into the papillary-reticular dermal interface (the layer between the papillary dermis and the reticular dermis).

Level IV: The cancer has spread into the reticular dermis (lower layer of the dermis).

Level V: The cancer has spread into the subcutaneous layer (below the skin).

Stage 0 (Melanoma in Situ)

Stage 0 melanoma: In stage 0, abnormal melanocytes are found in the epidermis. These abnormal melanocytes may become cancer and spread into nearby normal tissue. Stage 0 is also called melanoma in situ.

Stage I

Stage I is divided into two stages, IA and IB.

In stage IA, the tumor is not more than one millimeter thick (a sharp pencil point is about 1 mm), with no ulceration (break in the skin).

In stage IB, the tumor is either not more than one millimeter thick, with ulceration, OR more than one but not more than two millimeters thick, with no ulceration (a new crayon point is about 2 mm). Skin thickness is different on different parts of the body.

Stage II

Stage II is divided into stages IIA, IIB, and IIC.

In stage IIA, the tumor is either more than one but not more than two millimeters thick, with ulceration; OR more than two but not more than four millimeters thick (smaller than a new pencil eraser, which is about five mm), with no ulceration.

In stage IIB, the tumor is either more than two but not more than four millimeters thick, with ulceration; OR more than four millimeters thick, with no ulceration.

In stage IIC, the tumor is more than four millimeters thick, with ulceration.

Stage III

In stage III, the tumor may be any thickness, with or without ulceration. One or more of the following is true:

- Cancer has spread to one or more lymph nodes.

- Lymph nodes may be joined together (matted).
- Cancer may be in a lymph vessel between the primary tumor and nearby lymph nodes.
- Very small tumors may be found on or under the skin, not more than two centimeters away from where the cancer first started.

Stage IV

In stage IV, the cancer has spread to other places in the body, such as the lung, liver, brain, bone, soft tissue, or gastrointestinal (GI) tract. Cancer may also spread to places in the skin far away from where the cancer first started.

Recurrent Melanoma

Recurrent melanoma is cancer that has recurred (come back) after it has been treated. The cancer may come back in the original site or in other parts of the body, such as the lungs or liver.

Treatment Option Overview

Different types of treatment are available for patients with melanoma. Some treatments are standard (the currently used treatment), and some are being tested in clinical trials. Four types of standard treatment are used.

Surgery

Surgery to remove the tumor is the primary treatment of all stages of melanoma. The doctor may remove the tumor using the following operations:

- **Local excision:** Taking out the melanoma and some of the normal tissue around it. Or possibly a wide local excision, with or without removal of lymph nodes.
- **Lymphadenectomy:** A surgical procedure in which the lymph nodes are removed and examined to see whether they contain cancer.
- **Sentinel lymph node biopsy:** The removal of the sentinel lymph node (the first lymph node the cancer is likely to spread to from the tumor) during surgery. A radioactive substance and/or blue dye is injected near the tumor. The substance or dye

flows through the lymph ducts to the lymph nodes. The first lymph node to receive the substance or dye is removed for biopsy. A pathologist views the tissue under a microscope to look for cancer cells. If cancer cells are not found, it may not be necessary to remove more lymph nodes.

Skin grafting (taking skin from another part of the body to replace the skin that is removed) may be done to cover the wound caused by surgery.

Even if the doctor removes all the melanoma that can be seen at the time of the operation, some patients may be offered chemotherapy after surgery to kill any cancer cells that are left. Chemotherapy given after surgery, to lower the risk that the cancer will come back, is called adjuvant therapy.

Chemotherapy

Chemotherapy is a cancer treatment that uses drugs to stop the growth of cancer cells, either by killing the cells or by stopping them from dividing. When chemotherapy is taken by mouth or injected into a vein or muscle, the drugs enter the bloodstream and can reach cancer cells throughout the body (systemic chemotherapy). When chemotherapy is placed directly into the cerebrospinal fluid, an organ, or a body cavity such as the abdomen, the drugs mainly affect cancer cells in those areas (regional chemotherapy).

In treating melanoma, anticancer drugs may be given as a hyperthermic isolated limb perfusion. This technique sends anticancer drugs directly to the arm or leg in which the cancer is located. The flow of blood to and from the limb is temporarily stopped with a tourniquet, and a warm solution containing anticancer drugs is put directly into the blood of the limb. This allows the patient to receive a high dose of drugs in the area where the cancer occurred.

The way the chemotherapy is given depends on the type and stage of the cancer being treated.

Radiation Therapy

Radiation therapy is a cancer treatment that uses high-energy x-rays or other types of radiation to kill cancer cells or keep them from growing. There are two types of radiation therapy. External radiation therapy uses a machine outside the body to send radiation toward the cancer. Internal radiation therapy uses a radioactive substance sealed in needles, seeds, wires, or catheters that are placed directly into or near the cancer. The way the radiation therapy is given depends on the type and stage of the cancer being treated.

Biologic Therapy

Biologic therapy is a treatment that uses the patient's immune system to fight cancer. Substances made by the body or made in a laboratory are used to boost, direct, or restore the body's natural defenses against cancer. This type of cancer treatment is also called biotherapy or immunotherapy.

Clinical Trials

New types of treatment are being tested in clinical trials. A treatment clinical trial is a research study meant to help improve current treatments or obtain information on new treatments for patients with cancer. When clinical trials show that a new treatment is better than the standard treatment, the new treatment may become the standard treatment. Patients may want to think about taking part in a clinical trial. Some clinical trials are open only to patients who have not started treatment.

This summary section describes treatments that are being studied in clinical trials. It may not mention every new treatment being studied. For additional information, visit the National Cancer Institute's clinical trials website at www.cancer.gov/clinicaltrials.

Chemoimmunotherapy: Chemoimmunotherapy is the use of anticancer drugs combined with biologic therapy to boost the immune system to kill cancer cells.

Targeted therapy: Targeted therapy is a type of treatment that uses drugs or other substances to identify and attack specific cancer cells without harming normal cells. Monoclonal antibody therapy is a type of targeted therapy being studied in the treatment of melanoma.

Monoclonal antibody therapy is a cancer treatment that uses antibodies made in the laboratory, from a single type of immune system cell. These antibodies can identify substances on cancer cells or normal substances that may help cancer cells grow. The antibodies attach to the substances and kill the cancer cells, block their growth, or keep them from spreading. Monoclonal antibodies are given by infusion. They may be used alone or to carry drugs, toxins, or radioactive material directly to cancer cells. Monoclonal antibodies may be used in combination with chemotherapy as adjuvant therapy.

Vaccine therapy: Vaccine therapy is a type of biologic therapy. Cancer vaccines work by helping the immune system recognize and attack specific types of cancer cells. Vaccine therapy can also be a type of targeted therapy.

Follow-Up Tests

Some of the tests that were done to diagnose the cancer or to find out the stage of the cancer may be repeated. Some tests will be repeated in order to see how well the treatment is working. Decisions about whether to continue, change, or stop treatment may be based on the results of these tests. This is sometimes called re-staging.

Some of the tests will continue to be done from time to time after treatment has ended. The results of these tests can show if your condition has changed or if the cancer has recurred (come back). These tests are sometimes called follow-up tests or check-ups.

Chapter 50

Non-Melanoma Skin Cancer

The Skin

The skin is the body's largest organ. It protects against heat, light, injury, and infection. It helps control body temperature. It stores water and fat. The skin also makes vitamin D. The skin has two main layers (the layers of the skin are illustrated in Figure 49.1 in the previous chapter).

Epidermis: The epidermis is the top layer of the skin. It is mostly made of flat cells. These are squamous cells. Under the squamous cells in the deepest part of the epidermis are round cells called basal cells. Cells called melanocytes make the pigment (color) found in skin and are located in the lower part of the epidermis.

Dermis: The dermis is under the epidermis. It contains blood vessels, lymph vessels, and glands. Some of these glands make sweat, which helps cool the body. Other glands make sebum. Sebum is an oily substance that helps keep the skin from drying out. Sweat and sebum reach the surface of the skin through tiny openings called pores.

Understanding Skin Cancer

Skin cancer begins in cells, the building blocks that make up the skin. Normally, skin cells grow and divide to form new cells. Every day skin cells grow old and die, and new cells take their place.

Excerpted from "What You Need to Know About Skin Cancer," National Cancer Institute (www.cancer.gov), July 2009.

Sometimes, this orderly process goes wrong. New cells form when the skin does not need them, and old or damaged cells do not die when they should. These extra cells can form a mass of tissue called a growth or tumor.

Growths or tumors can be benign or malignant. Benign growths are not cancer. Benign growths are rarely life-threatening. Generally, benign growths can be removed. They usually do not grow back. Cells from benign growths do not invade the tissues around them. Cells from benign growths do not spread to other parts of the body.

Malignant growths are cancer. Malignant growths are generally more serious than benign growths. They may be life-threatening. However, the two most common types of skin cancer cause only about one out of every thousand deaths from cancer. Malignant growths often can be removed. But sometimes they grow back. Cells from malignant growths can invade and damage nearby tissues and organs. Cells from some malignant growths can spread to other parts of the body. The spread of cancer is called metastasis.

Types of Skin Cancer

Skin cancers are named for the type of cells that become cancerous. The two most common types of skin cancer are basal cell cancer and squamous cell cancer. These cancers usually form on the head, face, neck, hands, and arms. These areas are exposed to the sun. But skin cancer can occur anywhere.

Basal cell skin cancer grows slowly. It usually occurs on areas of the skin that have been in the sun. It is most common on the face. Basal cell cancer rarely spreads to other parts of the body.

Squamous cell skin cancer also occurs on parts of the skin that have been in the sun. But it also may be in places that are not in the sun. Squamous cell cancer sometimes spreads to lymph nodes and organs inside the body.

If skin cancer spreads from its original place to another part of the body, the new growth has the same kind of abnormal cells and the same name as the primary growth. It is still called skin cancer.

Risk Factors

Doctors cannot explain why one person develops skin cancer and another does not. However, we do know that skin cancer is not contagious. You cannot "catch" it from another person.

Research has shown that people with certain risk factors are more likely than others to develop skin cancer. A risk factor is something that may increase the chance of developing a disease. Studies have found the following risk factors for skin cancer.

Ultraviolet (UV) radiation: UV radiation comes from the sun, sunlamps, tanning beds, or tanning booths. A person's risk of skin cancer is related to lifetime exposure to UV radiation. Most skin cancer appears after age 50, but the sun damages the skin from an early age.

UV radiation affects everyone. But people who have fair skin that freckles or burns easily are at greater risk. These people often also have red or blond hair and light-colored eyes. But even people who tan can get skin cancer.

People who live in areas that get high levels of UV radiation have a higher risk of skin cancer. In the United States, areas in the south (such as Texas and Florida) get more UV radiation than areas in the north (such as Minnesota). Also, people who live in the mountains get high levels of UV radiation. UV radiation is present even in cold weather or on a cloudy day.

Actinic keratosis: Actinic keratosis is a type of flat, scaly growth on the skin. It is most often found on areas exposed to the sun, especially the face and the backs of the hands. The growths may appear as rough red or brown patches on the skin. They may also appear as cracking or peeling of the lower lip that does not heal. Without treatment, a small number of these scaly growths may turn into squamous cell cancer.

Bowen's disease: Bowen's disease is a type of scaly or thickened patch on the skin. It may turn into squamous cell skin cancer.

Other risk factors: Other risk factors for skin cancer include the following:

- Scars or burns on the skin
- Infection with certain human papillomaviruses
- Exposure to arsenic at work
- Chronic skin inflammation or skin ulcers
- Diseases that make the skin sensitive to the sun, such as xeroderma pigmentosum, albinism, and basal cell nevus syndrome
- Radiation Therapy
- Medical conditions or drugs that suppress the immune system
- Personal history of one or more skin cancers
- Family history of skin cancer

If you think you may be at risk for skin cancer, you should discuss this concern with your doctor. Your doctor may be able to suggest ways to reduce your risk and can plan a schedule for checkups.

Prevention

The best way to prevent skin cancer is to protect yourself from the sun. Also, protect children from an early age. Doctors suggest that people of all ages limit their time in the sun and avoid other sources of UV radiation:

- It is best to stay out of the midday sun (from mid-morning to late afternoon) whenever you can. You also should protect yourself from UV radiation reflected by sand, water, snow, and ice. UV radiation can go through light clothing, windshields, windows, and clouds.

- Wear long sleeves and long pants of tightly woven fabrics, a hat with a wide brim, and sunglasses that absorb UV.

- Use sunscreen lotions. Sunscreen may help prevent skin cancer, especially broad-spectrum sunscreen (to filter UVB and UVA rays) with a sun protection factor (SPF) of at least 15. But you still need to avoid the sun and wear clothing to protect your skin.

- Stay away from sunlamps and tanning booths.

Symptoms

A change on the skin is the most common sign of skin cancer. This may be a new growth, a sore that doesn't heal, or a change in an old growth. Not all skin cancers look the same. Skin changes to watch for include the following:

- Small, smooth, shiny, pale, or waxy lump
- Firm, red lump
- Sore or lump that bleeds or develops a crust or a scab
- Flat red spot that is rough, dry, or scaly and may become itchy or tender
- Red or brown patch that is rough and scaly
- Sometimes skin cancer is painful, but usually it is not

Checking your skin for new growths or other changes is a good idea. Keep in mind that changes are not a sure sign of skin cancer. Still, you should report any changes to your health care provider right away. You may need to see a dermatologist, a doctor who has special training in the diagnosis and treatment of skin problems.

Diagnosis

If you have a change on the skin, the doctor must find out whether it is due to cancer or to some other cause. Your doctor removes all or part of the area that does not look normal. The sample goes to a lab. A pathologist checks the sample under a microscope. This is a biopsy. A biopsy is the only sure way to diagnose skin cancer.

You may have the biopsy in a doctor's office or as an outpatient in a clinic or hospital. Where it is done depends on the size and place of the abnormal area on your skin. You probably will have local anesthesia.

There are four common types of skin biopsies:

- **Punch biopsy:** The doctor uses a sharp, hollow tool to remove a circle of tissue from the abnormal area.

- **Incisional biopsy:** The doctor uses a scalpel to remove part of the growth.

- **Excisional biopsy:** The doctor uses a scalpel to remove the entire growth and some tissue around it.

- **Shave biopsy:** The doctor uses a thin, sharp blade to shave off the abnormal growth.

You may want to ask your doctor these questions before having a biopsy:

- Which type of biopsy do you recommend for me?

- How will the biopsy be done?

- Will I have to go to the hospital?

- How long will it take? Will I be awake? Will it hurt?

- Are there any risks? What are the chances of infection or bleeding after the biopsy?

- What will my scar look like?

- How soon will I know the results? Who will explain them to me?

Staging Skin Cancer

If the biopsy shows that you have cancer, your doctor needs to know the extent (stage) of the disease. In very few cases, the doctor may check your lymph nodes to stage the cancer. The stage is based on the size of the growth, how deeply it has grown beneath the top layer of skin, and whether it has spread to nearby lymph nodes or to other parts of the body.

These are the stages of skin cancer:

Stage 0: The cancer involves only the top layer of skin. It is carcinoma in situ.

Stage I: The growth is two centimeters wide (three-quarters of an inch) or smaller.

Stage II: The growth is larger than two centimeters wide (three-quarters of an inch).

Stage III: The cancer has spread below the skin to cartilage, muscle, bone, or to nearby lymph nodes. It has not spread to other places in the body.

Stage IV: The cancer has spread to other places in the body.

Treatment Options

Sometimes all of the cancer is removed during the biopsy. In such cases, no more treatment is needed. If you do need more treatment, your doctor will describe your options.

Treatment for skin cancer depends on the type and stage of the disease, the size and place of the growth, and your general health and medical history. In most cases, the aim of treatment is to remove or destroy the cancer completely. Many skin cancers can be removed quickly and easily.

Your doctor may refer you to a specialist, or you may ask for a referral. Specialists who treat skin cancer include dermatologists, surgeons, and radiation oncologists. You may want to talk to your doctor about taking part in a clinical trial, a research study of new ways to treat cancer or prevent it from coming back.

Your doctor can describe your treatment choices and what to expect. You and your doctor can work together to develop a treatment plan that meets your needs.

Surgery is the usual treatment for people with skin cancer. In some cases, the doctor may suggest topical chemotherapy, photodynamic therapy, or radiation therapy.

Because skin cancer treatment may damage healthy cells and tissues, unwanted side effects sometimes occur. Side effects depend mainly on the type and extent of the treatment. Side effects may not be the same for each person. Before treatment starts, your doctor will tell you about possible side effects and suggest ways to help you manage them.

Surgery

Surgery to treat skin cancer may be done in one of several ways. The method your doctor uses depends on the size and place of the growth and other factors. Your doctor can further describe these types of surgery:

- **Excisional skin surgery** is a common treatment to remove skin cancer. After numbing the area, the surgeon removes the growth with a scalpel. The surgeon also removes a border of skin around the growth. This skin is the margin. The margin is examined under a microscope to be certain that all the cancer cells have been removed. The size of the margin depends on the size of the growth.

- **Mohs surgery** (also called Mohs micrographic surgery) is often used for skin cancer. The area of the growth is numbed. A specially trained surgeon shaves away thin layers of the growth. Each layer is immediately examined under a microscope. The surgeon continues to shave away tissue until no cancer cells can be seen under the microscope. In this way, the surgeon can remove all the cancer and only a small bit of healthy tissue.

- **Electrodesiccation and curettage** is often used to remove small basal cell skin cancers. The doctor numbs the area to be treated. The cancer is removed with a sharp tool shaped like a spoon. This tool is a curette. An electric current is sent into the treated area to control bleeding and kill any cancer cells that may be left. Electrodesiccation and curettage is usually a fast and simple procedure.

- **Cryosurgery** is often used for people who are not able to have other types of surgery. It uses extreme cold to treat early stage or very thin skin cancer. Liquid nitrogen creates the cold. The doctor applies liquid nitrogen directly to the skin growth. This treatment may cause swelling. It also may damage nerves, which can cause a loss of feeling in the damaged area.

- **Laser surgery** uses a narrow beam of light to remove or destroy cancer cells. It is most often used for growths that are on the outer layer of skin only.

Grafts are sometimes needed to close an opening in the skin left by surgery. The surgeon first numbs and then removes a patch of healthy skin from another part of the body, such as the upper thigh. The patch is then used to cover the area where skin cancer was removed. If you have a skin graft, you may have to take special care of the area until it heals.

The time it takes to heal after surgery is different for each person. You may be uncomfortable for the first few days. However, medicine can usually control the pain. Before surgery, you should discuss the plan for pain relief with your doctor or nurse. After surgery, your doctor can adjust the plan if you need more pain relief.

Surgery nearly always leaves some type of scar. The size and color of the scar depend on the size of the cancer, the type of surgery, and how your skin heals.

For any type of surgery, including skin grafts or reconstructive surgery, it is important to follow your doctor's advice on bathing, shaving, exercise, or other activities.

You may want to ask your doctor these questions about surgery:

- What kind of surgery will I have?

- Will I need a skin graft?

- What will the scar look like? Can anything be done to help reduce the scar? Will I need plastic surgery or reconstructive surgery?

- How will I feel after the operation?

- If I have pain, how will it be controlled?

- Will I have to stay in the hospital?

- Am I likely to have infection, swelling, blistering, or bleeding, or to get a scab where the cancer was removed?

Topical Chemotherapy

Chemotherapy uses anticancer drugs to kill skin cancer cells. When a drug is put directly on the skin, the treatment is topical chemotherapy. It is most often used when the skin cancer is too large for surgery. It is also used when the doctor keeps finding new cancers.

Most often, the drug comes in a cream or lotion. It is usually applied to the skin one or two times a day for several weeks. A drug called fluorouracil (5-FU) is used to treat basal cell and squamous cell cancers that are in the top layer of the skin only. A drug called imiquimod also is used to treat basal cell cancer only in the top layer of skin.

These drugs may cause your skin to turn red or swell. It also may itch, hurt, ooze, or develop a rash. It may be sore or sensitive to the sun. These skin changes usually go away after treatment is over. Topical chemotherapy usually does not leave a scar. If healthy skin becomes too red or raw when the skin cancer is treated, your doctor may stop treatment.

You may want to ask your doctor these questions about topical chemotherapy:

- Do I need to take special care when I put chemotherapy on my skin? What do I need to do? Will I be sensitive to the sun?

- When will treatment start? When will it end?

Photodynamic Therapy

Photodynamic therapy (PDT) uses a chemical along with a special light source, such as a laser light, to kill cancer cells. The chemical is a photosensitizing agent. A cream is applied to the skin or the chemical is injected. It stays in cancer cells longer than in normal cells. Several hours or days later, the special light is focused on the growth. The chemical becomes active and destroys nearby cancer cells.

PDT is used to treat cancer on or very near the surface of the skin. The side effects of PDT are usually not serious. PDT may cause burning or stinging pain. It also may cause burns, swelling, or redness. It may scar healthy tissue near the growth. If you have PDT, you will need to avoid direct sunlight and bright indoor light for at least six weeks after treatment.

You may want to ask your doctor these questions about PDT:

- Will I need to stay in the hospital while the chemical is in my body?

- Will I need to have the treatment more than once?

Radiation Therapy

Radiation therapy (also called radiotherapy) uses high-energy rays to kill cancer cells. The rays come from a large machine outside the body. They affect cells only in the treated area. This treatment is given at a hospital or clinic in one dose or many doses over several weeks.

Radiation is not a common treatment for skin cancer. But it may be used for skin cancer in areas where surgery could be difficult or leave a bad scar. You may have this treatment if you have a growth on your eyelid, ear, or nose. It also may be used if the cancer comes back after surgery to remove it.

Side effects depend mainly on the dose of radiation and the part of your body that is treated. During treatment your skin in the treated area may become red, dry, and tender. Your doctor can suggest ways to relieve the side effects of radiation therapy.

You may want to ask your doctor these questions about radiation therapy:

- How will I feel after the radiation?

- Am I likely to have infection, swelling, blistering, or bleeding, or to get a scar in the treated area?

- How should I take care of the treated area?

Getting a Second Opinion

Before you have treatment, you might want a second opinion about the diagnosis and treatment plan. Many insurance companies cover a second opinion if you or your doctor requests it. It may take some time and effort to gather medical records and arrange to see another doctor. Usually it is not a problem to take several weeks to get a second opinion. In most cases, the delay will not make treatment less effective. To make sure, you should discuss this delay with your doctor. Sometimes people with skin cancer need treatment right away.

There are a number of ways to find a doctor for a second opinion. Your doctor may refer you to one or more specialists. At cancer centers, several specialists often work together as a team.

You may want to ask the doctor these questions before treatment begins:

- What is the stage of the disease?

- What are my treatment choices? Which do you recommend for me? Why?

- What are the expected benefits of each kind of treatment?

- What are the risks and possible side effects of each treatment? What can we do to control my side effects?

- Will the treatment affect my appearance? If so, can a reconstructive surgeon or plastic surgeon help?

- Will treatment affect my normal activities? If so, for how long?

- What is the treatment likely to cost? Does my insurance cover this treatment?

- How often should I have checkups?

- Would a clinical trial (research study) be appropriate for me?

Follow-Up Care

Follow-up care after treatment for skin cancer is important. Your doctor will monitor your recovery and check for new skin cancer. New skin cancers are more common than having a treated skin cancer spread. Regular checkups help ensure that any changes in your health are noted and treated if needed. Between scheduled visits, you should check your skin regularly. You will find a guide for checking your skin below. You should contact the doctor if you notice anything unusual. It also is important to follow your doctor's advice about how to reduce your risk of developing skin cancer again.

How to Do a Skin Self-Exam

Your doctor or nurse may suggest that you do a regular skin self-exam to check for skin cancer, including melanoma.

The best time to do this exam is after a shower or bath. You should check your skin in a room with plenty of light. You should use a full-length mirror and a hand-held mirror. It's best to begin by learning where your birthmarks, moles, and other marks are and their usual look and feel.

Check for anything new:

- New mole (that looks different from your other moles)

- New red or darker color flaky patch that may be a little raised

- New flesh-colored firm bump

- Change in the size, shape, color, or feel of a mole

- Sore that does not heal

Check yourself from head to toe. Don't forget to check your back, scalp, genital area, and between your buttocks.

Look at your face, neck, ears, and scalp. You may want to use a comb or a blow dryer to move your hair so that you can see better. You also may want to have a relative or friend check through your hair. It may be hard to check your scalp by yourself. Look at the front and back of your body in the mirror. Then, raise your arms and look at your left and right sides.

Bend your elbows. Look carefully at your fingernails, palms, forearms (including the undersides), and upper arms. Examine the back, front, and sides of your legs. Also look around your genital area and between your buttocks.

Sit and closely examine your feet, including your toenails, your soles, and the spaces between your toes.

By checking your skin regularly, you will learn what is normal for you. It may be helpful to record the dates of your skin exams and to write notes about the way your skin looks. If your doctor has taken photos of your skin, you can compare your skin to the photos to help check for changes. If you find anything unusual, see your doctor.

Chapter 51

Merkel Cell Carcinoma

General Information about Merkel Cell Carcinoma

Merkel cells are found in the top layer of the skin. These cells are very close to the nerve endings that receive the sensation of touch. Merkel cell carcinoma, also called neuroendocrine carcinoma of the skin or trabecular cancer, is a very rare type of skin cancer that forms when Merkel cells grow out of control. Merkel cell carcinoma starts most often in areas of skin exposed to the sun, especially the head and neck, as well as the arms, legs, and trunk.

Merkel cell carcinoma tends to grow quickly and to metastasize (spread) at an early stage. It usually spreads first to nearby lymph nodes and then may spread to lymph nodes or skin in distant parts of the body, lungs, brain, bones, or other organs.

Risk Factors and Signs

Sun exposure and having a weak immune system can affect the risk of developing Merkel cell carcinoma. Anything that increases your risk of getting a disease is called a risk factor. Having a risk factor does not mean that you will get cancer; not having risk factors doesn't mean that you will not get cancer. People who think they may be at

Excerpted from PDQ® Cancer Information Summary. National Cancer Institute; Bethesda, MD. "Merkel Cell Carcinoma Treatment (PDQ) - Patient Version." Updated 09/2010. Available at: http://cancer.gov. Accessed October 24, 2010.

risk should discuss this with their doctor. Risk factors for Merkel cell carcinoma include the following:

- Being exposed to a lot of natural sunlight

- Being exposed to artificial sunlight, such as from tanning beds or psoralen and ultraviolet A (PUVA) therapy for psoriasis

- Having an immune system weakened by disease, such as chronic lymphocytic leukemia or HIV infection

- Taking drugs that make the immune system less active, such as after an organ transplant

- Having a history of other types of cancer

- Being older than 50 years, male, or white

Merkel cell carcinoma usually appears as a single painless lump on sun-exposed skin. This and other changes in the skin may be caused by Merkel cell carcinoma. Other conditions may cause the same symptoms. A doctor should be consulted if changes in the skin are seen.

Merkel cell carcinoma usually appears on sun-exposed skin as a single lump that has these characteristics:

- Fast-growing

- Painless

- Firm and dome-shaped or raised

- Red or violet in color

Detection and Diagnosis

Tests and procedures that examine the skin are used to detect (find) and diagnose Merkel cell carcinoma. The following tests and procedures may be used:

Physical exam and history: An exam of the body to check general signs of health, including checking for signs of disease, such as lumps or anything else that seems unusual. A history of the patient's health habits and past illnesses and treatments will also be taken.

Full-body skin exam: A doctor or nurse checks the skin for bumps or spots that look abnormal in color, size, shape, or texture. The size, shape, and texture of the lymph nodes will also be checked.

Biopsy: The removal of cells or tissues so they can be viewed under a microscope by a pathologist to check for signs of cancer.

Prognosis

Certain factors affect prognosis (chance of recovery) and treatment options. The prognosis and treatment options depend on the stage of the cancer (the size of the tumor and whether it has spread to the lymph nodes or other parts of the body), where the cancer is in the body, whether the cancer has just been diagnosed or has recurred (come back), and the patient's age and general health. Prognosis also depends on how deeply the tumor has grown into the skin.

Stages of Merkel Cell Carcinoma

After Merkel cell carcinoma has been diagnosed, tests are done to find out if cancer cells have spread to other parts of the body.

The process used to find out if cancer has spread to other parts of the body is called staging. The information gathered from the staging process determines the stage of the disease. It is important to know the stage in order to plan treatment. The following tests and procedures may be used in the staging process:

- **CT scan (CAT scan):** A procedure that makes a series of detailed pictures of areas inside the body, taken from different angles. The pictures are made by a computer linked to an x-ray machine. A dye may be injected into a vein or swallowed to help the organs or tissues show up more clearly. A CT scan of the chest and abdomen may be used to check for primary small cell lung cancer, or to find Merkel cell carcinoma that has spread. A CT scan of the head and neck may also be used to find Merkel cell carcinoma that has spread to the lymph nodes. This procedure is also called computed tomography, computerized tomography, or computerized axial tomography.

- **MRI (magnetic resonance imaging):** A procedure that uses a magnet, radio waves, and a computer to make a series of detailed pictures of areas inside the body. This procedure is also called nuclear magnetic resonance imaging (NMRI).

- **PET scan (positron emission tomography scan):** A procedure to find malignant tumor cells in the body. A small amount of radioactive glucose (sugar) is injected into a vein. The PET scanner rotates around the body and makes a picture of where glucose is being used in the body. Malignant tumor cells show up brighter in the picture because they are more active and take up more glucose than normal cells do.

673

- **Octreotide scan:** A type of radionuclide scan used to find carcinomas and other types of tumors. A small amount of radioactive octreotide (a hormone that attaches to carcinoid tumors) is injected into a vein and travels through the bloodstream. The radioactive octreotide attaches to the tumor and a special camera that detects radioactivity is used to show where the tumor cells are in the body.

- **Lymph node biopsy:** There are two main types of lymph node biopsy used to stage Merkel cell carcinoma.

- **Sentinel lymph node biopsy:** The removal of the sentinel lymph node during surgery. The sentinel lymph node is the first lymph node to receive lymphatic drainage from a tumor. It is the first lymph node the cancer is likely to spread to from the tumor. A radioactive substance and/or blue dye is injected near the tumor. The substance or dye flows through the lymph ducts to the lymph nodes. The first lymph node to receive the substance or dye is removed. A pathologist views the tissue under a microscope to look for cancer cells. If cancer cells are not found, it may not be necessary to remove more lymph nodes.

- **Lymph node dissection:** A surgical procedure in which the lymph nodes are removed and a sample of tissue is checked under a microscope for signs of cancer. For a regional lymph node dissection, some of the lymph nodes in the tumor area are removed. For a radical lymph node dissection, most or all of the lymph nodes in the tumor area are removed. This procedure is also called lymphadenectomy.

The following stages are used for Merkel cell carcinoma.

Stage 0 (Carcinoma in Situ): In stage 0, the tumor is a group of abnormal cells that remain in the place where they first formed and have not spread. These abnormal cells may become cancer and spread to lymph nodes or distant parts of the body.

Stage IA: In stage IA, the tumor is two centimeters or smaller at its widest point and no cancer is found when the lymph nodes are checked under a microscope.

Stage IB: In stage IB, the tumor is two centimeters or smaller at its widest point and no swollen lymph nodes are found by a physical exam or imaging tests.

Stage IIA: In stage IIA, the tumor is larger than two centimeters and no cancer is found when the lymph nodes are checked under a microscope.

Stage IIB: In stage IIB, the tumor is larger than two centimeters and no swollen lymph nodes are found by a physical exam or imaging tests.

Stage IIC: In stage IIC, the tumor may be any size and has spread to nearby bone, muscle, connective tissue, or cartilage. It has not spread to lymph nodes or distant parts of the body.

Stage IIIA: In stage IIIA, the tumor may be any size and may have spread to nearby bone, muscle, connective tissue, or cartilage. Cancer is found in the lymph nodes when they are checked under a microscope.

Stage IIIB: In stage IIIB, the tumor may be any size and may have spread to nearby bone, muscle, connective tissue, or cartilage. Cancer has spread to the lymph nodes near the tumor and is found by a physical exam or imaging test. The lymph nodes are removed and cancer is found in the lymph nodes when they are checked under a microscope. There may also be a second tumor, which is either:

- Between the primary tumor and nearby lymph nodes; or
- Farther away from the center of the body than the primary tumor is.

Stage IV: In stage IV, the tumor may be any size and has spread to distant parts of the body, such as the liver, lung, bone, or brain.

Recurrent Merkel Cell Carcinoma: Recurrent Merkel cell carcinoma is cancer that has recurred (come back) after it has been treated. The cancer may come back in the skin, lymph nodes, or other parts of the body. It is common for Merkel cell carcinoma to recur.

Treatment Option Overview

Different types of treatments are available for patients with Merkel cell carcinoma. Some treatments are standard (the currently used treatment), and some are being tested in clinical trials. A treatment clinical trial is a research study meant to help improve current treatments or obtain information on new treatments for patients with cancer. When clinical trials show that a new treatment is better than the standard treatment, the new treatment may become the standard treatment. Patients may want to think about taking part in a clinical trial. Some clinical trials are open only to patients who have not started treatment. Three types of standard treatment are used.

Surgery

One or more of the following surgical procedures may be used to treat Merkel cell carcinoma:

- **Wide local excision:** The cancer is cut from the skin along with some of the tissue around it. A sentinel lymph node biopsy may be done during the wide local excision procedure. If there is cancer in the lymph nodes, a lymph node dissection also may be done.

- **Lymph node dissection:** A surgical procedure in which the lymph nodes are removed and a sample of tissue is checked under a microscope for signs of cancer. For a regional lymph node dissection, some of the lymph nodes in the tumor area are removed; for a radical lymph node dissection, most or all of the lymph nodes in the tumor area are removed. This procedure is also called lymphadenectomy.

Even if the doctor removes all the cancer that can be seen at the time of the surgery, some patients may be given chemotherapy or radiation therapy after surgery to kill any cancer cells that are left. Treatment given after the surgery, to lower the risk that the cancer will come back, is called adjuvant therapy.

Radiation Therapy

Radiation therapy is a cancer treatment that uses high-energy x-rays or other types of radiation to kill cancer cells. There are two types of radiation therapy. External radiation therapy uses a machine outside the body to send radiation toward the cancer. Internal radiation therapy uses a radioactive substance sealed in needles, seeds, wires, or catheters that are placed directly into or near the cancer. The way the radiation therapy is given depends on the type and stage of the cancer being treated.

Chemotherapy

Chemotherapy is a cancer treatment that uses drugs to stop the growth of cancer cells, either by killing the cells or by stopping the cells from dividing. When chemotherapy is taken by mouth or injected into a vein or muscle, the drugs enter the bloodstream and can reach cancer cells throughout the body (systemic chemotherapy). When chemotherapy is placed directly into the cerebrospinal fluid, an organ, or a body cavity such as the abdomen, the drugs mainly affect cancer cells in those areas (regional chemotherapy). The way the chemotherapy is given depends on the type and stage of the cancer being treated. New types of treatment are being tested in clinical trials.

Clinical Trials

Patients may want to think about taking part in a clinical trial. For some patients, taking part in a clinical trial may be the best treatment choice. Clinical trials are part of the cancer research process. Clinical trials are done to find out if new cancer treatments are safe and effective or better than the standard treatment.

Many of today's standard treatments for cancer are based on earlier clinical trials. Patients who take part in a clinical trial may receive the standard treatment or be among the first to receive a new treatment.

Patients who take part in clinical trials also help improve the way cancer will be treated in the future. Even when clinical trials do not lead to effective new treatments, they often answer important questions and help move research forward.

Patients can enter clinical trials before, during, or after starting their cancer treatment.

Some clinical trials only include patients who have not yet received treatment. Other trials test treatments for patients whose cancer has not gotten better. There are also clinical trials that test new ways to stop cancer from recurring (coming back) or reduce the side effects of cancer treatment.

Clinical trials are taking place in many parts of the country. For more information about clinical trials, visit the National Cancer Institute's clinical trials website at www.cancer.gov/clinicaltrials.

Follow-Up Tests

Some of the tests that were done to diagnose the cancer or to find out the stage of the cancer may be repeated. Some tests will be repeated in order to see how well the treatment is working. Decisions about whether to continue, change, or stop treatment may be based on the results of these tests. This is sometimes called re-staging.

Some of the tests will continue to be done from time to time after treatment has ended. The results of these tests can show if your condition has changed or if the cancer has recurred (come back). These tests are sometimes called follow-up tests or check-ups.

Chapter 52

Bone Cancers

Chapter Contents

Section 52.1

Questions and Answers About Bone Cancer

Excerpted from "Bone Cancer: Questions and Answers,"
National Cancer Institute (www.cancer.gov), March 2008.

What is bone cancer?

Bone cancer is a malignant (cancerous) tumor of the bone that destroys normal bone tissue. Not all bone tumors are malignant. In fact, benign (noncancerous) bone tumors are more common than malignant ones. Both malignant and benign bone tumors may grow and compress healthy bone tissue, but benign tumors do not spread, do not destroy bone tissue, and are rarely a threat to life.

Malignant tumors that begin in bone tissue are called primary bone cancer. Cancer that metastasizes (spreads) to the bones from other parts of the body, such as the breast, lung, or prostate, is called metastatic cancer, and is named for the organ or tissue in which it began. Primary bone cancer is far less common than cancer that spreads to the bones.

Are there different types of primary bone cancer?

Yes. Cancer can begin in any type of bone tissue. Bones are made up of osteoid (hard or compact), cartilaginous (tough, flexible), and fibrous (threadlike) tissue, as well as elements of bone marrow (soft, spongy tissue in the center of most bones).

Common types of primary bone cancer include:

- Osteosarcoma, which arises from osteoid tissue in the bone. This tumor occurs most often in the knee and upper arm.

- Chondrosarcoma, which begins in cartilaginous tissue. Cartilage pads the ends of bones and lines the joints. Chondrosarcoma occurs most often in the pelvis (located between the hip bones), upper leg, and shoulder. Sometimes a chondrosarcoma contains cancerous bone cells. In that case, doctors classify the tumor as an osteosarcoma.

- The Ewing sarcoma family of tumors (ESFTs), which usually occur in bone but may also arise in soft tissue (muscle, fat, fibrous tissue, blood vessels, or other supporting tissue). Scientists think that ESFTs arise from elements of primitive nerve tissue in the bone or soft tissue. ESFTs occur most commonly along the backbone and pelvis and in the legs and arms.

Other types of cancer that arise in soft tissue are called soft tissue sarcomas. For more information about soft tissue sarcomas, see chapter 53.

What are the possible causes of bone cancer?

Although bone cancer does not have a clearly defined cause, researchers have identified several factors that increase the likelihood of developing these tumors. Osteosarcoma occurs more frequently in people who have had high-dose external radiation therapy or treatment with certain anticancer drugs; children seem to be particularly susceptible. A small number of bone cancers are due to heredity. For example, children who have had hereditary retinoblastoma (an uncommon cancer of the eye) are at a higher risk of developing osteosarcoma, particularly if they are treated with radiation. Additionally, people who have hereditary defects of bones and people with metal implants, which doctors sometimes use to repair fractures, are more likely to develop osteosarcoma. Ewing sarcoma is not strongly associated with any heredity cancer syndromes, congenital childhood diseases, or previous radiation exposure.

How often does bone cancer occur?

Primary bone cancer is rare. It accounts for much less than 1% of all cancers. About 2,300 new cases of primary bone cancer are diagnosed in the United States each year. Different types of bone cancer are more likely to occur in certain populations:

- Osteosarcoma occurs most commonly between ages 10 and 19. However, people over age 40 who have other conditions, such as Paget disease (a benign condition characterized by abnormal development of new bone cells), are at increased risk of developing this cancer.

- Chondrosarcoma occurs mainly in older adults (over age 40). The risk increases with advancing age. This disease rarely occurs in children and adolescents.

- ESFTs occur most often in children and adolescents under 19 years of age. Boys are affected more often than girls. These tumors are extremely rare in African American children.

What are the symptoms of bone cancer?

Pain is the most common symptom of bone cancer, but not all bone cancers cause pain. Persistent or unusual pain or swelling in or near a bone can be caused by cancer or by other conditions. It is important to see a doctor to determine the cause.

How is bone cancer diagnosed?

To help diagnose bone cancer, the doctor asks about the patient's personal and family medical history. The doctor also performs a physical examination and may order laboratory and other diagnostic tests. These tests may include:

- X-rays, which can show the location, size, and shape of a bone tumor. If x-rays suggest that an abnormal area may be cancer, the doctor is likely to recommend special imaging tests. Even if x-rays suggest that an abnormal area is benign, the doctor may want to do further tests, especially if the patient is experiencing unusual or persistent pain.

  - A bone scan, which is a test in which a small amount of radioactive material is injected into a blood vessel and travels through the bloodstream; it then collects in the bones and is detected by a scanner.

  - A computed tomography (CT or CAT) scan, which is a series of detailed pictures of areas inside the body, taken from different angles, that are created by a computer linked to an x-ray machine.

  - A magnetic resonance imaging (MRI) procedure, which uses a powerful magnet linked to a computer to create detailed pictures of areas inside the body without using x-rays.

  - A positron emission tomography (PET) scan, in which a small amount of radioactive glucose (sugar) is injected into a vein, and a scanner is used to make detailed, computerized pictures of areas inside the body where the glucose is used. Because cancer cells often use more glucose than normal cells, the pictures can be used to find cancer cells in the body.

- An angiogram, which is an x-ray of blood vessels.

- Biopsy (removal of a tissue sample from the bone tumor) to determine whether cancer is present. The surgeon may perform a needle biopsy or an incisional biopsy. During a needle biopsy, the surgeon makes a small hole in the bone and removes a sample of tissue from the tumor with a needle-like instrument. In an incisional biopsy, the surgeon cuts into the tumor and removes a sample of tissue. Biopsies are best done by an orthopedic oncologist (a doctor experienced in the treatment of bone cancer). A pathologist (a doctor who identifies disease by studying cells and tissues under a microscope) examines the tissue to determine whether it is cancerous.

- Blood tests to determine the level of an enzyme called alkaline phosphatase. A large amount of this enzyme is present in the blood when the cells that form bone tissue are very active—when children are growing, when a broken bone is mending, or when a disease or tumor causes production of abnormal bone tissue. Because high levels of alkaline phosphatase are normal in growing children and adolescents, this test is not a completely reliable indicator of bone cancer.

What are the treatment options for bone cancer?

Treatment options depend on the type, size, location, and stage of the cancer, as well as the person's age and general health. Treatment options for bone cancer include surgery, chemotherapy, radiation therapy, and cryosurgery.

- Surgery is the usual treatment for bone cancer. The surgeon removes the entire tumor with negative margins (no cancer cells are found at the edge or border of the tissue removed during surgery). The surgeon may also use special surgical techniques to minimize the amount of healthy tissue removed with the tumor. Dramatic improvements in surgical techniques and preoperative tumor treatment have made it possible for most patients with bone cancer in an arm or leg to avoid radical surgical procedures (removal of the entire limb). However, most patients who undergo limb-sparing surgery need reconstructive surgery to maximize limb function.

- Chemotherapy is the use of anticancer drugs to kill cancer cells. Patients who have bone cancer usually receive a combination of anticancer drugs. However, chemotherapy is not currently used to treat chondrosarcoma.

- Radiation therapy, also called radiotherapy, involves the use of high-energy x-rays to kill cancer cells. This treatment may be used in combination with surgery. It is often used to treat chondrosarcoma, which cannot be treated with chemotherapy, as well as ESFTs. It may also be used for patients who refuse surgery.

- Cryosurgery is the use of liquid nitrogen to freeze and kill cancer cells. This technique can sometimes be used instead of conventional surgery to destroy the tumor.

Is follow-up treatment necessary? What does it involve?

Yes. Bone cancer sometimes metastasizes, particularly to the lungs, or can recur (come back), either at the same location or in other bones in the body. People who have had bone cancer should see their doctor regularly and should report any unusual symptoms right away. Follow-up varies for different types and stages of bone cancer. Generally, patients are checked frequently by their doctor and have regular blood tests and x-rays. People who have had bone cancer, particularly children and adolescents, have an increased likelihood of developing another type of cancer, such as leukemia, later in life. Regular follow-up care ensures that changes in health are discussed and that problems are treated as soon as possible.

Are clinical trials (research studies) available for people with bone cancer?

Yes. Participation in clinical trials is an important treatment option for many people with bone cancer. To develop new treatments and better ways to use current treatments, the National Cancer Institute (NCI), a part of the National Institutes of Health, is sponsoring clinical trials in many hospitals and cancer centers around the country. Clinical trials are a critical step in the development of new methods of treatment. Before any new treatment can be recommended for general use, doctors conduct clinical trials to find out whether the treatment is safe for patients and effective against the disease.

Section 52.2

Osteosarcoma and Bone Fibrous Histiocytoma

Excerpted from PDQ® Cancer Information Summary. National Cancer Institute; Bethesda, MD. "Osteosarcoma and Malignant Fibrous Histiocytoma of Bone Treatment (PDQ) - Patient Version." Updated 07/2010. Available at: http://cancer.gov. Accessed October 23, 2010.a

General Information about Osteosarcoma and Malignant Fibrous Histiocytoma of Bone

Osteosarcoma and malignant fibrous histiocytoma (MFH) of the bone are diseases in which malignant (cancer) cells form in bone. Osteosarcoma usually starts in osteoblasts, which are a type of bone cell that grows into new bone tissue. Osteosarcoma is most common in teenagers and young adults. It commonly forms in the ends of the long bones of the body, which include bones of the arms and legs. In children and teenagers, it often develops around the knee. Rarely, osteosarcoma may be found in soft tissue or organs in the chest or abdomen.

Osteosarcoma is the most common type of bone cancer. Malignant fibrous histiocytoma (MFH) of bone is a rare tumor of the bone. It is treated like osteosarcoma.

Risk Factors and Signs

Anything that increases your risk of getting a disease is called a risk factor. Having a risk factor does not mean that you will get cancer; not having risk factors doesn't mean that you will not get cancer. People who think they may be at risk should discuss this with their doctor.

Risk factors for osteosarcoma include the following:

- Being a teen or young adult. Osteosarcoma and MFH often form during a growth spurt.
- Being male
- Past treatment with radiation therapy

- Past treatment with anticancer drugs called alkylating agents
- Having a certain change in the retinoblastoma gene
- Having certain conditions such as:
  - Hereditary retinoblastoma
  - Paget disease
  - Diamond-Blackfan anemia
  - Li-Fraumeni syndrome
  - Rothmund-Thomson syndrome
  - Bloom syndrome
  - Werner syndrome

Possible signs of osteosarcoma and MFH include pain and swelling over a bone or a bony part of the body. These and other symptoms may be caused by osteosarcoma or MFH. Other conditions may cause the same symptoms. A doctor should be consulted if any of the following problems occur:

- Swelling over a bone or bony part of the body
- Pain in a bone or joint
- A bone that breaks for no known reason

Detection and Diagnosis

Imaging tests are used to detect (find) osteosarcoma and MFH. Imaging tests are done before the biopsy. The following tests and procedures may be used:

- **Physical exam and history:** An exam of the body to check general signs of health, including checking for signs of disease, such as lumps or anything else that seems unusual. A history of the patient's health habits and past illnesses and treatments will also be taken.

- **X-ray:** An x-ray of the organs and bones inside the body. An x-ray is a type of energy beam that can go through the body and onto film, making a picture of areas inside the body.

- **CT scan (CAT scan):** A procedure that makes a series of detailed pictures of areas inside the body, taken from different angles. The pictures are made by a computer linked to an x-ray machine. A dye may be injected into a vein or swallowed to help the organs or tissues show up more clearly. This procedure is also called computed tomography, computerized tomography, or computerized axial tomography.

- **MRI (magnetic resonance imaging):** A procedure that uses a magnet, radio waves, and a computer to make a series of detailed pictures of areas inside the body. This procedure is also called nuclear magnetic resonance imaging (NMRI).

A biopsy is done to diagnose osteosarcoma. Cells and tissues are removed during a biopsy so they can be viewed under a microscope by a pathologist to check for signs of cancer. It is important that the biopsy be done by a surgeon who is an expert in treating cancer of the bone. It is best if that surgeon is also the one who removes the tumor. The biopsy and the surgery to remove the tumor are planned together. The way the biopsy is done affects which type of surgery can be done later.

The type of biopsy that is done will be based on the size of the tumor and where it is in the body. There are three types of biopsy that may be used:

- **Fine-needle aspiration (FNA) biopsy:** The removal of tissue or fluid using a thin needle.

- **Core biopsy:** The removal of tissue using a wide needle.

- **Incisional biopsy:** The removal of part of a lump or a sample of tissue that doesn't look normal.

The following tests may be done on the tissue that is removed:

- **Light and electron microscopy:** A laboratory test in which cells in a sample of tissue are viewed under regular and high-powered microscopes to look for certain changes in the cells.

- **Cytogenetic analysis:** A laboratory test in which cells in a sample of tissue are viewed under a microscope to look for certain changes in the chromosomes.

- **Immunocytochemistry study:** A laboratory test in which a substance such as an antibody, dye, or radioisotope is added to a sample of cancer cells to test for certain antigens. This type of study is used to tell the difference between different types of cancer.

Prognosis

Certain factors affect prognosis (chance of recovery) and treatment options. The prognosis (chance of recovery) is affected by certain factors before and after treatment.

The prognosis of untreated osteosarcoma and MFH depends on the following:

- Where the tumor is in the body and whether tumors formed in more than one bone
- The size of the tumor
- Whether the cancer has spread to other parts of the body and where it has spread
- The age of the patient
- The type of tumor (based on how the cancer cells look under a microscope)
- Whether the patient has certain genetic diseases

After osteosarcoma or MFH is treated, prognosis also depends on the following:

- How much of the cancer was killed by chemotherapy
- How much of the tumor was taken out by surgery
- Whether chemotherapy is delayed for more than three weeks after surgery takes place

Treatment options for osteosarcoma and MFH depend on the following:

- Where the tumor is in the body
- The size of the tumor
- The stage of the cancer
- Whether the bones are still growing
- The patient's age and general health
- The desire of the patient and family for the patient to be able to participate in activities such as sports or have a certain appearance
- Whether the cancer is newly diagnosed or has recurred (come back) after treatment

Stages of Osteosarcoma and Malignant Fibrous Histiocytoma of Bone

The process used to find out if cancer has spread to other parts of the body is called staging. For osteosarcoma and malignant fibrous histiocytoma (MFH), most patients are grouped according to whether cancer is found in only one part of the body or has spread. In addition to x-rays, CT scans, and MRI, which are also used for diagnosis and are described above, the following tests and procedures may be used:

Bone scan: A procedure to check if there are rapidly dividing cells, such as cancer cells, in the bone. A very small amount of radioactive material is injected into a vein and travels through the bloodstream. The radioactive material collects in the bones and is detected by a scanner.

PET scan (positron emission tomography scan): A procedure to find malignant tumor cells in the body. A small amount of radioactive glucose (sugar) is injected into a vein. The PET scanner rotates around the body and makes a picture of where glucose is being used in the body. Malignant tumor cells show up brighter in the picture because they are more active and take up more glucose than normal cells do.

Osteosarcoma and MFH are described as either localized or metastatic.

- Localized osteosarcoma or MFH has not spread out of the bone where the cancer started. There may be one or more areas of cancer in the bone that can be removed during surgery.

- Metastatic osteosarcoma or MFH has spread from the bone in which the cancer began to other parts of the body. The cancer most often spreads to the lungs. It may also spread to other bones.

Recurrent Osteosarcoma and Malignant Fibrous Histiocytoma of Bone

Recurrent osteosarcoma and malignant fibrous histiocytoma (MFH) of bone are cancers that have recurred (come back) after being treated. The cancer may come back in the bone or in other parts of the body. Osteosarcoma and MFH most often recur in the lung, bone, or both. When osteosarcoma recurs, it is usually within 18 months after treatment is completed.

Treatment Option Overview

Different types of treatment are available for children with osteosarcoma or malignant fibrous histiocytoma (MFH) of bone. Some treatments are standard (the currently used treatment), and some are being tested in clinical trials. A treatment clinical trial is a research study meant to help improve current treatments or obtain information on new treatments for patients with cancer. When clinical trials show that a new treatment is better than the standard treatment, the new treatment may become the standard treatment.

Children with osteosarcoma or MFH should have their treatment planned by a team of health care providers with expertise in treating cancer in children. Treatment will be overseen by a pediatric oncologist, a doctor who specializes in treating children with cancer. The pediatric oncologist works with other pediatric health care providers who are experts in treating osteosarcoma and MFH and who specialize in certain areas of medicine. These may include the following specialists:

- Orthopedic surgeon

- Radiation oncologist

- Rehabilitation specialist

- Pediatric nurse specialist

- Social worker

- Psychologist

Some cancer treatments cause side effects months or years after treatment has ended. Side effects from cancer treatment that begin during or after treatment and continue for months or years are called late effects. Late effects of cancer treatment may include physical problems; changes in mood, feelings, thinking, learning, or memory; and second cancers (new types of cancer).

Some late effects may be treated or controlled. It is important to talk with your child's doctors about the effects cancer treatment can have on your child.

Four types of standard treatment are used.

Surgery

Surgery to remove the entire tumor will be done when possible. Chemotherapy may be given first, to make the tumor smaller so less tissue and bone needs to be removed. This is called neoadjuvant chemotherapy.

The following types of surgery may be done:

- **Wide local excision:** Surgery to remove the cancer and some healthy tissue around it.

- **Limb-sparing surgery:** Removal of the tumor in a limb (arm or leg) without amputation, so the use and appearance of the limb is saved. Most patients with osteosarcoma in a limb can be treated with limb-sparing surgery. The tumor is removed by wide local excision. Tissue and bone that are removed may be replaced with a graft using tissue and bone taken from another part of the patient's body, or with an implant such as artificial bone. If a fracture is found at diagnosis or during chemotherapy before surgery, limb-sparing surgery may still be possible in some cases. If the surgeon is not able to remove all of the tumor and enough healthy tissue around it, an amputation may be done.

- **Amputation:** Surgery to remove part or all of an arm or leg. This may be done when it is not possible to remove all of the tumor in limb-sparing surgery. The patient may be fitted with a prosthesis (artificial limb) after amputation.

- **Rotationplasty:** Surgery to remove the tumor and the knee joint. The part of the leg that remains below the knee is then attached to the part of the leg that remains above the knee, with the foot facing backward and the ankle acting as a knee. A prosthesis may then be attached to the foot.

Studies have shown that survival is the same whether the first surgery done is a limb-sparing surgery or an amputation.

Even if the doctor removes all the cancer that can be seen at the time of the surgery, some patients may be given chemotherapy or radiation therapy after surgery to kill any cancer cells that are left. Treatment given after the surgery, to lower the risk that the cancer will come back, is called adjuvant therapy.

Chemotherapy

Chemotherapy is a cancer treatment that uses drugs to stop the growth of cancer cells, either by killing the cells or by stopping them from dividing. When chemotherapy is taken by mouth or injected into a vein or muscle, the drugs enter the bloodstream and can reach cancer cells throughout the body (systemic chemotherapy). When chemotherapy is placed directly into the cerebrospinal fluid, an organ, or a body cavity such as the abdomen, the drugs mainly affect cancer cells in those areas (regional chemotherapy). Combination chemotherapy is the use of more than one anticancer drug. The way the chemotherapy is given depends on the type and stage of the cancer being treated.

Radiation Therapy

Radiation therapy is a cancer treatment that uses high-energy x-rays or other types of radiation to kill cancer cells or keep them from growing. There are two types of radiation therapy. External radiation therapy uses a machine outside the body to send radiation toward the cancer. Internal radiation therapy uses a radioactive substance sealed in needles, seeds, wires, or catheters that are placed directly into or near the cancer. The way the radiation therapy is given depends on the type and stage of the cancer being treated.

Osteosarcoma and MFH cells are not killed easily by radiation therapy. It may be used when a small amount of cancer is left after surgery or used together with other treatments.

Samarium

Samarium is a radioactive drug that targets areas where bone cells are growing, such as tumor cells in bone. It helps relieve pain caused by cancer in the bone and it also kills blood cells in the bone marrow.

Treatment with samarium may be followed by stem cell transplant. Before treatment with samarium, stem cells (immature blood cells) are removed from the blood or bone marrow of the patient and are frozen and stored. After treatment with samarium is complete, the stored stem cells are thawed and given back to the patient through an infusion. These reinfused stem cells grow into (and restore) the body's blood cells.

Clinical Trials

New types of treatment are being tested in clinical trials. Patients may want to think about taking part in a clinical trial. For some patients, taking part in a clinical trial may be the best treatment choice. Clinical trials are part of the cancer research process. Clinical trials are done to find out if new cancer treatments are safe and effective or better than the standard treatment.

Many of today's standard treatments for cancer are based on earlier clinical trials. Patients who take part in a clinical trial may receive the standard treatment or be among the first to receive a new treatment.

Patients who take part in clinical trials also help improve the way cancer will be treated in the future. Even when clinical trials do not lead to effective new treatments, they often answer important questions and help move research forward.

Patients can enter clinical trials before, during, or after starting their cancer treatment. Some clinical trials only include patients who have not yet received treatment. Other trials test treatments for patients whose cancer has not gotten better. There are also clinical trials that test new ways to stop cancer from recurring (coming back) or reduce the side effects of cancer treatment.

One type of treatment that is being tested in clinical trials is biologic therapy. Biologic therapy is a treatment that uses the patient's immune system to fight cancer. Substances made by the body or made in a laboratory are used to boost, direct, or restore the body's natural defenses against cancer. This type of cancer treatment is also called biotherapy or immunotherapy.

Clinical trials are taking place in many parts of the country. For more information, visit the National Cancer Institute's clinical trials website at www.cancer.gov/clinicaltrials

Follow-Up Tests

Some of the tests that were done to diagnose the cancer or to find out the stage of the cancer may be repeated. Some tests will be repeated in order to see how well the treatment is working. Decisions about whether to continue, change, or stop treatment may be based on the results of these tests. This is sometimes called re-staging.

Some of the tests will continue to be done from time to time after treatment has ended. The results of these tests can show if your condition has changed or if the cancer has recurred (come back). These tests are sometimes called follow-up tests or check-ups.

Section 52.3

Ewing Sarcoma Family of Tumors

Excerpted from PDQ® Cancer Information Summary. National Cancer Institute; Bethesda, MD. "Ewing Sarcoma Family of Tumors Treatment (PDQ) - Patient Version." Updated 12/2009. Available at: http://cancer.gov. Accessed January 20, 2010.

General Information about Ewing Sarcoma Family of Tumors

Ewing sarcoma family of tumors is a group of tumors that form from a certain kind of cell in bone or soft tissue. This family of tumors includes the following:

Ewing tumor of bone: This type of tumor is found in the bones of the legs, arms, chest, trunk, back, or head. There are three types of Ewing tumor of bone:

- Classic Ewing sarcoma

- Primitive neuroectodermal tumor (PNET)

- Askin tumor (PNET of the chest wall)

Extraosseous Ewing sarcoma (tumor growing in tissue other than bone): This type of soft tissue tumor is found in the trunk, arms, legs, head, and neck. In some patients, the tumor may have spread by the time it is diagnosed. Ewing tumors usually occur in teenagers and are more common in boys and Caucasians. Possible signs of Ewing sarcoma family of tumors include swelling and pain near the tumor.

Signs and Symptoms

These and other symptoms may be caused by Ewing sarcoma family of tumors. Other conditions may cause the same symptoms. A doctor should be consulted if any of the following problems occur:

- Pain and/or swelling, most commonly in the arms, legs, chest, back, or pelvis (area between the hips)

- A lump (which may feel warm) in the arms, legs, chest, or pelvis
- Fever for no known reason
- A bone that breaks for no known reason
- Tests that examine the bone and soft tissue are used to diagnose and stage Ewing sarcoma family of tumors

Diagnosis

The following tests and procedures may be used to diagnose or stage Ewing sarcoma family of tumors.

Physical exam and history: An exam of the body to check general signs of health, including checking for signs of disease, such as lumps or anything else that seems unusual. A history of the patient's health habits and past illnesses and treatments will also be taken.

Complete blood count (CBC): A procedure in which a sample of blood is drawn and checked for the following:

- The number of red blood cells, white blood cells, and platelets
- The amount of hemoglobin (the protein that carries oxygen) in the red blood cells
- The portion of the blood sample made up of red blood cells

Blood chemistry studies: A procedure in which a blood sample is checked to measure the amounts of certain substances, such as lactate dehydrogenase (LDH), released into the blood by organs and tissues in the body. An unusual (higher or lower than normal) amount of a substance can be a sign of disease in the organ or tissue that makes it.

Sedimentation rate: A procedure in which a sample of blood is drawn and checked for the rate at which the red blood cells settle to the bottom of the test tube.

X-ray: An x-ray is a type of energy beam that can go through the body and onto film, making a picture of areas inside the body.

MRI (magnetic resonance imaging): A procedure that uses a magnet, radio waves, and a computer to make a series of detailed pictures of areas inside the body. This procedure is also called nuclear magnetic resonance imaging (NMRI).

CT scan (CAT scan): A procedure that makes a series of detailed pictures of areas inside the body, such as the chest, taken from different angles. The pictures are made by a computer linked to an x-ray machine. A dye may be injected into a vein or swallowed to help the organs or tissues show up more clearly. This procedure is also called computed tomography, computerized tomography, or computerized axial tomography.

Bone marrow aspiration and biopsy: The removal of bone marrow, blood, and a small piece of bone by inserting a hollow needle into the hipbone. Samples are removed from both hipbones. A pathologist views the bone marrow, blood, and bone under a microscope to look for signs of cancer.

Bone scan: A procedure to check if there are rapidly dividing cells, such as cancer cells, in the bone. A very small amount of radioactive material is injected into a vein and travels through the bloodstream. The radioactive material collects in the bones and is detected by a scanner.

PET scan (positron emission tomography scan): A procedure to find malignant tumor cells in the body. A small amount of radioactive glucose (sugar) is injected into a vein. The PET scanner rotates around the body and makes a picture of where glucose is being used in the body. Malignant tumor cells show up brighter in the picture because they are more active and take up more glucose than normal cells do.

Biopsy: A biopsy is done to diagnose Ewing sarcoma family of tumors. Cells and tissues are removed during a biopsy so they can be viewed under a microscope by a pathologist to check for signs of cancer. The specialists (pathologist, radiation oncologist, and surgeon) who will treat the patient usually work together to plan the biopsy. This is done so that the biopsy incision doesn't affect later treatment with surgery to remove the tumor and radiation therapy. It is helpful if the biopsy is done at the same center where treatment will be given.

Laboratory tests: The following tests may be done on the tissue that is removed:

- **Light and electron microscopy:** A laboratory test in which cells in a sample of tissue are viewed under regular and high-powered microscopes to look for certain changes in the cells.

- **Cytogenetic analysis:** A laboratory test in which cells in a sample of tissue are viewed under a microscope to look for certain changes in the chromosomes.

- **Reverse-transcription polymerase chain reaction test (RT-PCR):** A laboratory test in which cells in a sample of tissue are studied using chemicals to look for certain changes in the genes.

- **Immunohistochemistry study:** A laboratory test in which a substance such as an antibody, dye, or radioisotope is added to a sample of tissue to test for certain antigens. This type of study is used to tell the difference between different types of cancer.

Prognosis

Certain factors affect prognosis (chance of recovery) and treatment options. The prognosis depends on certain factors before and after treatment. Before treatment, prognosis depends on the following:

- Whether the tumor has spread to distant parts of the body

- Where in the body the tumor started

- How large the tumor is at diagnosis

- Whether the tumor has certain genetic changes

- The patient's age. Infants and patients aged younger than 15 years have a better prognosis than adolescents aged 15 years and older, young adults, or adults

- The patient's gender. Girls have a better prognosis than boys

- Whether the tumor has just been diagnosed or has recurred (come back)

After treatment, prognosis is affected by whether the tumor was completely removed by surgery and whether the cancer came back more than two years after the initial treatment.

Treatment options depend on the following:

- Where the tumor is found in the body and how large the tumor is.

- The patient's age and general health

- The effect the treatment will have on the patient's appearance and important body functions

- Whether the cancer has just been diagnosed or has recurred (come back)

- Decisions about surgery may depend on how well the initial treatment with chemotherapy or radiation therapy works

Stages of Ewing Sarcoma Family of Tumors

The process used to find out if cancer has spread from where it began to other parts of the body is called staging. There is no standard staging system for Ewing sarcoma family of tumors. The results of the tests and procedures done to diagnose Ewing sarcoma family of tumors are used to group the tumors into localized or metastatic.

Ewing sarcoma family of tumors are grouped based on whether the cancer has spread from the bone or soft tissue in which the cancer began.

Ewing sarcoma family of tumors is described as either localized or metastatic:

- In localized Ewing sarcoma family of tumors the cancer is found in the bone or soft tissue in which the cancer began and may have spread to nearby tissue, including lymph nodes.

- In metastatic Ewing sarcoma family of tumors. The cancer has spread from the bone or soft tissue in which the cancer began to other parts of the body. In Ewing tumor of bone, the cancer most often spreads to the lung, other bones, and bone marrow.

Recurrent Ewing Sarcoma Family of Tumors

Recurrent Ewing sarcoma family of tumors is cancer that has recurred (come back) after it has been treated. The cancer may come back in the tissues where it first started or in another part of the body.

Treatment Option Overview

Different types of treatments are available for children with Ewing sarcoma family of tumors. Some treatments are standard (the currently used treatment), and some are being tested in clinical trials. A treatment clinical trial is a research study meant to help improve current treatments or obtain information on new treatments for patients with cancer. When clinical trials show that a new treatment is better than the standard treatment, the new treatment may become the standard treatment.

Because cancer in children is rare, taking part in a clinical trial should be considered. Some clinical trials are open only to patients who have not started treatment.

Children with Ewing sarcoma family of tumors should have their treatment planned by a team of health care providers who are experts in treating cancer in children.

Treatment will be overseen by a pediatric oncologist, a doctor who specializes in treating children with cancer. The pediatric oncologist works with other health care providers who are experts in treating children with Ewing sarcoma family of tumors and who specialize in certain areas of medicine. These may include the following specialists:

- Surgical oncologist or orthopedic oncologist
- Radiation oncologist
- Pediatric nurse specialist
- Social worker
- Rehabilitation specialist
- Psychologist

Some cancer treatments cause side effects months or years after treatment has ended. Side effects from cancer treatment that begin during or after treatment and continue for months or years are called late effects. Late effects of cancer treatment may include physical problems; changes in mood, feelings, thinking, learning, or memory; and second cancers (new types of cancer).

Patients treated for Ewing sarcoma family of tumors have an increased risk of developing acute myeloid leukemia, myelodysplastic syndrome, and sarcomas in the area treated with radiation therapy. Some late effects may be treated or controlled. It is important to talk with your child's doctors about the effects cancer treatment can have on your child.

Three types of standard treatment are used.

Chemotherapy

Chemotherapy is part of the treatment for all patients with Ewing tumors. It is usually given first, to shrink the tumor before treatment with surgery or radiation therapy. It may also be given to kill any tumor cells that have spread to other parts of the body.

Chemotherapy is a cancer treatment that uses drugs to stop the growth of cancer cells, either by killing the cells or by stopping them from dividing. When chemotherapy is taken by mouth or injected into a vein or muscle, the drugs enter the bloodstream and can reach cancer cells throughout the body (systemic chemotherapy). When chemotherapy is placed directly into the spinal column, an organ, or a body cavity such as the abdomen, the drugs mainly affect cancer cells in those areas (regional chemotherapy). Combination chemotherapy is treatment using more than one anticancer drug. The way the chemotherapy is given depends on the type of the cancer being treated and whether it is found at the place it first formed only or whether it has spread to other parts of the body.

Surgery

Surgery is usually done to remove cancer that is left after chemotherapy or radiation therapy. When possible, the entire tumor is removed by surgery. Tissue and bone that are removed may be replaced with a graft using tissue and bone taken from another part of the patient's body or a donor, or with an implant such as artificial bone.

Radiation Therapy

Radiation therapy may be used to shrink the tumor before surgery so less tissue needs to be removed. It may also be used to kill tumor cells that are left after surgery or chemotherapy. Radiation therapy is a cancer treatment that uses high-energy x-rays or other types of radiation to kill cancer cells or keep them from growing. There are two types of radiation therapy. External radiation therapy uses a machine outside the body to send radiation toward the cancer. Internal radiation therapy uses a radioactive substance sealed in needles, seeds, wires, or catheters that are placed directly into or near the cancer. The way the radiation therapy is given depends on the type of the cancer being treated and whether it is found at the place it first formed only or whether it has spread to other parts of the body.

Clinical Trials

Patients may want to think about taking part in a clinical trial. For some patients, taking part in a clinical trial may be the best treatment choice. Clinical trials are part of the cancer research process. Clinical trials are done to find out if new cancer treatments are safe and effective or better than the standard treatment.

Many of today's standard treatments for cancer are based on earlier clinical trials. Patients who take part in a clinical trial may receive the standard treatment or be among the first to receive a new treatment.

Patients who take part in clinical trials also help improve the way cancer will be treated in the future. Even when clinical trials do not lead to effective new treatments, they often answer important questions and help move research forward.

Patients can enter clinical trials before, during, or after starting their cancer treatment. Some clinical trials only include patients who have not yet received treatment. Other trials test treatments for patients whose cancer has not gotten better. There are also clinical trials that test new ways to stop cancer from recurring (coming back) or reduce the side effects of cancer treatment.

Clinical trials are taking place in many parts of the country.

Two new types of treatment that are being tested in clinical trials are chemotherapy with stem cell transplant and targeted therapy. For more information about clinical trials, visit the National Cancer Institute's clinical trials website at www.cancer.gov/clinicaltrials.

Chemotherapy with stem cell transplant: Stem cell transplant is a way of replacing blood -forming cells destroyed by chemotherapy. Stem cells (immature blood cells) are removed from the blood or bone marrow of the patient or a donor and are frozen and stored. After chemotherapy is completed, the stored stem cells are thawed and given back to the patient through an infusion. These reinfused stem cells grow into (and restore) the body's blood cells.

Targeted therapy: Targeted therapy is a type of treatment that uses drugs or other substances to identify and attack specific cancer cells without harming normal cells. Angiogenesis inhibitors and monoclonal antibodies are two types of targeted therapies being studied in the treatment of Ewing sarcoma family of tumors.

Angiogenesis inhibitors are substances that block the growth of new blood vessels. In cancer treatment, angiogenesis inhibitors prevent the growth of new blood vessels needed for tumors to grow.

Monoclonal antibody therapy is a cancer treatment that uses antibodies made in the laboratory from a single type of immune system cell. These antibodies can identify substances on cancer cells or normal substances that may help cancer cells grow. The antibodies attach to the substances and kill the cancer cells, block their growth, or keep them from spreading. Monoclonal antibodies are given by infusion. They may be used alone or to carry drugs, toxins, or radioactive material directly to cancer cells.

Follow-Up Tests

Some of the tests that were done to diagnose the cancer or to find out the stage of the cancer may be repeated. Some tests will be repeated in order to see how well the treatment is working. Decisions about whether to continue, change, or stop treatment may be based on the results of these tests. This is sometimes called re-staging.

Some of the tests will continue to be done from time to time after treatment has ended. The results of these tests can show if your condition has changed or if the cancer has recurred (come back). These tests are sometimes called follow-up tests or check-ups.

Chapter 53

Soft Tissue Sarcomas

Chapter Contents

Section 53.1

Childhood Soft Tissue Sarcoma

Excerpted from PDQ® Cancer Information Summary. National Cancer In-
stitute; Bethesda, MD. "Childhood Soft Tissue Sarcomas Treatment (PDQ)
- Patient Version." Updated 07/2010. Available at: http://cancer.gov. Accessed
September 13, 2010; with supplemental information excerpted from PDQ®
Cancer Information Summary. National Cancer Institute; Bethesda, MD.
"Childhood Rhabdomyosarcoma Treatment (PDQ®) - Patient Version." Up-
dated 06/2010. Available at: http://cancer.gov. Accessed September 13, 2010.
Reviewed by David A. Cooke, MD, FACP, September 2010.

General Information about Childhood Soft Tissue Sarcoma

Childhood soft tissue sarcoma is a disease in which malignant
(cancer) cells form in soft tissues of the body. Soft tissues of the body
connect, support, and surround other body parts and organs. The soft
tissues include the following:

- Muscles

- Tendons (bands of tissue that connect muscles to bones)

- Synovial tissues (tissues around joints)

- Fat

- Blood vessels

- Lymph vessels

- Nerves

Soft tissue sarcoma may be found anywhere in the body. In children, the tumors form most often in the arms, legs, or trunk (chest
and abdomen).

There are many different types of soft tissue sarcomas. The cells
of each type of sarcoma look different under a microscope. The soft
tissue tumors are grouped based on the type of soft tissue cell where
they first formed.

Rhabdomyosarcoma is the most common type of childhood soft tissue sarcoma. It begins in muscles that surround bone. There are three main types of rhabdomyosarcoma:

- **Embryonal:** This type occurs most often in the head and neck area or in the genital or urinary organs. It is the most common type.

- **Alveolar:** This type occurs most often in the arms or legs, chest, abdomen, or genital or anal areas. It usually occurs during the teen years.

- **Anaplastic:** This type rarely occurs in children.

Other types of soft tissue sarcoma include the following:

- **Fibrous (connective) tissue tumors:** Fibromatoses (desmoid tumor); dermatofibrosarcoma., and fibrosarcoma

- **Fibrohistiocytic tumors:** Malignant fibrous histiocytoma (also called MFH, undifferentiated pleomorphic sarcoma, or spindle cell sarcoma); plexiform histiocytic tumor

- **Fat tissue tumors:** Liposarcoma

- **Smooth muscle tumors:** Leiomyosarcoma

- **Blood and lymph vessel tumors:** Angiosarcoma; lymphangiosarcoma; hemangiopericytoma; hemangioendothelioma

- **Peripheral nervous system tumors:** Malignant schwannoma (malignant peripheral nerve sheath tumor)

- **Bone and cartilage tumors:** Extraosseous osteosarcoma; Extraosseous myxoid chondrosarcoma; extraosseous mesenchymal chondrosarcoma

- **Tumors with more than one type of tissue:** Malignant mesenchymoma; malignant Triton tumor; malignant ectomesenchymoma.

- **Tumors of unknown origin** (the place where the tumor first formed is not known): Alveolar soft part sarcoma; epithelioid sarcoma; clear cell sarcoma (malignant melanoma of soft parts); synovial sarcoma; desmoplastic small round cell tumor

After rhabdomyosarcomas, the most common soft tissue sarcomas in children are in joint tissue, connective tissue, and nerve tissue.

Soft tissue sarcoma occurs in children and adults. Soft tissue sarcoma in children may respond differently to treatment, and may have a better outcome than soft tissue sarcoma in adults.

Risk Factors

Having certain diseases and inherited disorders can increase the risk of developing childhood soft tissue sarcoma. Risk factors for childhood soft tissue sarcoma include having the following inherited disorders:

- Li-Fraumeni syndrome and neurofibromatosis type 1 (NF1): Risk factors for rhabdomyosarcoma and other childhood soft tissue sarcomas

- Beckwith-Wiedemann syndrome, Costello syndrome, and Noonan syndrome: Risk factors for rhabdomyosarcoma

- Familial adenomatous polyposis (FAP): A risk factor for childhood soft tissue sarcomas other than rhabdomyosarcoma

High birth weight and larger than expected size at birth are linked with an increased risk of embryonal rhabdomyosarcoma. In most cases, the cause of rhabdomyosarcoma is not known.

Other risk factors for childhood soft tissue sarcomas include having AIDS (acquired immune deficiency syndrome) and Epstein-Barr virus infection, having retinoblastoma in both eyes, and past treatment with radiation therapy.

Signs and Symptoms

A sarcoma may appear as a painless lump under the skin, often on an arm, a leg, or the trunk. There may be no other symptoms at first. As the sarcoma grows larger and presses on nearby organs, nerves, muscles, or blood vessels, symptoms may occur, including pain or weakness. A doctor should be consulted if any of the following problems occur:

- A lump or swelling that keeps getting bigger or does not go away. It may be painful

- Bulging of the eye

- Headache

- Trouble urinating or having bowel movements

- Blood in the urine

- Bleeding in the nose, throat, vagina, or rectum

Diagnosis

Diagnostic tests and a biopsy are used to detect and diagnose childhood soft tissue sarcoma. The following tests and procedures may be used:

- **Physical exam and history:** An exam of the body to check general signs of health, including checking for signs of disease, such as lumps or anything else that seems unusual. A history of the patient's health habits and past illnesses and treatments will also be taken.

- **X-rays:** An x-ray is a type of energy beam that can go through the body onto film, making pictures of areas inside the body. A series of x-rays may be done to check the lump or painful area.

- **MRI (magnetic resonance imaging):** A procedure that uses a magnet, radio waves, and a computer to make a series of detailed pictures of areas inside the body. This procedure is also called nuclear magnetic resonance imaging (NMRI).

Additional diagnostic tests for rhabdomyosarcoma may include a CT scan (CAT scan), a bone scan, lumbar puncture (also called a spinal tap), and an ultrasound exam.

If these tests show there may be a soft tissue sarcoma, a biopsy is done. One of the following types of biopsies may be used:

- **Fine-needle aspiration (FNA) biopsy:** The removal of tissue or fluid using a thin needle. A pathologist views the tissue or fluid under a microscope to look for cancer cells.

- **Core biopsy:** The removal of tissue using a wide needle. A pathologist views the tissue under a microscope to look for cancer cells.

- **Incisional biopsy:** The removal of part of a lump or a sample of tissue. A pathologist views the tissue under a microscope to look for cancer cells.

- **Excisional biopsy:** The removal of an entire lump or area of tissue that doesn't look normal. A pathologist views the tissue under a microscope to look for cancer cells. An excisional biopsy may be used to completely remove smaller tumors that are near the surface of the skin.

In order to plan the best treatment, a large sample of tissue may be removed during the biopsy to find out the type of soft tissue sarcoma and do laboratory tests. Tissue samples will be taken from the primary tumor, lymph nodes, and other areas that may have a tumor. A pathologist views the tissue under a microscope to look for cancer cells and to find out the type and grade of the tumor. The grade of a tumor depends on how abnormal the cancer cells look under a microscope and how quickly the cells are dividing. High-grade tumors usually grow and spread more quickly than low-grade tumors.

Because soft tissue sarcomas can be hard to diagnose and rhabdomyosarcoma treatment depends on the type, patients should ask to have biopsy samples checked by a pathologist who has pertinent experience in diagnosing soft tissue sarcomas.

One or more of the following laboratory tests may be done to study the tissue samples:

- **Bone marrow aspiration and biopsy:** The removal of bone marrow, blood, and a small piece of bone by inserting a hollow needle into the hipbone. Samples are removed from both hipbones. A pathologist views the bone marrow, blood, and bone under a microscope to look for signs of cancer.

- **Cytogenetic analysis:** A laboratory test in which cells in a sample of tissue are viewed under a microscope to look for certain changes in the chromosomes.

- **Immunohistochemistry study:** A laboratory test in which a substance such as an antibody, dye, or radioisotope is added to a sample of cancer tissue to test for certain antigens. This type of study is used to tell the difference between different types of cancer.

- **Immunocytochemistry study**: A laboratory test that uses different substances to stain (color) cells in a sample of tissue. This is used to tell the difference between the different types of soft tissue sarcoma.

- **Light and electron microscopy:** A laboratory test in which cells in a sample of tissue are viewed under regular and high-powered microscopes to look for certain changes in the cells.

Stages of Childhood Rhabdomyosarcoma

After childhood rhabdomyosarcoma has been diagnosed, treatment is based on the stage of the cancer and whether cancer remains after surgery to remove the tumor. Childhood rhabdomyosarcoma is staged by using three different ways to describe the cancer: A staging system, a grouping system, and a risk group.

Staging System

The staging system is based on the size of the tumor, where it is in the body, and whether it has spread to other parts of the body:

Stage 1: In stage 1, cancer is any size, has not spread to lymph nodes, and is found in only one of the following "favorable" sites:

- Eye or area around the eye.

- Head and neck (but not in the tissue next to the brain and spinal cord).

- Gallbladder and bile ducts.

- In the testes or vagina (but not in the kidney, bladder, or prostate).

Rhabdomyosarcoma that occurs in a "favorable" site has a better prognosis. If the site where cancer occurs is not one of the favorable sites listed above, it is said to be an "unfavorable" site.

Stage 2: In stage 2, cancer is found in any one area not included in stage 1. The tumor is five centimeters or smaller and has not spread to lymph nodes.

Stage 3: In stage 3, cancer is found in any one area not included in stage 1 and one of the following is true:

- The tumor is five centimeters or smaller and cancer has spread to nearby lymph nodes.

- The tumor is larger than five centimeters and cancer may have spread to nearby lymph nodes.

Stage 4: In stage 4, the tumor may be any size and cancer may have spread to nearby lymph nodes. Cancer has also spread to distant parts of the body such as the lung, bone marrow, or bone.

Grouping System

The grouping system is based on whether the cancer has spread and how much cancer remains after surgery to remove the tumor:

Group I: Cancer was found only in the place where it started and it was completely removed by surgery. Tissue was taken from the edges of where the tumor was removed. The tissue was checked under a microscope by a pathologist and no cancer cells were seen.

Group II: Group II is divided into groups IIA, IIB, and IIC.

- **IIA:** Cancer was removed by surgery but cancer cells were seen when the tissue, taken from the edges of where the tumor was removed, was viewed under a microscope by a pathologist.

- **IIB:** Cancer had spread to nearby lymph nodes and the cancer and lymph nodes were removed by surgery.

- **IIC:** Cancer had spread to nearby lymph nodes and the cancer and lymph nodes were removed by surgery. Tissue was taken from the edges of where the tumor was removed. The tissue was checked under a microscope by a pathologist and no cancer cells were seen.

Group III: Cancer was partly removed by surgery and there are cancer cells (a lump or mass) remaining that can be seen by x-ray or other imaging test. Cancer has not spread to distant parts of the body.

Group IV: Cancer had spread to distant parts of the body at the time of diagnosis.

Risk Group

The risk group is based on the staging system and the grouping system and is used to plan treatment. The risk group describes the chance that rhabdomyosarcoma will recur (come back).

Low-risk childhood rhabdomyosarcoma is one of the following:

- An embryonal tumor of any size that is found in a "favorable" site. There may be tumor remaining after surgery that can be seen without a microscope. The cancer may have spread to nearby lymph nodes.

- An embryonal tumor of any size that is not found in one of the "favorable" sites listed above. There may be tumor remaining after surgery that can be seen only with a microscope. The cancer may have spread to nearby lymph nodes.

Intermediate-risk childhood rhabdomyosarcoma is one of the following:

- An embryonal tumor of any size that is not found in one of the "favorable" sites. There is tumor remaining after surgery, that can be seen with or without a microscope. The cancer may have spread to nearby lymph nodes.

- An alveolar tumor of any size in a "favorable" or "unfavorable" site. There may be tumor remaining after surgery that can be seen with or without a microscope. The cancer may have spread to nearby lymph nodes.

High-risk childhood rhabdomyosarcoma may be the embryonal type or the alveolar type. It may have spread to nearby lymph nodes and has spread to one or more distant parts of the body.

Recurrent childhood rhabdomyosarcoma is cancer that has recurred (come back) after it has been treated. The cancer may come back in the same place or in other parts of the body.

Stages of Other Childhood Soft Tissue Sarcomas

There is no standard staging system for childhood soft tissue sarcoma. Two methods that are commonly used for staging are based on the amount of tumor remaining after surgery to remove the tumor and/or the grade and size of the tumor and whether it has spread to the lymph nodes or other parts of the body.

Sentinel lymph node biopsy may be used to stage childhood soft tissue sarcoma. This is the removal of the sentinel lymph node during surgery. The sentinel lymph node is the first lymph node to receive lymphatic drainage from a tumor. It is the first lymph node the cancer is likely to spread to from the tumor. A radioactive substance and/or blue dye is injected near the tumor. The substance or dye flows through the lymph ducts to the lymph nodes. The first lymph node to receive the substance or dye is removed. A pathologist views the tissue under a microscope to look for cancer cells. If cancer cells are not found, it may not be necessary to remove more lymph nodes.

Another staging test is a CT scan (CAT scan), a procedure that makes a series of detailed pictures of areas inside the body, taken from different angles. The pictures are made by a computer linked to an x-ray machine. A dye may be injected into a vein or swallowed to help the organs or tissues show up more clearly. This procedure is also called computed tomography, computerized tomography, or computerized axial tomography.

The results of the sentinel lymph node biopsy and CT scan are viewed together with the results of the diagnostic tests and initial surgery to determine the stage of the soft tissue sarcoma.

Amount of Tumor Remaining

One method used to stage childhood soft tissue sarcoma is based on how much cancer remains after surgery to remove the tumor and whether the cancer has spread:

In nonmetastatic childhood soft tissue sarcoma, the cancer has been partly or completely removed by surgery and has not spread to other parts of the body.

- **Group I:** The tumor has been completely removed by surgery.

- **Group II:** After surgery to remove the tumor, there are remaining cancer cells that can be seen only with a microscope.

- **Group III:** After surgery, there is tumor remaining that can be seen with the eye.

Metastatic childhood soft tissue sarcoma is considered Group IV. The cancer has spread from where it started to other parts of the body (metastasis).

Tumor Size and Spread

Another method used to stage childhood soft tissue sarcoma is based on the size of the tumor and whether cancer has spread to lymph nodes or other parts of the body. Sometimes the stages used for adult soft tissue sarcoma are used for childhood soft tissue sarcoma:

- **Stage I:** The tumor is any size, low-grade (likely to grow and spread slowly), and may be either superficial (close to the skin's surface) or deep.

- **Stage II:** The tumor is high-grade (likely to grow and spread quickly) and either five centimeters or smaller and either superficial (close to the skin's surface) or deep; or larger than five centimeters and superficial.

- **Stage III:** The tumor is high-grade, larger than five centimeters, and deep.

- **Stage IV:** The tumor is any size, any grade, and has spread to nearby lymph nodes and/or to other parts of the body.

- **Recurrent and progressive childhood soft tissue sarcoma:** Cancer has recurred (come back) after it has been treated. The cancer may come back in the same place or in other parts of the body. Progressive childhood soft tissue sarcoma is cancer that did not respond to treatment.

Rhabdomyosarcoma Treatment Option Overview

Different types of treatments are available for children with rhabdomyosarcoma. Some treatments are standard (the currently used treatment), and some are being tested in clinical trials. Because rhabdomyosarcoma can form in many different parts of the body, many different kinds of treatments are used. Treatment will be overseen by a pediatric oncologist, a doctor who specializes in treating children with cancer. The pediatric oncologist works with other health care providers who are experts in treating children with rhabdomyosarcoma and who specialize in certain areas of medicine.

Surgery, radiation therapy, and chemotherapy are the three types of standard treatment. Radiation therapy is a cancer treatment that uses high-energy x-rays or other types of radiation to kill cancer cells or stop them from growing. Chemotherapy is a cancer treatment that uses drugs to stop the growth of cancer cells, either by killing the cells or by stopping them from dividing.

Surgery

Surgery (removing the cancer in an operation) is used to treat childhood rhabdomyosarcoma. A type of surgery called wide local excision is often done. A wide local excision is the removal of tumor and some of the normal tissue around it, including the lymph nodes. When an extra amount of normal tissue is removed from around the tumor, it is called an en bloc removal of a cuff of normal tissue. A second surgery may be needed to remove all the cancer. Whether surgery is done and the type of surgery done depends on where in the body the tumor started, the effect the surgery will have on the way the child will look, the effect the surgery will have on the child's important body functions, and how the tumor responded to chemotherapy or radiation therapy that may have been given first. For most children with rhabdomyosarcoma, complete removal of the tumor by surgery is not possible.

Rhabdomyosarcoma can form in many different places in the body and the surgery will be different for each site. Surgery to treat rhabdomyosarcoma of the eye or genital areas is usually a biopsy. Chemotherapy, and sometimes radiation therapy, may be given before surgery to shrink large tumors.

Even if the doctor removes all the cancer that can be seen at the time of the surgery, patients will be given chemotherapy, with or without radiation therapy, after surgery to kill any cancer cells that are left. Treatment given after the surgery, to lower the risk that the cancer will come back, is called adjuvant therapy.

Treatment Option Overview for Other Childhood Soft Tissue Sarcomas

Different types of treatments are available for patients with childhood soft tissue sarcoma. Some treatments are standard (the currently used treatment), and some are being tested in clinical trials. Seven types of standard treatment are used, they include radiation therapy and chemotherapy, plus the five listed below.

Surgery

Surgery to completely remove the soft tissue sarcoma is done whenever possible. If the tumor is very large, radiation therapy or chemotherapy may be given first, to make the tumor smaller and decrease the amount of tissue that needs to be removed during surgery. The following types of surgery may be used:

- **Wide local excision:** Removal of the tumor along with some normal tissue around it.

- **Amputation:** Surgery to remove part or all of a limb or appendage, such as the arm or hand.

- **Limb-sparing surgery**: Removal of the tumor in an arm or leg without amputation, so the use and appearance of the limb is saved. Radiation therapy or chemotherapy may be given first to shrink the tumor. The tumor is then removed in a wide local excision. Tissue and bone that are removed may be replaced with a graft using tissue and bone taken from another part of the patient's body, or with an implant such as artificial bone.

- **Lymphadenectomy:** Removal of the lymph nodes that contain cancer.

A second surgery may be needed to remove any remaining cancer cells and check the area around where the tumor was removed for cancer cells and then remove them.

Even if the doctor removes all the cancer that can be seen at the time of the surgery, some patients may be given radiation therapy or chemotherapy after surgery to kill any cancer cells that are left. Treatment given after the surgery, to lower the risk that the cancer will come back, is called adjuvant therapy.

Hormone Therapy

Hormone therapy is a cancer treatment that removes hormones or blocks their action and stops cancer cells from growing. Hormones are substances made by glands in the body and circulated in the bloodstream. Some hormones can cause certain cancers to grow. If tests show that the cancer cells have places where hormones can attach (receptors), drugs, surgery, or radiation therapy is used to reduce the production of hormones or block them from working. Antiestrogens (drugs that block estrogen) may be used to treat childhood soft tissue sarcoma.

Watchful Waiting

Watchful waiting is closely monitoring a patient's condition without giving any treatment until symptoms appear or change. Watchful waiting may be done when complete removal of the tumor is not possible, no other treatments are available, and the tumor does not place any vital organs in danger.

Nonsteroidal Anti-Inflammatory Drugs

Nonsteroidal anti-inflammatory drugs (NSAIDs) are drugs (such as aspirin, ibuprofen, and naproxen) that are commonly used to decrease fever, swelling, pain, and redness. In the treatment of soft tissue sarcomas, an NSAID called sulindac may be used to help block the growth of cancer cells.

Liver Transplant

The liver is removed and replaced with a healthy one from a donor.

Clinical Trials

For some patients, taking part in a clinical trial may be the best treatment choice. Clinical trials are part of the cancer research process. Clinical trials are done to find out if new cancer treatments are safe and effective or better than the standard treatment.

New types of treatment for rhabdomyosarcoma and other childhood soft tissue sarcomas are being tested in clinical trials. This summary may not mention every new treatment being studied. Information about clinical trials is available from the National Cancer Institute website (www.cancer.gov).

High-Dose Chemotherapy with Stem Cell Transplant

High-dose chemotherapy with stem cell transplant is a way of giving high doses of chemotherapy and replacing blood-forming cells destroyed by the cancer treatment. Stem cells (immature blood cells) are removed from the blood or bone marrow of the patient or a donor and are frozen and stored. After the chemotherapy is completed, the stored stem cells are thawed and given back to the patient through an infusion. These reinfused stem cells grow into (and restore) the body's blood cells.

Immunotherapy

Immunotherapy is a treatment that uses the patient's immune system to fight cancer. Substances made by the body or made in a laboratory are used to boost, direct, or restore the body's natural defenses against cancer. This type of cancer treatment is also called biologic therapy or biotherapy.

Targeted Therapy

Targeted therapy is a treatment that uses drugs or other substances to identify and attack specific cancer cells without harming normal cells. Imatinib (Gleevec) is a type of targeted therapy called a tyrosine kinase inhibitor. It finds and blocks an abnormal protein on cancer cells that causes them to divide and grow. Other targeted therapies being studied in clinical trials include angiogenesis inhibitors. In cancer treatment, angiogenesis inhibitors prevent the growth of new blood vessels needed for tumors to grow.

Follow-Up Tests

Some of the tests that were done to diagnose the cancer or to find out the stage of the cancer may be repeated. Some tests will be repeated in order to see how well the treatment is working. Decisions about whether to continue, change, or stop treatment may be based on the results of these tests. This is sometimes called re-staging.

Some of the tests will continue to be done from time to time after treatment has ended. The results of these tests can show if your condition has changed or if the cancer has recurred (come back). These tests are sometimes called follow-up tests or check-ups.

Section 53.2

Adult Soft Tissue Sarcoma

Excerpted from PDQ® Cancer Information Summary. National Cancer Institute; Bethesda, MD. "Adult Soft Tissue Sarcoma Treatment (PDQ) - Patient Version." Updated 09/2009. Available at: http://cancer.gov. Accessed January 20, 2010.

General Information about Adult Soft Tissue Sarcoma

Adult soft tissue sarcoma is a disease in which malignant (cancer) cells form in the soft tissues of the body (muscles, tendons, fat, blood vessels, lymph vessels, nerves, and tissues around joints). Adult soft tissue sarcomas can form almost anywhere in the body, but are most common in the legs, abdomen, arms, and trunk.

There are many types of soft tissue sarcoma. One type that forms in the wall of the stomach, intestines, or rectum is called a gastrointestinal stromal tumor (GIST). The cells of each type of sarcoma look different under a microscope, based on the type of soft tissue in which the cancer began.

Risk Factors

Risk factors for soft tissue sarcoma include the following inherited disorders:

- Retinoblastoma.
- Neurofibromatosis type 1 (von Recklinghausen disease or NF1).
- Tuberous sclerosis.
- Familial adenomatous polyposis (FAP).
- Li-Fraumeni syndrome.
- Werner syndrome.
- Basal cell nevus syndrome.

Other risk factors for soft tissue sarcoma include past treatment with radiation therapy during childhood or for retinoblastoma, breast cancer, lymphoma, or cervical cancer.

Signs and Symptoms

A sarcoma may appear as a painless lump under the skin, often on an arm or a leg. Sarcomas that begin in the abdomen may not cause symptoms until they become very large. As the sarcoma grows larger and presses on nearby organs, nerves, muscles, or blood vessels, symptoms may include pain or trouble breathing. Other conditions may cause the same symptoms that soft tissue sarcomas do. A doctor should be consulted if any of these problems occur.

Diagnosis

If a soft tissue sarcoma is suspected, a biopsy will be done. The type of biopsy that is done will be based on the size and location of the tumor. An incisional biopsy, one of two types of biopsy that may be used, involves the removal of part of a lump or a sample of tissue. The other type, a core biopsy, involves the removal of tissue using a wide needle.

Samples will be taken from the primary tumor, lymph nodes, and other suspicious areas. A pathologist views the tissue under a microscope to look for cancer cells and to find out the grade of the tumor. The grade of a tumor depends on how abnormal the cancer cells look under a microscope and how quickly the cells are dividing. High-grade tumors usually grow and spread more quickly than low-grade tumors. Because soft tissue sarcoma can be hard to diagnose, patients should ask to have biopsy samples checked by a pathologist who has experience in diagnosing soft tissue sarcoma.

The treatment options and prognosis (chance of recovery) depend on the type of soft tissue sarcoma, the size, grade, and stage of the tumor, where the tumor is in the body, whether the entire tumor is removed by surgery, the patient's age and general health, and whether the cancer has recurred (come back).

Stages of Adult Soft Tissue Sarcoma

The process used to find out if cancer has spread within the soft tissue or to other parts of the body is called staging. Staging of soft tissue sarcoma is also based on the grade and size of the tumor, whether it is superficial (close to the skin's surface) or deep, and whether it has spread to the lymph nodes or other parts of the body. The information gathered from the staging process determines the stage of the disease. It is important to know the stage in order to plan treatment.

Tests and procedures may be used in the staging process include a physical exam and history, x-rays, laboratory tests, CT scan (CAT scan), and MRI (magnetic resonance imaging). The results of these tests are viewed together with the results of the tumor biopsies to determine the stage of the soft tissue sarcoma. The following stages are used for adult soft tissue sarcoma:

- **Stage I:** The tumor is any size, low-grade (likely to grow and spread slowly), and may be either superficial (close to the skin's surface) or deep.

- **Stage II:** The tumor is high-grade (likely to grow and spread quickly) and either five centimeters or smaller and can be superficial (close to the skin's surface) or deep; or larger than five centimeters and superficial.

- **Stage III:** The tumor is high-grade, larger than five centimeters, and deep.

- **Stage IV:** The tumor is any size, any grade, and has spread to nearby lymph nodes or to other parts of the body.

- **Recurrent adult soft tissue sarcoma:** Cancer that has recurred (come back) after it has been treated. The cancer may come back in the same soft tissue or in other parts of the body.

Treatment Option Overview

Different types of treatments are available for patients with adult soft tissue sarcoma. Some treatments are standard (the currently used treatment), and some are being tested in clinical trials. A treatment clinical trial is a research study meant to help improve current treatments or obtain information on new treatments for patients with cancer. When clinical trials show that a new treatment is better than the standard treatment, the new treatment may become the standard treatment. Patients may want to think about taking part in a clinical trial. Some clinical trials are open only to patients who have not started treatment.

Three types of standard treatment are used:

Surgery

Surgery is the most common treatment for adult soft tissue sarcoma. For some soft-tissue sarcomas, removal of the tumor in surgery may be the only treatment needed. The following surgical procedures may be used:

- **Mohs microsurgery:** A procedure in which the tumor is cut from the skin in thin layers. During surgery, the edges of the tumor and each layer of tumor removed are viewed through a microscope to check for cancer cells. Layers continue to be removed until no more cancer cells are seen. This type of surgery removes as little normal tissue as possible and is often used where appearance is important, such as on the skin.

- **Wide local excision:** Removal of the tumor along with some normal tissue around it.

- **Limb-sparing surgery:** Removal of the tumor in an arm or leg without amputation, so the use and appearance of the limb is saved. Radiation therapy or chemotherapy may be given first to shrink the tumor. The tumor is then removed in a wide local excision. Tissue and bone that are removed may be replaced with a graft using tissue and bone taken from another part of the patient's body, or with an implant such as artificial bone.

- **Amputation:** Surgery to remove part or all of a limb or appendage, such as an arm or leg.

- **Lymphadenectomy:** Removal of the lymph nodes that contain cancer.

Radiation therapy or chemotherapy may be given before or after surgery to remove the tumor. When given before surgery, radiation therapy or chemotherapy will make the tumor smaller and reduce the amount of tissue that needs to be removed during surgery. Treatment given before surgery is called neoadjuvant therapy. When given after surgery, radiation therapy or chemotherapy will kill any remaining cancer cells. Treatment given after the surgery, to lower the risk that the cancer will come back, is called adjuvant therapy.

Radiation Therapy

Radiation therapy is a cancer treatment that uses high-energy x-rays or other types of radiation to kill cancer cells or keep them from growing. There are two types of radiation therapy. External radiation therapy uses a machine outside the body to send radiation toward the cancer. Internal radiation therapy uses a radioactive substance sealed in needles, seeds, wires, or catheters that are placed directly into or near the cancer. The way the radiation therapy is given depends on the type and stage of the cancer being treated.

Fast neutron radiation therapy is a type of high-energy external radiation therapy. A radiation therapy machine aims tiny, invisible particles, called neutrons, at the cancer cells to kill them. Fast neutron radiation therapy uses a higher-energy radiation than the x-ray type of radiation therapy. This allows the same amount of radiation to be given in fewer treatments.

Chemotherapy

Chemotherapy is a cancer treatment that uses drugs to stop the growth of cancer cells, either by killing the cells or by stopping them from dividing. When chemotherapy is taken by mouth or injected into a vein or muscle, the drugs enter the bloodstream and can reach cancer cells throughout the body (systemic chemotherapy). When chemotherapy is placed directly into the spinal column, an organ, or a body cavity such as the abdomen, the drugs mainly affect cancer cells in those areas (regional chemotherapy). The way the chemotherapy is given depends on the type and stage of the cancer being treated.

Clinical Trials

For some patients, taking part in a clinical trial may be the best treatment choice. Clinical trials are part of the cancer research process. Clinical trials are done to find out if new cancer treatments are safe and effective or better than the standard treatment. High-dose chemotherapy with stem cell transplant and targeted therapy (a type of treatment that uses drugs or other substances to find and attack specific cancer cells without harming normal cells) are two new treatments being studied for soft tissue sarcomas. Information about clinical trials is available from the National Cancer Institute website (www.cancer.gov).

Follow-Up Tests

Some of the tests that were done to diagnose the cancer or to find out the stage of the cancer may be repeated. Some tests will be repeated in order to see how well the treatment is working. Decisions about whether to continue, change, or stop treatment may be based on the results of these tests. This is sometimes called re-staging.

Some of the tests will continue to be done from time to time after treatment has ended. The results of these tests can show if your condition has changed or if the cancer has recurred (come back). These tests are sometimes called follow-up tests or check-ups.

Section 53.3

Synovial Sarcoma

Excerpted from "Synovial Sarcoma: Questions and Answers," a fact sheet produced by the National Cancer Institute, May 29, 2005. Reviewed by David A. Cooke, MD, FACP, September 2010.

What is synovial sarcoma?

Synovial sarcoma is a type of soft tissue sarcoma. Soft tissue sarcomas are cancers of the muscle, fat, fibrous tissue, blood vessels, or other supporting tissue of the body, including synovial tissue. Synovial tissue lines the cavities of joints, such as the knee or elbow, tendons (tissues that connect muscle to bone), and bursae (fluid-filled, cushioning sacs in the spaces between tendons, ligaments, and bones). Although synovial sarcoma does not have a clearly defined cause, genetic factors are believed to influence the development of this disease.

How often does synovial sarcoma occur?

Synovial sarcoma is rare. It accounts for between 5% and 10% of the approximately 10,000 new soft tissue sarcomas reported each year. Synovial sarcoma occurs mostly in young adults, with a median age of 26.5. Approximately 30% of patients with synovial sarcoma are younger than 20. This disease occurs more often in men than in women.

Where does synovial sarcoma develop?

About 50% of synovial sarcomas develop in the legs, especially the knees. The second most common location is the arms. Less frequently, the disease develops in the trunk, head and neck region, or the abdomen. It is common for synovial cancer to recur (come back), usually within the first two years after treatment. Half of the cases of synovial sarcoma metastasize (spread to other areas of the body) to the lungs, lymph nodes, or bone marrow.

What are the symptoms of synovial sarcoma?

Synovial sarcoma is a slow-growing tumor. Because it grows slowly, a person may not have or notice symptoms for some time, resulting in a delay in diagnosis. The most common symptoms of synovial sarcoma are swelling or a mass that may be tender or painful. The tumor may limit range of motion or press against nerves and cause numbness. The symptoms of synovial sarcoma can be mistaken for those of inflammation of the joints, the bursae, or synovial tissue. These noncancerous conditions are called arthritis, bursitis, and synovitis, respectively.

How is synovial sarcoma diagnosed?

The doctor may remove tissue for examination under a microscope. This is called a biopsy. The tumor tissue may be tested for certain antigen and antibody interactions common to synovial sarcoma. This is called immunohistochemical analysis. Tissue may be examined using an ultramicroscope and electron microscope (a procedure called ultrastructural findings). Genetic testing may also be used. This involves testing tissue tested for a specific chromosome abnormality common to synovial sarcoma.

How is synovial sarcoma treated?

The type of treatment depends on the age of the patient, the location of the tumor, its size, its grade (how abnormal the cancer cells look under a microscope and how likely the tumor will quickly grow and spread), and the extent of the disease. The most common treatment is surgery to remove the entire tumor with negative margins (no cancer cells are found at the edge or border of the tissue removed during surgery). If the first surgery does not obtain negative tissue margins, a second surgery may be needed.

The patient may also receive radiation therapy before or after surgery to control the tumor or decrease the chance of recurrence (cancer coming back). The use of intraoperative radiation therapy (radiation aimed directly at the tumor during surgery) and brachytherapy (radioactive material sealed in needles, wires, seeds, or catheters, and placed directly into or near a tumor) are under study.

Patients may also receive chemotherapy alone or in combination with radiation therapy.

Are clinical trials (research studies) available?

Yes. Participation in clinical trials is an important treatment option for many people with synovial sarcoma. Studies are in progress to determine the effectiveness of biological therapies (treatment to stimulate or restore the ability of the immune system to fight cancer), including monoclonal antibodies, and chemotherapy with hyperthermia (kills tumor cells by heating them to several degrees above body temperature).

People interested in taking part in a clinical trial should talk with their doctor. Information about clinical trials is available from the National Cancer Institute's Cancer Information Service (CIS) 800-4-CANCER and in the NCI booklet "Taking Part in Cancer Treatment Research Studies," which can be found online at http://www.cancer.gov/publications. Further information about clinical trials is available at http://www.cancer.gov/clinicaltrials.

Chapter 54

Germ Cell Tumors

Chapter Contents

Section 54.1

Ovarian Germ Cell Tumors

Excerpted from PDQ® Cancer Information Summary. National Cancer Institute; Bethesda, MD. "Ovarian Germ Cell Tumors Treatment (PDQ) - Patient Version." Updated 01/2010. Available at: http://cancer.gov. Accessed October 23, 2010.

General Information about Ovarian Germ Cell Tumors

Germ cell tumors begin in the reproductive cells (egg or sperm) of the body. Ovarian germ cell tumors usually occur in teenage girls or young women and most often affect just one ovary.

The ovaries are a pair of organs in the female reproductive system. They are located in the pelvis, one on each side of the uterus (the hollow, pear-shaped organ where a fetus grows). Each ovary is about the size and shape of an almond. The ovaries produce eggs and female hormones (chemicals that control the way certain cells or organs function).

Ovarian germ cell tumor is a general name that is used to describe several different types of cancer. The most common ovarian germ cell tumor is called dysgerminoma.

Detection and Diagnosis

Ovarian germ cell tumors can be difficult to diagnose (find) early. Often there are no symptoms in the early stages, but tumors may be found during regular gynecologic examinations (checkups). A woman who has swelling of the abdomen without weight gain in other places should see a doctor. A woman who no longer has menstrual periods (who has gone through menopause) should also see a doctor if she has bleeding from the vagina.

Tests that examine the ovaries, pelvic area, blood, and ovarian tissue are used to detect and diagnose ovarian germ cell tumor. The following tests and procedures may be used.

Pelvic exam: An exam of the vagina, cervix, uterus, fallopian tubes, ovaries, and rectum. The doctor or nurse inserts one or two lubricated, gloved fingers of one hand into the vagina and the other hand is placed over the lower abdomen to feel the size, shape, and position of the uterus and ovaries. A speculum is also inserted into the vagina and the doctor or nurse looks at the vagina and cervix for signs of disease. A Pap test or Pap smear of the cervix is usually done. The doctor or nurse also inserts a lubricated, gloved finger into the rectum to feel for lumps or abnormal areas.

Laparotomy: A surgical procedure in which an incision (cut) is made in the wall of the abdomen to check the inside of the abdomen for signs of disease. The size of the incision depends on the reason the laparotomy is being done. Sometimes organs are removed or tissue samples are taken for biopsy.

Lymphangiogram: A procedure used to x-ray the lymph system. A dye is injected into the lymph vessels in the feet. The dye travels upward through the lymph nodes and lymph vessels, and x-rays are taken to see if there are any blockages. This test helps find out whether cancer has spread to the lymph nodes.

CT scan (CAT scan): A procedure that makes a series of detailed pictures of areas inside the body, taken from different angles. The pictures are made by a computer linked to an x-ray machine. A dye may be injected into a vein or swallowed to help the organs or tissues show up more clearly. This procedure is also called computed tomography, computerized tomography, or computerized axial tomography.

Serum tumor marker test: A procedure in which a sample of blood is checked to measure the amounts of certain substances released into the blood by organs, tissues, or tumor cells in the body. Certain substances are linked to specific types of cancer when found in increased levels in the blood. These are called tumor markers. An increased level of alpha fetoprotein (AFP) or human chorionic gonadotropin (HCG) in the blood may be a sign of ovarian germ cell tumor.

Prognosis

Certain factors affect prognosis (chance of recovery). The prognosis and treatment options depend on the following:

- The type of cancer
- The size of the tumor
- The stage of cancer (whether it affects part of the ovary, involves the whole ovary, or has spread to other places in the body)
- The way the cancer cells look under a microscope
- The patient's general health

Ovarian germ cell tumors are generally curable if found and treated early.

Stages of Ovarian Germ Cell Tumors

The process used to find out whether cancer has spread within the ovary or to other parts of the body is called staging. The information gathered from the staging process determines the stage of the disease. It is important to know the stage in order to plan treatment. Certain tests are used in the staging process.

Many of the tests used to diagnose ovarian germ cell tumor are also used to determine the stage of the disease. Unless a doctor is sure the cancer has spread from the ovaries to other parts of the body, surgery is required to determine the stage of cancer in an operation called a laparotomy. The doctor must cut into the abdomen and carefully look at all the organs to see if they contain cancer. The doctor will cut out small pieces of tissue and look at them under a microscope to see whether they contain cancer. The doctor may also wash the abdominal cavity with fluid and then look at the fluid under a microscope to see if it contains cancer cells. Usually the doctor will remove the cancer and other organs that contain cancer during the laparotomy.

The following stages are used for ovarian germ cell tumors.

Stage I

In stage I, cancer is found in one or both of the ovaries and has not spread. Stage I is divided into stage IA, stage IB, and stage IC.

Stage IA: Cancer is found in a single ovary.

Stage IB: Cancer is found in both ovaries.

Stage IC: Cancer is found in one or both ovaries and one of the following is true:

- Cancer is found on the outside surface of one or both ovaries.

- The capsule (outer covering) of the tumor has ruptured (broken open).

- Cancer cells are found in the fluid of the peritoneal cavity (the body cavity that contains most of the organs in the abdomen) or in washings of the peritoneum (tissue lining the peritoneal cavity).

Stage II

In stage II, cancer is found in one or both ovaries and has spread into other areas of the pelvis. Stage II is divided into stage IIA, stage IIB, and stage IIC.

Stage IIA: Cancer has spread to the uterus and/or the fallopian tubes (the long slender tubes through which eggs pass from the ovaries to the uterus).

Stage IIB: Cancer has spread to other tissue within the pelvis.

Stage IIC: Cancer has spread to the uterus and/or fallopian tubes and/or other tissue within the pelvis and cancer cells are found in the fluid of the peritoneal cavity (the body cavity that contains most of the organs in the abdomen) or in washings of the peritoneum (tissue lining the peritoneal cavity).

Stage III

In stage III, cancer is found in one or both ovaries and has spread to other parts of the abdomen. (Cancer that has spread to the surface of the liver is also considered stage III disease.) Stage III is divided into stage IIIA, stage IIIB, and stage IIIC as follows:

Stage IIIA: The tumor is found only in the pelvis, but cancer cells have spread to the surface of the peritoneum (tissue that lines the abdominal wall and covers most of the organs in the abdomen).

Stage IIIB: Cancer has spread to the peritoneum but is two centimeters or smaller in diameter.

Stage IIIC: Cancer has spread to the peritoneum and is larger than two centimeters in diameter and/or has spread to lymph nodes in the abdomen.

Stage IV

In stage IV, cancer is found in one or both ovaries and has metastasized (spread) beyond the abdomen to other parts of the body. Cancer that has spread to tissues in the liver is also considered stage IV disease.

Recurrent Ovarian Germ Cell Tumors

Recurrent ovarian germ cell tumor is cancer that has recurred (come back) after it has been treated. The cancer may come back in the other ovary or in other parts of the body.

Treatment Option Overview

Different types of treatment are available for patients with ovarian germ cell tumor. Some treatments are standard (the currently used treatment), and some are being tested in clinical trials. Three types of standard treatment are used:

Surgery

Surgery is the most common treatment of ovarian germ cell tumor. A doctor may take out the cancer using one of the following types of surgery.

Unilateral salpingo-oophorectomy: A surgical procedure to remove one ovary and one fallopian tube.

Total hysterectomy: A surgical procedure to remove the uterus, including the cervix. If the uterus and cervix are taken out through the vagina, the operation is called a vaginal hysterectomy. If the uterus and cervix are taken out through a large incision (cut) in the abdomen, the operation is called a total abdominal hysterectomy. If the uterus and cervix are taken out through a small incision (cut) in the abdomen using a laparoscope, the operation is called a total laparoscopic hysterectomy.

Bilateral salpingo-oophorectomy: A surgical procedure to remove both ovaries and both fallopian tubes.

Tumor debulking: A surgical procedure in which as much of the tumor as possible is removed. Some tumors may not be able to be completely removed.

Chemotherapy

Chemotherapy is a cancer treatment that uses drugs to stop the growth of cancer cells, either by killing the cells or by stopping the cells from dividing. When chemotherapy is taken by mouth or injected into a vein or muscle, the drugs enter the bloodstream and can reach cancer cells throughout the body (systemic chemotherapy). When chemotherapy is placed directly in the spinal column, an organ, or a body cavity such as the abdomen, the drugs mainly affect cancer cells in those areas. The way the chemotherapy is given depends on the type and stage of the cancer being treated.

Radiation Therapy

Radiation therapy is a cancer treatment that uses high-energy x-rays or other types of radiation to kill cancer cells. There are two types of radiation therapy. External radiation therapy uses a machine outside the body to send radiation toward the cancer. Internal radiation therapy uses a radioactive substance sealed in needles, seeds, wires, or catheters that are placed directly into or near the cancer. The way the radiation therapy is given depends on the type and stage of the cancer being treated.

Even if the doctor removes all the cancer that can be seen at the time of the operation, some patients may be offered chemotherapy or radiation after surgery to kill any cancer cells that are left. Treatment given after the surgery, to lower the risk that the cancer will come back, is called adjuvant therapy.

Following radiation or chemotherapy, an operation called a second-look laparotomy is sometimes done. This is similar to the laparotomy that is done to determine the stage of the cancer. During the second-look operation, the doctor will take samples of lymph nodes and other tissues in the abdomen to see if any cancer is left.

Clinical Trials

Patients may want to think about taking part in a clinical trial. For some patients, taking part in a clinical trial may be the best treatment choice. Clinical trials are part of the cancer research process. Clinical trials are done to find out if new cancer treatments are safe and effective or better than the standard treatment.

Many of today's standard treatments for cancer are based on earlier clinical trials. Patients who take part in a clinical trial may receive the standard treatment or be among the first to receive a new treatment.

Patients who take part in clinical trials also help improve the way cancer will be treated in the future. Even when clinical trials do not lead to effective new treatments, they often answer important questions and help move research forward.

Patients can enter clinical trials before, during, or after starting their cancer treatment. Some clinical trials only include patients who have not yet received treatment. Other trials test treatments for patients whose cancer has not gotten better. There are also clinical trials that test new ways to stop cancer from recurring (coming back) or reduce the side effects of cancer treatment.

Two treatments being studied for ovarian germ cell tumors are high-dose chemotherapy with bone marrow transplant and combination chemotherapy.

- High-dose chemotherapy with bone marrow transplant is a method of giving very high doses of chemotherapy and replacing blood-forming cells destroyed by the cancer treatment. Stem cells (immature blood cells) are removed from the bone marrow of the patient or a donor and are frozen and stored. After the chemotherapy is completed, the stored stem cells are thawed and given back to the patient through an infusion. These reinfused stem cells grow into (and restore) the body's blood cells.

- Combination chemotherapy is the use of more than one chemotherapy drug to fight cancer.

For more information about clinical trials, visit the National Cancer Institute's clinical trials website at www.cancer.gov/clinicaltrials.

Follow-Up Tests

Some of the tests that were done to diagnose the cancer or to find out the stage of the cancer may be repeated. Some tests will be repeated in order to see how well the treatment is working. Decisions about whether to continue, change, or stop treatment may be based on the results of these tests. This is sometimes called re-staging.

Some of the tests will continue to be done from time to time after treatment has ended. The results of these tests can show if your condition has changed or if the cancer has recurred (come back). These tests are sometimes called follow-up tests or check-ups.

Section 54.2

Extragonadal Germ Cell Tumors

Excerpted from PDQ® Cancer Information Summary. National Cancer Institute; Bethesda, MD. "Extragonadal Germ Cell Tumors Treatment (PDQ) - Patient Version." Updated 06/2008. Available at: http://cancer.gov. Accessed January 20, 2010.

General Information about Extragonadal Germ Cell Tumors

"Extragonadal" means outside of the gonads (sex organs). When cells that are meant to form sperm in the testicles or eggs in the ovaries travel to other parts of the body, they may grow into extragonadal germ cell tumors. These tumors may begin to grow anywhere in the body but usually begin in organs such as the pineal gland in the brain, in the mediastinum, or in the abdomen.

Extragonadal germ cell tumors can be benign (noncancer) or malignant (cancer). Benign extragonadal germ cell tumors are called benign teratomas. These are more common than malignant extragonadal germ cell tumors and often are very large.

Malignant extragonadal germ cell tumors are divided into two types, nonseminoma and seminoma. Nonseminomas tend to grow and spread more quickly than seminomas. They usually are large and cause symptoms. If untreated, malignant extragonadal germ cell tumors may spread to the lungs, lymph nodes, bones, liver, or other parts of the body.

Risk Factors and Signs

Age and gender can affect the risk of developing extragonadal germ cell tumors. Anything that increases your chance of getting a disease is called a risk factor. Having a risk factor does not mean that you will get cancer; not having risk factors doesn't mean that you will not get cancer. People who think they may be at risk should discuss this with their doctor. Risk factors for malignant extragonadal germ cell tumors include the following:

- Being male
- Being age 20 or older
- Having Klinefelter syndrome

Malignant extragonadal germ cell tumors may cause symptoms as they grow into nearby areas. Other conditions may cause the same symptoms. A doctor should be consulted if any of the following problems occur:

- Chest pain
- Breathing problems
- Cough
- Fever
- Headache
- Change in bowel habits
- Feeling very tired
- Trouble walking
- Trouble in seeing or moving the eyes

Detection and Diagnosis

Imaging and blood tests are used to detect and diagnose extragonadal germ cell tumors. The following tests and procedures may be used:

Physical exam and history: An exam of the body to check general signs of health, including checking for signs of disease, such as lumps or anything else that seems unusual. The testicles may be checked for lumps, swelling, or pain. A history of the patient's health habits and past illnesses and treatments will also be taken.

Chest x-ray: An x-ray of the organs and bones inside the chest. An x-ray is a type of energy beam that can go through the body and onto film, making a picture of areas inside the body.

Serum tumor marker test: A procedure in which a sample of blood is examined to measure the amounts of certain substances released into the blood by organs, tissues, or tumor cells in the body. Certain substances are linked to specific types of cancer when found in increased levels in the blood. These are called tumor markers. The following three tumor markers are used to detect extragonadal germ cell tumor.

- Alpha-fetoprotein (AFP)
- Beta-human chorionic gonadotropin (ß-hCG)
- Lactate dehydrogenase (LDH)

Blood levels of the tumor markers help determine if the tumor is a seminoma or nonseminoma.

CT scan (CAT scan): A procedure that makes a series of detailed pictures of areas inside the body, taken from different angles. The pictures are made by a computer linked to an x-ray machine. A dye may be injected into a vein or swallowed to help the organs or tissues show up more clearly. This procedure is also called computed tomography, computerized tomography, or computerized axial tomography.

Ultrasound exam: A procedure in which high-energy sound waves (ultrasound) are bounced off internal tissues or organs, such as the testicles, and make echoes. The echoes form a picture of body tissues called a sonogram. The picture can be printed to be looked at later.

Biopsy: The removal of cells or tissues so they can be viewed under a microscope by a pathologist to check for signs of cancer. The type of biopsy used depends on where the extragonadal germ cell tumor is found.

- Excisional biopsy is the removal of an entire lump of tissue.
- Incisional biopsy is the removal of part of a lump or sample of tissue.
- Core biopsy is the removal of tissue using a wide needle.
- Fine-needle aspiration (FNA) biopsy is the removal of tissue or fluid using a thin needle.

Prognosis

Certain factors affect prognosis and treatment options. The prognosis and treatment options depend on the following:

- Whether the tumor is nonseminoma or seminoma
- The size of the tumor and where it is in the body
- The blood levels of AFP, ß-hCG, and LDH
- Whether the tumor has spread to other parts of the body
- The way the tumor responds to initial treatment

- Whether the tumor has just been diagnosed or has recurred (come back)

Stages of Extragonadal Germ Cell Tumors

After an extragonadal germ cell tumor has been diagnosed, tests are done to find out if cancer cells have spread to other parts of the body.

The extent or spread of cancer is usually described as stages. For extragonadal germ cell tumors, prognostic groups are used instead of stages. The tumors are grouped according to how well the cancer is expected to respond to treatment. It is important to know the prognostic group in order to plan treatment. The following prognostic groups are used for extragonadal germ cell tumors:

Good Prognosis

A nonseminoma extragonadal germ cell tumor is in the good prognosis group if the tumor is in the back of the abdomen; and the tumor has not spread to organs other than the lungs; and the levels of tumor markers AFP and ß-hCG are normal and LDH is slightly above normal.

A seminoma extragonadal germ cell tumor is in the good prognosis group if the tumor has not spread to organs other than the lungs; and the level of AFP is normal; ß-hCG and LDH may be at any level.

Intermediate Prognosis

A nonseminoma extragonadal germ cell tumor is in the intermediate prognosis group if the tumor is in the back of the abdomen; and the tumor has not spread to organs other than the lungs; and the level of any one of the tumor markers (AFP, ß -hCG, or LDH) is more than slightly above normal.

A seminoma extragonadal germ cell tumor is in the intermediate prognosis group if the tumor has spread to organs other than the lungs; and the level of AFP is normal; ß-hCG and LDH may be at any level.

Poor Prognosis

A nonseminoma extragonadal germ cell tumor is in the poor prognosis group if the tumor is in the chest; or the tumor has spread to organs other than the lungs; or the level of any one of the tumor markers (AFP, ß-hCG, or LDH) is high.

Seminoma extragonadal germ cell tumor does not have a poor prognosis group.

Treatment Option Overview

Different types of treatments are available for patients with extragonadal germ cell tumors. Some treatments are standard (the currently used treatment), and some are being tested in clinical trials. Three types of standard treatment are used.

Radiation Therapy

Radiation therapy is a cancer treatment that uses high-energy x-rays or other types of radiation to kill cancer cells or keep them from growing. There are two types of radiation therapy. External radiation therapy uses a machine outside the body to send radiation toward the cancer. Internal radiation therapy uses a radioactive substance sealed in needles, seeds, wires, or catheters that are placed directly into or near the cancer. The way the radiation therapy is given depends on the type and stage of the cancer being treated.

Chemotherapy

Chemotherapy is a cancer treatment that uses drugs to stop the growth of cancer cells, either by killing the cells or by stopping them from dividing. When chemotherapy is taken by mouth or injected into a vein or muscle, the drugs enter the bloodstream and can reach cancer cells throughout the body (systemic chemotherapy). When chemotherapy is placed directly in the spinal column, an organ, or a body cavity such as the abdomen, the drugs mainly affect cancer cells in those areas (regional chemotherapy). The way the chemotherapy is given depends on the type and stage of the cancer being treated.

Surgery

Patients who have benign tumors or tumor remaining after chemotherapy or radiation therapy may need to have surgery.

Clinical Trials

A treatment clinical trial is a research study meant to help improve current treatments or obtain information on new treatments for patients with cancer. When clinical trials show that a new treatment is better than the standard treatment, the new treatment may become the standard treatment. Patients may want to think about taking part in a clinical trial. Some clinical trials are open only to patients who have not started treatment.

One type of treatment being studied for extragonadal germ cell tumors is high-dose chemotherapy with stem cell transplant. High-dose chemotherapy with stem cell transplant is a method of giving high doses of chemotherapy and replacing blood-forming cells destroyed by the cancer treatment. Stem cells (immature blood cells) are removed from the blood or bone marrow of the patient or a donor and are frozen and stored. After the chemotherapy is completed, the stored stem cells are thawed and given back to the patient through an infusion. These reinfused stem cells grow into (and restore) the body's blood cells.

For more information about clinical trials, visit the National Cancer Institute's clinical trials website at www.cancer.gov/clinicaltrials.

Follow-Up Tests

Some of the tests that were done to diagnose the cancer or to find out the stage of the cancer may be repeated. Some tests will be repeated in order to see how well the treatment is working. Decisions about whether to continue, change, or stop treatment may be based on the results of these tests. This is sometimes called re-staging.

Some of the tests will continue to be done from time to time after treatment has ended. The results of these tests can show if your condition has changed or if the cancer has recurred (come back). These tests are sometimes called follow-up tests or check-ups.

After initial treatment for extragonadal germ cell tumors, blood levels of AFP and other tumor markers continue to be checked to find out how well the treatment is working.

Section 54.3

Childhood Extracranial Germ Cell Tumors

Excerpted from PDQ® Cancer Information Summary. National Cancer Institute; Bethesda, MD. "Childhood Extracranial Germ Cell Tumors Treatment (PDQ) - Patient Version." Updated 04/2010. Available at: http://cancer .gov. Accessed October 24, 2010.

General Information about Childhood Extracranial Germ Cell Tumors

Childhood extracranial germ cell tumors form from developing sperm or egg cells that travel to parts of the body other than the brain.

As a fetus develops, certain cells form sperm in the testicles or eggs in the ovaries. Sometimes these cells travel to other parts of the body and grow into germ cell tumors. This section is about germ cell tumors that form in parts of the body that are extracranial (outside the brain). Extracranial germ cell tumors are most common in teenagers 15 to 19 years old.

Extracranial germ cell tumors may be benign (noncancer) or malignant (cancer). Extracranial germ cell tumors are grouped into mature teratomas, immature teratomas, or malignant germ cell tumors.

- Mature teratomas are the most common type of extracranial germ cell tumor. The cells of mature teratomas look very much like normal cells. Mature teratomas are benign and not likely to become cancer.

- Immature teratomas have cells that look very different from normal cells. They are more likely to become cancer.

- Malignant germ cell tumors are cancer. There are three types of malignant germ cell tumors:

  - **Yolk sac tumors:** Tumors that make a hormone called alpha-fetoprotein (AFP).

  - **Germinomas:** Tumors that make a hormone called beta-human chorionic gonadotropin (ß-hCG).

  - **Choriocarcinomas:** Tumors that make a hormone called beta-human chorionic gonadotropin (ß-hCG).

Malignant extracranial germ cell tumors are grouped into gonadal and extragonadal. Gonadal germ cell tumors form in the testicles or ovaries.

Gonadal Germ Cell Tumors

Testicular germ cell tumors: Testicular germ cell tumors usually occur before the age of four years or in teenagers and young adults. Testicular germ cell tumors in teenagers and young adults are different from those that form in early childhood. They are more like testicular cancer in adults. Testicular germ cell tumors are divided into two main types, nonseminoma and seminoma.

- **Nonseminoma:** These tumors are usually large and cause symptoms. They tend to grow and spread more quickly than seminomas.

- **Seminoma:** These tumors make a hormone called beta-human chorionic gonadotropin (ß-hCG). They are more sensitive to radiation therapy than nonseminomas.

Boys older than 14 years with testicular germ cell tumors are treated in pediatric cancer centers, but the treatment is similar to that used in adults.

Ovarian germ cell tumors: Ovarian germ cell tumors form in egg-making cells in an ovary. These tumors are more common in teenage girls and young women. Most ovarian germ cell tumors are benign teratomas. (For more information about ovarian germ cell tumors, see section 54.1).

Extragonadal Extracranial Germ Cell Tumors

Extragonadal germ cell tumors form in areas other than the testicles or ovaries. Most germ cell tumors that are not in the testicles, ovaries, or brain, form along the midline of the body. This includes the following:

- Sacrum (the large, triangle-shaped bone in the lower spine that forms part of the pelvis)

- Coccyx (the small bone at the bottom of the spine, also called the tailbone)

- Mediastinum (the area between the lungs)

- Back of the abdomen

- Neck

In younger children, extragonadal extracranial germ cell tumors usually occur at birth or in early childhood. Most of these tumors are teratomas in the sacrum or coccyx.

In older children, teenagers, and young adults, extragonadal extracranial germ cell tumors are often in the mediastinum.

Risk Factors and Signs

The cause of most childhood extracranial germ cell tumors is unknown. Anything that increases your risk of getting a disease is called a risk factor. Having a risk factor does not mean that you will get cancer; not having risk factors doesn't mean that you will not get cancer. People who think they may be at risk should discuss this with their doctor. Possible risk factors for extracranial germ cell tumors include the following.

- Having certain genetic syndromes may increase the risk of developing childhood germ cell tumors: Klinefelter syndrome may increase the risk of developing germ cell tumors in the mediastinum. Swyer syndrome may increase the risk of developing germ cell tumors in the testes or ovaries.

- Having an undescended testicle may increase the risk of developing a testicular germ cell tumor.

Signs of childhood extracranial germ cell tumors depend on the type of tumor and where it is in the body. Different tumors may cause the following signs and symptoms. Other conditions may cause these same symptoms. A doctor should be consulted if any of these problems occur:

- Most tumors of the sacrum and coccyx can be seen as a lump.

- A testicular tumor may cause a painless lump in the testicles.

- An ovarian germ cell tumor may cause a pain or a lump in the abdomen, fever, constipation, no menstruation, or unusual vaginal bleeding.

Detection and Diagnosis

Imaging studies and blood tests are used to detect (find) and diagnose childhood extracranial germ cell tumors. The following tests and procedures may be used:

Physical exam and history: An exam of the body to check general signs of health, including checking for signs of disease, such as lumps or anything else that seems unusual. The testicles may be checked for lumps, swelling, or pain. A history of the patient's health habits and past illnesses and treatments will also be taken.

Serum tumor marker test: A procedure in which a sample of blood is checked to measure the amounts of certain substances released into the blood by organs, tissues, or tumor cells in the body. Certain substances are linked to specific types of cancer when found in increased levels in the blood. These are called tumor markers.

Most malignant germ cell tumors release tumor markers. The following tumor markers are used to detect extracranial germ cell tumors:

- Alpha-fetoprotein (AFP)

- Beta-human chorionic gonadotropin (ß-hCG)

For testicular germ cell tumors, blood levels of the tumor markers help show if the tumor is a seminoma or nonseminoma.

Blood chemistry studies: A procedure in which a blood sample is checked to measure the amounts of certain substances released into the blood by organs and tissues in the body. An unusual (higher or lower than normal) amount of a substance can be a sign of disease in the organ or tissue that makes it.

Cytogenetic analysis: A laboratory test in which cells in a sample of tissue are viewed under a microscope to look for certain changes in the chromosomes.

Immunohistochemistry study: A laboratory test in which a substance such as an antibody, dye, or radioisotope is added to a sample of cancer tissue to test for certain antigens. This type of study is used to tell the difference between different types of cancer.

Chest x-ray: An x-ray of the organs and bones inside the chest. An x-ray is a type of energy beam that can go through the body and onto film, making a picture of areas inside the body.

CT scan (CAT scan): A procedure that makes a series of detailed pictures of areas inside the body, taken from different angles. The pictures are made by a computer linked to an x-ray machine. A dye may be injected into a vein or swallowed to help the organs or tissues show up more clearly. This procedure is also called computed tomography, computerized tomography, or computerized axial tomography.

Ultrasound exam: A procedure in which high-energy sound waves (ultrasound) are bounced off internal tissues or organs and make echoes. The echoes form a picture of body tissues called a sonogram. The picture can be printed to be looked at later.

Biopsy: The removal of cells or tissues so they can be viewed under a microscope by a pathologist to check for signs of cancer. In some cases, the tumor is removed during surgery and then a biopsy is done.

Prognosis

Certain factors affect prognosis and treatment options. The prognosis and treatment options depend on the following:

- The type of germ cell tumor
- Where the tumor first began to grow
- The stage of the cancer (whether it has spread to nearby areas or to other places in the body)
- Whether the tumor can be completely removed by surgery
- The patient's age and general health
- Whether the cancer has just been diagnosed or has recurred (come back)

The prognosis for childhood extracranial germ cell tumors, especially ovarian germ cell tumors, is good.

Stages of Childhood Extracranial Germ Cell Tumors

After a childhood extracranial germ cell tumor has been diagnosed, tests are done to find out if cancer cells have spread from where the tumor started to nearby areas or to other parts of the body. The process used to find out if cancer has spread from where the tumor started to other parts of the body is called staging. The information gathered from the staging process determines the stage of the disease. It is important to know the stage in order to plan treatment. In some cases, staging may follow surgery to remove the tumor. The following procedures may be used:

- **MRI (magnetic resonance imaging):** A procedure that uses a magnet, radio waves, and a computer to make a series of detailed pictures of areas inside the body. This procedure is also called nuclear magnetic resonance imaging.

- **Bone scan:** A procedure to check if there are rapidly dividing cells, such as cancer cells, in the bone. A very small amount of radioactive material is injected into a vein and travels through the bloodstream. The radioactive material collects in the bones and is detected by a scanner.

- **Thoracentesis:** The removal of fluid from the space between the lining of the chest and the lung, using a needle. A pathologist views the fluid under a microscope to look for cancer cells.

- **Paracentesis:** The removal of fluid from the space between the lining of the abdomen and the organs in the abdomen, using a needle. A pathologist views the fluid under a microscope to look for cancer cells.

The results from tests and procedures used to detect and diagnose childhood extracranial germ cell tumor may also be used in staging.

The following stages are commonly used for most childhood extracranial germ cell tumors:

Stage I: In stage I, the cancer is in one place and can be completely removed by surgery.

Stage II: In stage II, the cancer has spread to nearby tissues or lymph nodes and is not completely removed by surgery. The cancer remaining after surgery can be seen with a microscope only.

Stage III: In stage III, the cancer has spread to nearby tissues and lymph nodes; is found in fluid in the abdomen or around the lungs; and is not completely removed by surgery. The remaining cancer can be seen without a microscope.

Stage IV: In stage IV, the cancer has spread to other places in the body, such as the lung, liver, brain, bone, and distant lymph nodes.

Recurrent Childhood Extracranial Germ Cell Tumors

Recurrent childhood extracranial germ cell tumor is cancer that has recurred (come back) after it has been treated. The cancer may come back in the same place or in other parts of the body.

The number of patients who have tumors that come back is small. Most recurrent germ cell tumors occur within three years of surgery. About half of the teratomas that recur in the sacrum or coccyx are malignant, so follow-up is important.

Treatment Option Overview

Different types of treatments are available for children with extracranial germ cell tumors. Some treatments are standard (the currently used treatment), and some are being tested in clinical trials..

Children with extracranial germ cell tumors should have their treatment planned by a team of health care providers who are experts in treating cancer in children.

Treatment will be overseen by a pediatric oncologist, a doctor who specializes in treating children with cancer. The pediatric oncologist works with other health care providers who are experts in treating children with extracranial germ cell tumors and who specialize in certain areas of medicine. These may include the following specialists:

- Pediatric surgeon
- Pediatric hematologist
- Radiation oncologist
- Endocrinologist
- Pediatric nurse specialist
- Rehabilitation specialist
- Psychologist
- Social worker
- Geneticist

Some cancer treatments cause side effects months or years after treatment has ended. Side effects from cancer treatment that begin during or after treatment and continue for months or years are called late effects. Late effects of cancer treatment may include physical problems; changes in mood, feelings, thinking, learning, or memory; and second cancers (new types of cancer). For example, late effects of surgery to remove tumors in the sacrum or coccyx include constipation, loss of bowel and bladder control, and scars.

Some late effects may be treated or controlled. It is important to talk with your child's doctors about the effects cancer treatment can have on your child.

Three types of standard treatment are used.

Surgery

Surgery to completely remove the tumor is done whenever possible. If the tumor is very large, chemotherapy may be given first, to make

745

the tumor smaller and decrease the amount of tissue that needs to be removed during surgery. The following types of surgery may be used:

- **Resection:** Surgery to remove tissue or part or all of an organ. If cancer is in the coccyx, the entire coccyx is removed.

- **Tumor debulking:** A surgical procedure in which as much of the tumor as possible is removed. Some tumors may not be able to be completely removed.

- **Radical inguinal orchiectomy:** Surgery to remove one or both testicles through an incision (cut) in the groin.

- **Unilateral salpingo-oophorectomy:** Surgery to remove one ovary and one fallopian tube.

Watchful Waiting

Watchful waiting is closely monitoring a patient's condition without giving any treatment until symptoms appear or change. For childhood extracranial germ cell tumors, this includes physical exams, imaging tests, and tumor marker tests.

Chemotherapy

Chemotherapy is a cancer treatment that uses drugs to stop the growth of cancer cells, either by killing the cells or by stopping them from dividing. When chemotherapy is taken by mouth or injected into a vein or muscle, the drugs enter the bloodstream and can reach cancer cells throughout the body (systemic chemotherapy). When chemotherapy is placed directly into the spinal column, an organ, or a body cavity such as the abdomen, the drugs mainly affect cancer cells in those areas (regional chemotherapy). Combination chemotherapy is treatment using more than one anticancer drug. The way the chemotherapy is given depends on the type and stage of the cancer being treated.

Clinical Trials

A treatment clinical trial is a research study meant to help improve current treatments or obtain information on new treatments for patients with cancer. When clinical trials show that a new treatment is better than the standard treatment, the new treatment may become the standard treatment.

Because cancer in children is rare, taking part in a clinical trial should be considered. Some clinical trials are open only to patients who have not started treatment.

New types of treatment are being tested in clinical trials. Patients may want to think about taking part in a clinical trial. For more information about clinical trials, visit the National Cancer Institute's clinical trials website at www.cancer.gov/clinicaltrials.

Follow-Up Tests

Some of the tests that were done to diagnose the cancer or to find out the stage of the cancer may be repeated. Some tests will be repeated in order to see how well the treatment is working. Decisions about whether to continue, change, or stop treatment may be based on the results of these tests. This is sometimes called re-staging.

Some of the tests will continue to be done from time to time after treatment has ended. The results of these tests can show if your condition has changed or if the cancer has recurred (come back). These tests are sometimes called follow-up tests or check-ups.

For childhood extracranial germ cell tumors, alpha-fetoprotein (AFP) tests are done to see if treatment is working. Continued high levels of AFP may mean the cancer is still growing. For at least three years after surgery, follow-up will include regular physical exams, imaging tests, and tumor marker tests.

Chapter 55

Carcinoma of Unknown Primary Origin

Basic Information about Carcinoma of Unknown Primary

Carcinoma of unknown primary (CUP) is a disease in which cancer (malignant) cells are found somewhere in the body, but the place where they first started growing (the origin or primary site) cannot be found. This occurs in about 2 to 4% of cancer patients.

Actually, CUP can be described as a group of different types of cancer all of which have become known by the place or places in the body where the cancer has spread (metastasized) from another part of the body. Because all of these diseases are not alike, chance of recovery (prognosis) and choice of treatment may be different for each patient.

If CUP is suspected, a doctor will order several tests, one of which may be a biopsy. This means a small piece of tissue is cut from the tumor and looked at under a microscope. The doctor may also do a complete history and physical examination, and order chest x-rays along with blood, urine, and stool tests. A cancer can be called CUP when the doctor cannot tell from the test results where the cancer began.

Excerpted from PDQ® Cancer Information Summary. National Cancer Institute; Bethesda, MD. "Carcinoma of Unknown Primary Treatment (PDQ) - Patient Version." Updated 08/2009. Available at: http://cancer.gov. Accessed January 20, 2010.

The pattern of how CUP has spread may also give the doctor information to help determine where it started. For example, lung metastases are more common when cancer begins above the diaphragm (the thin muscle under the lungs that helps the breathing process). Most large studies have shown that CUP often starts in the lungs or pancreas. Less often, it may start in the colon, rectum, breast, or prostate.

An important part of trying to find out where the cancer started is to see how the cancer cells look under a microscope (histology). Other special tests may also be done that help the doctor find out where the cancer started and choose the best type of treatment.

Stages of Carcinoma of Unknown Primary

When cancer is diagnosed, more tests are usually done to find out if cancer cells have spread to other parts of the body. This is called staging. But, when CUP is diagnosed, the number and type of tests done may be different for each patient. The treatment options in this summary are based on whether the cancer has just been found (newly diagnosed) or the cancer has come back after it has been treated (recurrent).

The treatment options are also based on where the cancer is found, where the doctor thinks the cancer started, what the cancer cells look like under a microscope, and other factors. A doctor may find that the cancer fits into one of the following groups:

- **Cancer in the cervical lymph nodes:** Cancer in the small, bean-shaped organs that make and store infection-fighting cells (lymph nodes) in the neck area

- **Poorly differentiated carcinomas:** The cancer cells look very different from normal cells

- **Metastatic melanoma to a single nodal site:** Cancer of the cells that color the skin (melanocytes) that has spread to lymph nodes in only one part of the body

- **Isolated axillary metastasis:** Cancer that has spread only to lymph nodes in the area of the armpits

- **Inguinal node metastasis:** Cancer that has spread to lymph nodes in the groin area

- **Multiple involvement:** Cancer that has spread to several different areas of the body

Treatment Option Overview

Different types of treatment are available for patients with carcinoma of unknown primary (CUP). Some treatments are standard (the currently used treatment), and some are being tested in clinical trials. Surgery, radiation therapy, chemotherapy, and hormone therapy are some of the standard treatments that are used:

Surgery: Surgery is a common treatment for CUP. A doctor may remove the cancer and some of the healthy tissue around it. Different operations are used depending on where the cancer is found. If the cancer has spread to lymph nodes, the lymph nodes may be removed (lymph node dissection). If the nodes involved are in the groin, this operation is called a superficial groin dissection. If the cancer has spread to lymph nodes and also to some surrounding areas, the doctor may have to remove a larger portion of tissue around the nodes. When muscles, nerves, and other tissue in the neck are removed, this is called a radical neck dissection.

Radiation therapy: Radiation therapy uses x-rays or other high-energy rays to kill cancer cells and shrink tumors. Radiation may be used alone or before or after surgery.

Chemotherapy: Chemotherapy uses drugs to kill cancer cells. Chemotherapy may be taken by mouth or it may be put into the body by a needle in a vein or muscle. Chemotherapy is called a systemic treatment because the drugs enter the bloodstream, travel through the body, and can kill cancer cells throughout the body. Chemotherapy may be used alone or after surgery. Therapy given after an operation when there are no cancer cells that can be seen is called adjuvant therapy.

Hormone therapy: Hormone therapy is used to stop the hormones in the body that help cancer cells grow. This may be done by using drugs that change the way hormones work or by surgery that takes out organs that make hormones, such as the testicles (orchiectomy).

Clinical Trials

A treatment clinical trial is a research study meant to help improve current treatments or obtain information on new treatments for patients with cancer. When clinical trials show that a new treatment is better than the standard treatment, the new treatment may become the standard treatment. Patients may want to think about taking part in a clinical trial. Some clinical trials are open only to patients who have not started treatment.

For some patients, taking part in a clinical trial may be the best treatment choice. Clinical trials are part of the cancer research process. Clinical trials are done to find out if new cancer treatments are safe and effective or better than the standard treatment.

Many of today's standard treatments for cancer are based on earlier clinical trials. Patients who take part in a clinical trial may receive the standard treatment or be among the first to receive a new treatment.

Patients who take part in clinical trials also help improve the way cancer will be treated in the future. Even when clinical trials do not lead to effective new treatments, they often answer important questions and help move research forward.

Some clinical trials only include patients who have not yet received treatment. Other trials test treatments for patients whose cancer has not gotten better. There are also clinical trials that test new ways to stop cancer from recurring (coming back) or reduce the side effects of cancer treatment.

Check with your doctor for clinical trials that may be right for you. You can also check the National Cancer Institute's clinical trials website, available online at www.cancer.gov/clinicaltrials.

Part Three

Cancer-Related Tests
and Treatments

Chapter 56

Cancer Screening and Early Detection

It's hard to say why one person gets cancer and another does not. It may seem that cancer can't be avoided, but there are things that you can do to reduce your risk of the disease. You can start by living a healthy lifestyle and taking charge of your health.

Early Detection and Screening

Early detection means finding cancer at an early stage. When cancer is found early, it is often easier to treat. Recognizing symptoms and getting regular checkups help detect cancer early. Be aware of your body and don't ignore any changes. The sooner you report symptoms to your doctor, the sooner a problem can be dealt with.

Screening is the early detection of cancer by testing or checking for disease when you don't have any symptoms. Many types of cancer don't have a screening test, but some cancers can be found before you've even noticed that something might be wrong. Screening tests can help find cancer at its earliest, most treatable stages. Some screening tests can also help detect precancerous conditions that can be treated before cancer develops. If a screening test shows something unusual, follow-up tests will be needed.

The information in this chapter is excerpted from "Early Detection and Screening: Facts for Women," Canadian Cancer Society, 2007; and "Early Detection and Screening: Facts for Men," Canadian Cancer Society, 2007. © 2007 Canadian Cancer Society. Revised July 2008. To view the complete text of these documents along with additional information, visit http://www.cancer.ca.

It's important to know that no screening test for cancer is 100% accurate. For example, a screening test can sometimes show cancer when there isn't, or not show cancer when there is. But overall, screening tests save lives.

Recommended Cancer Screening for Women

Breast Cancer

Breast cancer starts in the cells of the breast tissue. Breast tissue in women covers an area larger than just the breast. It extends up to the collarbone and from the armpit across to the breastbone in the center of the chest.

Breast cancer is the most commonly diagnosed cancer in women in Canada. It can also be found in men, but this is very rare.

Breast cancer can happen at any age, but most cases occur in women over the age of 50. Many women are alive and well today because their breast cancer was found and treated early.

What you can do: The most reliable tests used to find breast cancer early are:

- **mammography:** A low-dose x-ray of the breasts.

- **clinical breast examination (CBE):** A physical examination of the breasts by a trained healthcare professional.

Breast screening programs vary among the provinces and territories. Your doctor can tell you more about the screening tests or programs in your area.

Table 56.1. Breast Cancer Screening

If you are:	What to do:
40 or older	Have a CBE by a trained healthcare professional at least every two years
40 to 49	Talk to your doctor about your risk of breast cancer, along with the benefits and risks of mammography
50 to 69	Have a mammogram every two years
70 or older	Talk to your doctor about how often you should get tested for breast cancer

Some women have a higher-than-average risk for breast cancer. Talk to your doctor about your risk and a personal plan of testing. It may make sense to consider getting tested earlier or more often if:

- you have had breast cancer before.

- you have a history of breast biopsies showing certain breast changes, such as an increased number of abnormal cells which are not cancerous (atypical hyperplasia).

- you have a family history of breast cancer (especially in a mother, sister, or daughter diagnosed before menopause or if hereditary mutations are present in certain genes, such as BRCA1 or BRCA2).

You can also be aware of how your breasts normally look and feel so that you can notice any changes, even if you are getting tested regularly. Keep in mind that your breasts may feel different at different times of your menstrual cycle. They might become lumpy just before your period. Breast tissue changes with age, too. Learning what is normal for you will help you know what changes to see your doctor about.

What to watch for: For most women, finding a lump in their breast is the most common sign of breast cancer. If it's painful, it's usually a symptom of a benign condition, but it should be checked by your doctor. Most lumps are not cancer. These signs and symptoms may be caused by breast cancer or another breast problem. See your doctor if you have:

- a lump or swelling in the armpit;

- changes in breast size or shape;

- dimpling or puckering of the skin—sometimes called orange peel skin;

- redness, swelling, and increased warmth in the affected breast;

- inverted nipple—nipple turns inwards;

- crusting or scaling on the nipple.

Cervical Cancer

Cervical cancer starts in the cells of the cervix. It usually grows very slowly. Before cervical cancer develops, the cells of the cervix start to change and become abnormal. These abnormal cells are precancerous, meaning they are not cancer. Precancerous changes in the cervix are called cervical dysplasia.

Cervical dysplasia and cervical cancer in its early stages often do not cause any symptoms. Having screening tests regularly can help find dysplasia or cervical cancer before symptoms develop. Both can usually be treated successfully when diagnosed early.

You are at higher risk of developing cervical cancer if you became sexually active at a young age or have had multiple sexual partners. These factors increase your risk of being exposed to HPV (the human papillomavirus). HPV is a group of viruses that can be passed easily from person to person through sexual contact. HPV infections are common and usually go away without treatment, because the immune system gets rid of the virus. Only certain types of HPV can cause changes to cells in the cervix that may lead to cervical cancer.

What you can do: Once you become sexually active, have a Pap test every one to three years (depending on the screening guidelines in your province and your previous test results). A Pap test is a laboratory examination of cells taken from the cervix to detect changes. It can detect changes early before cancer develops.

Continue to have a Pap test even if you have stopped having sex.

Talk to your doctor about whether to continue having a Pap test if you have had a hysterectomy (removal of the uterus, cervix, and sometimes the ovaries).

When you have a Pap test, you might also have a pelvic exam. This is a physical examination of the organs within the pelvis through the vagina. The doctor puts a gloved finger into the vagina to check the cervix and pelvic organs for anything that seems unusual. It doesn't check for cervical cancer but may uncover other problems.

Use a condom during sex to help avoid an HPV infection.

Consider the HPV vaccine if you are between 9 and 26 years of age. It protects against some of the HPV infections that cause more than 70% of cervical cancer cases and most types of genital warts. The vaccine should be used along with cervical cancer screening, not instead of screening.

What to watch for: These signs and symptoms may be caused by cervical cancer or by other health problems. See your doctor if you have:

- abnormal bleeding or bloodstained discharge from the vagina between periods;

- unusually long or heavy periods;

- bleeding after sexual intercourse;

- watery discharge from the vagina;

- increased amount of discharge from the vagina;

- bleeding from the vagina after menopause.

Recommended Cancer Screening for Men

Prostate Cancer

Prostate cancer starts in the cells of the prostate gland. It is the most common cancer in Canadian men and is diagnosed most often in men over the age of 65. Men with a family history of prostate cancer or men who are of African ancestry are at higher risk of developing the disease at a younger age.

What you can do: If you are 50 or older, talk to your doctor about the risks and benefits of testing for prostate cancer.

If you are at higher risk for prostate cancer because of your family history or African ancestry, discuss the possibility of starting testing at a younger age.

These tests may be used for the early detection of prostate cancer:

- **Digital rectal exam (DRE)**: A physical exam of the prostate gland through the rectum. The doctor inserts a gloved finger into the rectum to feel the prostate for lumps or anything else that seems unusual.

- **Prostate-specific antigen (PSA) test:** A blood test that measures prostate-specific antigen, a substance made by the prostate.

The PSA and DRE tests can help detect prostate cancer early, but they can also cause "false alarms" or miss prostate cancer that is present. In some cases, these tests can detect prostate cancer that may not pose a serious threat to your health. It is important to talk to your doctor about your personal risk of developing prostate cancer and about the benefits and risks of testing.

What to watch for: These signs and symptoms may be caused by prostate cancer or by other health problems, such as an inflamed or enlarged prostate. See your doctor if you have:

- the need to urinate often, especially at night;

- an intense need to urinate;

- difficulty in starting or stopping the urine flow;

- an inability to urinate;

- weak, decreased, or interrupted urine stream;

- a feeling that the bladder hasn't completely emptied;

- burning or pain during urination;

- blood in the urine or semen;

- painful ejaculation.

Testicular Cancer

Testicular cancer starts in the cells of a testicle. While testicular cancer is quite rare, men between the ages of 15 and 49 are at increased risk of developing it. Treatment for testicular cancer is usually successful, especially if the cancer is found early.

What you can do: Become familiar with your testicles and check them regularly. The best time to do it is after a warm bath or shower, when the testicles descend and the muscles of the scrotum are relaxed. See your doctor right away if you notice anything unusual.

Have regular medical checkups by your doctor that include testicular examination.

What to watch for: These signs and symptoms may be caused by testicular cancer or by other health problems. See your doctor if you have:

- a lump on the testicle;

- a painful testicle;

- a feeling of heaviness or dragging in the lower abdomen or scrotum;

- a dull ache in the lower abdomen and groin.

Recommended Screening for Men and Women

Colorectal Cancer

Most colorectal cancers start in the cells that line the inside of the colon and the rectum. It is the third most common cancer in Canada for both men and women. Colorectal cancer often grows slowly and in a predictable way. It may not cause any symptoms in its early stages because the lower abdomen (below the stomach area) has lots of room for a tumor to grow and expand. Screening tests help find colorectal cancer before symptoms develop. It can usually be treated successfully when diagnosed early.

What you can do: If you are 50 or older, have a fecal occult blood test (FOBT) at least every two years. This test checks your stool for blood that can be seen only with a microscope. Having blood in the stool doesn't always mean that you have cancer. It could have other causes—for example, polyps (non-cancerous tissue growth), ulcers, or even hemorrhoids.

If the FOBT shows traces of blood in the stool, follow-up tests may include a:

- **colonoscopy:** A test that lets the doctor look at the lining of the entire colon using a thin, flexible tube with a light and camera at the end.

- **sigmoidoscopy:** A test that lets the doctor look at the lining of the rectum and lower part of the colon using a thin, flexible tube with a light and camera at the end.

- **double-contrast barium enema:** An x-ray of the colon and rectum that uses a special dye (called barium) that helps the doctor see the lining of the colon more clearly.

Some men and women have a higher than average risk for colorectal cancer. Talk to your doctor about when and how often you should have tests if you have:

- a parent, brother, sister, or child with colorectal cancer (especially if the relative was diagnosed before the age of 45);

- a personal history of colorectal cancer;

- already been diagnosed with inflammatory bowel disease or polyps

- an inherited condition such as familial adenomatous polyposis (PAP) or hereditary non-polyposis colon cancer (HNCC).

What to watch for: These signs and symptoms may be caused by colorectal cancer or by other health problems. See your doctor if you have:

- general discomfort in the abdomen (bloating, fullness, cramps);

- a change in bowel habits, such as diarrhea or constipation, for no apparent reason;

- blood in the stool (either bright red or very dark);

- stools that are narrower than usual;

- an urgent need to have a bowel movement;

- a feeling that the bowel hasn't completely emptied;

- nausea or vomiting;

- fatigue (feeling very tired);

- weight loss.

Skin Cancer

The different types of skin cancer (basal cell, squamous cell, and melanoma) begin in different kinds of cells in the skin. Basal cell and squamous cell skin cancers are very common in Canada, but both types can usually be treated easily and successfully.

What you can do: The best way to prevent skin cancer is to protect yourself from the sun. Here are a few tips on how to stay safe in the sun:

- Protect yourself and your family particularly between 11:00 a.m. and 4:00 p.m. when the sun's rays are at their strongest, or at any time of the day when the UV Index is 3 or higher. Stay in the shade—under trees, an awning, or an umbrella—and try to plan outdoor activities before 11:00 a.m. or after 4:00 p.m.

- Cover your arms, legs, and head. Choose clothing that is loose-fitting, tightly woven, and lightweight. Don't forget your hat to protect your head, face, ears, and neck.

- Use a sunscreen with a sun protection factor (SPF) of 15 or higher. Don't forget to apply sunscreen on cloudy days and during the winter.

- Wear sunglasses to help prevent damage to your eyes. Choose glasses with even shading, medium to dark lenses, and UVA and UVB protection.

- Avoid using indoor tanning equipment. Just like the sun, tanning lights and sun lamps give off ultraviolet rays that can cause sunburn, damage skin, and increase the risk of skin cancer.

- Check your skin regularly. Get to know the skin you're in and report any changes to your doctor.

What to watch for: These signs and symptoms may be caused by skin cancer or by other skin problems. See your doctor if you have:

- changes in the shape, color, or size of birthmarks or moles;

- patches of skin the bleed, itch, or become red and bumpy.

Reducing Your Risk of Cancer

There is a lot of health information out there—some of it is confusing or even conflicting. What we do know is that you can help reduce your chances of getting cancer by making healthy choices every day. At least half of all cancers can be prevented through healthy living and policies that protect the health of Canadians. You can:

- Be a non-non smoker and avoid secondhand smoke.

- Eat five to ten servings of vegetables and fruit a day. Choose high-fiber, lower-fat foods. If you drink alcohol, limit your intake to less than one drink a day.

- Be physically active regularly. This will also help you maintain a healthy body weight.

- Protect yourself and your family from the sun, particularly between 11:00 a.m. and 4:00 p.m. when the sun's rays are strongest, or any time of the day when the UV Index is 3 or higher. Check your skin regularly and report any changes to your doctor.

- Follow cancer screening guidelines. Knowing your family's history of cancer will help you and your doctor decide on a personal plan of testing.

- Visit your doctor or other healthcare provider if you notice a change in your normal state of health.

- Follow health and safety instructions both at home and at work when using, storing, and disposing of hazardous materials.

Chapter 57

Common Medical Procedures and Tests

Chapter Contents

Section 57.1

Medical Tests and Procedures for Cancer Patients

Excerpted and adapted from "Young People with Cancer: A Handbook for Parents," National Cancer Institute, July 31, 2003. Revised by David A. Cooke, MD, FACP, September 2010.

Medical tests and procedures are not only used to diagnose cancer, but also to see how well the treatment is working and to make sure that the treatment is causing as little damage to normal cells as possible. Many of these tests will be repeated from time to time throughout treatment.

Knowing about the tests before they are done can help you cope. You may want to ask your doctor these questions before any testing is done:

- Which tests will I have?

- What procedures are involved with the test? (An IV? An oral contrast?)

- Where and how is each test done?

- Will the tests be painful? If so, what can be done to reduce the pain?

- Who will do the tests?

- What information does the doctor expect to get from the tests?

- How soon will the results be known? What do the results mean?

- Will the tests be covered by insurance?

The following information provides facts about some common medical procedures used during the diagnosis and treatment of cancer.

Biopsy

A biopsy determines if a tumor is not cancerous (benign) or cancerous (malignant). If the biopsy is "positive," cancer is present. If it is "negative," cancer cells were not seen.

A doctor removes part or all of the tumor or part of the bone marrow. A pathologist, a doctor who specializes in recognizing changes caused by disease in humans, looks at the tissue under a microscope.

Bone marrow aspiration or bone marrow biopsy is a special type of biopsy. It examines the bone marrow under a microscope to see if leukemia is present or if the treatment is working. For other cancers, this test tells whether the disease has spread to the bone marrow.

Blood Studies

A sample of blood is usually obtained through a needle inserted in a vein or by pricking the tip of the finger and squeezing out a few drops of blood. Sometimes blood is obtained via tubes (catheters) that have been surgically placed through the chest and into one of the major blood vessels leading to the heart.

Tumor markers: This type of test searches for substances that may increase in the blood of a person with cancer. It can help to diagnose cancer and to find out how well the patient is responding to treatment. For more information about tumor markers, see Section 57.4.

Complete blood count (CBC): A CBC test checks the white blood cells, hemoglobin, hematocrit, and platelet count in a sample blood.

White blood cell (WBC) count: A WBC count measures the number of WBCs in the blood and is also used to find certain types of immature cells—called blast cells—typical of leukemia. WBCs protect the body from infection. Chemotherapy and other treatments can lower the number of WBCs, increasing the risk of infection. If the test reveals a low WBC count, treatment may need to be delayed until the count goes up.

Hemoglobin: Hemoglobin is the substance in red blood cells that carries oxygen to the body's tissues. Low hemoglobin indicates anemia. Anemia can cause the patient to look pale and feel weak and tired. It may be a side effect of chemotherapy or a sign that the cancer has returned.

Hematocrit: Hematocrit determines the size, function, and number of red blood cells. A low hematocrit also may mean that anemia is present.

Neutrophils: This test may also be called ANC—absolute neutrophil count. This blood study tests for the body's ability to fight bacterial infections.

Platelet count: This test measures the number of platelets. Platelets help the blood clot. A low platelet count, which may be due to side effects of medicine or to infection, or may mean that leukemia is present, could cause one to bleed or bruise easily.

Flow cytometry: A specialized test used frequently in cancer testing, particularly when cancers such as leukemia and lymphoma are suspected. Flow cytometry can give information about individual cell types in a sample and may be able to distinguish whether cells show cancer characteristics.

Lumbar Puncture

A lumbar puncture, also called a spinal tap, obtains a sample of spinal fluid—the liquid that surrounds the brain and spinal cord. The doctor looks at the fluid under the microscope to see if any infection or cancer cells are present. It is also used to give anticancer drugs directly to the brain and spinal cord. The patient, in a curled position, lies on one side or sits. A needle is inserted between the small bones of the spine into the fluid space around the spinal cord. A sample of the spinal fluid is taken. This test can be somewhat painful.

Imaging Tests

Imaging tests take pictures of areas inside the body to see what is happening. Tests are generally not painful, but the equipment may be frightening to some patients, especially children. Some machines make loud noises. The following descriptions provide a brief overview of the most commonly used imaging tests. Additional information follows in the next section.

Angiograms: An angiogram obtains an x-ray of the blood vessels and shows changes in the blood vessels and in nearby organs. Clogged blood vessels or blood vessels that have moved may mean that a tumor is present. A special dye is injected into an artery and travels through the blood vessels. Then a series of x-rays is taken. The dye makes the blood vessels show up on an x-ray.

Ultrasound: Ultrasound obtains a picture of part of the body by using sound waves. The waves echo or bounce off tissues and organs, making pictures called sonograms. Tumors have different echoes than normal tissues, making it possible to "see" abnormal growths. A small hand-held device called a transducer is used to send the sound waves to a site in the body. The transducer is rubbed firmly back and forth over the site after the skin has been lubricated with a special gel.

Radioisotope scanning: This test studies the liver, brain, bones, kidneys, and other organs of the body. The patient either swallows or has an injection of a mild, radioactive material that is not harmful. After a short wait, a scanning device is passed over the body to detect where the radioactive material collects in the body and allows the doctor to locate tumors. The patient will not be radioactive during or after these tests. PET (positron emission tomography) scanning is a form of radioisotope scanning which is being used with increasing frequency to help distinguish benign from malignant tumors, and to get additional information about a tumor's growth.

CT scan (computerized tomography scan; also called a CAT scan): This test obtains a three-dimensional picture of organs and tissues; ordinary x-rays give a two-dimensional view. Using pencil-like x-ray beams to scan parts of the body, a CT also gives better pictures of soft tissues than does an x-ray. It provides precise and very useful details about the location, size, and type of tumor. While the patient lies still, a large machine moves back and forth, taking pictures. The scan can take as little as five minutes or as long as 90 minutes, depending upon the equipment used and the area of the body that is being scanned. Sometimes a special dye is injected into a vein before the scan.

If the patient has a central venous line in the chest, it generally cannot be used during a CT scan of the chest. The IV may be moved to the hand.

MRI (magnetic resonance imaging): An MRI creates pictures of areas inside the body that cannot be seen using other imaging methods. MRI uses a strong magnet linked to a computer. Because an MRI can see through the bone, it can provide clearer pictures of tumors located near the bone. The patient lies on a flat surface, which is pushed into a long, round chamber. The machine makes a loud thumping noise, followed by other rhythmic beats. The test takes 15–90 minutes, during which the patient must lie still. Sometimes a special dye is injected into a vein before the test.

Combination imaging: Devices which perform more than one kind of imaging at a time are becoming common. For example, combination CT scan/PET scan machines can allow doctors to precisely overlay both kinds of images and get more detailed information about tumors.

Section 57.2

Cancer Imaging

From "Cancer Imaging Program," an undated document
produced by the National Cancer Institute (www.cancer.gov).
Revised by David A. Cooke, MD, FACP, September 2010.

Cancer may be difficult to detect, but for some types of cancer, the earlier it is detected, the better are the chances of treating it effectively. Imaging techniques—methods of producing pictures of the body—have become an important element of early detection for many cancers. But imaging is not simply used for detection. Imaging is also important for determining the stage (telling how advanced the cancer is) and the precise locations of cancer to aid in directing surgery and other cancer treatments, or to check if a cancer has returned.

Uses of Imaging

Imaging, by itself, is not a treatment but can help in making better decisions about treatments. The same imaging technique can help doctors find cancer, tell how far a cancer has spread, guide delivery of specific treatments, or find out if a treatment is working.

Screening for cancer: Imaging can be used to determine if a person has any suspicious areas or abnormalities that might be cancerous. Mammograms are an example of a familiar imaging tool used to screen for breast cancer. Screening for cancer is usually recommended for people who are at increased risk (due to their family history, lifestyle, or age) for developing a particular type of cancer.

Diagnosis/staging: Imaging can be used to find out where a cancer is located in the body, if it has spread, and how much is present. Used in this way, imaging can help determine what stage (how advanced) the cancer is, and if the cancer is in, around, or near important organs and blood vessels. If a biopsy (taking a small amount of the tumor for laboratory examination) is necessary, imaging may be used to help guide doctors to the tumor and take a sample of it.

Guiding cancer treatments: Imaging can be used to make cancer treatments less invasive by narrowly focusing treatments on the tumors. For instance, ultrasound, MRI, or CT scans may be used to determine exact tumor locations so that therapy procedures can be focused on the tumor, minimizing damage to surrounding tissue.

Determining if a treatment is working: Imaging can be used to see if a tumor is shrinking or if the tumor has changed and is using less of the body's resources than before treatment. For example, in some current cancer treatment trials, x-rays, MRIs, and CT scans are done at intervals to see if a treatment is working and the tumor is shrinking. Positron emission tomography (PET) and other nuclear medicine techniques are used to monitor the ways the tumor uses the body's resources. Magnetic resonance spectroscopy is used to study chemical changes in the tumor.

Monitoring for cancer recurrence: Imaging can be used to see if a previously treated cancer has returned or if the cancer is spreading to other locations.

X-Ray Imaging

X-ray imaging is perhaps the most familiar type of imaging. Images produced by x-rays are due to the different absorption rates of different tissues. Calcium in bones absorbs x-rays the most, so bones look white on a film recording of the x-ray image, called a radiograph. Fat and other soft tissues absorb less, and look gray. Air absorbs least, so lungs look black on a radiograph. The most familiar use of x-rays is checking for broken bones, but x-rays are also used in cancer diagnosis. For example, chest radiographs and mammograms are often used for early cancer detection or to see if cancer has spread to the lungs or other areas in the chest. Mammograms use x-rays to look for tumors or suspicious areas in the breasts.

CT Scans

A computed tomography scan (CT scan, also called a CAT scan) uses computer-controlled x-rays to create images of the body. However a radiograph and a CT scan show different types of information. Although an experienced radiologist can get a sense for the approximate three-dimensional location of a tumor from a radiograph, in general, a plain radiograph is two-dimensional.

An arm or chest radiograph looks all the way through a body without being able to tell how deep anything is. A CT scan is three-dimensional.

By imaging and looking at several three-dimensional slices of a body (like slices of bread) a doctor could not only tell if a tumor is present, but roughly how deep it is in the body. A CT scan can be three dimensional because the information about how much of the x-rays are passing through a body is collected not just on a flat piece of film, but on a computer.

The data from a CT scan can be enhanced to be more vivid than a plain radiograph. For both plain radiographs and CT scans, the patient may be given a contrast agent to drink and/or by injection to more clearly show the boundaries between organs or between organs and tumors.

Recent technical advances in CT scanning dramatically increased its speed and effectiveness by a process called multi-slice or helical (spiral) scanning. While conventional CT scans take pictures of slices of the body that are a few millimeters apart, the newer spiral CT scan takes continuous pictures of the body in a rapid spiral motion, so that there are no gaps in the pictures collected.

Additional information about CT scans is included in Section 57.3.

Nuclear Imaging (PET and SPECT)

Nuclear imaging uses low doses of radioactive substances linked to compounds used by the body's cells or compounds that attach to tumor cells. Using special detection equipment, the radioactive substances can be traced in the body to see where and when they concentrate. Two major instruments of nuclear imaging used for cancer imaging are PET and SPECT scanners.

PET Scan

The positron emission tomography (PET) scan creates computerized images of chemical changes, such as sugar metabolism, that take place in tissue. Typically, the patient is given an injection of a substance that consists of a combination of a sugar and a small amount of radioactively labeled sugar. The radioactive sugar can help in locating a tumor, because cancer cells take up or absorb sugar more avidly than other tissues in the body.

After receiving the radioactive sugar, the patient lies still for about 60 minutes while the radioactively labeled sugar circulates throughout the body. If a tumor is present, the radioactive sugar will accumulate in the tumor. The patient then lies on a table, which gradually moves through the PET scanner six to seven times during a 45–60-minute period. The PET scanner is used to detect the distribution of the sugar in the tumor and in the body. By the combined matching of a CT scan with PET images, there is an improved capacity to discriminate normal from abnormal tissues. A computer translates this information into the images that are interpreted by a radiologist.

PET scans may play a role in determining whether a mass is cancerous. However, PET scans are more accurate in detecting larger and more aggressive tumors than they are in locating tumors that are smaller than 8 mm and/or less aggressive. They may also detect cancer when other imaging techniques show normal results. PET scans may be helpful in evaluating and staging recurrent disease (cancer that has come back). PET scans are beginning to be used to check if a treatment is working—if a tumor cells are dying and thus using less sugar.

SPECT Scan

Similar to PET, single photon emission computed tomography (SPECT) uses radioactive tracers and a scanner to record data that a computer constructs into two- or three-dimensional images. A small amount of a radioactive drug is injected into a vein and a scanner is used to make detailed images of areas inside the body where the radioactive material is taken up by the cells. SPECT can give information about blood flow to tissues and chemical reactions (metabolism) in the body.

In this procedure, antibodies (proteins that recognize and stick to tumor cells) can be linked to a radioactive substance. If a tumor is present, the antibodies will stick to it. Then a SPECT scan can be done to detect the radioactive substance and reveal where the tumor is located.

Ultrasound

Ultrasound uses sound waves with frequencies above those humans can hear. A transducer sends sound waves traveling into the body which are reflected back from organs and tissues, allowing a picture to be made of the internal organs. Ultrasound can show tumors, and can also guide doctors doing biopsies or treating tumors.

Magnetic Resonance Imaging (MRI)

Magnetic resonance imaging (MRI) uses radio waves in the presence of a strong magnetic field that surrounds the opening of the MRI machine where the patient lies to get tissues to emit radio waves of their own.

Different tissues (including tumors) emit a more or less intense signal based on their chemical makeup, so a picture of the body organs can be displayed on a computer screen. Much like CT scans, MRI can produce three-dimensional images of sections of the body, but MRI is sometimes more sensitive than CT scans for distinguishing soft tissues.

Digital Mammography

Conventional mammography uses x-rays to look for tumors or suspicious areas in the breasts. Digital mammography also uses x-rays, but the data is collected on computer instead of on a piece of film. This means that the image can be computer-enhanced, or areas can be magnified. Some institutions now use computer programs to examine mammograms in addition to human readings, theoretically detecting suspicious areas that human error might miss. Experts continue to debate whether digital mammography is superior to conventional film mammography.

Colonoscopy

Virtual Colonoscopy

Virtual colonoscopy (VC) (also called computerized tomographic colonography; CTC) uses x rays and computers to produce two- and three-dimensional images of the colon (large intestine) from the lowest part, the rectum, all the way to the lower end of the small intestine and display them on a screen. The procedure is used to diagnose colon and bowel disease, including polyps, diverticulosis, and cancer. VC can be performed with computed tomography (CT), sometimes called a CAT scan, or with magnetic resonance imaging (MRI).

While preparations for VC vary, the patient is usually asked to take laxatives or other oral agents at home the day before the procedure to clear stool from the colon. A suppository to cleanse rectum of any remaining fecal matter may also be used.

VC takes place in the radiology department of a hospital or medical center. The examination takes about 10 minutes and does not require sedatives. The procedure involves these steps:

- The doctor asks the patient to lie on his or her back on a table.

- A thin tube is inserted into the rectum, and air is pumped through the tube to inflate the colon for better viewing.

- The table moves through the scanner to produce a series of two-dimensional cross-sections along the length of the colon. A computer program puts these images together to create a three-dimensional picture that can be viewed on the video screen.

- The patient is asked to hold his or her breath during the scan to avoid distortion on the images.

- The scanning procedure is then repeated with the patient lying on his or her stomach.

- After the examination, the information from the scanner must be processed to create the computer picture or image of the colon. A radiologist evaluates the results to identify any abnormalities.

The patient typically may resume normal activity after the procedure, although the doctor may ask the patient to wait while the test results are analyzed. If abnormalities are found and a conventional colonoscopy is needed, it may be performed the same day.

Conventional Colonoscopy

In a conventional colonoscopy, the doctor inserts a colonoscope—a long, flexible, lighted tube—into the patient's rectum and slowly guides it up through the colon. Pain medication and a mild sedative help the patient stay relaxed and comfortable during the 30- to 60-minute procedure. A tiny camera in the scope transmits an image of the lining of the colon, so the doctor can examine it on a video monitor. If an abnormality is detected, the doctor can remove it or take tissue samples using tiny instruments passed through the scope.

Advantages of Virtual Colonoscopy

VC may be more comfortable than conventional colonoscopy for some people because it does not use a colonoscope. As a result, no sedation is needed, and you can return to your usual activities or go home after the procedure without the aid of another person. VC provides clearer, more detailed images than a conventional x-ray using a barium enema, sometimes called a lower gastrointestinal (GI) series. It also takes less time than either a conventional colonoscopy or a lower GI series.

Disadvantages of Virtual Colonoscopy

The doctor cannot take tissue samples or remove polyps during VC, so a conventional colonoscopy must be performed if abnormalities are found. Also, VC does not show as much detail as a conventional colonoscopy, so polyps smaller than 10 millimeters in diameter may not show up on the images. While virtual colonoscopy does not involve inserting a colonoscope, current methods do require the colon to be inflated with air during the test. Some patients consider this more uncomfortable than conventional colonoscopy. Virtual colonoscopy also typically requires the same bowel cleansing prep as conventional colonoscopy, and many find the prep to be the most unpleasant part of either procedure.

Image-Guided Brain Surgery

This "hi-tech" concept has become a reality in the last several years. A conventional video image of a patient lying on the operating table is combined with MRI scans to locate key structural components of the brain and tumor. This allows the surgeon to see into the brain of a patient in a new way—virtually. Using this virtual image, the surgeon can make the best plan to enter the brain and remove the tumor, avoiding important brain structures and blood vessels.

Once the surgery is underway, taking new MRI images of the patient's brain allows the surgeon to check his or her progress, see if the position of anything has changed, and look for remaining pieces of the tumor. This new technology helps make brain surgery safer and less damaging, can help reduce the time spent in surgery, reduce blood loss, allows for removal of all the accessible tumor in one operation and sometimes allows operations that before would have been considered too risky.

Section 57.3

Questions and Answers about Computed Tomography (CT)

From "Computed Tomography (CT): Questions and Answers,"
National Cancer Institute (www.cancer.gov), September 8, 2003.
Revised by David A. Cooke, MD, FACP, September 2010.

What is computed tomography?

Computed tomography (CT) is a diagnostic procedure that uses special x-ray equipment to obtain cross-sectional pictures of the body. The CT computer displays these pictures as detailed images of organs, bones, and other tissues. This procedure is also called CT scanning, computerized tomography, or computerized axial tomography (CAT).

How is CT used in cancer?

Computed tomography is used in several ways:

- To detect or confirm the presence of a tumor

- To provide information about the size and location of the tumor and whether it has spread

- To guide a biopsy (the removal of cells or tissues for examination under a microscope)

- To help plan radiation therapy or surgery

- To determine whether the cancer is responding to treatment

What can a person expect during the CT procedure?

During a CT scan, the person lies very still on a table. The table slowly passes through the center of a large x-ray machine. The person might hear whirring sounds during the procedure. People may be asked to hold their breath at times, to prevent blurring of the pictures.

Often, a contrast agent, or "dye," may be given by mouth, injected into a vein, given by enema, or given in all three ways before the CT scan is done. The contrast dye can highlight specific areas inside the body, resulting in a clearer picture.

Computed tomography scans do not cause any pain. However, lying in one position during the procedure may be slightly uncomfortable. The length of the procedure depends on the size of the area being x-rayed; CT scans take from five minutes to 90 minutes to complete. Newer equipment generally performs scans much faster than older CT machines. For most people, the CT scan is performed on an outpatient basis at a hospital or a doctor's office, without an overnight hospital stay.

Are there risks associated with a CT scan?

Some people may be concerned about the amount of radiation they receive during a CT scan. It is true that the radiation exposure from a CT scan can be higher than from a regular x-ray, and concerns have been raised recently over potential cancer risk from this. However, it is not known whether having a CT scan actually increases cancer risk. In some cases, not having the procedure can be more risky than having it, especially if cancer is suspected. People considering CT must weigh the risks and benefits.

In very rare cases, contrast agents can cause allergic reactions. Some people experience mild itching or hives (small bumps on the skin). Symptoms of a more serious allergic reaction include shortness of breath and swelling of the throat or other parts of the body. People should tell the technologist immediately if they experience any of these symptoms, so they can be treated promptly. Rarely, contrast agents can lead to kidney damage or failure, but this is usually in people who already have kidney problems. If you have known kidney problems, be sure your doctor is aware of this before having a CT scan.

What is spiral CT?

A spiral (or helical) CT scan is a newer kind of CT. During a spiral CT, the x-ray machine rotates continuously around the body, following a spiral path to make cross-sectional pictures of the body. Spiral CT can be used to make three-dimensional pictures of areas inside the body. It may detect small abnormal areas better than conventional CT, and it is faster, so the test takes less time than a conventional CT. Most CT scan equipment produced in the past five years are spiral CT machines.

What is total or whole body CT? Should a person have one?

A total or whole body CT scan creates images of nearly the entire body—from the chin to below the hips. This test has not been shown to have any value as a screening tool. ("Screening" means checking for signs of a disease when a person has no symptoms.)

The American College of Radiology (as well as most doctors) does not recommend scanning a person's body on the chance of finding signs of any sort of disease. In most cases abnormal findings do not indicate a serious health problem; however, a person must often undergo more tests to find this out. The additional tests can be expensive, inconvenient, and uncomfortable. The disadvantages of total body CT almost always outweigh the benefits.

For more information about whole body scanning, please visit the U.S. Food and Drug Administration's website at http://www.fda.gov/cdrh/ct/screening.html.

What is virtual endoscopy?

Virtual endoscopy is a new technique that uses spiral CT. It allows doctors to see inside organs and other structures without surgery or special instruments. One type of virtual endoscopy, known as CT colonography or virtual colonoscopy, is under study as a screening technique for colon cancer.

What is combined PET/CT scanning?

Combined PET/CT scanning joins two imaging tests, CT and positron emission tomography (PET), into one procedure. A PET scan creates colored pictures of chemical changes (metabolic activity) in tissues. Because cancerous tumors usually are more active than normal tissue, they appear different on a PET scan.

Combining CT with PET scanning may provide a more complete picture of a tumor's location and growth or spread than either test alone. Researchers hope that the combined procedure will improve health care professionals' ability to diagnose cancer, determine how far it has spread, and follow patients' responses to treatment. The combined PET/CT scan may also reduce the number of additional imaging tests and other procedures a patient needs. However, this new technology is currently available only at some facilities.

Section 57.4

Tumor Markers

From "Tumor Markers: Questions and Answers," National Cancer
Institute (www.cancer.gov), February 3, 2006. Revised by
David A. Cooke, MD, FACP, September 2010.

What are tumor markers?

Tumor markers are substances produced by tumor cells or by other cells of the body in response to cancer or certain benign (noncancerous) conditions. These substances can be found in the blood, in the urine, in the tumor tissue, or in other tissues. Different tumor markers are found in different types of cancer, and levels of the same tumor marker can be altered in more than one type of cancer. In addition, tumor marker levels are not altered in all people with cancer, especially if the cancer is early stage. Some tumor marker levels can also be altered in patients with noncancerous conditions.

To date, researchers have identified more than a dozen substances that seem to be expressed abnormally when some types of cancer are present. Some of these substances are also found in other conditions and diseases. Scientists have not found markers for every type of cancer.

What are risk markers?

Some people have a greater chance of developing certain types of cancer because of a change, known as a mutation or alteration, in specific genes. The presence of such a change is sometimes called a risk marker. Tests for risk markers can help the doctor to estimate a person's chance of developing a certain cancer. Risk markers can indicate that cancer is more likely to occur, whereas tumor markers can indicate the presence of cancer.

How are tumor markers used in cancer care?

Tumor markers are used in the detection, diagnosis, and management of some types of cancer. Although an abnormal tumor marker level may suggest cancer, this alone is usually not enough to diagnose cancer. Therefore, measurements of tumor markers are usually combined with other tests, such as a biopsy, to diagnose cancer.

Tumor marker levels may be measured before treatment to help doctors plan appropriate therapy. In some types of cancer, tumor marker levels reflect the stage (extent) of the disease.

Tumor marker levels also may be used to check how a patient is responding to treatment. A decrease or return to a normal level may indicate that the cancer is responding to therapy, whereas an increase may indicate that the cancer is not responding. After treatment has ended, tumor marker levels may be used to check for recurrence (cancer that has returned).

How and when are tumor markers measured?

The doctor takes a blood, urine, or tissue sample and sends it to the laboratory, where various methods are used to measure the level of the tumor marker.

If the tumor marker is being used to determine whether a treatment is working or if there is recurrence, the tumor marker levels are often measured over a period of time to see if the levels are increasing or decreasing. Usually these "serial measurements" are more meaningful than a single measurement. Tumor marker levels may be checked at the time of diagnosis; before, during, and after therapy; and then periodically to monitor for recurrence.

Can tumor markers be used as a screening test for cancer?

Screening tests are a way of detecting cancer early, before there are any symptoms. For a screening test to be helpful, it should have high sensitivity and specificity. Sensitivity refers to the test's ability to identify people who have the disease. Specificity refers to the test's ability to identify people who do not have the disease. Most tumor markers are not sensitive or specific enough to be used for cancer screening.

Even commonly used tests may not be completely sensitive or specific. For example, prostate-specific antigen (PSA) levels are often used to screen men for prostate cancer, but this is controversial. Elevated PSA levels can be caused by prostate cancer or benign conditions, and most men with elevated PSA levels turn out not to have prostate cancer. Moreover, studies so far question whether the benefits of PSA screening outweigh the risks of follow-up diagnostic tests and cancer treatments. Screening may lead to unnecessary treatment of non-aggressive cancers which do not affect health or life expectancy. This is discussed in the following section on research in the field.

Another tumor marker, CA 125, is sometimes used to screen women who have an increased risk for ovarian cancer. However, most experts feel CA 125 is too unreliable for screening. The reasons for this view are discussed in the next section. Mostly, CA 125 is used to monitor response to treatment and check for recurrence in women with ovarian cancer.

What research is being done in this field?

Scientists continue to study tumor markers and their possible role in the early detection and diagnosis of cancer. The National Cancer Institute (NCI) is currently conducting the Prostate, Lung, Colorectal, and Ovarian Cancer screening trial, or PLCO trial, to determine if certain screening tests reduce the number of deaths from these cancers. The PLCO trial is actually many different studies looking at different ways to prevent or screen for these four types of cancer. Recently, PLCO researchers announced the results of trials studying the use of PSA to screen for prostate cancer and CA 125 to screen for ovarian cancer.

Results of the PLCO trial for prostate cancer screening were published in 2009. This study found that screening men with the PSA blood test did not reduce the risk of death from prostate cancer over a seven to ten year period.

Results of a European study, the ERSPC (European Randomized Study of Screening for Prostate Cancer), were published in 2009 at the same time as the PLCO results. This study compared men who were screened over a 10–12 year period with those who were not. It found that men who were screened were 20% less likely to die of prostate cancer over this period. However, it also found that only one out of every 48 men who underwent cancer treatment as a result of PSA testing actually lived longer because of it.

Results of the PLCO trial for ovarian cancer screening were also published in 2009. This study concluded that screening for ovarian cancer using the CA125 blood test and ultrasound did not reduce deaths from ovarian cancer. Screening found very few early-stage cancers; most cancers found through screening were advanced cancers that respond poorly to treatment. Additionally, the trial found that ovarian cancer screening resulted in many women undergoing unnecessary surgeries.

Cancer researchers are turning to proteomics (the study of protein shape, function, and patterns of expression) in hopes of developing better cancer screening and treatment options. Proteomics technology is being used to search for proteins that may serve as markers of disease in its early stages or to predict the effectiveness of treatment or the chance of the disease returning after treatment has ended.

Scientists are also evaluating patterns of gene expression (the step required to translate what is in the genes to proteins) for their ability to predict a patient's prognosis (likely outcome or course of disease) or response to therapy. NCI's Early Detection Research Network is developing a number of genomic- and proteomic-based biomarkers, some of which are being validated.

Chapter 58

Surgical Procedures and Cancer

Chapter Contents

Section 58.1

What You Need to Know about Surgery

Excerpted from "Having Surgery? What You Need to Know," Agency for
Healthcare Research and Quality (www.ahrq.gov), October 2005.
Reviewed by David A. Cooke, MD, FACP, September 2010.

Making Decisions

Are you facing surgery? You are not alone. Every year, more than 15
million Americans have surgery. Most operations are not emergencies
and are considered elective surgery. This means that you have time to
learn about your operation to be sure it is the best treatment for you.
You also have time to work with your surgeon to make the surgery as
safe as possible.

Get the Basic Facts

Why do I need an operation?

There are many reasons to have surgery. Some operations can relieve or prevent pain. Others can reduce a symptom of a problem or
improve some body function. Some surgeries are done to find a problem.
Surgery can also save your life.

Your doctor will tell you the purpose of the procedure. Make sure
you understand how the proposed operation will help fix your medical
problem. For example, if something is going to be repaired or removed,
find out why it needs to be done.

What operation are you recommending?

Ask your surgeon to explain the surgery and how it is done. Your
surgeon can draw a picture or a diagram and explain the steps in the
surgery.

Ask if there is more than one way of doing the operation. One way
may require more extensive surgery than another. Some operations
that once needed large incisions (cuts in the body) can now be done
using much smaller incisions (laparoscopic surgery). These incisions

let doctors insert a thin tube with a camera (a laparoscope) into the body to help them see. Then they use small tools to do the surgery. Because laparoscopic surgery is done using a few small cuts, you will have only a few small scars instead of a large scar. Usually, you will recover from this type of surgery more quickly.

Some surgeries require that you stay in the hospital for one or more days. Others let you come in and go home on the same day. Ask why your surgeon wants to do the operation one way over another.

Are there alternatives to surgery?

Sometimes, surgery is not the only answer to a medical problem. Medicines or treatments other than surgery, such as a change in diet or special exercises, might help you just as well—or more. Ask your surgeon or primary care doctor about the benefits and risks of these other choices. You need to know as much as possible about these benefits and risks to make the best decision.

One alternative to surgery may be watchful waiting. During a watchful wait, your doctor and you check to see if your problem gets better or worse over time. If it gets worse, you may need surgery right away. If it gets better, you may be able to wait to have surgery or not have it at all.

How much will the operation cost?

Even if you have health insurance, there may be some costs for you to pay. This may depend on your choice of surgeon or hospital. Ask what your surgeon's fee is and what it covers. Surgical fees often also include some visits after the operation. You also will get a bill from the hospital for your care and from the other doctors who gave you care during your surgery.

Before you have the operation, call your insurance company. They can tell you how much of the costs your insurance will pay and what share you will have to pay. If you are covered by Medicare, call 800-MEDICARE (800-633-4227) to find out your share of surgery costs.

Learn about the Benefits and Risks

What are the benefits of having the operation?

Ask your surgeon what you will gain by having the operation. Ask how long the benefits will last. For some procedures, it is not unusual for the benefits to last for a short time only. You may need a second operation at a later date. For other procedures, the benefits may last a lifetime.

When finding out about the benefits of the operation, be realistic. Sometimes patients expect too much and are disappointed with the outcome or results. Ask your doctor if there is anything you can read to help you understand the procedure and its likely results.

What are the risks of having the operation?

All operations have some risk. This is why you need to weigh the benefits of the operation against the risks of complications or side effects. Complications are unplanned events linked to the operation. Typical complications are infection, too much bleeding, reaction to anesthesia, or accidental injury. Some people have a greater risk of complications because of other medical conditions.

There also may be side effects after the operation. Often, your surgeon can tell you what side effects to expect. For example, there may be swelling and some soreness around the incision. There is almost always some pain with surgery. Ask your surgeon how much pain there will be and what the doctors and nurses will do to help stop the pain. Controlling the pain will help you to be more comfortable while you heal. Controlling the pain will also help you get well faster and improve the results of your operation.

What if I don't have this operation?

Based on what you learn about the benefits and risks of the operation, you might decide not to have it. Ask your surgeon what you will gain—or lose—by not having the operation now. Could you be in more pain? Could your condition get worse? Could the problem go away?

Where can I get a second opinion?

Getting a second opinion from another doctor is a very good way to make sure that having the operation is the best choice for you. You can ask your primary care doctor for the name of another surgeon who could review your medical file. If you consult another doctor, make sure to get your records from the first doctor so that your tests do not have to be repeated.

Many health insurance plans ask patients to get a second opinion before they have certain operations that are not for an emergency. If your plan does not require a second opinion, you may still ask to have one. Check with your insurance company to see if they will pay for a second opinion. You should discuss your insurance questions with your health insurance company or your employee benefits office. If you are eligible for Medicare, they will pay for a second opinion.

Find Out More about Your Operation

What kind of anesthesia will I need?

Anesthesia is used so that surgery can be performed without unnecessary pain. Your surgeon can tell you whether the operation calls for local, regional, or general anesthesia and why this form of anesthesia is best for your procedure.

Local anesthesia numbs only a part of your body and only for a short period of time. For example, when you go to the dentist, you may get a local anesthetic called Novocain. It numbs the gum area around a tooth. Not all procedures done with local anesthesia are painless. Regional anesthesia numbs a larger portion of your body—for example, the lower part of your body—for a few hours. In most cases, you will be awake during the operation with regional anesthesia. General anesthesia numbs your entire body. You will be asleep during the whole operation if you have general anesthesia.

Anesthesia is quite safe for most patients. It is usually given by a specialized doctor (anesthesiologist) or nurse (nurse anesthetist). Both are highly skilled and have been trained to give anesthesia.

If you decide to have an operation, ask to meet with the person who will give you anesthesia. It is okay to ask what his or her qualifications are. Ask what the side effects and risks of having anesthesia are in your case. Be sure to tell him or her what medical problems you have—including allergies and what medicines you have been taking. These medicines may affect your response to the anesthesia. Be sure to include both prescription and over-the-counter medicines, like vitamins and supplements.

How long will it take me to recover?

Your surgeon can tell you how you might feel and what you will be able to do—or not do—the first few days, weeks, or months after surgery. Ask how long you will be in the hospital. Find out what kind of supplies, equipment, and help you will need when you go home. Knowing what to expect can help you get better faster.

Ask how long it will be before you can go back to work or start regular exercise again. You do not want to do anything that will slow your recovery. For example, lifting a 10-pound bag of potatoes may not seem to be "too much" a week after your operation, but it could be. You should follow your surgeon's advice to make sure you recover fully as soon as possible.

Making Sure Your Surgery is Safe

Check with your insurance company to find out if you may choose a surgeon or hospital or if you must use ones selected by the insurer. Ask your doctor about which hospital has the best care and results for your condition if you have more than one hospital to choose from. Studies show that for some types of surgery, numbers count—using a surgeon or hospital that does more of a particular type of surgery can improve your chance of a good result. If you do have a choice of surgeon or hospital, ask the surgeon the following questions:

What are your qualifications?

You will want to know that your surgeon is experienced and qualified to perform the operation. Many surgeons have taken special training and passed exams given by a national board of surgeons. Ask if your surgeon is "board certified" in surgery. Some surgeons also have the letters F.A.C.S. after their name. This means they are Fellows of the American College of Surgeons and have passed another review by surgeons of their surgical skills.

How much experience do you have doing this operation?

One way to reduce the risks of surgery is to choose a surgeon who has been well trained to do the surgery and has plenty of experience doing it. You can ask your surgeon about his or her recent record of successes and complications with this surgery. If it is easier for you, you can discuss the surgeon's qualifications with your primary care doctor.

At which hospital will the operation be done?

Most surgeons work at one or two local hospitals. Find out where your surgery will be done and how often the same operation is done there. Research shows that patients often do better when they have surgery in hospitals with more experience in the operation. Ask your doctor about the success rate at the hospitals you can choose between. The success rate is the number of patients who improve divided by all patients having that operation at a hospital. If your surgeon suggests using a hospital with a lower success rate for your surgery, find out why.

Ask the surgeon how long you will be in the hospital. Until recently, most patients who had surgery stayed in the hospital overnight for one or more days. Today, many patients have surgery done as an outpatient in a doctor's office, a special surgical center, or a day surgery unit of a hospital. These patients have an operation and go home the same day. Outpatient surgery is less expensive because you do not have to pay for staying in a hospital room. Ask whether your operation will be done in the hospital or in an outpatient setting, and ask which of these is the usual way the surgery is done. If your doctor recommends that you stay overnight in the hospital (have inpatient surgery) for an operation that is usually done as outpatient surgery—or recommends outpatient surgery that is usually done as inpatient surgery—ask why. You want to be in the right place for your operation.

Have the surgeon mark the site he or she will operate on. Rarely, surgeons will make a mistake and operate on the wrong part of the body. A number of groups of surgeons now urge their members to use a marking pen to show the place that they will operate on. The surgeons do this by writing directly on the patient's skin on the day of surgery. Don't be afraid to ask your surgeon to do this to make your surgery safer.

Section 58.2

Lasers in Cancer Treatment

From "Lasers in Cancer Treatment: Questions and Answers," National Cancer Institute (www.cancer.gov), September 10, 2004. Reviewed by David A. Cooke, MD, FACP, September 2010.

What is laser light?

The term "laser" stands for light amplification by stimulated emission of radiation. Ordinary light, such as that from a light bulb, has many wavelengths and spreads in all directions. Laser light, on the other hand, has a specific wavelength. It is focused in a narrow beam and creates a very high-intensity light. This powerful beam of light may be used to cut through steel or to shape diamonds. Because lasers can focus very accurately on tiny areas, they can also be used for very precise surgical work or for cutting through tissue (in place of a scalpel).

What is laser therapy, and how is it used in cancer treatment?

Laser therapy uses high-intensity light to treat cancer and other illnesses. Lasers can be used to shrink or destroy tumors. Lasers are most commonly used to treat superficial cancers (cancers on the surface of the body or the lining of internal organs) such as basal cell skin cancer and the very early stages of some cancers, such as cervical, penile, vaginal, vulvar, and non-small cell lung cancer.

Lasers also may be used to relieve certain symptoms of cancer, such as bleeding or obstruction. For example, lasers can be used to shrink or destroy a tumor that is blocking a patient's trachea (windpipe) or esophagus. Lasers also can be used to remove colon polyps or tumors that are blocking the colon or stomach.

Laser therapy can be used alone, but most often it is combined with other treatments, such as surgery, chemotherapy, or radiation therapy. In addition, lasers can seal nerve endings to reduce pain after surgery and seal lymph vessels to reduce swelling and limit the spread of tumor cells.

How is laser therapy given to the patient?

Laser therapy is often given through a flexible endoscope (a thin, lighted tube used to look at tissues inside the body). The endoscope is fitted with optical fibers (thin fibers that transmit light). It is inserted through an opening in the body, such as the mouth, nose, anus, or vagina. Laser light is then precisely aimed to cut or destroy a tumor.

Laser-induced interstitial thermotherapy (LITT) (or interstitial laser photocoagulation) also uses lasers to treat some cancers. LITT is similar to a cancer treatment called hyperthermia, which uses heat to shrink tumors by damaging or killing cancer cells. During LITT, an optical fiber is inserted into a tumor. Laser light at the tip of the fiber raises the temperature of the tumor cells and damages or destroys them. LITT is sometimes used to shrink tumors in the liver.

Photodynamic therapy (PDT) is another type of cancer treatment that uses lasers. In PDT, a certain drug, called a photosensitizer or photosensitizing agent, is injected into a patient and absorbed by cells all over the patient's body. After a couple of days, the agent is found mostly in cancer cells. Laser light is then used to activate the agent and destroy cancer cells. Because the photosensitizer makes the skin and eyes sensitive to light for approximately six weeks, patients are advised to avoid direct sunlight and bright indoor light during that time.

What types of lasers are used in cancer treatment?

Three types of lasers are used to treat cancer: carbon dioxide ($CO2$) lasers, argon lasers, and neodymium:yttrium-aluminum-garnet (Nd:YAG) lasers. Each of these can shrink or destroy tumors and can be used with endoscopes. $CO2$ and argon lasers can cut the skin's surface without going into deeper layers. Thus, they can be used to remove superficial cancers, such as skin cancer. In contrast, the Nd:YAG laser is more commonly applied through an endoscope to treat internal organs, such as the uterus, esophagus, and colon. Nd:YAG laser light can also travel through optical fibers into specific areas of the body during LITT. Argon lasers are often used to activate the drugs used in PDT.

What are the advantages of laser therapy?

Lasers are more precise than standard surgical tools (scalpels), so they do less damage to normal tissues. As a result, patients usually have less pain, bleeding, swelling, and scarring. With laser therapy, operations are usually shorter. In fact, laser therapy can often be done on an outpatient basis. It takes less time for patients to heal after laser surgery, and they are less likely to get infections. Patients should consult with their health care provider about whether laser therapy is appropriate for them.

What are the disadvantages of laser therapy?

Laser therapy also has several limitations. Surgeons must have specialized training before they can do laser therapy, and strict safety precautions must be followed. Also, laser therapy is expensive and requires bulky equipment. In addition, the effects of laser therapy may not last long, so doctors may have to repeat the treatment for a patient to get the full benefit.

Section 58.3

Cryosurgery in Cancer Treatment

From "Cryosurgery in Cancer Treatment: Questions and Answers," National Cancer Institute (www.cancer.gov), September 10, 2003. Reviewed by David A. Cooke, MD, FACP, September 2010.

What is cryosurgery?

Cryosurgery (also called cryotherapy) is the use of extreme cold produced by liquid nitrogen (or argon gas) to destroy abnormal tissue. Cryosurgery is used to treat external tumors, such as those on the skin. For external tumors, liquid nitrogen is applied directly to the cancer cells with a cotton swab or spraying device.

Cryosurgery is also used to treat tumors inside the body (internal tumors and tumors in the bone). For internal tumors, liquid nitrogen or argon gas is circulated through a hollow instrument called a cryoprobe, which is placed in contact with the tumor. The doctor uses ultrasound or MRI to guide the cryoprobe and monitor the freezing of the cells, thus limiting damage to nearby healthy tissue. (In ultrasound, sound waves are bounced off organs and other tissues to create a picture called a sonogram.) A ball of ice crystals forms around the probe, freezing nearby cells. Sometimes more than one probe is used to deliver the liquid nitrogen to various parts of the tumor. The probes may be put into the tumor during surgery or through the skin (percutaneously). After cryosurgery, the frozen tissue thaws and is either naturally absorbed by the body (for internal tumors), or it dissolves and forms a scab (for external tumors).

What types of cancer can be treated with cryosurgery?

Cryosurgery is used to treat several types of cancer, and some precancerous or noncancerous conditions. In addition to prostate and liver tumors, cryosurgery can be an effective treatment for the following:

- Retinoblastoma (a childhood cancer that affects the retina of the eye). Doctors have found that cryosurgery is most effective when the tumor is small and only in certain parts of the retina.

- Early-stage skin cancers (both basal cell and squamous cell carcinomas).

- Precancerous skin growths known as actinic keratosis.

- Precancerous conditions of the cervix known as cervical intraepithelial neoplasia (abnormal cell changes in the cervix that can develop into cervical cancer).

Cryosurgery is also used to treat some types of low-grade cancerous and noncancerous tumors of the bone. It may reduce the risk of joint damage when compared with more extensive surgery, and help lessen the need for amputation. The treatment is also used to treat AIDS-related Kaposi sarcoma when the skin lesions are small and localized.

Researchers are evaluating cryosurgery as a treatment for a number of cancers, including breast, colon, and kidney cancer. They are also exploring cryotherapy in combination with other cancer treatments, such as hormone therapy, chemotherapy, radiation therapy, or surgery.

In what situations can cryosurgery be used to treat prostate cancer? What are the side effects?

Cryosurgery can be used to treat men who have early-stage prostate cancer that is confined to the prostate gland. It is less well established than standard prostatectomy and various types of radiation therapy. Long-term outcomes are not known. Because it is effective only in small areas, cryosurgery is not used to treat prostate cancer that has spread outside the gland, or to distant parts of the body.

Some advantages of cryosurgery are that the procedure can be repeated, and it can be used to treat men who cannot have surgery or radiation therapy because of their age or other medical problems.

Cryosurgery for the prostate gland can cause side effects. These side effects may occur more often in men who have had radiation to the prostate. Cryosurgery may obstruct urine flow or cause incontinence (lack of control over urine flow); often, these side effects are temporary. Many men become impotent (loss of sexual function). In some cases, the surgery has caused injury to the rectum.

In what situations can cryosurgery be used to treat liver cancer?

Cryosurgery may be used to treat primary liver cancer that has not spread. It is used especially if surgery is not possible due to factors such as other medical conditions. The treatment also may be used for cancer that has spread to the liver from another site (such as the colon or rectum). In some cases, chemotherapy and/or radiation therapy may be given before or after cryosurgery. Cryosurgery in the liver may cause damage to the bile ducts and/or major blood vessels, which can lead to hemorrhage (heavy bleeding) or infection.

Does cryosurgery have any complications or side effects?

Cryosurgery does have side effects, although they may be less severe than those associated with surgery or radiation therapy. The effects depend on the location of the tumor. Cryosurgery for cervical intraepithelial neoplasia has not been shown to affect a woman's fertility, but it can cause cramping, pain, or bleeding. When used to treat skin cancer (including Kaposi sarcoma), cryosurgery may cause scarring and swelling; if nerves are damaged, loss of sensation may occur, and, rarely, it may cause a loss of pigmentation and loss of hair in the treated area. When used to treat tumors of the bone, cryosurgery may lead to the destruction of nearby bone tissue and result in fractures, but these effects may not be seen for some time after the initial treatment and can often be delayed with other treatments. In rare cases, cryosurgery may interact badly with certain types of chemotherapy. Although the side effects of surgery may be less severe than those associated with conventional surgery or radiation, more studies are needed to determine the long-term effects.

What are the advantages of cryosurgery?

Cryosurgery offers advantages over other methods of cancer treatment. It is less invasive than surgery, involving only a small incision or insertion of the cryoprobe through the skin. Consequently, pain, bleeding, and other complications of surgery are minimized. Cryosurgery is less expensive than other treatments and requires shorter recovery time and a shorter hospital stay, or no hospital stay at all. Sometimes cryosurgery can be done using only local anesthesia.

Because physicians can focus cryosurgical treatment on a limited area, they can avoid the destruction of nearby healthy tissue. The treatment can be safely repeated and may be used along with standard treatments such as surgery, chemotherapy, hormone therapy, and radiation. Cryosurgery may offer an option for treating cancers that are considered inoperable or that do not respond to standard treatments. Furthermore, it can be used for patients who are not good candidates for conventional surgery because of their age or other medical conditions.

What are the disadvantages of cryosurgery?

The major disadvantage of cryosurgery is the uncertainty surrounding its long-term effectiveness. While cryosurgery may be effective in treating tumors the physician can see by using imaging tests (tests that produce pictures of areas inside the body), it can miss microscopic cancer spread. Furthermore, because the effectiveness of the technique is still being assessed, insurance coverage issues may arise.

What does the future hold for cryosurgery?

Additional studies are needed to determine the effectiveness of cryosurgery in controlling cancer and improving survival. Data from these studies will allow physicians to compare cryosurgery with standard treatment options such as surgery, chemotherapy, and radiation. Moreover, physicians continue to examine the possibility of using cryosurgery in combination with other treatments.

Where is cryosurgery currently available?

Cryosurgery is widely available in gynecologists' offices for the treatment of cervical neoplasias. A limited number of hospitals and cancer centers throughout the country currently have skilled doctors and the necessary technology to perform cryosurgery for other noncancerous, precancerous, and cancerous conditions. Individuals can consult with their doctors or contact hospitals and cancer centers in their area to find out where cryosurgery is being used.

Chapter 59

Chemotherapy

What is chemotherapy?

Chemotherapy (also called chemo) is a type of cancer treatment that uses drugs to destroy cancer cells.

How does chemotherapy work?

Chemotherapy works by stopping or slowing the growth of cancer cells, which grow and divide quickly. But it can also harm healthy cells that divide quickly, such as those that line your mouth and intestines or cause your hair to grow. Damage to healthy cells may cause side effects. Often, side effects get better or go away after chemotherapy is over.

What does chemotherapy do?

Depending on your type of cancer and how advanced it is, chemotherapy can be used for different purposes:

- **Cure cancer:** When chemotherapy destroys cancer cells to the point that your doctor can no longer detect them in your body and they will not grow back.

- **Control cancer:** When chemotherapy keeps cancer from spreading, slows its growth, or destroys cancer cells that have spread to other parts of your body.

Excerpted from "Chemotherapy and You: Support for People with Cancer," National Cancer Institute (www.cancer.gov), June 29, 2007.

- **Ease cancer symptoms (also called palliative care):** When chemotherapy shrinks tumors that are causing pain or pressure.

How is chemotherapy used?

Sometimes, chemotherapy is used as the only cancer treatment. But more often, you will get chemotherapy along with surgery, radiation therapy, or biological therapy. Chemotherapy can help with the following:

- Make a tumor smaller before surgery or radiation therapy. This is called neoadjuvant chemotherapy.

- Destroy cancer cells that may remain after surgery or radiation therapy. This is called adjuvant chemotherapy.

- Help radiation therapy and biological therapy work better.

- Destroy cancer cells that have come back (recurrent cancer) or spread to other parts of your body (metastatic cancer).

How does my doctor decide which chemotherapy drugs to use?

This choice depends on these factors:

- The type of cancer you have. Some types of chemotherapy drugs are used for many types of cancer. Other drugs are used for just one or two types of cancer.

- Whether you have had chemotherapy before

- Whether you have other health problems, such as diabetes or heart disease

Where do I go for chemotherapy?

You may receive chemotherapy during a hospital stay, at home, or in a doctor's office, clinic, or outpatient unit in a hospital (which means you do not have to stay overnight). No matter where you go for chemotherapy, your doctor and nurse will watch for side effects and make any needed drug changes.

How often will I receive chemotherapy?

Treatment schedules for chemotherapy vary widely. How often and how long you get chemotherapy depends on several factors:

- Your type of cancer and how advanced it is
- The goals of treatment (whether chemotherapy is used to cure your cancer, control its growth, or ease the symptoms)
- The type of chemotherapy
- How your body reacts to chemotherapy

You may receive chemotherapy in cycles. A cycle is a period of chemotherapy treatment followed by a period of rest. For instance, you might receive one week of chemotherapy followed by three weeks of rest. These four weeks make up one cycle. The rest period gives your body a chance to build new healthy cells.

Can I miss a dose of chemotherapy?

It is not good to skip a chemotherapy treatment. But sometimes your doctor or nurse may change your chemotherapy schedule. This can be due to side effects you are having. If this happens, your doctor or nurse will explain what to do and when to start treatment again.

How is chemotherapy given?

Chemotherapy may be given in many ways:

- **Injection:** The chemotherapy is given by a shot in a muscle in your arm, thigh, or hip or right under the skin in the fatty part of your arm, leg, or belly.
- **Intra-arterial (IA):** The chemotherapy goes directly into the artery that is feeding the cancer.
- **Intraperitoneal (IP):** The chemotherapy goes directly into the peritoneal cavity (the area that contains organs such as your intestines, stomach, liver, and ovaries).
- **Intravenous (IV):** The chemotherapy goes directly into a vein.
- **Topically:** The chemotherapy comes in a cream that you rub onto your skin.
- **Orally:** The chemotherapy comes in pills, capsules, or liquids that you swallow.

Chemotherapy is often given through a thin needle that is placed in a vein on your hand or lower arm. Your nurse will put the needle in at the start of each treatment and remove it when treatment is over.

Let your doctor or nurse know right away if you feel pain or burning while you are getting IV chemotherapy. IV chemotherapy is often given through catheters or ports, sometimes with the help of a pump.

- **Catheters:** A catheter is a soft, thin tube. A surgeon places one end of the catheter in a large vein, often in your chest area. The other end of the catheter stays outside your body. Most catheters stay in place until all your chemotherapy treatments are done. Catheters can also be used for drugs other than chemotherapy and to draw blood. Be sure to watch for signs of infection around your catheter.

- **Ports:** A port is a small, round disc made of plastic or metal that is placed under your skin. A catheter connects the port to a large vein, most often in your chest. Your nurse can insert a needle into your port to give you chemotherapy or draw blood. This needle can be left in place for chemotherapy treatments that are given for more than one day. Be sure to watch for signs of infection around your port.

- **Pumps:** Pumps are often attached to catheters or ports. They control how much and how fast chemotherapy goes into a catheter or port. Pumps can be internal or external. External pumps remain outside your body. Most people can carry these pumps with them. Internal pumps are placed under your skin during surgery.

How will I feel during chemotherapy?

Chemotherapy affects people in different ways. How you feel depends on how healthy you are before treatment, your type of cancer, how advanced it is, the kind of chemotherapy you are getting, and the dose. Doctors and nurses cannot know for certain how you will feel during chemotherapy.

Some people do not feel well right after chemotherapy. The most common side effect is fatigue, feeling exhausted and worn out. You can prepare for fatigue by taking these steps:

- Asking someone to drive you to and from chemotherapy
- Planning time to rest on the day of and day after chemotherapy
- Getting help with meals and childcare the day of and at least one day after chemotherapy

Can I work during chemotherapy?

Many people can work during chemotherapy, as long as they match their schedule to how they feel. Whether or not you can work may depend on what kind of work you do. If your job allows, you may want to see if you can work part-time or work from home on days you do not feel well.

Many employers are required by law to change your work schedule to meet your needs during cancer treatment. Talk with your employer about ways to adjust your work during chemotherapy. You can learn more about these laws by talking with a social worker.

Can I take over-the-counter and prescription drugs while I get chemotherapy?

This depends on the type of chemotherapy you get and the other types of drugs you plan to take. Take only drugs that are approved by your doctor or nurse. Tell your doctor or nurse about all the over-the-counter and prescription drugs you take, including laxatives, allergy medicines, cold medicines, pain relievers, aspirin, and ibuprofen.

One way to let your doctor or nurse know about these drugs is by bringing in all your pill bottles. Your doctor or nurse needs to know the name of each drug, the reason you take it, how much you take, and how often you take it. Talk to your doctor or nurse before you take any over-the-counter or prescription drugs, vitamins, minerals, dietary supplements, or herbs.

Can I take vitamins, minerals, dietary supplements, or herbs while I get chemotherapy?

Some of these products can change how chemotherapy works. For this reason, it is important to tell your doctor or nurse about all the vitamins, minerals, dietary supplements, and herbs that you take before you start chemotherapy. During chemotherapy, talk with your doctor before you take any of these products.

How will I know if my chemotherapy is working?

Your doctor will give you physical exams and medical tests (such as blood tests and x-rays). He or she will also ask you how you feel.

You cannot tell if chemotherapy is working based on its side effects. Some people think that severe side effects mean that chemotherapy is working well. Or that no side effects mean that chemotherapy is not working. The truth is that side effects have nothing to do with how well chemotherapy is fighting your cancer.

How much does chemotherapy cost?

It is hard to say how much chemotherapy will cost. It depends the types and doses of chemotherapy used, how long and how often chemotherapy is given, and whether you get chemotherapy at home, in a clinic or office, or during a hospital stay. It also depends on the part of the country where you live.

Does my health insurance pay for chemotherapy?

Talk with your health insurance plan about what costs it will pay for. Questions to ask include the following:

- What will my insurance pay for?
- Do I or does the doctor's office need to call my insurance company before each treatment for it to be paid for?
- What do I have to pay for?
- Can I see any doctor I want or do I need to choose from a list of preferred providers?
- Do I need a written referral to see a specialist?
- Is there a co-pay (money I have to pay) each time I have an appointment?
- Is there a deductible (certain amount I need to pay) before my insurance pays?
- Where should I get my prescription drugs?
- Does my insurance pay for all my tests and treatments, whether I am an inpatient or outpatient?

How can I best work with my insurance plan?

- Read your insurance policy before treatment starts to find out what your plan will and will not pay for.
- Keep records of all your treatment costs and insurance claims.
- Send your insurance company all the paperwork it asks for. This may include receipts from doctors' visits, prescriptions, and lab work. Be sure to also keep copies for your own records.
- As needed, ask for help with the insurance paperwork. You can ask a friend, family member, social worker, or local group such as a senior center.

If your insurance does not pay for something you think it should, find out why the plan refused to pay. Then talk with your doctor or nurse about what to do next. He or she may suggest ways to appeal the decision or other actions to take.

What are clinical trials and are they an option for me?

Cancer clinical trials (also called cancer treatment studies or research studies) test new treatments for people with cancer. These can be studies of new types of chemotherapy, other types of treatment, or new ways to combine treatments. The goal of all these clinical trials is to find better ways to help people with cancer.

Your doctor or nurse may suggest you take part in a clinical trial. You can also suggest the idea. Before you agree to be in a clinical trial, learn about these details:

- **Benefits:** All clinical trials offer quality cancer care. Ask how this clinical trial could help you or others. For instance, you may be one of the first people to get a new treatment or drug.

- **Risks:** New treatments are not always better or even as good as standard treatments. And even if this new treatment is good, it may not work well for you.

- **Payment:** Your insurance company may or may not pay for treatment that is part of a clinical trial. Before you agree to be in a trial, check with your insurance company to make sure it will pay for this treatment.

What are some tips for meeting with your doctor or nurse?

Make a list of your questions before each appointment. Some people keep a "running list" and write down new questions as they think of them. Make sure to have space on this list to write down the answers from your doctor or nurse.

- Bring a family member or trusted friend to your medical visits. This person can help you understand what the doctor or nurse says and talk with you about it after the visit is over.

- Ask all your questions. There is no such thing as a stupid question. If you do not understand an answer, keep asking until you do.

- Take notes. You can write them down or use a tape recorder. Later, you can review your notes and remember what was said.

- Ask for printed information about your type of cancer and chemotherapy.

- Let your doctor or nurse know how much information you want to know, when you want to learn it, and when you have learned enough. Some people want to learn everything they can about cancer and its treatment. Others only want a little information. The choice is yours.

- Find out how to contact your doctor or nurse in an emergency. This includes who to call and where to go.

What are some questions to ask?

Ask these questions about your cancer:

- What kind of cancer do I have?
- What is the stage of my cancer?

Ask these questions about chemotherapy:

- Why do I need chemotherapy?
- What is the goal of this chemotherapy?
- What are the benefits of chemotherapy?
- What are the risks of chemotherapy?
- Are there other ways to treat my type of cancer?
- What is the standard care for my type of cancer?
- Are there any clinical trials for my type of cancer?

Ask these questions about your treatment:

- How many cycles of chemotherapy will I get? How long is each treatment? How long between treatments?
- What types of chemotherapy will I get?
- How will these drugs be given?
- Where do I go for this treatment?
- How long does each treatment last?
- Should someone drive me to and from treatments?

Ask these questions about side effects:

- What side effects can I expect right away?
- What side effects can I expect later?

- How serious are these side effects?

- How long will these side effects last?

- Will all the side effects go away when treatment is over?

- What can I do to manage or ease these side effects?

- What can my doctor or nurse do to manage or ease these side effects?

- When should I call my doctor or nurse about these side effects?

What feelings can I expect during chemotherapy?

At some point during chemotherapy, you may feel anxious, depressed, afraid, angry, frustrated, helpless, or lonely. It is normal to have a wide range of feelings while going through chemotherapy. After all, living with cancer and getting treatment can be stressful. You may also feel fatigue, which can make it harder to cope with your feelings.

How can I cope with my feelings during chemotherapy?

Relax: Find some quiet time and think of yourself in a favorite place. Breathe slowly or listen to soothing music. This may help you feel calmer and less stressed.

Exercise: Many people find that light exercise helps them feel better. There are many ways for you to exercise, such as walking, riding a bike, and doing yoga. Talk with your doctor or nurse about ways you can exercise.

Talk with others: Talk about your feelings with someone you trust. Choose someone who can focus on you, such as a close friend, family member, chaplain, nurse, or social worker. You may also find it helpful to talk with someone else who is getting chemotherapy.

Join a support group: Cancer support groups provide support for people with cancer. These groups allow you to meet others with the same problems. You will have a chance to talk about your feelings and listen to other people talk about theirs. You can find out how others cope with cancer, chemotherapy, and side effects. Your doctor, nurse, or social worker may know about support groups near where you live. Some support groups also meet online (over the Internet), which can be helpful if you cannot travel.

Talk to your doctor or nurse about things that worry or upset you: You may want to ask about seeing a counselor. Your doctor may also suggest that you take medication if you find it very hard to cope with your feelings.

What are side effects?

Side effects are problems caused by cancer treatment. Some common side effects from chemotherapy are fatigue, nausea, vomiting, decreased blood cell counts, hair loss, mouth sores, and pain.

What causes side effects?

Chemotherapy is designed to kill fast-growing cancer cells. But it can also affect healthy cells that grow quickly. These include cells that line your mouth and intestines, cells in your bone marrow that make blood cells, and cells that make your hair grow. Chemotherapy causes side effects when it harms these healthy cells.

Will I get side effects from chemotherapy?

You may have a lot of side effects, some, or none at all. This depends on the type and amount of chemotherapy you get and how your body reacts. Before you start chemotherapy, talk with your doctor or nurse about which side effects to expect.

How long do side effects last?

How long side effects last depends on your health and the kind of chemotherapy you get. Most side effects go away after chemotherapy is over. But sometimes it can take months or even years for them to go away.

Sometimes, chemotherapy causes long-term side effects that do not go away. These may include damage to your heart, lungs, nerves, kidneys, or reproductive organs. Some types of chemotherapy may cause a second cancer years later. Ask your doctor or nurse about your chance of having long-term side effects.

What can be done about side effects?

Doctors have many ways to prevent or treat chemotherapy side effects and help you heal after each treatment session. Talk with your doctor or nurse about which ones to expect and what to do about them. Make sure to let your doctor or nurse know about any changes you notice, they may be signs of a side effect.

Chapter 60

Radiation Therapy

What is radiation therapy?

Radiation therapy (also called radiotherapy) is a cancer treatment that uses high doses of radiation to kill cancer cells and stop them from spreading. At low doses, radiation is used as an x-ray to see inside your body and take pictures (such as x-rays of your teeth or broken bones). Radiation used in cancer treatment works in much the same way, except that it is given at higher doses.

How is radiation therapy given?

Radiation therapy can be external beam (when a machine outside your body aims radiation at cancer cells) or internal (when radiation is put inside your body, in or near the cancer cells). Sometimes people get both forms of radiation therapy.

Who gets radiation therapy?

Many people with cancer need radiation therapy. In fact, more than half (about 60%) of people with cancer get radiation therapy. Sometimes, radiation therapy is the only kind of cancer treatment people need.

Excerpted from "Radiation Therapy and You: Support for People with Cancer," National Cancer Institute (www.cancer.gov), April 20, 2007.

What does radiation therapy do to cancer cells?

Given in high doses, radiation kills or slows the growth of cancer cells. Radiation therapy is used for these reasons:

- **Treat cancer:** Radiation can be used to cure, stop, or slow the growth of cancer.

- **Reduce symptoms:** When a cure is not possible, radiation may be used to shrink cancer tumors in order to reduce pressure. Radiation therapy used in this way can treat problems such as pain, or it can prevent problems such as blindness or loss of bowel and bladder control.

How long does radiation therapy take to work?

Radiation therapy does not kill cancer cells right away. It takes days or weeks of treatment before cancer cells start to die. Then, cancer cells keep dying for weeks or months after radiation therapy ends.

What does radiation therapy do to healthy cells?

Radiation not only kills or slows the growth of cancer cells, it can also affect nearby healthy cells. The healthy cells almost always recover after treatment is over. But sometimes people may have side effects that do not get better or are severe. Doctors try to protect healthy cells during treatment by taking these precautions:

- Using as low a dose of radiation as possible. The radiation dose is balanced between being high enough to kill cancer cells yet low enough to limit damage to healthy cells.

- Spreading out treatment over time. You may get radiation therapy once a day for several weeks or in smaller doses twice a day. Spreading out the radiation dose allows normal cells to recover while cancer cells die.

- Aiming radiation at a precise part of your body. New techniques, such as intensity-modulated radiation therapy (IMRT) and 3-D conformal radiation therapy, allow your doctor to aim higher doses of radiation at your cancer while reducing the radiation to nearby healthy tissue.

- Using medicines. Some drugs can help protect certain parts of your body, such as the salivary glands that make saliva (spit).

Does radiation therapy hurt?

No, radiation therapy does not hurt while it is being given. But the side effects that people may get from radiation therapy can cause pain or discomfort. Talk to your doctor about managing side effects.

Is radiation therapy used with other types of cancer treatment?

Yes, radiation therapy is often used with other cancer treatments. Here are some examples:

Radiation therapy and surgery: Radiation may be given before, during, or after surgery. Doctors may use radiation to shrink the size of the cancer before surgery, or they may use radiation after surgery to kill any cancer cells that remain. Sometimes, radiation therapy is given during surgery so that it goes straight to the cancer without passing through the skin. This is called intraoperative radiation.

Radiation therapy and chemotherapy: Radiation may be given before, during, or after chemotherapy. Before or during chemotherapy, radiation therapy can shrink the cancer so that chemotherapy works better. Sometimes, chemotherapy is given to help radiation therapy work better. After chemotherapy, radiation therapy can be used to kill any cancer cells that remain.

Who is on my radiation therapy team?

Many people help with your radiation treatment and care. This group of health care providers is often called the "radiation therapy team." They work together to provide care that is just right for you. Your radiation therapy team can include the following people:

Radiation oncologist: This is a doctor who specializes in using radiation therapy to treat cancer. He or she prescribes how much radiation you will receive, plans how your treatment will be given, closely follows you during your course of treatment, and prescribes care you may need to help with side effects. He or she works closely with the other doctors, nurses, and health care providers on your team. After you are finished with radiation therapy, your radiation oncologist will see you for follow-up visits. During these visits, this doctor will check for late side effects and assess how well the radiation has worked.

Nurse practitioner: This is a nurse with advanced training. He or she can take your medical history, do physical exams, order tests, manage side effects, and closely watch your response to treatment. After you are finished with radiation therapy, your nurse practitioner may see you for follow-up visits to check for late side effects and assess how well the radiation has worked.

Radiation nurse: This person provides nursing care during radiation therapy, working with all the members of your radiation therapy team. He or she will talk with you about your radiation treatment and help you manage side effects.

Radiation therapist: This person works with you during each radiation therapy session. He or she positions you for treatment and runs the machines to make sure you get the dose of radiation prescribed by your radiation oncologist.

Other health care providers: Your team may also include a dietitian, physical therapist, social worker, and others.

You: You are the most important part of the radiation therapy team. Your role is to a arrive on time for all radiation therapy sessions, ask questions and talk about your concerns, let someone on your radiation therapy team know when you have side effects, and tell your doctor or nurse if you are in pain. Follow the advice of your doctors and nurses about how to care for yourself at home, such as taking care of your skin, drinking liquids, eating foods that they suggest, and keeping your weight the same.

Is radiation therapy expensive?

Yes, radiation therapy costs a lot of money. It uses complex machines and involves the services of many health care providers. The exact cost of your radiation therapy depends on the cost of health care where you live, what kind of radiation therapy you get, and how many treatments you need.

Talk with your health insurance company about what services it will pay for. Most insurance plans pay for radiation therapy for their members. To learn more, talk with the business office where you get treatment.

Should I follow a special diet while I am getting radiation therapy?

Your body uses a lot of energy to heal during radiation therapy. It is important that you eat enough calories and protein to keep your weight the same during this time. Ask your doctor or nurse if you need a special diet while you are getting radiation therapy. You might also find it helpful to speak with a dietitian. Ask your doctor, nurse, or dietitian if you need a special diet while you are getting radiation therapy.

Can I go to work during radiation therapy?

Some people are able to work full-time during radiation therapy. Others can only work part-time or not at all. How much you are able to work depends on how you feel. Ask your doctor or nurse what you may expect based on the treatment you are getting.

You are likely to feel well enough to work when you start radiation therapy. As time goes on, do not be surprised if you are more tired, have less energy, or feel weak. Once you have finished your treatment, it may take a few weeks or many months for you to feel better.

You may get to a point during your radiation therapy when you feel too sick to work. Talk with your employer to find out if you can go on medical leave. Make sure that your health insurance will pay for treatment when you are on medical leave.

What happens when radiation therapy is over?

Once you have finished radiation therapy, you will need follow-up care for the rest of your life. Follow-up care refers to checkups with your radiation oncologist or nurse practitioner after your course of radiation therapy is over. During these checkups, your doctor or nurse will see how well the radiation therapy worked, check for other signs of cancer, look for late side effects, and talk with you about your treatment and care. Your doctor or nurse will take these steps:

- Examine you and review how you have been feeling. Your doctor or nurse practitioner can prescribe medicine or suggest other ways to treat any side effects you may have.

- Order lab and imaging tests. These may include blood tests, x-rays, or CT, MRI, or PET scans.

- Discuss treatment. Your doctor or nurse practitioner may suggest that you have more treatment, such as extra radiation treatments, chemotherapy, or both.

- Answer your questions and respond to your concerns. It may be helpful to write down your questions ahead of time and bring them with you.

After radiation therapy is over, what symptoms should I look for?

You have gone through a lot with cancer and radiation therapy. Now you may be even more aware of your body and how you feel each day. Pay attention to changes in your body and let your doctor or nurse know if you have symptoms such as these:

- A pain that does not go away

- New lumps, bumps, swellings, rashes, bruises, or bleeding

- Appetite changes, nausea, vomiting, diarrhea, or constipation

- Weight loss that you cannot explain

- A fever, cough, or hoarseness that does not go away

- Any other symptoms that worry you

Make a list of questions and problems you want to discuss with your doctor or nurse. Be sure to bring this list to your follow-up visits.

What is external beam radiation therapy?

External beam radiation therapy comes from a machine that aims radiation at your cancer. The machine is large and may be noisy. It does not touch you, but rotates around you, sending radiation to your body from many directions.

External beam radiation therapy is a local treatment, meaning that the radiation is aimed only at a specific part of your body. For example, if you have lung cancer, you will get radiation to your chest only and not the rest of your body.

How often will I get external beam radiation therapy?

Most people get external beam radiation therapy once a day, five days a week, Monday through Friday. Treatment lasts for two to ten weeks, depending on the type of cancer you have and the goal of your treatment. The time between your first and last radiation therapy sessions is called a course of treatment.

Radiation is sometimes given in smaller doses twice a day (hyper-fractionated radiation therapy). Your doctor may prescribe this type of treatment if he or she feels that it will work better. Although side effects may be more severe, there may be fewer late side effects. Doctors are doing research to see which types of cancer are best treated this way.

Where do I go for external beam radiation therapy?

Most of the time, you will get external beam radiation therapy as an outpatient. This means that you will have treatment at a clinic or radiation therapy center and will not have to stay in the hospital.

What happens before my first external beam radiation treatment?

If you are getting radiation to the head, you may need a mask. You will have a one to two-hour meeting with your doctor or nurse before you begin radiation therapy. At this time, you will have a physical exam, talk about your medical history, and maybe have imaging tests. Your doctor or nurse will discuss external beam radiation therapy, its benefits and side effects, and ways you can care for yourself during and after treatment. You can then choose whether to have external beam radiation therapy.

If you agree to have external beam radiation therapy, you will be scheduled for a treatment planning session called a simulation. These tasks may be performed during the simulation:

- A radiation oncologist and radiation therapist will define your treatment area (also called a treatment port or treatment field). This refers to the places in your body that will get radiation. You will be asked to lie very still while x-rays or scans are taken to define the treatment area.

- The radiation therapist will then put small marks (tattoos or dots of colored ink) on your skin to mark the treatment area. You will need these marks throughout the course of radiation therapy. The radiation therapist will use them each day to make sure you are in the correct position. Tattoos are about the size of a freckle and will remain on your skin for the rest of your life. Ink markings will fade over time. Be careful not to remove them and make sure to tell the radiation therapist if they fade or lose color.

- You may need a body mold. This is a plastic or plaster form that helps keep you from moving during treatment. It also helps make sure that you are in the exact same position each day of treatment.

- If you are getting radiation to the head, you may need a mask. The mask has air holes, and holes can be cut for your eyes, nose, and mouth. It attaches to the table where you will lie to receive your treatments. The mask helps keep your head from moving so that you are in the exact same position for each treatment.

What should I wear when I get external beam radiation therapy?

Wear clothes that are comfortable and made of soft fabric, such as cotton. Choose clothes that are easy to take off, since you may need to change into a hospital gown or show the area that is being treated. Do not wear clothes that are tight, such as close-fitting collars or waistbands, near your treatment area. Also, do not wear jewelry, adhesive bandages, powder, lotion, or deodorant in or near your treatment area, and do not use deodorant soap before your treatment.

What happens during treatment sessions?

- You may be asked to change into a hospital gown or robe.

- You will go to a treatment room where you will receive radiation.

- Depending on where your cancer is, you will either sit in a chair or lie down on a treatment table. The radiation therapist will use your body mold and skin marks to help you get into position.

- You may see colored lights pointed at your skin marks. These lights are harmless and help the therapist position you for treatment each day.

- You will need to stay very still so the radiation goes to the exact same place each time. You can breathe as you always do and do not have to hold your breath.

The radiation therapist will leave the room just before your treatment begins. He or she will go to a nearby room to control the radiation machine and watch you on a TV screen or through a window. You are not alone, even though it may feel that way. The radiation therapist can see you on the screen or through the window. He or she can hear and talk with you through a speaker in your treatment room. Make sure to tell the therapist if you feel sick or are uncomfortable. He or she can stop the radiation machine at any time. You cannot feel, hear, see, or smell radiation.

Your entire visit may last from 30 minutes to one hour. Most of that time is spent setting you in the correct position. You will get radiation for only one to five minutes. If you are getting IMRT, your treatment may last longer. Your visit may also take longer if your treatment team needs to take and review x-rays.

Will external beam radiation therapy make me radioactive?

No, external beam radiation therapy does not make people radioactive. You may safely be around other people, even babies and young children.

How can I relax during my treatment sessions?

- Bring something to read or do while in the waiting room.
- Ask if you can listen to music or books on tape.
- Meditate, breathe deeply, use imagery, or find other ways to relax.

What is internal radiation therapy?

Internal radiation therapy is a form of treatment where a source of radiation is put inside your body. One form of internal radiation therapy is called brachytherapy. In brachytherapy, the radiation source is a solid in the form of seeds, ribbons, or capsules, which are placed in your body in or near the cancer cells. This allows treatment with a high dose of radiation to a smaller part of your body. Internal radiation can also be in a liquid form. You receive liquid radiation by drinking it, by swallowing a pill, or through an IV. Liquid radiation travels throughout your body, seeking out and killing cancer cells.

Brachytherapy may be used with people who have cancers of the head, neck, breast, uterus, cervix, prostate, gall bladder, esophagus, eye, and lung. Liquid forms of internal radiation are most often used with people who have thyroid cancer or non-Hodgkin lymphoma. You may also get internal radiation along with other types of treatment, including external beam radiation, chemotherapy, or surgery.

What happens before my first internal radiation treatment?

You will have a one to two-hour meeting with your doctor or nurse before you begin internal radiation therapy. At this time, you will have a physical exam, talk about your medical history, and maybe have imaging tests. Your doctor will discuss the type of internal radiation therapy that is best for you, its benefits and side effects, and ways you can care for yourself during and after treatment. You can then choose whether to have internal radiation therapy.

How is brachytherapy put in place?

Most brachytherapy is put in place through a catheter, which is a small, stretchy tube. Sometimes, it is put in place through a larger device called an applicator. When you decide to have brachytherapy, your doctor will place the catheter or applicator into the part of your body that will be treated.

What happens when the catheter or applicator is put in place?

You will most likely be in the hospital when your catheter or applicator is put in place. Here is what to expect:

- You will either be put to sleep or the area where the catheter or applicator goes will be numbed. This will help prevent pain when it is put in.

- Your doctor will place the catheter or applicator in your body.

- If you are awake, you may be asked to lie very still while the catheter or applicator is put in place.

- Tell your doctor or nurse if you are in pain. If you feel any discomfort, tell your doctor or nurse so he or she can give you medicine to help manage the pain.

What happens after the catheter or applicator is placed in my body?

Once your treatment plan is complete, radiation will be placed inside the catheter or applicator. The radiation source may be kept in place for a few minutes, many days, or the rest of your life. How long the radiation is in place depends on which type of brachytherapy you get, your type of cancer, where the cancer is in your body, your health, and other cancer treatments you have had.

What are the types of brachytherapy?

There are three types of brachytherapy:

Low-dose rate (LDR) implants: In this type of brachytherapy, radiation stays in place for one to seven days. You are likely to be in the hospital during this time. Once your treatment is finished, your doctor will remove the radiation sources and your catheter or applicator.

High-dose rate (HDR) implants: In this type of brachytherapy, the radiation source is in place for 10 to 20 minutes at a time and then taken out. You may have treatment twice a day for two to five days or once a week for two to five weeks. The schedule depends on your type of cancer. During the course of treatment, your catheter or applicator may stay in place, or it may be put in place before each treatment. You may be in the hospital during this time, or you may make daily trips to the hospital to have the radiation source put in place. Like LDR implants, your doctor will remove your catheter or applicator once you have finished treatment.

Permanent implants: After the radiation source is put in place, the catheter is removed. The implants always stay in your body, while the radiation gets weaker each day. You may need to limit your time around other people when the radiation is first put in place. Be extra careful not to spend time with children or pregnant women. As time goes by, almost all the radiation will go away, even though the implant stays in your body.

What happens while the radiation is in place?

Your body will give off radiation once the radiation source is in place. With brachytherapy, your body fluids (urine, sweat, and saliva) will not give off radiation. With liquid radiation, your body fluids will give off radiation for a while.

Your doctor or nurse will talk with you about safety measures that you need to take. If the radiation you receive is a very high dose, safety measures may include the following:

- Staying in a private hospital room to protect others from radiation coming from your body.

- Being treated quickly by nurses and other hospital staff. They will provide all the care you need, but they may stand at a distance and talk with you from the doorway to your room.

Your visitors will also need to follow safety measures, which may include steps such as these:

- Not being allowed to visit when the radiation is first put in

- Needing to check with the hospital staff before they go to your room

- Keeping visits short (30 minutes or less each day). The length of visits depends on the type of radiation being used and the part of your body being treated.

- Standing by the doorway rather than going into your hospital room

- Not having visits from children younger than 18 and pregnant women

You may also need to follow safety measures once you leave the hospital, such as not spending much time with other people. Your doctor or nurse will talk with you about the safety measures you should follow when you go home.

What happens when the catheter is taken out after treatment with LDR or HDR implants?

- You will get medicine for pain before the catheter or applicator is removed.

- The area where the catheter or applicator was might be tender for a few months.

- There is no radiation in your body after the catheter or applicator is removed. It is safe for people to be near you—even young children and pregnant women.

- For one to two weeks, you may need to limit activities that take a lot of effort. Ask your doctor what kinds of activities are safe for you.

What feelings can I expect during radiation therapy?

At some point during radiation therapy, you may feel anxious, depressed, afraid, angry, frustrated, helpless, or alone. It is normal to have these kinds of feelings. Living with cancer and going through treatment is stressful. You may also feel fatigue, which can make it harder to cope with these feelings.

How can I cope with my feelings during radiation therapy?

There are many things you can do to cope with your feelings during treatment. Here are some things that have worked for other people:

Relax and meditate: You might try thinking of yourself in a favorite place, breathing slowly while paying attention to each breath, or listening to soothing music. These kinds of activities can help you feel calmer and less stressed.

Exercise: Many people find that light exercise (such as walking, biking, yoga, or water aerobics) helps them feel better. Talk with your doctor or nurse about types of exercise that you can do.

Talk with others: Talk about your feelings with someone you trust. You may choose a close friend, family member, chaplain, nurse, social worker, or psychologist. You may also find it helpful to talk to someone else who is going through radiation therapy.

Join a support group: Cancer support groups are meetings for people with cancer. These groups allow you to meet others facing the same problems. You will have a chance to talk about your feelings and listen to other people talk about theirs. You can learn how others cope with cancer, radiation therapy, and side effects. Your doctor, nurse, or social worker can tell you about support groups near where you live. Some support groups also meet over the internet, which can be helpful if you cannot travel or find a meeting in your area.

Talk to your doctor or nurse about things that worry or upset you: You may want to ask about seeing a counselor. Your doctor may also suggest that you take medicine if you find it very hard to cope with these feelings.

What are some side effects of radiation therapy?

Side effects are problems that can happen as a result of treatment. They may happen with radiation therapy because the high doses of radiation used to kill cancer cells can also damage healthy cells in the treatment area. Side effects are different for each person. Some people have many side effects; others have hardly any. Side effects may be more severe if you also receive chemotherapy before, during, or after your radiation therapy.

Talk to your radiation therapy team about your chances of having side effects. The team will watch you closely and ask if you notice any problems. If you do have side effects or other problems, your doctor or nurse will talk with you about ways to manage them.

Common side effects: Many people who get radiation therapy have skin changes and some fatigue. Other side effects depend on the part of your body being treated.

Skin changes may include dryness, itching, peeling, or blistering. These changes occur because radiation therapy damages healthy skin cells in the treatment area. You will need to take special care of your skin during radiation therapy.

Fatigue is often described as feeling worn out or exhausted. There are many ways to manage fatigue.

Depending on the part of your body being treated, you may also have symptoms such as the following:

- Diarrhea

- Hair loss in the treatment area

- Mouth problems

- Nausea and vomiting

- Sexual changes

- Swelling

- Trouble swallowing

- Urinary and bladder changes

Most of these side effects go away within two months after radiation therapy is finished. Late side effects may first occur six or more months after radiation therapy is over. They vary by the part of your body that was treated and the dose of radiation you received. Late side effects may include infertility, joint problems, lymphedema, mouth problems, and secondary cancer. Everyone is different, so talk to your doctor or nurse about whether you might have late side effects and what signs to look for.

Chapter 61

Bone Marrow Transplantation and Peripheral Blood Stem Cell Transplantation

What are bone marrow and hematopoietic stem cells?

Bone marrow is the soft, sponge-like material found inside bones. It contains immature cells known as hematopoietic or blood-forming stem cells. (Hematopoietic stem cells are different from embryonic stem cells. Embryonic stem cells can develop into every type of cell in the body.) Hematopoietic stem cells divide to form more blood-forming stem cells, or they mature into one of three types of blood cells: White blood cells, which fight infection; red blood cells, which carry oxygen; and platelets, which help the blood to clot. Most hematopoietic stem cells are found in the bone marrow, but some cells, called peripheral blood stem cells (PBSCs), are found in the bloodstream. Blood in the umbilical cord also contains hematopoietic stem cells. Cells from any of these sources can be used in transplants.

What are bone marrow transplantation and peripheral blood stem cell transplantation?

Bone marrow transplantation (BMT) and peripheral blood stem cell transplantation (PBSCT) are procedures that restore stem cells that have been destroyed by high doses of chemotherapy and/or radiation therapy. There are three types of transplants:

Excerpted from "Bone Marrow Transplantation and Peripheral Blood Stem Cell Transplantation," National Cancer Institute, October 29, 2008.

- In autologous transplants, patients receive their own stem cells.

- In syngeneic transplants, patients receive stem cells from their identical twin.

- In allogeneic transplants, patients receive stem cells from their brother, sister, or parent. A person who is not related to the patient (an unrelated donor) also may be used.

Why are BMT and PBSCT used in cancer treatment?

One reason BMT and PBSCT are used in cancer treatment is to make it possible for patients to receive very high doses of chemotherapy and/or radiation therapy. To understand more about why BMT and PBSCT are used, it is helpful to understand how chemotherapy and radiation therapy work.

Chemotherapy and radiation therapy generally affect cells that divide rapidly. They are used to treat cancer because cancer cells divide more often than most healthy cells. However, because bone marrow cells also divide frequently, high-dose treatments can severely damage or destroy the patient's bone marrow. Without healthy bone marrow, the patient is no longer able to make the blood cells needed to carry oxygen, fight infection, and prevent bleeding. BMT and PBSCT replace stem cells destroyed by treatment. The healthy, transplanted stem cells can restore the bone marrow's ability to produce the blood cells the patient needs.

In some types of leukemia, the graft-versus-tumor (GVT) effect that occurs after allogeneic BMT and PBSCT is crucial to the effectiveness of the treatment. GVT occurs when white blood cells from the donor (the graft) identify the cancer cells that remain in the patient's body after the chemotherapy and/or radiation therapy (the tumor) as foreign and attack them.

What types of cancer are treated with BMT and PBSCT?

BMT and PBSCT are most commonly used in the treatment of leukemia and lymphoma. They are most effective when the leukemia or lymphoma is in remission (the signs and symptoms of cancer have disappeared). BMT and PBSCT are also used to treat other cancers such as neuroblastoma (cancer that arises in immature nerve cells and affects mostly infants and children) and multiple myeloma. Researchers are evaluating BMT and PBSCT in clinical trials (research studies) for the treatment of various types of cancer.

How are the donor's stem cells matched to the patient's stem cells in allogeneic or syngeneic transplantation?

To minimize potential side effects, doctors most often use transplanted stem cells that match the patient's own stem cells as closely as possible. People have different sets of proteins, called human leukocyte-associated (HLA) antigens, on the surface of their cells. The set of proteins, called the HLA type, is identified by a special blood test.

In most cases, the success of allogeneic transplantation depends in part on how well the HLA antigens of the donor's stem cells match those of the recipient's stem cells. The higher the number of matching HLA antigens, the greater the chance that the patient's body will accept the donor's stem cells. In general, patients are less likely to develop a complication known as graft-versus-host disease (GVHD) if the stem cells of the donor and patient are closely matched.

Close relatives, especially brothers and sisters, are more likely than unrelated people to be HLA-matched. However, only 25 to 35% of patients have an HLA-matched sibling. The chances of obtaining HLA-matched stem cells from an unrelated donor are slightly better, approximately 50%. Among unrelated donors, HLA-matching is greatly improved when the donor and recipient have the same ethnic and racial background. Although the number of donors is increasing overall, individuals from certain ethnic and racial groups still have a lower chance of finding a matching donor. Large volunteer donor registries can assist in finding an appropriate unrelated donor.

Because identical twins have the same genes, they have the same set of HLA antigens. As a result, the patient's body will accept a transplant from an identical twin. However, identical twins represent a small number of all births, so syngeneic transplantation is rare.

How is bone marrow obtained for transplantation?

The stem cells used in BMT come from the liquid center of the bone, called the marrow. In general, the procedure for obtaining bone marrow, which is called "harvesting," is similar for all three types of BMTs (autologous, syngeneic, and allogeneic). The donor is given either general anesthesia, which puts the person to sleep during the procedure, or regional anesthesia, which causes loss of feeling below the waist. Needles are inserted through the skin over the pelvic (hip) bone or, in rare cases, the sternum (breastbone), and into the bone marrow to draw the marrow out of the bone. Harvesting the marrow takes about an hour.

The harvested bone marrow is then processed to remove blood and bone fragments. Harvested bone marrow can be combined with a preservative and frozen to keep the stem cells alive until they are needed. This technique is known as cryopreservation. Stem cells can be cryopreserved for many years.

How are PBSCs obtained for transplantation?

The stem cells used in PBSCT come from the bloodstream. A process called apheresis or leukapheresis is used to obtain PBSCs for transplantation. For four or five days before apheresis, the donor may be given a medication to increase the number of stem cells released into the bloodstream. In apheresis, blood is removed through a large vein in the arm or a central venous catheter (a flexible tube that is placed in a large vein in the neck, chest, or groin area). The blood goes through a machine that removes the stem cells. The blood is then returned to the donor and the collected cells are stored. Apheresis typically takes four to six hours. The stem cells are then frozen until they are given to the recipient.

How are umbilical cord stem cells obtained for transplantation?

Stem cells also may be retrieved from umbilical cord blood. For this to occur, the mother must contact a cord blood bank before the baby's birth. The cord blood bank may request that she complete a questionnaire and give a small blood sample.

Cord blood banks may be public or commercial. Public cord blood banks accept donations of cord blood and may provide the donated stem cells to another matched individual in their network. In contrast, commercial cord blood banks will store the cord blood for the family, in case it is needed later for the child or another family member.

After the baby is born and the umbilical cord has been cut, blood is retrieved from the umbilical cord and placenta. This process poses minimal health risk to the mother or the child. If the mother agrees, the umbilical cord blood is processed and frozen for storage by the cord blood bank. Only a small amount of blood can be retrieved from the umbilical cord and placenta, so the collected stem cells are typically used for children or small adults.

Are any risks associated with donating bone marrow?

Because only a small amount of bone marrow is removed, donating usually does not pose any significant problems for the donor. The most serious risk associated with donating bone marrow involves the use of anesthesia during the procedure.

The area where the bone marrow was taken out may feel stiff or sore for a few days, and the donor may feel tired. Within a few weeks, the donor's body replaces the donated marrow; however, the time required for a donor to recover varies. Some people are back to their usual routine within two or three days, while others may take up to three to four weeks to fully recover their strength.

Are any risks associated with donating PBSCs?

Apheresis usually causes minimal discomfort. During apheresis, the person may feel lightheadedness, chills, numbness around the lips, and cramping in the hands. Unlike bone marrow donation, PBSC donation does not require anesthesia. The medication that is given to stimulate the release of stem cells from the marrow into the bloodstream may cause bone and muscle aches, headaches, fatigue, nausea, vomiting, and/or difficulty sleeping. These side effects generally stop within two to three days of the last dose of the medication.

How does the patient receive the stem cells during the transplant?

After being treated with high-dose anticancer drugs and/or radiation, the patient receives the stem cells through an intravenous (IV) line just like a blood transfusion. This part of the transplant takes one to five hours.

Are any special measures taken when the cancer patient is also the donor (autologous transplant)?

The stem cells used for autologous transplantation must be relatively free of cancer cells. The harvested cells can sometimes be treated before transplantation in a process known as "purging" to get rid of cancer cells. This process can remove some cancer cells from the harvested cells and minimize the chance that cancer will come back. Because purging may damage some healthy stem cells, more cells are obtained from the patient before the transplant so that enough healthy stem cells will remain after purging.

What happens after the stem cells have been transplanted to the patient?

After entering the bloodstream, the stem cells travel to the bone marrow, where they begin to produce new white blood cells, red blood cells, and platelets in a process known as "engraftment." Engraftment usually occurs within about two to four weeks after transplantation. Doctors monitor it by checking blood counts on a frequent basis. Complete recovery of immune function takes much longer, however—up to several months for autologous transplant recipients and one to two years for patients receiving allogeneic or syngeneic transplants. Doctors evaluate the results of various blood tests to confirm that new blood cells are being produced and that the cancer has not returned. Bone marrow aspiration (the removal of a small sample of bone marrow through a needle for examination under a microscope) can also help doctors determine how well the new marrow is working.

What are the possible side effects of BMT and PBSCT?

The major risk of both treatments is an increased susceptibility to infection and bleeding as a result of the high-dose cancer treatment. Doctors may give the patient antibiotics to prevent or treat infection. They may also give the patient transfusions of platelets to prevent bleeding and red blood cells to treat anemia. Patients who undergo BMT and PBSCT may experience short-term side effects such as nausea, vomiting, fatigue, loss of appetite, mouth sores, hair loss, and skin reactions.

Potential long-term risks include complications of the pretransplant chemotherapy and radiation therapy, such as infertility (the inability to produce children); cataracts (clouding of the lens of the eye, which causes loss of vision); secondary (new) cancers; and damage to the liver, kidneys, lungs, and/or heart.

With allogeneic transplants, a complication known as graft-versus-host disease (GVHD) sometimes develops. GVHD occurs when white blood cells from the donor (the graft) identify cells in the patient's body (the host) as foreign and attack them. The most commonly damaged organs are the skin, liver, and intestines. This complication can develop within a few weeks of the transplant (acute GVHD) or much later (chronic GVHD). To prevent this complication, the patient may receive medications that suppress the immune system. Additionally, the donated stem cells can be treated to remove the white blood cells that cause GVHD in a process called "T-cell depletion." If GVHD develops, it can be very serious and is treated with steroids or other immunosuppressive agents. GVHD can be difficult to treat, but some studies suggest that patients with leukemia who develop GVHD are less likely to have the cancer come back. Clinical trials are being conducted to find ways to prevent and treat GVHD.

The likelihood and severity of complications are specific to the patient's treatment and should be discussed with the patient's doctor.

What is a "mini-transplant"?

A "mini-transplant" (also called a non-myeloablative or reduced-intensity transplant) is a type of allogeneic transplant. This approach is being studied in clinical trials for the treatment of several types of cancer, including leukemia, lymphoma, multiple myeloma, and other cancers of the blood.

A mini-transplant uses lower, less toxic doses of chemotherapy and/or radiation to prepare the patient for an allogeneic transplant. The use of lower doses of anticancer drugs and radiation eliminates some, but not all, of the patient's bone marrow. It also reduces the number of cancer cells and suppresses the patient's immune system to prevent rejection of the transplant.

Unlike traditional BMT or PBSCT, cells from both the donor and the patient may exist in the patient's body for some time after a mini-transplant. Once the cells from the donor begin to engraft, they may cause the graft-versus-tumor (GVT) effect and work to destroy the cancer cells that were not eliminated by the anticancer drugs and/or radiation. To boost the GVT effect, the patient may be given an injection of the donor's white blood cells. This procedure is called a "donor lymphocyte infusion."

What is a "tandem transplant"?

A "tandem transplant" is a type of autologous transplant. This method is being studied in clinical trials for the treatment of several types of cancer, including multiple myeloma and germ cell cancer. During a tandem transplant, a patient receives two sequential courses of high-dose chemotherapy with stem cell transplant. Typically, the two courses are given several weeks to several months apart. Researchers hope that this method can prevent the cancer from recurring (coming back) at a later time.

How do patients cover the cost of BMT or PBSCT?

Advances in treatment methods, including the use of PBSCT, have reduced the amount of time many patients must spend in the hospital by speeding recovery. This shorter recovery time has brought about a reduction in cost. However, because BMT and PBSCT are complicated technical procedures, they are very expensive. Many health insurance companies cover some of the costs of transplantation for certain types of cancer. Insurers may also cover a portion of the costs if special care is required when the patient returns home.

There are options for relieving the financial burden associated with BMT and PBSCT. A hospital social worker is a valuable resource in planning for these financial needs. Federal government programs and local service organizations may also be able to help.

What are the costs of donating bone marrow, PBSCs, or umbilical cord blood?

Persons willing to donate bone marrow or PBSCs must have a sample of blood drawn to determine their HLA type. This blood test usually costs $65 to $96. The donor may be asked to pay for this blood test, or the donor center may cover part of the cost. Community groups and other organizations may also provide financial assistance. Once a donor is identified as a match for a patient, all of the costs pertaining to the retrieval of bone marrow or PBSCs is covered by the patient or the patient's medical insurance.

A woman can donate her baby's umbilical cord blood to public cord blood banks at no charge. However, commercial blood banks do charge varying fees to store umbilical cord blood for the private use of the patient or his or her family.

The National Marrow Donor Program® (NMDP), a federally funded nonprofit organization, was created to improve the effectiveness of the search for donors. The NMDP maintains an international registry of volunteers willing to be donors for all sources of blood stem cells used in transplantation: Bone marrow, peripheral blood, and umbilical cord blood. For more information, call 800-627-7692 or visit www.marrow.org.

Chapter 62

Biological Therapies

What is biological therapy?

Biological therapy (sometimes called immunotherapy, biotherapy, or biological response modifier therapy) is a relatively new addition to the family of cancer treatments that also includes surgery, chemotherapy, and radiation therapy. Biological therapies use the body's immune system, either directly or indirectly, to fight cancer or to lessen the side effects that may be caused by some cancer treatments.

What is the immune system and what are its components?

The immune system is a complex network of cells and organs that work together to defend the body against attacks by "foreign" or "non-self" invaders. This network is one of the body's main defenses against infection and disease. The immune system works against diseases, including cancer, in a variety of ways. For example, the immune system may recognize the difference between healthy cells and cancer cells in the body and works to eliminate cancerous cells. However, the immune system does not always recognize cancer cells as "foreign." Also, cancer may develop when the immune system breaks down or does not function adequately. Biological therapies are designed to repair, stimulate, or enhance the immune system's responses.

Excerpted from "Biological Therapies for Cancer: Questions and Answers," National Cancer Institute (www.cancer.gov), June 13, 2006.

Immune system cells include the following:

- Lymphocytes are a type of white blood cell found in the blood and many other parts of the body. Types of lymphocytes include B cells, T cells, and natural killer cells.

- B cells (B lymphocytes) mature into plasma cells that secrete proteins called antibodies (immunoglobulins). Antibodies recognize and attach to foreign substances known as antigens, fitting together much the way a key fits a lock. Each type of B cell makes one specific antibody, which recognizes one specific antigen.

- T cells (T lymphocytes) work primarily by producing proteins called cytokines. Cytokines allow immune system cells to communicate with each other and include lymphokines, interferons, interleukins, and colony-stimulating factors. Some T cells, called cytotoxic T cells, release pore-forming proteins that directly attack infected, foreign, or cancerous cells. Other T cells, called helper T cells, regulate the immune response by releasing cytokines to signal other immune system defenders.

- Natural killer cells (NK cells) produce powerful cytokines and pore-forming proteins that bind to and kill many foreign invaders, infected cells, and tumor cells. Unlike cytotoxic T cells, they are poised to attack quickly, upon their first encounter with their targets.

- Phagocytes are white blood cells that can swallow and digest microscopic organisms and particles in a process known as phagocytosis. There are several types of phagocytes, including monocytes, which circulate in the blood, and macrophages, which are located in tissues throughout the body.

What are biological response modifiers and how can they be used to treat cancer?

Some antibodies, cytokines, and other immune system substances can be produced in the laboratory for use in cancer treatment. These substances are often called biological response modifiers (BRMs). They alter the interaction between the body's immune defenses and cancer cells to boost, direct, or restore the body's ability to fight the disease. BRMs include interferons, interleukins, colony-stimulating factors, monoclonal antibodies, vaccines, gene therapy, and nonspecific immunomodulating agents.

Researchers continue to discover new BRMs, to learn more about how they function, and to develop ways to use them in cancer therapy. Biological therapies may be used for these purposes:

- Stop, control, or suppress processes that permit cancer growth
- Make cancer cells more recognizable and, therefore, more susceptible to destruction by the immune system
- Boost the killing power of immune system cells, such as T cells, NK cells, and macrophages
- Alter the growth patterns of cancer cells to promote behavior like that of healthy cells
- Block or reverse the process that changes a normal cell or a precancerous cell into a cancerous cell
- Enhance the body's ability to repair or replace normal cells damaged or destroyed by other forms of cancer treatment, such as chemotherapy or radiation
- Prevent cancer cells from spreading to other parts of the body

Some BRMs are a standard part of treatment for certain types of cancer, while others are being studied in clinical trials (research studies). BRMs are being used alone or in combination with each other. They are also being used with other treatments, such as radiation therapy and chemotherapy.

What are interferons?

Interferons (IFNs) are types of cytokines that occur naturally in the body. They were the first cytokines produced in the laboratory for use as BRMs. There are three major types of interferons—interferon alpha, interferon beta, and interferon gamma; interferon alpha is the type most widely used in cancer treatment.

Researchers have found that interferons can improve the way a cancer patient's immune system acts against cancer cells. In addition, interferons may act directly on cancer cells by slowing their growth or promoting their development into cells with more normal behavior. Researchers believe that some interferons may also stimulate NK cells, T cells, and macrophages, boosting the immune system's anticancer function.

The U.S. Food and Drug Administration (FDA) has approved the use of interferon alpha for the treatment of certain types of cancer, including hairy cell leukemia, melanoma, chronic myeloid leukemia, and AIDS-related Kaposi's sarcoma. Studies have shown that interferon alpha may also be effective in treating other cancers such as kidney cancer and non-Hodgkin lymphoma. Researchers are exploring combinations of interferon alpha and other BRMs or chemotherapy in clinical trials to treat a number of cancers.

What are interleukins?

Like interferons, interleukins (ILs) are cytokines that occur naturally in the body and can be made in the laboratory. Many interleukins have been identified; interleukin-2 (IL-2 or aldesleukin) has been the most widely studied in cancer treatment. IL-2 stimulates the growth and activity of many immune cells, such as lymphocytes, that can destroy cancer cells. The FDA has approved IL-2 for the treatment of metastatic kidney cancer and metastatic melanoma.

Researchers continue to study the benefits of interleukins to treat a number of other cancers, including leukemia, lymphoma, and brain, colorectal, ovarian, breast, and prostate cancers.

What are colony-stimulating factors?

Colony-stimulating factors (CSFs) (sometimes called hematopoietic growth factors) usually do not directly affect tumor cells; rather, they encourage bone marrow stem cells to divide and develop into white blood cells, platelets, and red blood cells. Bone marrow is critical to the body's immune system because it is the source of all blood cells.

Stimulation of the immune system by CSFs may benefit patients undergoing cancer treatment. Because anticancer drugs can damage the body's ability to make white blood cells, red blood cells, and platelets, patients receiving anticancer drugs have an increased risk of developing infections, becoming anemic, and bleeding more easily. By using CSFs to stimulate blood cell production, doctors can increase the doses of anticancer drugs without increasing the risk of infection or the need for transfusion with blood products. As a result, researchers have found CSFs particularly useful when combined with high-dose chemotherapy.

Some examples of CSFs and their use in cancer therapy are as follows:

- G-CSF (filgrastim) and GM-CSF (sargramostim) can increase the number of white blood cells, thereby reducing the risk of infection in patients receiving chemotherapy. G-CSF and GM-CSF can also stimulate the production of stem cells in preparation for stem cell or bone marrow transplants.

- Erythropoietin (epoetin) can increase the number of red blood cells and reduce the need for red blood cell transfusions in patients receiving chemotherapy.

- Interleukin-11 (oprelvekin) helps the body make platelets and can reduce the need for platelet transfusions in patients receiving chemotherapy.

Researchers are studying CSFs in clinical trials to treat a large variety of cancers, including lymphoma, leukemia, multiple myeloma, melanoma, and cancers of the brain, lung, esophagus, breast, uterus, ovary, prostate, kidney, colon, and rectum.

What are monoclonal antibodies?

Researchers are evaluating the effectiveness of certain antibodies made in the laboratory called monoclonal antibodies (MOABs or MoABs). These antibodies are produced by a single type of cell and are specific for a particular antigen. Researchers are examining ways to create MOABs specific to the antigens found on the surface of various cancer cells.

To create MOABs , scientists first inject human cancer cells into mice. In response, the mouse immune system makes antibodies against these cancer cells. The scientists then remove the mouse plasma cells that produce antibodies, and fuse them with laboratory-grown cells to create "hybrid" cells called hybridomas. Hybridomas can indefinitely produce large quantities of these pure antibodies, or MOABs.

MOABs may be used in cancer treatment in a number of ways:

- MOABs that react with specific types of cancer may enhance a patient's immune response to the cancer.

- MOABs can be programmed to act against cell growth factors, thus interfering with the growth of cancer cells.

- MOABs may be linked to anticancer drugs, radioisotopes (radio-active substances), other BRMs, or other toxins. When the antibodies latch onto cancer cells, they deliver these poisons directly to the tumor, helping to destroy it.

- MOABs carrying radioisotopes may also prove useful in diagnosing certain cancers, such as colorectal, ovarian, and prostate.

Rituxan® (rituximab) and Herceptin® (trastuzumab) are examples of MOABs that have been approved by the FDA. Rituxan is used for the treatment of non-Hodgkin lymphoma. Herceptin is used to treat metastatic breast cancer in patients with tumors that produce excess amounts of a protein called HER-2. In clinical trials, researchers are testing MOABs to treat lymphoma, leukemia, melanoma, and cancers of the brain, breast, lung, kidney, colon, rectum, ovary, prostate, and other areas.

What are cancer vaccines?

Cancer vaccines are another form of biological therapy currently under study. Vaccines for infectious diseases, such as measles, mumps, and tetanus, are injected into a person before the disease develops. These vaccines are effective because they expose the body's immune cells to weakened forms of antigens that are present on the surface of the infectious agent. This exposure causes the immune system to increase production of plasma cells that make antibodies specific to the infectious agent. The immune system also increases production of T cells that recognize the infectious agent. These activated immune cells remember the exposure, so that the next time the agent enters the body, the immune system is already prepared to respond and stop the infection.

Researchers are developing vaccines that may encourage the patient's immune system to recognize cancer cells. Cancer vaccines are designed to treat existing cancers (therapeutic vaccines) or to prevent the development of cancer (prophylactic vaccines). Therapeutic vaccines are injected in a person after cancer is diagnosed. These vaccines may stop the growth of existing tumors, prevent cancer from recurring, or eliminate cancer cells not killed by prior treatments. Cancer vaccines given when the tumor is small may be able to eradicate the cancer. On the other hand, prophylactic vaccines are given to healthy individuals before cancer develops. These vaccines are designed to stimulate the immune system to attack viruses that can cause cancer. By targeting these cancer-causing viruses, doctors hope to prevent the development of certain cancers.

Early cancer vaccine clinical trials involved mainly patients with melanoma. Therapeutic vaccines are also being studied in the treatment of many other types of cancer, including lymphoma, leukemia, and cancers of the brain, breast, lung, kidney, ovary, prostate, pancreas, colon, and rectum. Researchers are also studying prophylactic vaccines to prevent cancers of the cervix and liver. Moreover, scientists are investigating ways that cancer vaccines can be used in combination with other BRMs.

What is gene therapy?

Gene therapy is an experimental treatment that involves introducing genetic material into a person's cells to fight disease. Researchers are studying gene therapy methods that can improve a patient's immune response to cancer. For example, a gene may be inserted into an immune cell to enhance its ability to recognize and attack cancer cells. In another approach, scientists inject cancer cells with genes that cause the cancer cells to produce cytokines and stimulate the immune system. A number of clinical trials are currently studying gene therapy and its potential application to the biological treatment of cancer.

What are nonspecific immunomodulating agents?

Nonspecific immunomodulating agents are substances that stimulate or indirectly augment the immune system. Often, these agents target key immune system cells and cause secondary responses such as increased production of cytokines and immunoglobulins. Two nonspecific immunomodulating agents used in cancer treatment are bacillus Calmette-Guerin (BCG) and levamisole.

BCG, which has been widely used as a tuberculosis vaccine, is used in the treatment of superficial bladder cancer following surgery. BCG may work by stimulating an inflammatory, and possibly an immune, response. A solution of BCG is instilled in the bladder and stays there for about two hours before the patient is allowed to empty the bladder by urinating. This treatment is usually performed once a week for six weeks.

Levamisole is sometimes used along with fluorouracil (5-FU) chemotherapy in the treatment of stage III (Dukes-C) colon cancer following surgery. Levamisole may act to restore depressed immune function.

Do biological therapies have any side effects?

Like other forms of cancer treatment, biological therapies can cause a number of side effects, which can vary widely from agent to agent and patient to patient. Rashes or swelling may develop at the site where the BRMs are injected. Several BRMs, including interferons and interleukins, may cause flu-like symptoms including fever, chills, nausea, vomiting, and appetite loss. Fatigue is another common side effect of some BRMs. Blood pressure may also be affected. The side effects of IL-2 can often be severe, depending on the dosage given. Patients need to be closely monitored during treatment with high doses of IL-2. Side effects of CSFs may include bone pain, fatigue, fever, and appetite loss. The side effects of MOABs vary, and serious allergic reactions may occur. Cancer vaccines can cause muscle aches and fever.

Chapter 63

Molecularly Targeted Therapies

What are targeted cancer therapies?

Targeted cancer therapies are drugs or other substances that block the growth and spread of cancer by interfering with specific molecules involved in tumor growth and progression. Because scientists often call these molecules "molecular targets," targeted cancer therapies are sometimes called "molecularly targeted drugs," "molecularly targeted therapies," or other similar names. By focusing on molecular and cellular changes that are specific to cancer, targeted cancer therapies may be more effective than other types of treatment, including chemotherapy and radiotherapy, and less harmful to normal cells.

Many targeted cancer therapies have been approved by the U.S. Food and Drug Administration (FDA) for the treatment of specific types of cancer. Others are being studied in clinical trials (research studies with people), and many more are in preclinical testing (research studies with animals).

Targeted cancer therapies are being studied for use alone, in combination with other targeted therapies, and in combination with other cancer treatments, such as chemotherapy.

How do targeted cancer therapies work?

Targeted cancer therapies interfere with cancer cell division (proliferation) and spread in different ways. Many of these therapies focus

Excerpted from "Targeted Cancer Therapies," National Cancer Institute (www.cancer.gov), June 21, 2010.

on proteins that are involved in cell signaling pathways, which form a complex communication system that governs basic cellular functions and activities, such as cell division, cell movement, how a cell responds to specific external stimuli, and even cell death. By blocking signals that tell cancer cells to grow and divide uncontrollably, targeted cancer therapies can help stop cancer progression and may induce cancer cell death through a process known as apoptosis. Other targeted therapies can cause cancer cell death directly, by specifically inducing apoptosis, or indirectly, by stimulating the immune system to recognize and destroy cancer cells and/or by delivering toxic substances to them.

The development of targeted therapies, therefore, requires the identification of good targets—that is, targets that are known to play a key role in cancer cell growth and survival. (It is for this reason that targeted therapies are often referred to as the product of "rational drug design.")

For example, most cases of chronic myeloid leukemia (CML) are caused by the formation of a gene called BCR-ABL. This gene is formed when pieces of chromosome 9 and chromosome 22 break off and trade places. One of the changed chromosomes resulting from this switch contains part of the ABL gene from chromosome 9 coupled, or fused, to part of the BCR gene from chromosome 22. The protein normally produced by the ABL gene (Abl) is a signaling molecule that plays an important role in controlling cell proliferation and usually must interact with other signaling molecules to be active. However, Abl signaling is always active in the protein (Bcr-Abl) produced by the BCR-ABL fusion gene. This activity promotes the continuous proliferation of CML cells. Therefore, Bcr-Abl represents a good molecule to target.

How are targeted therapies developed?

Once a target has been identified, a therapy must be developed. Most targeted therapies are either small-molecule drugs or monoclonal antibodies. Small-molecule drugs are typically able to diffuse into cells and can act on targets that are found inside the cell. Most monoclonal antibodies usually cannot penetrate the cell's plasma membrane and are directed against targets that are outside cells or on the cell surface.

Candidates for small-molecule drugs are usually identified in studies known as drug screens—laboratory tests that look at the effects of thousands of test compounds on a specific target, such as Bcr-Abl. The best candidates are then chemically modified to produce numerous closely related versions, and these are tested to identify the most effective and specific drugs.

Monoclonal antibodies, by contrast, are prepared first by immunizing animals (typically mice) with purified target molecules. The immunized animals will make many different types of antibodies against the target. Next, spleen cells, each of which makes only one type of antibody, are collected from the immunized animals and fused with myeloma cells. Cloning of these fusion cells results in cultures of cells that produce large amounts of a single type of antibody, or a monoclonal antibody. These antibodies are then tested to find the ones that react best with the target.

Before they can be used in humans, monoclonal antibodies are "humanized" by replacing as much of the nonhuman portion of the molecule as possible with human portions. This is done through genetic engineering. Humanizing is necessary to prevent the human immune system from recognizing the monoclonal antibody as "foreign" and destroying it before it has a chance to interact with and inactivate its target molecule.

What was the first target for targeted cancer therapy?

The first molecular target for targeted cancer therapy was the cellular receptor for the female sex hormone estrogen, which many breast cancers require for growth. When estrogen binds to the estrogen receptor (ER) inside cells, the resulting hormone-receptor complex activates the expression of specific genes, including genes involved in cell growth and proliferation. Research has shown that interfering with estrogen's ability to stimulate the growth of breast cancer cells that have these receptors (ER-positive breast cancer cells) is an effective treatment approach.

Several drugs that interfere with estrogen binding to the ER have been approved by the FDA for the treatment of ER-positive breast cancer. Drugs called selective estrogen receptor modulators (SERMs), including tamoxifen and toremifene (Fareston®), bind to the ER and prevent estrogen binding. Another drug, fulvestrant (Faslodex®), binds to the ER and promotes its destruction, thereby reducing ER levels inside cells.

Another class of targeted drugs that interfere with estrogen's ability to promote the growth of ER-positive breast cancers is called aromatase inhibitors (AIs). The enzyme aromatase is necessary to produce estrogen in the body. Blocking the activity of aromatase lowers estrogen levels and inhibits the growth of cancers that need estrogen to grow. AIs are used mostly in women who have reached menopause because the ovaries of premenopausal women can produce enough aromatase to override the inhibition. Three AIs have been approved by the FDA for the treatment of ER-positive breast cancer: Anastrozole (Arimidex®), exemestane (Aromasin®), and letrozole (Femara®).

What are some other targeted therapies?

Targeted cancer therapies have been developed that interfere with a variety of other cellular processes. FDA-approved targeted therapies are listed below:

Some targeted therapies block specific enzymes and growth factor receptors involved in cancer cell proliferation. These drugs are also called signal transduction inhibitors.

- Imatinib mesylate (Gleevec®) is approved to treat gastrointestinal stromal tumor (a rare cancer of the gastrointestinal tract) and certain kinds of leukemia. It targets several members of a class of proteins called tyrosine kinase enzymes that participate in signal transduction. These enzymes are overactive in some cancers, leading to uncontrolled growth. It is a small-molecule drug, which means that it can pass through cell membranes and reach targets inside the cell.

- Dasatinib (Sprycel®) is approved to treat some patients with CML or acute lymphoblastic leukemia. It is a small-molecule inhibitor of several tyrosine kinase enzymes.

- Nilotinib (Tasigna®) is approved to treat some patients with CML. It is another small-molecule tyrosine kinase inhibitor.

- Trastuzumab (Herceptin®) is approved for the treatment of certain types of breast cancer. It is a monoclonal antibody that binds to the human epidermal growth factor receptor 2 (HER-2). HER-2, a receptor with tyrosine kinase activity, is expressed at high levels in some breast cancers and also some other types of cancer. The mechanism by which trastuzumab acts is not completely understood, but one likely possibility is that by binding to HER-2 on the surface of tumor cells that express high levels of HER-2, it prevents HER-2 from sending growth-promoting signals. Trastuzumab may have other effects as well, such as inducing the immune system to attack cells that express high levels of HER-2.

- Lapatinib (Tykerb®) is approved for the treatment of certain types of advanced or metastatic breast cancer. This small-molecule drug inhibits several tyrosine kinases, including the tyrosine kinase activity of HER-2. Lapatinib treatment prevents HER-2 signals from activating cell growth.

- Gefitinib (Iressa®) is approved to treat patients with advanced non-small cell lung cancer. Its use is restricted to patients who, in the opinion of their treating physician, are currently benefiting, or have previously benefited, from gefitinib treatment. This small-molecule drug inhibits the tyrosine kinase activity of the epidermal growth factor receptor (EGFR), which is overproduced by many types of cancer cells.

- Erlotinib (Tarceva®) is approved to treat metastatic non-small cell lung cancer and pancreatic cancer that cannot be removed by surgery or has metastasized. This small-molecule drug inhibits the tyrosine kinase activity of EGFR.

- Cetuximab (Erbitux®) is a monoclonal antibody that is approved for treating some patients with squamous cell carcinoma of the head and neck or colorectal cancer. It binds to the external portion of EGFR, thereby preventing the receptor from being activated by growth signals, which may inhibit signal transduction and lead to antiproliferative effects.

- Panitumumab (Vectibix®) is approved to treat some patients with metastatic colon cancer. This monoclonal antibody attaches to EGFR and prevents it from sending growth signals.

- Temsirolimus (Torisel®) is approved to treat patients with advanced renal cell carcinoma. This small-molecule drug is a specific inhibitor of a serine/threonine kinase called mTOR that is activated in tumor cells and stimulates their growth and proliferation.

- Everolimus (Afinitor®) is approved to treat patients with advanced kidney cancer whose disease has progressed after treatment with other therapies. This small-molecule drug binds to a protein called immunophilin FK binding protein-12, forming a complex that in turn binds to and inhibits the mTOR kinase.

Other targeted therapies modify the function of proteins that regulate gene expression and other cellular functions.

- Vorinostat (Zolinza®) is approved for the treatment of CTCL that has persisted, progressed, or recurred during or after treatment with other medicines. This small-molecule drug inhibits the activity of a group of enzymes called histone deacetylases (HDACs), which remove small chemical groups called acetyl groups from many different proteins, including proteins that regulate gene expression. By altering the acetylation of these proteins, HDAC inhibitors can induce tumor cell differentiation, cell cycle arrest, and apoptosis.

843

- Romidepsin (Istodax®) is approved for the treatment of cutaneous T-cell lymphoma (CTCL) in patients who have received at least one prior systemic therapy. This small-molecule drug inhibits members of one class of HDACs and induces tumor cell apoptosis.

- Bexarotene (Targretin®) is approved for the treatment of some patients with CTCL. This drug belongs to a class of compounds called retinoids, which are chemically related to vitamin A. Bexarotene binds selectively to, and thereby activates, retinoid X receptors. Once activated, these nuclear proteins act in concert with retinoic acid receptors to regulate the expression of genes that control cell growth, differentiation, survival, and death.

- Alitretinoin (Panretin®) is approved for the treatment of cutaneous lesions in patients with AIDS-related Kaposi sarcoma. This retinoid binds to both retinoic acid receptors and retinoid X receptors.

- Tretinoin (Vesanoid®) is approved for the induction of remission in certain patients with acute promyelocytic leukemia. This retinoid binds to and thereby activates retinoic acid receptors.

Some targeted therapies induce cancer cells to undergo apoptosis (cell death).

- Bortezomib (Velcade®) is approved to treat some patients with multiple myeloma. It is also approved for the treatment of some patients with mantle cell lymphoma. Bortezomib causes cancer cells to die by interfering with the action of a large cellular structure called the proteasome, which degrades proteins. Proteasomes control the degradation of many proteins that regulate cell proliferation. By blocking this process, bortezomib causes cancer cells to die. Normal cells are affected too, but to a lesser extent.

- Pralatrexate (Folotyn®) is approved for the treatment of some patients with peripheral T-cell lymphoma. Pralatrexate is an antifolate, which is a type of molecule that interferes with DNA synthesis. Other antifolates, such as methotrexate, are not considered targeted therapies because they interfere with DNA synthesis in all dividing cells. However, pralatrexate appears to selectively accumulate in cells that express RFC-1, a protein that may be overexpressed by some cancer cells.

- Other targeted therapies block the growth of blood vessels to tumors (angiogenesis). To grow beyond a certain size, tumors must obtain a blood supply to get the oxygen and nutrients needed for continued growth. Treatments that interfere with angiogenesis may block tumor growth.

- Bevacizumab (Avastin®) is a monoclonal antibody that is approved for the treatment of glioblastoma. It is also approved for some patients with non-small cell lung cancer, metastatic breast cancer, and metastatic colorectal cancer. Bevacizumab binds to the vascular endothelial growth factor (VEGF). This prevents VEGF from interacting with its receptors on endothelial cells, a step that is necessary for the initiation of new blood vessel growth.

- Sorafenib (Nexavar®) is a small-molecule inhibitor of tyrosine kinases that is approved for the treatment of advanced renal cell carcinoma and some cases of hepatocellular carcinoma. One of the kinases that sorafenib inhibits is involved in the signaling pathway that is initiated when VEGF binds to its receptors. As a result, new blood vessel development is halted. Sorafenib also blocks an enzyme that is involved in cell growth and division.

- Sunitinib (Sutent®) is another small-molecule tyrosine kinase inhibitor that is approved for the treatment of patients with metastatic renal cell carcinoma or gastrointestinal stromal tumor that is not responding to imatinib. It blocks kinases involved in VEGF signaling, thereby inhibiting angiogenesis and cell proliferation.

- Pazopanib (Votrient®) is approved for the treatment of patients with advanced renal cell carcinoma. Pazopanib is a small-molecule inhibitor of several tyrosine kinases, including VEGF receptors, c-kit, and platelet-derived growth factor receptor.

Some targeted therapies act by helping the immune system to destroy cancer cells.

- Rituximab (Rituxan®) is a monoclonal antibody that is approved to treat certain types of B-cell non-Hodgkin lymphoma. It recognizes a molecule called CD20 that is found on B cells. When rituximab binds to these cells, it triggers an immune response that results in their destruction. Rituximab may also induce apoptosis.

- Alemtuzumab (Campath®) is approved to treat patients with B-cell chronic lymphocytic leukemia. It is a monoclonal antibody that is directed against CD52, a protein found on the surface of normal and malignant B and T cells and many other cells of the immune system. Binding of alemtuzumab to CD52 triggers an immune response that destroys the cells.

- Ofatumumab (Arzerra®) is approved for the treatment of some patients with chronic lymphocytic leukemia (CLL) that does not respond to treatment with fludarabine and alemtuzumab. This monoclonal antibody is directed against the B-cell CD20 cell surface antigen.

Another class of targeted therapies includes monoclonal antibodies that deliver toxic molecules to cancer cells specifically.

- Tositumomab and 131I-tositumomab (Bexxar®) is approved to treat certain types of B-cell non-Hodgkin lymphoma. It is a mixture of monoclonal antibodies that recognize the CD20 molecule. Some of the antibodies in the mixture are linked to a radioactive substance called iodine-131. The 131I-tositumomab component delivers radioactive energy to CD20-expressing B cells specifically, reducing collateral damage to normal cells of the type that is seen with traditional radiotherapy. In addition, the binding of tositumomab to the CD20-expressing B cells triggers the immune system to destroy these cells.

- Ibritumomab tiuxetan (Zevalin®) is approved to treat some patients with B-cell non-Hodgkin lymphoma. It is a monoclonal antibody directed against CD20 that is linked to a molecule that can bind radioisotopes such as indium-111 or yttrium-90. The radiolabeled forms of Zevalin deliver a high dose of radioactivity to cells that express CD20.

- Denileukin diftitox (Ontak®) is approved for the treatment of some patients with CTCL. Denileukin diftitox consists of interleukin-2 (IL-2) protein sequences fused to diphtheria toxin. The drug binds to cell surface IL-2 receptors, which are found on certain immune cells and some cancer cells, directing the cytotoxic action of the diphtheria toxin to these cells.

What impact will targeted therapies have on cancer treatment?

Targeted cancer therapies give doctors a better way to tailor cancer treatment, especially when a target is present in some but not all tumors of a particular type, as is the case for HER-2. Eventually, treatments may be individualized based on the unique set of molecular targets produced by the patient's tumor. Targeted cancer therapies also hold the promise of being more selective for cancer cells than normal cells, thus harming fewer normal cells, reducing side effects, and improving quality of life.

Nevertheless, targeted therapies have some limitations. Chief among these is the potential for cells to develop resistance to them. In some patients who have developed resistance to imatinib, for example, a mutation in the BCR-ABL gene has arisen that changes the shape of the protein so that it no longer binds this drug as well. In most cases, another targeted therapy that could overcome this resistance is not available. It is for this reason that targeted therapies may work best in combination, either with other targeted therapies or with more traditional therapies.

Chapter 64

Photodynamic Therapy for Cancer

What is photodynamic therapy?

Photodynamic therapy (PDT) is a treatment that uses a drug, called a photosensitizer or photosensitizing agent, and a particular type of light. When photosensitizers are exposed to a specific wavelength of light, they produce a form of oxygen that kills nearby cells.

Each photosensitizer is activated by light of a specific wavelength. This wavelength determines how far the light can travel into the body. Thus, doctors use specific photosensitizers and wavelengths of light to treat different areas of the body with PDT.

How is PDT used to treat cancer?

In the first step of PDT for cancer treatment, a photosensitizing agent is injected into the bloodstream. The agent is absorbed by cells all over the body but stays in cancer cells longer than it does in normal cells. Approximately 24 to 72 hours after injection, when most of the agent has left normal cells but remains in cancer cells, the tumor is exposed to light. The photosensitizer in the tumor absorbs the light and produces an active form of oxygen that destroys nearby cancer cells.

In addition to directly killing cancer cells, PDT appears to shrink or destroy tumors in two other ways. The photosensitizer can damage blood vessels in the tumor, thereby preventing the cancer from

From "Photodynamic Therapy for Cancer," National Cancer Institute (www.can cer.gov), May 12, 2004. Reviewed by David A. Cooke, MD, FACP, September 2010.

receiving necessary nutrients. In addition, PDT may activate the immune system to attack the tumor cells.

The light used for PDT can come from a laser or other sources of light. Laser light can be directed through fiber optic cables (thin fibers that transmit light) to deliver light to areas inside the body. For example, a fiber optic cable can be inserted through an endoscope (a thin, lighted tube used to look at tissues inside the body) into the lungs or esophagus to treat cancer in these organs. Other light sources include light-emitting diodes (LEDs), which may be used for surface tumors, such as skin cancer.

PDT is usually performed as an outpatient procedure. PDT may also be repeated and may be used with other therapies, such as surgery, radiation, or chemotherapy.

What types of cancer are currently treated with PDT?

To date, the U.S. Food and Drug Administration (FDA) has approved the photosensitizing agent called porfimer sodium, or Photofrin®, for use in PDT to treat or relieve the symptoms of esophageal cancer and non-small cell lung cancer. Porfimer sodium is approved to relieve symptoms of esophageal cancer when the cancer obstructs the esophagus or when the cancer cannot be satisfactorily treated with laser therapy alone. Porfimer sodium is used to treat non-small cell lung cancer in patients for whom the usual treatments are not appropriate, and to relieve symptoms in patients with non-small cell lung cancer that obstructs the airways. In 2003, the FDA approved porfimer sodium for the treatment of precancerous lesions in patients with Barrett esophagus (a condition that can lead to esophageal cancer).

What are the limitations of PDT?

The light needed to activate most photosensitizers cannot pass through more than about one-third of an inch of tissue (one centimeter). For this reason, PDT is usually used to treat tumors on or just under the skin or on the lining of internal organs or cavities. PDT is also less effective in treating large tumors, because the light cannot pass far into these tumors. PDT is a local treatment and generally cannot be used to treat cancer that has spread (metastasized).

Does PDT have any complications or side effects?

Porfimer sodium makes the skin and eyes sensitive to light for approximately six weeks after treatment. Thus, patients are advised to avoid direct sunlight and bright indoor light for at least six weeks.

Photosensitizers tend to build up in tumors and the activating light is focused on the tumor. As a result, damage to healthy tissue is minimal. However, PDT can cause burns, swelling, pain, and scarring in nearby healthy tissue. Other side effects of PDT are related to the area that is treated. They can include coughing, trouble swallowing, stomach pain, painful breathing, or shortness of breath; these side effects are usually temporary.

What does the future hold for PDT?

Researchers continue to study ways to improve the effectiveness of PDT and expand it to other cancers. Clinical trials (research studies) are under way to evaluate the use of PDT for cancers of the brain, skin, prostate, cervix, and peritoneal cavity (the space in the abdomen that contains the intestines, stomach, and liver). Other research is focused on the development of photosensitizers that are more powerful, more specifically target cancer cells, and are activated by light that can penetrate tissue and treat deep or large tumors. Researchers are also investigating ways to improve equipment and the delivery of the activating light.

Chapter 65

Cancer and Complementary and Alternative Medicine (CAM)

Chapter Contents

Section 65.1

Thinking about CAM

From "Thinking about Complementary and Alternative Medicine,"
National Cancer Institute (www.cancer.gov), June 8, 2005. Reviewed by
David A. Cooke, MD, FACP, September 2010.

Many Choices

You have many choices to make before, during, and after your cancer
treatment. One choice you may be thinking about is complementary
and alternative medicine. We call this CAM, for short.

People with cancer may use CAM to help cope with the side effects of
cancer treatments, such as nausea, pain, and fatigue. They may use CAM
to comfort themselves and ease the worries of cancer treatment and related stress or feel that they are doing something more to help with their
own care. They may also use CAM to try to treat or cure their cancer.

It's natural to want to fight your cancer in any way you can. There
is a lot of information available, and new methods for treating cancer
are always being tested, so it may be hard to know where to start.
This information may help you understand what you find and make it
easier to decide whether CAM is right for you. Many people try CAM
therapies during cancer care. CAM does not work for everyone, but
some methods may help you manage stress, nausea, pain, or other
symptoms or side effects.

The most important message of this chapter is to talk to your doctor
before you try anything new. This will help ensure that nothing gets
in the way of your cancer treatment.

What is complementary and alternative medicine (CAM)?

CAM is any medical system, practice, or product that is not thought
of as standard care. Standard medical care is care that is based on
scientific evidence. For cancer, it includes chemotherapy, radiation,
biological therapy, and surgery.

Complementary medicine is used along with standard medical
treatments. One example is using acupuncture to help with side effects of cancer treatment.

Alternative medicine is used in place of standard medical treatments. One example is using a special diet to treat cancer instead of a method that a cancer specialist (an oncologist) suggests.

Integrative medicine is a total approach to care that involves the patient's mind, body, and spirit. It combines standard medicine with the CAM practices that have shown the most promise. For example, some people learn to use relaxation as a way to reduce stress during chemotherapy.

What are the types of CAM?

We are learning about CAM therapies every day, but there is still more to learn. Consumers may use the terms "natural," "holistic," "home remedy," or "Eastern medicine" to refer to CAM. However, experts use five categories to describe it. These are listed below with a few examples for each.

Mind-body medicines: These are based on the belief that your mind is able to affect your body. Here are some examples:

- **Meditation:** Focused breathing or repetition of words or phrases to quiet the mind;

- **Biofeedback:** Using simple machines, the patient learns how to affect certain body functions that are normally out of one's awareness (such as heart rate);

- **Hypnosis:** A state of relaxed and focused attention in which the patient concentrates on a certain feeling, idea, or suggestion to aid in healing;

- **Yoga:** Systems of stretches and poses, with special attention given to breathing;

- **Imagery:** Imagining scenes, pictures, or experiences to help the body heal;

- **Creative outlets:** Such as art, music, or dance.

Biologically based practices: This type of CAM uses things found in nature. This includes dietary supplements and herbal products. Some examples include the use of vitamins, herbs, foods, or special diets.

The topic of nutrition is worthy of a special note: It's common for people with cancer to have questions about different foods to eat during treatment. Yet it's important to know that there is no one food or special diet that has been proven to control cancer. Too much of any one food is not helpful—and may even be harmful. Because of nutrition needs you may have, it's best to talk with the doctor in charge of your treatment about the foods you should be eating.

Manipulative and body-based practices: These are based on working with one or more parts of the body. Massage, the manipulation of tissues with hands or special tools, is one example. Chiropractic care, a type of manipulation of the joints and skeletal system, is another. Reflexology, using pressure points in the hands or feet to affect other parts of the body, is also an example of a body-based practice.

Energy medicine: Energy medicine involves the belief that the body has energy fields that can be used for healing and wellness. Therapists use pressure or move the body by placing their hands in or through these fields. Some examples include the following:

- **Tai chi** (pronounced: ty-CHEE): Involves slow, gentle movements with a focus on the breath and concentration

- **Reiki** (pronounced: RAY-kee): Balancing energy either from a distance or by placing hands on or near the patient

- **Therapeutic touch**: Moving hands over energy fields of the body

Whole medical systems: These are healing systems and beliefs that have evolved over time in different cultures and parts of the world.

- **Ayurvedic medicine** (eye-yer-VAY-dik): A system from India emphasizing balance among body, mind, and spirit.

- **Chinese medicine:** Based on the view that health is a balance in the body of two forces called yin and yang. Acupuncture is a common practice in Chinese medicine that involves stimulating specific points on the body to promote health, or to lessen disease symptoms and treatment side effects.

- **Homeopathy:** Uses very small doses of substances to trigger the body to heal itself.

- **Naturopathic medicine:** Uses different methods that help the body naturally heal itself.

Talk with Your Doctor before You Use CAM

Some people with cancer are afraid that their doctor won't understand or approve of the use of CAM. But doctors know that people with cancer want to take an active part in their care. They want the best for their patients and often are willing to work with them.

Talk to your doctor to make sure that all aspects of your cancer care work together. This is important because things that seem safe, such as certain foods or pills, may interfere with your cancer treatment.

What questions should I ask my doctor about CAM?

If you think CAM might be helpful, as your doctor what types of CAM might help with concerns such as these:

- What type of CAM might help me cope, reduce my stress, and feel better?
- What type of CAM might help me feel less tired?
- What type of CAM might help me deal with cancer symptoms, such as pain, or side effects of treatment, such as nausea?

If you decide to try a CAM therapy, ask questions such as these:

- Will it interfere with my treatment or medicines?
- Can you help me understand these articles I found about CAM?
- Can you suggest a CAM practitioner for me to talk to?
- Will you work with my CAM practitioner?

A Natural Product Does Not Mean a Safe Product

Here are some important facts about dietary supplements such as herbs and vitamins:

- They may affect how well other medicines work in your body. Herbs and some plant-based products may keep medicines from doing what they are supposed to do. These medicines can be ones your doctor prescribes for you, or even ones you buy off the shelf at the store. For example, the herb St. John's wort, which some people with cancer use for depression, may cause certain anti-cancer drugs not to work as well as they should.

- Herbal supplements can act like drugs in your body. They may be harmful when taken by themselves, with other substances, or in large doses. For example, some studies have shown that kava, an herb that has been used to help with stress and anxiety, may cause liver damage.

- Vitamins can also take strong action in your body. For example, high doses of vitamins, even vitamin C, may affect how chemotherapy and radiation work. Too much of any vitamin is not safe—even in a healthy person.

Tell your doctor if you are taking any dietary supplements, no matter how safe you think they are. This is very important. Even though there are ads or claims that something has been used for years, they do not prove that it is safe or effective. It is still important to be careful.

Supplements do not have to be approved by the federal government before being sold to the public. Also, a prescription is not needed to buy them. Therefore, it's up to consumers to decide what is best for them.

Choose Practitioners with Care

CAM practitioners are people who have training in CAM therapies. Choosing one should be done with the same care as choosing a doctor. Here are some things to remember when choosing a practitioner:

- Ask your doctor or nurse to suggest someone or speak with someone who knows about CAM.

- Ask whether someone at your cancer center or doctor's office can help you find a CAM practitioner. There may be a social worker or physical therapist who can help you.

- Ask whether your hospital keeps lists of centers or has staff who can suggest people.

- Contact CAM professional organizations to get names of practitioners who are certified. This means that they have proper training in their field.

- Contact local health and wellness organizations.

- Ask about each practitioner's training and experience.

- Ask whether the practitioner has a license to practice in your state. If you want to confirm the answer, ask what organization gives out the licenses. Then, you may choose to follow up with a phone call.

- Call your health care plan to see if it covers this therapy.

What general questions should I ask the CAM practitioner?

- What types of CAM do you practice?

- What are your training and qualifications?

- Do you see other patients with my type of cancer?

- Will you work with my doctor?

What questions about the therapy should I ask the CAM practitioner?

- How can this help me?
- Do you know of studies that prove it helps?
- What are the risks and side effects?
- Will this interfere with my cancer treatment?
- How long will I be on the therapy?
- What will it cost?
- Do you have information that I can read about it?
- Are there any reasons why I should not use it?

What questions should I ask myself?

- Do I feel comfortable with this person?
- Do I like how the office looks and feels?
- Do I like the staff?
- Does this person support standard cancer treatments?
- How far am I willing to travel for treatment?
- Is it easy to get an appointment?
- Are the hours good for me?
- Will insurance cover the cost of CAM? (Call your health plan or insurer to see whether they cover CAM therapies. Many are not covered.)

Getting Information from Trusted Sources

There is a lot of information on CAM, so it's important to go to sources you can trust. Be careful of products advertised by people or companies that make claims that they have a "cure" or do not give specific information about how well their product works. Be careful when companies make claims only about positive results that have few side effects or say they have clinical studies—but provide no proof or copies of the studies. Just remember, if it sounds too good to be true, it probably is.

Often patients and families have been able to find answers to many of their questions about CAM on the internet. Many websites are good resources for CAM information. However, some may be unreliable or misleading. If you find information on a website, ask these questions:

- Who runs and pays for the site?
- Does it list any credentials?
- Does it represent an organization that is well-known and respected?
- What is the purpose of the site, and who is it for?
- Is the site selling or promoting something?
- Where does the information come from?
- Is the information based on facts or only on someone's feelings or opinions?
- How is the information chosen? Is there a review board or is the content reviewed by experts?
- How current is the information?
- Does the site tell when it was last updated?
- How does the site choose which other sites to link you to?

Books are another source of information about CAM therapies. Some books are better than others and contain trustworthy content, while others do not. If you go to the library, ask the staff for suggestions. Or if you live near a college or university, there may be a medical library available. Local bookstores may also have people on staff who can help you.

It's important to know that information is always changing and that new research results are reported every day. Be aware that if a book is written by only one person, you may only be getting that one person's view. Here are some questions to ask about information in books:

- Is the author an expert on this subject?
- Do you know anyone else who has read the book?
- Has the book been reviewed by other experts?
- Was it published in the past five years?
- Does the book offer different points of view, or does it seem to hold one opinion?
- Has the author researched the topic in full?
- Are the references listed in the back?

If you want to look for magazine articles you can trust, ask your librarian to help you look for medical journals, books, and other research that has been done by experts. Articles in popular magazines are usually not written by experts. Rather, the authors speak with experts, gather information, and then write the article. If claims about CAM are made in magazine articles, remember these points:

- The authors may not have expert knowledge in this area.
- They may not say where they found their information.
- The articles have not been reviewed by experts.
- The publisher may have ties to advertisers or other organizations. Therefore, the article may be one-sided.

When you read these articles, you can use the same process that the magazine writer uses: Speak with experts, ask lots of questions, and then decide if the therapy is right for you.

Section 65.2

Dietary Supplements and Cancer Treatment

"Dietary Supplements and Cancer Treatment: A Risky Mixture,"
by Sharon Reynolds, *NCI Cancer Bulletin*, National Cancer Institute,
August 11, 2009.

Patients undergoing cancer treatment often experience not only pain and discomfort from their disease, but also the potentially debilitating side effects caused by their treatments.

Some patients who do not receive adequate palliative care to lessen these side effects, or those driven to do anything possible to feel better while fighting their disease, may turn to dietary supplements advertised as having anticancer effects or being supportive of general health, frequently without consulting a health care professional.

Some herbal medicines and dietary supplements have negative interactions with prescribed cancer treatments.

These supplements are often herbs or other natural products. "A common, false belief is that 'if it's natural, it must be safe,'" said Dr. Barrie Cassileth, chief of the Integrative Medicine Service at the Memorial Sloan-Kettering Cancer Center. "But herbs and other dietary supplements are biologically active compounds, and they frequently have negative interactions with prescription pharmaceuticals."

Furthermore, as a growing number of studies have shown, commonly used herbs and supplements can interact with cancer chemotherapy or radiation therapy, causing potentially life-threatening effects.

Widespread Use

In a systematic review published by Dr. Cassileth and a colleague in 1998, the use of complementary and alternative medicine (CAM) by cancer patients, including herbs and other dietary supplements, ranged from 7% to 64% in 21 different studies, with the average being about 31%.

CAM use has most likely increased during years since that study. In a 2004 study from the Mayo Clinic Comprehensive Cancer Center, more than 80% of patients enrolled in early phase chemotherapy trials concurrently used supplemental vitamins, herbs, or minerals, which were often explicitly not allowed as part of the trial protocols.

A study from a Midwestern oncology clinic published in 2005 showed that 65% of patients receiving chemotherapy had also taken dietary supplements, not including vitamins. Twenty-five percent of these had used one or more herbal therapies that are thought to have negative interactions with chemotherapy drugs. The majority of the patients did not consult a health care professional prior to supplement use.

Dangerous Interactions

"We tell patients that if you are on any chemotherapy or undergoing radiation, or planning for it in the future: no herbs, no antioxidants, no dietary supplements, across the board. Particularly herbal agents, because they can interact with and decrease the level of chemotherapy or any medication that enters your body," explained Dr. Cassileth.

These effects are due to pharmacokinetic interactions—what happens when biologically active compounds in an herb alter the way a chemotherapy drug is absorbed, distributed in the body, metabolized, or eliminated. These interactions can happen for many reasons, including interference with the enzymes in the liver that normally break down the drugs, or interactions with the transporters that carry drugs across cell membranes. St. John's wort, garlic extract, and Echinacea are examples of commonly used herbal products thought to pharmacokinetically interact with chemotherapy drugs.

Pharmacokinetic interactions can have two potentially disastrous consequences. One is that less chemotherapy drug circulates in the bloodstream than is needed, leading to treatment failure. The other is the opposite effect: if the chemotherapy drugs are not broken down and removed from the body as expected, severe side effects can occur as a result of an overdose.

Unwanted Protection for Cancer Cells

Even antioxidant supplements such as vitamin E have the potential to interfere with treatment. Radiation therapy and some types of chemotherapy work by generating free radicals that damage cells' DNA. Antioxidants can block this therapeutic effect.

"People are taking high-dose antioxidant supplements thinking they're only going to protect normal cells, but both preclinical and clinical data show that they may protect both normal and tumor cells," explained Dr. Brian Lawenda, a radiation oncologist from the Naval Medical Center in San Diego.

In 2008, Dr. Lawenda and his colleagues performed a review of results from the published randomized clinical trials testing antioxidants with radiation therapy or chemotherapy, and they concluded that the use of high doses of "supplemental antioxidants during chemotherapy and radiation therapy should be discouraged because of the possibility of tumor protection and reduced survival."

A Silver Lining?

Even though doctors now caution patients not to mix and match over-the-counter supplements with cancer treatment, the bioactivity of herbs and other natural products are of interest to some cancer researchers looking for ways to enhance chemotherapy. While many herbs have been shown to interfere with chemotherapy, some may actually improve its efficacy.

"The interaction between certain complementary approaches and conventional treatment is an area of special interest to the Office of Cancer Complementary and Alternative Medicine (OCCAM)," said Dr. Jeffrey White, director of OCCAM. "We're looking for ways to use natural products to improve the therapeutic index of conventional therapy."

In addition to supporting ongoing clinical trials testing several traditional Chinese medicines in combination with the chemotherapy drugs irinotecan, capecitabine, and gemcitabine, OCCAM recently released two program announcements (PA-09-167 and PA-09-168) that will provide funding for researchers interested in testing synergistic interactions between natural products and traditional therapies.

Part Four

Recurrent and Advanced Cancer

Chapter 66

Metastatic Cancer

What is cancer?

Cancer is a group of many related diseases. All cancers begin in cells, the building blocks that make up tissues. Cancer that arises from organs and solid tissues is called a solid tumor. Cancer that begins in blood cells is called leukemia, multiple myeloma, or lymphoma.

Normally, cells grow and divide to form new cells as the body needs them. When cells grow old and die, new cells take their place. Sometimes this orderly process goes wrong. New cells form when the body does not need them, and old cells do not die when they should.

The extra cells form a mass of tissue, called a growth or tumor. Tumors can be either benign (not cancerous) or malignant (cancerous). Benign tumors do not spread to other parts of the body, and they are rarely a threat to life. Malignant tumors can spread (metastasize) and may be life threatening.

What is primary cancer?

Cancer can begin in any organ or tissue of the body. The original tumor is called the primary cancer or primary tumor. It is usually named for the part of the body or the type of cell in which it begins.

Excerpted from "Metastatic Cancer: Questions and Answers," National Cancer Institute (www.cancer.gov), September 1, 2004. Reviewed by David A. Cooke, MD, FACP, September 2010.

What is metastasis, and how does it happen?

Metastasis means the spread of cancer. Cancer cells can break away from a primary tumor and enter the bloodstream or lymphatic system (the system that produces, stores, and carries the cells that fight infections). That is how cancer cells spread to other parts of the body.

When cancer cells spread and form a new tumor in a different organ, the new tumor is a metastatic tumor. The cells in the metastatic tumor come from the original tumor. This means, for example, that if breast cancer spreads to the lungs, the metastatic tumor in the lung is made up of cancerous breast cells (not lung cells). In this case, the disease in the lungs is metastatic breast cancer (not lung cancer). Under a microscope, metastatic breast cancer cells generally look the same as the cancer cells in the breast.

Where does cancer spread?

Cancer cells can spread to almost any part of the body. Cancer cells frequently spread to lymph nodes (rounded masses of lymphatic tissue) near the primary tumor (regional lymph nodes). This is called lymph node involvement or regional disease. Cancer that spreads to other organs or to lymph nodes far from the primary tumor is called metastatic disease. Doctors sometimes also call this distant disease.

The most common sites of metastasis from solid tumors are the lungs, bones, liver, and brain. Some cancers tend to spread to certain parts of the body. For example, lung cancer often metastasizes to the brain or bones, and colon cancer frequently spreads to the liver. Prostate cancer tends to spread to the bones. Breast cancer commonly spreads to the bones, lungs, liver, or brain. However, each of these cancers can spread to other parts of the body as well.

Because blood cells travel throughout the body, leukemia, multiple myeloma, and lymphoma cells are usually not localized when the cancer is diagnosed. Tumor cells may be found in the blood, several lymph nodes, or other parts of the body such as the liver or bones. This type of spread is not referred to as metastasis.

Are there symptoms of metastatic cancer?

Some people with metastatic cancer do not have symptoms. Their metastases are found by x-rays and other tests performed for other reasons.

When symptoms of metastatic cancer occur, the type and frequency of the symptoms will depend on the size and location of the metastasis.

For example, cancer that spreads to the bones is likely to cause pain and can lead to bone fractures. Cancer that spreads to the brain can cause a variety of symptoms, including headaches, seizures, and unsteadiness. Shortness of breath may be a sign of lung involvement. Abdominal swelling or jaundice (yellowing of the skin) can indicate that cancer has spread to the liver.

Sometimes a person's primary cancer is discovered only after the metastatic tumor causes symptoms. For example, a man whose prostate cancer has spread to the bones in his pelvis may have lower back pain (caused by the cancer in his bones) before he experiences any symptoms from the primary tumor in his prostate.

How does a doctor know whether a cancer is a primary or a metastatic tumor?

To determine whether a tumor is primary or metastatic, a pathologist examines a sample of the tumor under a microscope. In general, cancer cells look like abnormal versions of cells in the tissue where the cancer began. Using specialized diagnostic tests, a pathologist is often able to tell where the cancer cells came from. Markers or antigens found in or on the cancer cells can indicate the primary site of the cancer.

Metastatic cancers may be found before or at the same time as the primary tumor, or months or years later. When a new tumor is found in a patient who has been treated for cancer in the past, it is more often a metastasis than another primary tumor.

Is it possible to have a metastatic tumor without having a primary cancer?

No. A metastatic tumor always starts from cancer cells in another part of the body. In most cases, when a metastatic tumor is found first, the primary tumor can be found. The search for the primary tumor may involve lab tests, x-rays, and other procedures. However, in a small number of cases, a metastatic tumor is diagnosed but the primary tumor cannot be found, in spite of extensive tests. The pathologist knows the tumor is metastatic because the cells are not like those in the organ or tissue in which the tumor is found. Doctors refer to the primary tumor as unknown or occult (hidden), and the patient is said to have cancer of unknown primary origin (CUP). Because diagnostic techniques are constantly improving, the number of cases of CUP is going down.

What treatments are used for metastatic cancer?

When cancer has metastasized, it may be treated with chemotherapy, radiation therapy, biological therapy, hormone therapy, surgery, cryosurgery, or a combination of these. The choice of treatment generally depends on the type of primary cancer, the size and location of the metastasis, the patient's age and general health, and the types of treatments the patient has had in the past. In patients with CUP, it is possible to treat the disease even though the primary tumor has not been located. The goal of treatment may be to control the cancer, or to relieve symptoms or side effects of treatment.

Are new treatments for metastatic cancer being developed?

Yes, many new cancer treatments are under study. To develop new treatments, the National Cancer Institute (NCI) sponsors clinical trials (research studies) with cancer patients in many hospitals, universities, medical schools, and cancer centers around the country. Clinical trials are a critical step in the improvement of treatment. Before any new treatment can be recommended for general use, doctors conduct studies to find out whether the treatment is both safe for patients and effective against the disease. The results of such studies have led to progress not only in the treatment of cancer, but in the detection, diagnosis, and prevention of the disease as well. Patients interested in taking part in a clinical trial should talk with their doctor.

Chapter 67

Recurrent Cancer

Adjusting to the News

Maybe in the back of your mind, you feared that your cancer might return. Now you might be thinking, "How can this be happening to me again? Haven't I been through enough?"

You may be feeling shocked, angry, sad, or scared. Many people have these feelings. But you have something now that you didn't have before—experience. You've lived through cancer once. You know a lot about what to expect and hope for.

Also remember that treatments may have improved since you had your first cancer. New drugs or methods may help with your treatment or in managing side effects. In fact, cancer is now often thought of as a chronic disease, one which people manage for many years.

Why and Where Cancer Returns

When cancer comes back, doctors call it a recurrence (or recurrent cancer). A recurrent cancer starts with cancer cells that the first treatment didn't fully remove or destroy. Some may have been too small to be seen in follow-up. This doesn't mean that the treatment you received was wrong. And it doesn't mean that you did anything wrong, either. It just means that a small number of cancer cells survived the treatment. These cells grew over time into tumors or cancer that your doctor can now detect.

Excerpted from "When Cancer Returns," National Cancer Institute (www.cancer .gov), August 23, 2005. Reviewed by David A. Cooke, MD, FACP, September 2010.

When cancer comes back, it doesn't always show up in the same part of the body. For example, if you had colon cancer, it may come back in your liver. But the cancer is still called colon cancer. When the original cancer spreads to a new place, it is called a metastasis.

It is possible to develop a completely new cancer that has nothing to do with your original cancer. But this doesn't happen very often. Recurrences are more common.

Doctors define recurrent cancers by where they develop. There are different types of recurrence:

- **Local recurrence:** This means that the cancer is in the same place as the original cancer or is very close to it.

- **Regional recurrence:** This is when tumors grow in lymph nodes or tissues near the place of the original cancer.

- **Distant recurrence:** In these cases, the cancer has spread (metastasized) to organs or tissues far from the place of the original cancer.

Local cancer may be easier to treat than regional or distant cancer. But this can be different for each patient. Talk with your doctor about your options.

Taking Control: Your Care and Treatment

Cancer that returns can affect all parts of your life. You may feel weak and no longer in control. But you don't have to feel that way. You can take part in your care and in making decisions. You can also talk with your health care team and loved ones as you decide about your care. This may help you feel a sense of control and well-being.

Talking with Your Health Care Team

Many people have a treatment team of health providers who work together to help them. This team may include doctors, nurses, oncology social workers, dietitians, or other specialists. Some people don't like to ask about treatment choices or side effects. They think that doctors don't like being questioned. But this is not true. Most doctors want their patients to be involved in their own care. They want patients to discuss concerns with them.

Here are a few topics you may want to discuss with your health care team:

- **Pain or other symptoms:** Be honest and open about how you feel. Tell your doctors if you have pain and where. Tell them what you expect in the way of pain relief.

- **Communication:** Some people want to know details about their care. Others prefer to know as little as possible. Some people with cancer want their family members to make most of their decisions. What would you prefer? Decide what you want to know, how much you want to know, and when you've heard enough. Choose what is most comfortable for you. Then tell your doctor and family members. Ask that they follow through with your wishes.

- **Family wishes:** Some family members may have trouble dealing with cancer. They don't want to know how far the disease has advanced. Find out from your family members how much they want to know. And be sure to tell your doctors and nurses. Do this as soon as possible. It will help avoid conflicts or distress among your loved ones.

Other Tips for Talking with Your Health Care Team

- Speak openly about your needs, questions, and concerns. Don't be embarrassed to ask your doctor to repeat or explain something.

- Keep a file or notebook of all the papers and test results that your doctor has given you. Take this file to your visits. Also keep records or a diary of all your visits. List the drugs and tests you have taken. Then you can refer to your records when you need to. Many patients say this is helpful, especially when you meet with a new doctor for the first time.

- Write down your questions before you see your doctors so you will remember them.

- Ask a family member or friend to go to the doctor's office with you. They can help you ask questions to get a clear sense of what to expect. This can be an emotional time. You may have trouble focusing on what the doctor says. It may be easier for someone else to take notes. Then you can review them later.

- Ask your doctor if it's okay to tape-record your talks.

- Tell your doctor if you want to get dressed before talking about your results. Wearing a gown or robe is distracting for some patients. They find it harder to focus on what the doctor is saying.

Treatment Choices

There are many treatment choices for recurrent cancer. Your treatment will depend partly on the type of cancer and the treatment you had before. It will also depend on where the cancer has recurred.

- A local recurrence may be best treated by surgery or radiation therapy. This means that the doctor removes the tumor or destroys it with radiation.

- A distant recurrence may need chemotherapy, biological therapy, or radiation therapy.

It's important to ask your doctor questions about all your treatment choices. You may want to get a second opinion as well. You may also want to ask whether a clinical trial is an option for you.

Second Opinions

Some patients worry that doctors will be offended if they ask for a second opinion. Usually the opposite is true. Most doctors welcome a second opinion. And many health insurance companies will pay for them.

If you get a second opinion, the doctor may agree with your first doctor's treatment plan. Or the second doctor may suggest another approach. Either way, you have more information and perhaps a greater sense of control. You can feel more confident about the decisions you make, knowing that you've looked at your options.

Clinical Trials

Treatment clinical trials are research studies that try to find better ways to treat cancer. Every day, cancer researchers learn more about treatment options from clinical trials.

Each study has rules about who can take part. These rules include the person's age and type of cancer. They also cover earlier treatments and where the cancer has returned.

Clinical trials have both benefits and risks. Your doctor should tell you about them before you make any decisions about taking part.

There are different phases of clinical trials:

- Phase I trials test what dose of a treatment is safe and how it should be given.

- Phase II trials discover how cancer responds to a new drug or treatment.

874

- Phase III trials compare an accepted cancer treatment (standard treatment) with a new treatment that researchers hope is better.

Taking part in a clinical trial could help you and others who get cancer in the future. But insurance and managed care plans do not always cover the costs. What they cover varies by plan and by study. If you want to learn more about clinical trials, talk with your health care team.

Making Your Wishes Known

When cancer returns, the treatment goals may change, or they may be the same as they were for your first cancer. But for many people, it's the second cancer diagnosis that finally prompts them to make their wishes known. Although it can be tough to think about, and maybe even tougher to talk about, having recurrent cancer may prompt you to make certain decisions about what you want done for you if you are unable to speak for yourself.

Everyone should make a will and talk about end-of-life choices with loved ones. This is one of the most important things you can do. Also, think about giving someone you trust some rights to make medical decisions for you. You give these rights through legal documents called advance directives. These papers tell your loved ones and doctors what to do if you can't tell them yourself. They let you decide ahead of time how you want to be treated. These papers may include a living will and a durable power of attorney for health care.

Setting up an advance directive is not the same as giving up. Making such decisions at this time keeps you in control. You are making your wishes known for all to follow. This can help you worry less about the future and live each day to the fullest.

It's hard to talk about these issues. But it often comforts family members to know what you want. And it saves them from having to bring up the subject themselves. You may also gain peace of mind. You are making these hard choices for yourself instead of leaving them to your loved ones.

Make copies of your advance directives. Give them to your family members, your health care team, and your hospital medical records department. That way, everyone will know your decisions.

Advance Directives

- A living will lets people know what kind of medical care you want if you are unable to speak for yourself.

- A durable power of attorney for health care names a person to make medical decisions for you if you can't make them yourself. This person is called a health care proxy.

Other Legal Papers

- A will tells how you want to divide your money and property among your heirs. (Heirs are usually the family members who survive you. You may also name other people as heirs in your will.)

- A trust appoints a person you choose to manage your money for you.

- Power of attorney appoints a person to make financial decisions for you when you can't make them yourself.

You do not always need a lawyer present to fill out these papers. But you may need a notary public. Each state has its own laws about advance directives. Check with your lawyer or social worker about the laws in your state.

Managing Treatment Side Effects

Comfort Care

You have a right to comfort care both during and after treatment. This kind of care is often called palliative (PAL-ee-yuh-tiv) care. It includes treating or preventing cancer symptoms and the side effects caused by treatment. Comfort care can also mean getting help with emotional and spiritual problems during and after cancer treatment.

People once thought of palliative care as a way to comfort those dying of cancer. Doctors now offer this care to all cancer patients, beginning when the cancer is diagnosed. You should receive palliative care through treatment, survival, and advanced disease. Your oncologist may be able to help you. But a palliative care specialist may be the best person to treat some problems. Ask your doctor or nurse if there is a specialist you can go to.

Pain Control

Having cancer doesn't always mean that you'll have pain. But if you do, you shouldn't accept pain as normal. Your doctor can control pain with medicines and other treatments. Managing your pain helps you sleep and eat better. It makes it easier to enjoy your family and friends, and to focus on the things you enjoy.

Have regular talks with your health care team about your pain. Let them know what kind of pain it is, where it is, and how bad it is. These talks are important because pain can change throughout your illness. And your pain may show where cancer has returned after remission. Many hospitals have doctors who are experts in treating pain. Tell your doctor if you would like to talk to a pain specialist.

People with cancer often need strong medicine to help control their pain. Don't be afraid to ask for pain medicine or for larger doses if you need them. People with cancer hardly ever get addicted to these drugs. Sadly, fears of addiction sometimes prevent people from taking medicine for pain. The same fears also prompt family members to encourage loved ones to "hold off" between doses. But people in pain get the most relief when they take their medicines and treatments on a regular schedule.

Many people have found some types of complementary and alternative medicine (CAM) helpful. But talk with your health care team before trying any of them. Make sure they are safe and won't interfere with your cancer treatment.

- Acupuncture is a form of Chinese medicine that stimulates certain points on the body using small needles. It may help treat nausea and control pain. Before using acupuncture, ask your health care team if it is safe for your type of cancer.

- Imagery is imagining scenes, pictures, or experiences to feel calmer or perhaps to help the body to heal.

- Relaxation techniques include deep breathing and exercises to relax your muscles.

- Hypnosis is a state of relaxed and focused attention. One focuses on a certain feeling, idea, or suggestion.

- Biofeedback is the use of a special machine to help the patient learn how to control certain body functions. These are things that we are normally not aware of (such as heart rate).

- Massage therapy brings relaxation and a sense of well-being by the gentle rubbing of different body parts or muscles. Before you try this, you need to check with your doctor. Massage is not recommended for some kinds of cancer.

These methods may also help manage stress. Again, talk to your health care team before using anything new, no matter how safe it may seem. Ask your health care team for more information about where to get these treatments.

Fatigue

Fatigue is more than feeling tired. Fatigue is exhaustion—not being able to do even the small things you used to do. A number of things can cause fatigue. Besides cancer treatment, they include anxiety, stress, and changes in your diet or sleeping patterns. If you are having some of these problems, tell your doctor or nurse at your next visit. Ask about medicines that can help with fatigue. Eating a well-balanced diet and planning your days and doing only what is important to you can also help. Take short breaks every day to rest and relax and take naps. Don't be afraid to ask others for help.

Nutrition and Nausea and Vomiting

For some patients, it's hard to eat the foods they normally enjoy. For others, it's hard to eat anything at all. If you are having trouble eating or digesting food, talk with your doctor or other healthcare providers. They may suggest a special diet or other ways of getting the nutrition you need. You may find it helpful to see a dietitian.

Nausea and vomiting can both be problems for cancer patients. Untreated nausea and vomiting can make you feel very tired. They can also make it hard to get treatments or to care for yourself. There are many drugs to help you control nausea and vomiting. Ask your doctor which medicines might work best for you.

You also may find it helpful to make these changes to your diet:

- Eat small amounts of food five to six times a day.

- Avoid foods that are sweet, fatty, salty, spicy, or have strong smells. These may make nausea and vomiting worse.

- Have as much liquid as possible. You'll want to keep your body from getting too dry (dehydrated). Broth, ice cream, water, juices, herb teas, and watermelon are good choices.

Sleep Problems

Illness, pain, stress, drugs, and being in the hospital can cause sleep problems such as having trouble falling asleep, sleeping only for short amounts of time, waking up in the middle of the night, or having trouble getting back to sleep. To help with your sleep problem, you may want to try:

- Reducing noise, dimming lights, making the room warmer or cooler, and using pillows to support your body

- Dressing in loose, soft clothing

- Going to the bathroom before bed

- Eating a high-protein snack two hours before bedtime (such as peanut butter, cheese, nuts, or some sliced chicken or turkey)

- Avoiding caffeine (coffee, tea, cola, hot cocoa)

- Keeping regular sleep hours

- Avoiding naps longer than 15–30 minutes

- Talking with your health care team about drugs to help you sleep.

Physical Therapy

Sometimes people with cancer feel pain in different parts of their body. Others feel weak and tired. And some feel stiffer than they used to. So it can become hard to move different body parts. If you are having any of these problems, your health care team may suggest you see a physical therapist. The therapist may use heat, cold, massage, pressure, or exercises to help you. Physical therapy may reduce tiredness and help your body function better. It may help with strength and balance as well. It also may help with stiffness and other side effects of radiation therapy.

Setting Goals

Cancer treatment can take up a lot of your time and energy. It helps to plan something that takes your mind off the disease each day. Aim for small goals each day:

- Exercising

- Completing tasks you've been wanting to do

- Making phone calls

- Having lunch with a friend

- Reading one chapter of a book or doing a puzzle

- Listening to music or a relaxation tape

Many people with cancer also set longer-term goals. They say that they do much better if they set goals or look forward to something special. It could be an anniversary, the birth of a child or grandchild, a wedding, a graduation, or a vacation. But if you set a long-term goal, make sure you are realistic about how you will achieve it.

Remember, too, that being flexible is important. You may have to change your plans if your energy level drops. You may have to adjust your goals if the cancer causes new challenges. Whatever your goals, try to spend your time in a way that you enjoy.

Family and Friends

Your loved ones may need time to adjust to the news that your cancer has returned. They need to come to terms with their own feelings. These may include confusion, shock, helplessness, anger, and other feelings.

Let family members and friends know that they can offer comfort just by being themselves, listening and not trying to solve problems, and being at ease with you. Being able to comfort you can help them cope with their feelings.

Bear in mind that not everyone can handle the return of cancer. Sometimes a friend or family member can't face the idea that you might not get better. Some people may not know what to say or do for you. As a result, relationships may change, but not because of you. They may change because others can't cope with their own feelings and pain. If you can, remind your loved ones that you are still the same person you always were. Let them know if it's all right to ask questions or tell you how they feel. Sometimes just reminding them to be there for you is enough.

It's also okay if you don't feel comfortable talking about your cancer. Some topics are hard to talk about with people you are close to. In this case, you may want to talk with a member of your health care team or a trained counselor. You might want to attend a support group where people meet to share common concerns.

Looking for Meaning

At different times in life, it's natural for people to look for meaning in their lives. And many people with recurrent cancer find this search for meaning important. They want to understand their purpose in life. They often reflect on what they have gone through. Some look for a sense of peace or a bond with others. Some seek to forgive themselves or others for past actions. Some look for answers and strength through religion or spirituality.

Being spiritual means different things to different people. It's a very personal issue. Everyone has their own beliefs about the meaning of life. Some people find it through religion or faith. Some find it by teaching or through volunteer work. Others find it in other ways. Having cancer may cause you to think about what you believe—about God, an afterlife, or the connections between living things. This can bring a sense of peace, a lot of questions, or both.

You may have already given a lot of thought to these issues. Still, you might find comfort by exploring more deeply what is meaningful to you. You could do this with someone close to you, a member of your faith or spiritual community, a counselor, or a trusted friend. Or you may find that talking to others at gatherings and services at places of worship is helpful.

Or you may just want to take time for yourself. You may want to reflect on your experiences and relationships. Writing in a journal or reading also helps some people find comfort and meaning. Others find that prayer or meditation helps them.

Many people also find that cancer changes their values. The things you own and your daily duties may seem less important. You may decide to spend more time with loved ones or helping others. You may want to do more things outdoors or learn something new.

A Time to Reflect

This is a hard time in your life. Living with cancer is tough, especially when it has come back. You battled the disease once, and now you must face it again. But you're more experienced this time around.

Use this knowledge to your advantage. Try to remember what you did before to cope. Reflect on what you might have done differently. By looking back in this way, the hope is that you may find new strength. And that this strength can help carry you through each day, and through the coming weeks and months.

Chapter 68

End-of-Life Care

Overview

Thinking about and planning for the end-of-life can be a difficult time for patients and their families. Each person will have unique needs and will cope in different ways. This time is easier when patients, families, and health care providers talk openly about end-of-life plans. For many patients and their families, this can be a time of personal growth. These events often give people the chance to find out more about themselves and appreciate what is most important to them.

This summary discusses care during the last days and last hours of life, including treatment of common symptoms and ethical questions that may come up. It may help patients and their families prepare for the kinds of decisions that may be needed during this time.

Making end-of-life plans can lower the stress on both the patient and the family. When treatment choices and plans are discussed before the last days of life, it can lower the stress on both the patient and the family. Knowing the patient's wishes can help make it easier for family members to make major decisions for the patient during a very emotional time. It is most helpful if end-of life planning and decision-making begin soon after diagnosis and continue during the course of the disease. Having these decisions in writing can make the patient's wishes clear to both the family and the health care team. When it is

Excerpted from PDQ® Cancer Information Summary. National Cancer Institute; Bethesda, MD. "Last Days of Life (PDQ) - Patient Version." Updated 08/2010. Available at: http://cancer.gov. Accessed October 5, 2010.

a child who is terminally ill, having these discussions with the child's doctor may reduce the time the child spends in the hospital and help the parents feel more prepared for the child's end of life.

End-of-life planning usually includes making choices about the following:

- The goals of care (for example, whether to use certain medicines during the last days of life)

- Where the patient wants to spend his or her final days

- Which treatments for end-of-life care the patient wishes to receive

- What type of palliative care and hospice care the patient wishes to receive

Palliative care relieves symptoms and can improve the quality of life for patients and their families. The goal of palliative care is to improve the patient's and the family's quality of life by preventing and relieving suffering. This includes treating physical symptoms such as pain, and dealing with emotional, social, and spiritual concerns.

When palliative treatment is given at the end of life, care is taken to make sure the patient's wishes about treatments he or she wants to receive are followed.

Hospice programs provide care given by experts on end-of-life issues. Hospice is a program that gives care to people who are near the end of life and have stopped treatment to cure or control their cancer. Hospice care is usually meant for patients who are not expected to live longer than six months. Hospice care focuses on quality of life rather than length of life. The goal of hospice is to help patients live each day to the fullest by making them comfortable and relieving their symptoms. This may include palliative care to control pain and other symptoms so the patient can be as alert and comfortable as possible. Services to help and support the emotional, social, and spiritual needs of patients and their families are also an important part of hospice care.

Hospice programs are designed to keep a patient at home with family and friends, but hospice programs also provide services in hospice centers and in some hospitals and nursing home facilities. The hospice team includes doctors, nurses, spiritual advisors, social workers, nutritionists, and volunteers. Team members are specially trained on issues that occur at the end-of-life. After the patient's death, the hospice program continues to offer support, including grief or bereavement counseling.

Managing Symptoms

Common symptoms at the end of life include pain, feeling very tired, coughing, shortness of breath, rattle, delirium, and fever. Bleeding may also occur.

Pain

Pain medicines can be given in several ways. In the last days, a patient may not be able to swallow pain medicine. When patients cannot take medicines by mouth, the pain medicine may be given by placing it under the tongue or into the rectum, by injection or infusion, or by placing a patch on the skin. These methods can be used at home with a doctor's order.

Pain during the final hours of life can usually be controlled. Opioid analgesics work very well to relieve pain and are commonly used at the end of life. Some patients worry that the use of opioids may cause death to occur sooner, but studies have shown no link between opioid use and early death.

Myoclonic Jerking

Myoclonic jerks are sudden muscle twitches or jerks that cannot be controlled by the person having them. A hiccup is one type of myoclonic jerk. Myoclonic jerking often occurs in the arms or legs. Taking very high doses of an opioid for a long time may cause this side effect, but it can have other causes as well. In patients taking opioids, it may begin with jerking movements that happen once in a while and then begin to happen more often. Rarely, there is constant jerking of different muscle groups all over the body.

When opioids are the cause of myoclonic jerking, changing to another opioid may help. Different patients respond to opioids in different ways and certain opioids may be more likely than others to cause myoclonic jerking in some people.

When the patient is very near death, medicine to stop the myoclonic jerking may be given instead of changing the opioid. When myoclonic jerking is severe, drugs may be used to calm the patient down, relieve anxiety, and help the patient sleep.

Fatigue

Fatigue (feeling very tired) can have many causes at the end of life. These include physical and mental changes and side effects of treatments. Drugs that increase brain activity, alertness, attention, and energy may be helpful.

Shortness of Breath

Feeling short of breath is common during the final days or weeks of life. Shortness of breath or not being able to catch your breath is often caused by advanced cancer. Other causes include the following:

- Build-up of fluid in the abdomen

- Loss of muscle strength

- Hypoxemia (a condition in which there is not enough oxygen in the blood)

- Chronic obstructive pulmonary disease (COPD)

- Pneumonia

- Infection

The use of opioids and other methods can help the patient breathe more easily. Very low doses of an opioid may relieve shortness of breath in patients who are not taking opioids for pain. Higher doses may be needed in patients who are taking opioids for pain or who have severe shortness of breath.

Other methods that may help patients who feel short of breath include the following:

- Treating anxiety caused by shortness of breath

- Directing a cool fan towards the patient's face

- Having the patient sit up

- Having the patient do breathing and relaxation exercises, if able

- Using acupuncture or acupressure

- Giving antibiotics if shortness of breath is caused by an infection

- Giving extra oxygen if shortness of breath is caused by hypoxemia

In rare cases, shortness of breath may not be relieved by any of these treatments. Sedation with drugs may be needed, to help the patient feel more comfortable.

Some patients have spasms of the air passages in the lungs along with shortness of breath. Bronchodilators (drugs that open up small airways in the lungs) or steroid drugs (which relieve swelling and inflammation) may relieve these spasms.

Cough

Chronic coughing at the end of life may add to a patient's discomfort. Repeated coughing can cause pain and loss of sleep, increase tiredness, and make shortness of breath worse. At the end of life, the decision may be to treat the symptoms of the cough rather than finding and treating the cause. The following types of drugs may be used to make the patient as comfortable as possible:

- Opioids to stop the coughing
- Corticosteroids to shrink swollen lymph vessels
- Antibiotics to treat infection
- Bronchodilators to decrease wheezing and coughing from chronic obstructive pulmonary disease
- Diuretics to relieve coughing caused by congestive heart failure

Also, the doctor may look at drugs the patient is already taking, as some drugs (such as ACE inhibitors for high blood pressure or heart failure) can cause cough.

Death Rattle

Rattle occurs when saliva or other fluids build up in the throat and airways in a patient who is too weak to clear the throat. There are two types of rattle. Death rattle is caused by saliva pooling at the back of the throat. The other kind of rattle is caused by fluid in the airways from an infection, a tumor, or excess fluid in body tissues.

Drugs may be given to decrease the amount of saliva in the mouth or to dry the upper airway. Since most patients with rattle are unable to swallow, these drugs are usually given in patches on the skin or by infusion.

Non-drug treatments for rattle include changing the patient's position and giving less fluid. Raising the head of the bed, propping the patient up with pillows, or turning the patient to either side may help relieve rattle. If the rattle is caused by fluid at the back of the throat, excess fluid may be gently removed from the mouth using a suction tube. If the rattle is caused by fluid in the airways, the fluid is usually not removed by suction. Suctioning causes severe physical and mental stress on the patient.

At the end of life, the body needs less food and fluid. Reducing food and fluids can lessen the excess fluid in the body and greatly relieve rattle.

Death rattle is a sign that death may occur in hours or days. Rattle can be very upsetting for those at the bedside. It does not seem to be painful for the patient.

Delirium

Delirium is common during the final days of life. Some patients may be confused, nervous, and restless, and have hallucinations (see or hear things not really there). Other patients may be quiet and withdrawn.

Delirium can be caused by the direct effects of cancer, such as a growing tumor in the brain. Other causes include the following:

- A higher- or lower-than-normal amount of certain chemicals in the blood that keep the heart, kidneys, nerves, and muscles working the way they should
- Side effects of drugs or drug interactions (changes in the way a drug acts in the body when taken with certain other drugs, herbal medicine, or foods)
- Stopping the use of certain drugs or alcohol
- Dehydration (the loss of needed water from the body)
- A full bladder or constipation
- Shortness of breath

Delirium may be controlled by finding and treating the cause. Depending on the cause of the delirium, treatment may include the following:

- Giving drugs to fix the level of certain chemicals in the blood
- Stopping or lowering the dose of the drugs that are causing delirium
- Stopping drugs that may cause drug interactions but are no longer useful at the end of life, such as drugs to lower cholesterol
- Treating dehydration by putting fluids into the bloodstream

For some patients in the last hours of life, the decision may be to treat only the symptoms of delirium and make the patient as comfortable as possible. There are drugs that work very well to relieve these symptoms.

Hallucinations that are not related to delirium often occur at the end of life. It is common for dying patients to have hallucinations that include loved ones who have already died. It is normal for family members to feel distress when these hallucinations occur. Speaking with clergy, the hospital chaplain, or other religious advisors is often helpful.

Fever

Fever and infections are common at the end-of-life. Because patients often have many medical problems at the end of life, it can be hard to know the cause of a fever and if treatment will help the patient. Patients near the end of life may choose not to treat the cause of the fever but only to receive comfort measures, such as acetaminophen.

Hemorrhage

Sudden hemorrhage (heavy bleeding) may occur in patients who have certain cancers or disorders.

Hemorrhage (a lot of bleeding in a short time) is rare but may occur in the last hours or minutes of life. Blood vessels may be damaged by certain cancers or cancer treatments. Radiation therapy, for example, can weaken blood vessels in the area that was treated. Tumors can also damage blood vessels. Patients with the following conditions are at risk for this symptom:

- Head and neck cancers
- Stomach cancer
- Esophageal cancer
- Leukemias and other blood cancers
- Blood clotting disorders

The patient should talk with the doctor about any concerns he or she has about the chance of hemorrhage. Making the patient comfortable is the main goal of care during hemorrhage at the end of life.

When hemorrhage occurs during cancer care, it is treated with bandages and medicines or with treatments such as radiation therapy, surgery, and blood transfusions. When sudden bleeding occurs at the end of life, however, patients usually die soon afterwards. Resuscitation (restarting the heart) usually will not work. The main goal of care is to help the patient be calm and comfortable and to support family members. If hemorrhage occurs, it can be very upsetting for family members. It is helpful if the family talks about the feelings this causes and asks questions about it.

The following steps can be taken when bleeding occurs in the last hours of life:

- Cover the area with dark-colored towels so the blood is not seen
- Change towels and keep the area clean
- Speak calmly to the patient and to family members
- Let the patient know if loved ones are there

Fast-acting drugs may help calm the patient during this time.

Ethical Issues

Choices about care and treatment at the end of life should be made while the patient is able to make them.

In addition to decisions about treating symptoms at the end-of-life, it is also helpful for patients to decide if and when they want this treatment to stop. A patient may wish to receive all possible treatments, only some treatments, or no treatment at all. These decisions may be written down ahead of time in an advance directive, such as a living will. Advance directive is the general term for different types of legal documents that describe the treatment or care a patient wishes to receive or not receive when he or she is no longer able to speak their wishes.

The patient may also name a healthcare proxy to make these decisions when he or she becomes unable to do so. Having advance directives in place makes it easier for family members and caregivers when very important decisions have to be made in the last days, such as whether to give nutrition support, restart the heart, help with breathing, or give sedatives.

When the patient does not make choices about end-of-life care, or does not share his choices with family members, health care proxies, or the health care team, treatment may be given near death against the patient's wishes. As a result, studies show that the patient's quality of life may be worse and the family's grieving process may be more difficult.

Studies have shown that cancer patients who have end-of-life discussions with their doctors choose to have fewer procedures, such as resuscitation or the use of a ventilator. They are also less likely to be in intensive care, and the cost of their health care is lower during their final week of life. Reports from their caregivers show that these patients live as long as patients who choose to have more procedures and that they have a better quality of life in their last days.

Nutrition Support

Nutrition support can improve health and boost healing during cancer treatment. The goals of nutrition therapy for patients during the last hours of life are different from the goals for patients in active cancer treatment and recovery. In the final days of life, patients often lose the desire to eat or drink and may refuse food or fluids that are offered to them. Also, procedures used to put feeding tubes in place and problems that can occur with these types of feedings may be hard on a patient.

Making plans for nutrition support in the last days is helpful.

The goal of end-of-life care is to prevent suffering and relieve symptoms. If nutrition support causes the patient more discomfort than help, then nutrition support near the end of life may be stopped. The needs and best interests of each patient guide the decision to give nutrition support. When decisions and plans about nutrition support are made by the patient, doctors and family members can be sure they are doing what the patient wants.

If the patient cannot swallow, two types of nutrition support are commonly used:

- Enteral nutrition uses a tube inserted into the stomach or intestine.

- Parenteral nutrition uses an intravenous (IV) catheter inserted into a vein.

Each type of nutrition support has benefits and risks.

Resuscitation

An important decision for the patient to make is whether to have cardiopulmonary resuscitation (CPR) (trying to restart the heart and breathing when it stops). It is best if patients talk with their family, doctors, and caregivers about their wishes for CPR as early as possible (for example, when being admitted to the hospital or when active cancer treatment is stopped). A do-not-resuscitate (DNR) order is written by a doctor to tell other health professionals not to perform CPR at the moment of death, so that the natural process of dying occurs. If the patient wishes, he or she can ask the doctor to write a DNR order. The patient can ask that the DNR order be changed or removed at any time.

Ventilator Use

Ventilator use may keep the patient alive after normal breathing stops. A ventilator is a machine that helps patients breathe. Sometimes, using a ventilator will not improve the patient's condition, but will keep the patient alive longer. If the goal of care is to help the patient live longer, a ventilator may be used, according to the patient's wishes. If ventilator support stops helping the patient or is no longer what the patient wants, the patient, family, and health care team may decide to turn the ventilator off.

Some patients may want to be allowed to die when breathing gets difficult or stops. It is important for the patient to tell family members and health care providers, before breathing becomes difficult, of his or her wishes about being kept alive with a ventilator.

Before a ventilator is turned off, family members will be given information about what to expect.

Family members will be given information about how the patient may respond when the ventilator is removed and about pain relief or sedation to keep the patient comfortable. Family members will be given time to contact other loved ones who wish to be there. Chaplains or social workers may be called to give help and support to the family.

Sedation

The decision whether to sedate a patient at the end of life is a difficult one. Sedation may be considered for a patient's comfort or for a physical condition such as uncontrolled pain. Palliative sedation may be temporary. A patient's thoughts and feelings about end-of-life sedation may depend greatly on his or her own culture and beliefs. Some patients who become anxious facing the end of life may want to be sedated. Other patients may wish to have no procedures, including sedation, just before death.

It is important for the patient to tell family members and health care providers of his or her wishes about sedation at the end of life. When patients make their wishes about sedation known ahead of time, doctors and family members can be sure they are doing what the patient would want. Families may need support from the health care team and mental health professionals while palliative sedation is used.

Care in the Final Hours

Knowing what to expect in the final days or hours may be comforting to the family.

Most people are not familiar with the signs that death is near. Knowing what to expect can prepare them for the death of their loved one and make this time less stressful and confusing. Health care providers can give family members information about the changes they may see in their loved one in the final hours and how they may help their loved one through it.

In the final days to hours of life, patients often lose the desire to eat or drink, and may refuse food and fluids that are offered to them. The family may give ice chips or swab the mouth and lips to keep them moist. Forcing food and fluids can make the patient uncomfortable or cause choking. Family members may find other ways to show their love for the patient, such as massage.

Patients near death may not respond to others. Patients may withdraw and spend more time sleeping. They may answer questions slowly or not at all, seem confused, and show little interest in their surroundings. Most patients are still able to hear after they are no longer able to speak. It may give some comfort if family members continue to touch and talk to the patient, even if the patient does not respond.

A number of physical changes are common when the patient is near death. Some of the following physical changes may occur in the patient at the end of life:

- The patient may feel tired or weak.
- The patient may pass less urine and it may be dark in color.
- The patient's hands and feet may become blotchy, cold, or blue. Caregivers can use blankets to keep the patient warm. Electric blankets or heating pads should not be used.
- The heart rate may go up or down and become irregular.
- Blood pressure usually goes down.
- Breathing may become irregular, with very shallow breathing, short periods of not breathing, or deep, rapid breathing.

Patients and their families may have cultural or religious beliefs and customs that are important at the time of death. After the patient dies, family members and caregivers may wish to stay with the patient a while. There may be certain customs or rituals that are important to the patient and family at this time. These might include rituals for coping with death, handling the patient's body, making final arrangements for the body, and honoring the death. The patient and family members should let the health care team know about any customs or rituals they want performed after the patient's death.

Health care providers, hospice staff, social workers, or spiritual leaders can explain the steps that need to be taken once death has occurred, including contacting a funeral home.

Grief and Loss

Grief is a normal reaction to the loss of a loved one. People who feel unable to cope with their loss may be helped by grief counseling or grief therapy with trained professionals.

Part Five

Cancer Research

Chapter 69

How to Find a Cancer Treatment Trial

Introduction

This chapter will help you to look for a cancer treatment clinical trial that might benefit you. It is not intended to provide medical advice. You, your health care team, and your loved ones are in the best position to decide whether a clinical trial is right for you.

This chapter will help you to with these steps:

- Gathering the information you need to begin your search for a clinical trial

- Identifying sources of clinical trial listings

- Learning about clinical trials that may be of benefit to you

- Asking questions that will help you decide whether or not to participate in a particular trial

A Word about Timing

Many treatment trials will only take patients who have not yet been treated for their condition. Researchers conducting these trials are hoping to find an improved "first-line" treatment option for that type of cancer.

From "How to Find a Cancer Treatment Trial: A 10-Step Guide," National Cancer Institute (www.cancer.gov), May 8, 2009.

If you are newly diagnosed with cancer, the time to consider joining a clinical trial is before you've had surgery, chemotherapy, radiation, or other forms of treatment (tests to diagnose your cancer are okay). However, don't delay treatment if waiting could harm you. Talk with your doctor about how quickly you need to make a treatment decision.

If you have received one or more forms of treatment and are looking for a new treatment option, there also are many clinical trial options for you. You may want to look for trials that are testing a new follow-up treatment that may prevent the return of your cancer. Or, if your first treatment failed to work, you may want to look for trials of new "second-line" or even "third-line" treatments.

Before You Start: Steps 1–3

This section will help you to have a better understanding of clinical trials and gather information you will need in order to locate clinical trials that are appropriate for you.

Before You Start: Step 1

Understand clinical trials: This chapter assumes you already know what clinical trials are and why you might want to join one. If you need to, review your understanding of clinical trials before you continue the steps in this chapter.

Before You Start: Step 2

Talk with your doctor: When considering clinical trials, your best starting point is your doctor and other members of your health care team.

Your primary care physician, cancer doctor (oncologist), surgeon, or other health care provider might know about a clinical trial you should consider. He or she can help you determine whether a clinical trial might be a good option.

In some cases, your doctor may be reluctant to discuss clinical trials as a treatment option for you. Some doctors are unfamiliar with clinical trials, cautious about turning your care over to another medical team, or wary of the extra time that joining a clinical trial might require of them and their staff. If so, you may wish to get a second opinion about your treatment options and clinical trials.

Remember, you do not always need a referral from your doctor to join a clinical trial. If you are eligible to join a trial (discussed in Step

3), the final decision is up to you. However, be sure to consider the professional opinions of your doctor. He or she may present very specific reasons why a clinical trial may not be beneficial for you right now.

Before You Start: Step 3

Complete the Details Checklist: Before you begin looking for a clinical trial, you must know certain details about your cancer diagnosis. You will need to compare these details with the eligibility criteria of any trial in which you are interested. Eligibility criteria are the guidelines for who can and cannot participate in a particular study.

To help you gather the details of your diagnosis so you will know which trials you may be eligible to join, complete the Details Checklist show in Figure 69.1. It asks questions about your diagnosis and provides room to write down your answers. Keep this form with you during your search for a clinical trial. If you would like to print this form from your own computer or need additional copies, visit www.cancer.gov/clinicaltrials/finding/treatment-trial-guide and click on the link given near the end of the document.

To get the information you need for the form ask a nurse or social worker at your doctor's office for help. Explain to them that you are interested in looking for a clinical trial that may benefit you and that you need these details before starting to look. They will be able to review your medical records and help you fill out the form.

Searching for a Trial: Steps 4–6

You have learned what clinical trials are and how they work, talked with your doctor about your interest in clinical trials, and prepared a checklist of key details about your diagnosis. You are now ready to search for clinical trials.

This section will help you to find and search trustworthy lists of ongoing clinical trials, compare your Details Checklist with a trial's eligibility criteria, as provided in the trial's description (also called a protocol summary), and identify those trials that might be good options for you.

Searching for a Trial: Step 4

It is important to understand the possible biases and limitations of any clinical trials website. If you would like to learn more about this topic, you can look for the National Cancer Institute's fact sheet,

Cancer Details Checklist

Fill out this Cancer Details Checklist as completely as possible before you start looking for a clinical trial. It will help you know which clinical trials you may be eligible to join.

See Step 3 for information about how to obtain the details you need for the checklist.

1. What kind of cancer do you have?
Write down the full medical name.

2. Where did the cancer first start?
Many cancers spread to the bones, liver, or elsewhere. However, the type of cancer you have is determined by where it started. For example, breast cancer that spreads to the bone is still breast cancer.

3. What is the cancer's cell type?
This information will be in your pathology report.

4. If you have a solid tumor, what size is it?

5. If you have a solid tumor, where is it located?
If the tumor has spread, list all locations.

6. What is the stage of your cancer?
The stage describes the extent of cancer in the body and whether it has spread from the site where it started. There are different staging systems for different cancers.

7. Have you had cancer before that is different from the one you have now? If so, answer questions 1-6 for the other cancer, as well.

Figure 69.1. Cancer Details Checklist, continued on next page. (Source: National Cancer Institute; if you need additional copies of this form, visit www.cancer.gov/clinicaltrials/finding/treatment-trial-guide and click on the link given at the end of the document.)

_____
_____
_____
_____

8. What is your current performance status score?
This is an assessment by your doctor of how well you are able to perform ordinary tasks and carry out daily activities. Several different scoring methods can be used to describe performance status.

_____
_____
_____
_____
_____

9. Have you been treated for your current cancer? If not, what treatment(s) have been recommended to you?

_____
_____
_____
_____
_____
_____

10. If you have been treated for your current cancer, please list the treatments you have received (for example: type of surgery, chemotherapy, immunotherapy, or radiation therapy).

_____
_____
_____
_____

11. What are your bone marrow function test results? These blood tests show whether your blood cell count is normal.

a) White blood cell count:

_____
_____
_____

b) Platelet count:

_____
_____
_____

c) Hemoglobin/hematocrit:

_____
_____
_____

12. What are your renal function test results?

a) Bilirubin:

_____
_____
_____

b) Transaminases:

_____
_____
_____

13. What are your renal function test results? This blood test checks whether your kidneys are functioning normally.

a) Serum creatinine

_____
_____
_____

"How to Evaluate Health Information on the Internet: Questions And Answers," available through the NCI website (www.cancer.gov).

Search the PDQ® Clinical Trials Database: There are many nonprofit and for-profit resources in the United States that offer lists of cancer clinical trials. Unfortunately, no single list is complete. Clinical trials are run by many different organizations, so it is hard to collect information about all of them in one place.

However, the majority of trials listed in most resources are obtained from the Physician Data Query (PDQ) clinical trials database, which is maintained by the U.S. National Cancer Institute (NCI).

The NCI is the U.S. government's chief agency for cancer research and is part of the National Institutes of Health. The PDQ clinical trials database contains a list of more than 2,000 cancer clinical trials worldwide.

The U.S. National Library of Medicine maintains a database called ClinicalTrials.gov that includes trials for many diseases and conditions, including cancer. The PDQ and ClinicalTrials.gov databases contain the same cancer treatment trial listings. The main difference is in how information is searched and displayed. You may prefer one way over another.

Important: Get a copy of the protocol summary: Steps 4 and 5 describe where to look for cancer clinical trials. Whichever resource you use, be sure to get a copy of the protocol summary for each trial you are interested in

What is a protocol? It is the action plan for the trial. The protocol explains what will be done in the trial, how, and why. The protocol should also list the location(s) where the trial will enroll participants.

Both PDQ and ClinicalTrials.gov (Step 4) provide detailed summaries of the official protocols for each trial listed on their websites. Other resources (Step 5) may or may not provide protocol summaries.

How to search PDQ: You can search PDQ by telephone. Make a free telephone call—in English or Spanish—within the United States to the National Cancer Institute's Cancer Information Service (CIS) at 800-4-CANCER (800-422-6237). All calls to the CIS are strictly confidential.

When you call the CIS, be ready with the details of your Details Checklist from Step 3.

The CIS is staffed with understanding and knowledgeable information specialists who will search PDQ for you. They can send you the search results and protocol summaries by e-mail, fax, or regular mail. The CIS can also provide you with reliable information about your type of cancer and the current standard therapy for treating it.

You can also search PDQ through the NCI website. You can look for trials yourself using the PDQ search form on the NCI website (www .cancer.gov/clinicaltrials). Remember to print out the protocol summaries for each trial you may be interested in.

If you would like help searching PDQ while you're online, consider using LiveHelp. Through LiveHelp, you can communicate confidentially and in real time with a CIS information specialist from the National Cancer Institute. The service is available Monday through Friday from 9:00 a.m. to 11:00 p.m. Eastern time.

Searching for a Trial: Step 5

Search other resources: While PDQ and ClinicalTrials.gov have the most complete listing of cancer trials, you might want to check a few other resources, as well. Why? Because some may include a few trials not found in the federal databases or you may prefer their way of assisting you in your search.

TrialCheck®: TrialCheck is operated and maintained by the Coalition of Cancer Cooperative Groups (CCCG). The CCCG is made up of groups of doctors and other health professionals that carry out many of the large cancer clinical trials in the United States funded by the National Cancer Institute.

TrialCheck maintains comprehensive data on thousands of cancer clinical trials and contains a copyrighted cancer clinical trials screening questionnaire that will identify trials appropriate for a patient's individual medical condition.

To search TrialCheck, visit http://www.cancertrialshelp.org/ trialcheck.

Third-party clinical trial websites: There are a number of clinical trial websites that are not operated by funders, sponsors, or the organizations carrying out the trials. Some of these websites are operated by private companies—these may be funded through fees that industry sponsors pay to have their trials listed or according to how many participants the website refers to them. Keep the following points in mind:

- Most third-party clinical trials websites list or link to trials in PDQ or ClinicalTrials.gov.

- They may include a few more trials than you'll find in the federal databases, but they may also include fewer.

- Unlike the federal databases, these sites may not regularly update their content or links.

- Unlike the federal databases, these sites might require you to register to search for trials or to obtain contact information about the trials that interest you.

Industry-sponsored cancer trials: Pharmaceutical and biotechnology companies sponsor many of the cancer clinical trials being carried out in the United States. Some of these trials are listed in the federal databases (PDQ and ClinicalTrials.gov), but many are not.

Federal law requires that U.S. researchers submit to ClinicalTrials .gov all phase II, III, and IV trials of therapies for serious or life-threatening illnesses (including cancer) conducted as part of the approval process overseen by the U.S. Food and Drug Administration. However, this law is difficult to enforce and for business reasons, some drug companies have preferred to keep details about their clinical trials from the public.

If you are aware of an experimental cancer treatment and know the company that manufactures it, search the internet to find the website of the company. Find the company's customer service telephone number. When you call, ask to speak to the company's clinical trials department. Tell them you are looking for a trial that you might be eligible to join.

Cancer advocacy groups: Cancer advocacy groups work on behalf of people diagnosed with cancer and their loved ones. They provide education, support, financial assistance, and advocacy to help patients and families who are dealing with cancer. These organizations recognize that clinical trials are important to the cancer treatment process and, thus, work to educate and empower people to find information and access to treatment.

Because they work hard to know about the latest research advances in cancer treatment, these groups will sometimes have information about certain key government-sponsored trials, as well as some potentially significant trials sponsored by pharmaceutical companies or cancer care centers.

Contact the advocacy group for the type of cancer you are interested in and ask what they can tell you about ongoing clinical trials. The nonprofit Marti Nelson Cancer Foundation maintains a partial list of such groups on its CancerActionNow.org website.

Fee-based private search services: A number of private services will, for a fee, locate clinical trials for you. While having someone search for you may ease your stress, it is important to keep in mind that several of the resources mentioned earlier provide elements of this kind of service for free. Also, be sure to ask the following questions:

- What list or lists of clinical trials does the service search? Are those lists likely to provide you with an unbiased and largely complete source of options?

- Does the service receive any money for directing patients to certain trials or for including certain trials in their list?

Searching for a Trial: Step 6

Make a list of potential trials: At this point you have created a Details Checklist, identified one or more trials you might be interested in, and obtained a protocol summary for each one. This section will help you take a closer look at the protocol summaries and narrow your list to those trials you would like to get more information about.

Take a closer look: Now it's time to take a closer look at the protocol summaries you have obtained for the trials you're interested in. You should remove from your list those trials you aren't actually able to join and come up with one or more top possibilities.

What follows are some key questions to consider about each trial. However, don't worry if you cannot answer all of these questions just yet. The idea is to narrow the list if you can, but don't give up on one that you're not sure of.

Ideally, you should consult your doctor during this process, especially if you find the protocol summaries difficult to understand. But you can probably do Step 6 yourself if the protocol summary is relatively complete and easy to understand.

- **Trial objective:** What is the main purpose of the trial? Is it to improve your chances of a cure? To slow the rate at which your cancer may grow or return? To lessen the severity of treatment side effects? To establish whether a new treatment is safe and well tolerated? Read this information carefully to learn whether the trial's main objective matches your goals for treatment.

- **Eligibility criteria:** Do your diagnosis and current overall state of health match the eligibility criteria (sometimes referred to as enrollment or entry criteria)? This may tell you whether you could qualify for the trial. If you're not sure, keep the trial on your list for now.

- **Trial location:** Is the location of the clinical trial manageable for you? Some trials are available at more than one site. Look carefully at how often you will need to receive treatment during the course of the trial, and decide how far and how often you are willing to travel. You will also need to ask if the sponsoring organization will provide for some or all of your travel expenses.

- **Study duration:** How long will the study run? Not all protocol summaries list this information. If they do, consider the time commitment and whether it will work for you and your family.

If, after considering these questions, you are still interested in one or more of the clinical trials you have found, then you are ready for Step 7.

After Finding a Trial: Steps 7–10

Now that you have found one or more clinical trials for which you think you are eligible and that may be a good treatment option for you, it is time to make a telephone call to each trial's contact person so you can ask a few more crucial questions. Then, you will be ready to make a final treatment decision.

After Finding a Trial: Step 7

Contact the Clinical Trial Team: There are several ways to contact the Clinical Trial Team. You may want to contact the trial team directly. The protocol summary should include the name and telephone number of someone you can contact for more information. You do not need to talk to the lead researcher (called the "protocol chair" or "principal investigator") at this time, even if that is the name that is included with the telephone number. Instead, call the number and ask to speak with the "trial coordinator," the "referral coordinator," or the "protocol assistant." This person can answer questions from potential patients and their doctors. It is also this person's job to determine whether you are likely to be eligible to join the trial. (A final determination would be made only after you had gone in for a first appointment.)

You may prefer to ask your doctor or other health care team member to contact the trial team for you. Because the clinical trial coordinator will ask questions related to your diagnosis, you may want to ask your doctor or someone else on your health care team to contact the clinical trial team for you.

The trial team may contact you. If you have used some a third-party website and identified a trial that interests you, you may have provided your name, phone number, and e-mail address so that the clinical trial team can contact you.

You will need to refer to your Details Checklist (Step 3) during the conversation, so keep that handy.

After Finding a Trial: Step 8

Ask questions about the trial: Whether you or someone from your health care team calls the clinical trial coordinator, this is the time to get answers to questions that will help you decide whether or not to join this particular clinical trial.

It will be helpful if you can talk about your diagnosis in a manner that is brief and to the point. Before you make the call, rehearse with a family member or friend how you will present the key details of your diagnosis (Details Checklist). This will make you more comfortable when you are talking with the clinical trial coordinator and will enable you to answer his or her questions smoothly.

Questions to Ask the Trial Coordinator

1. Is the trial still open? On occasion, clinical trial listings will be out-of-date and will include trials that have actually closed to further enrollment.

2. Am I eligible for this trial? The trial coordinator will ask you many, if not all, of the questions listed on your Details Checklist (Step 3). This is the time to confirm that you are indeed a candidate for this trial, although a final decision will likely await your first appointment with the clinical trial team (Step 10).

3. Why do researchers think the new treatment might be effective? Results from earlier clinical trials will highlight the potential effectiveness of the treatment you may receive. The strength of the earlier evidence may influence your decision. You or someone who knows how to read the medical literature may also want to use a web-based service such as PubMed to explore any previously published evidence related to the trial you're interested in (PubMed is available online at http://www.ncbi.nlm.nih.gov/pubmed).

4. What are the risks and benefits associated with the treatments I may receive? Every treatment has risks. Be sure you understand what risks and side-effects are associated with any of the treatments you might receive as a participant in this trial. Likewise, ask for a detailed description of how the treatments may benefit you.

5. Who will monitor my care and safety? Primary responsibility for the care and safety of patients in a cancer clinical trial rests with the clinical trial health care team. In addition,

clinical trials are governed by safety and ethical regulations set by the federal government and the institution or organization sponsoring and carrying out the trial, including a group called the Institutional Review Board (IRB). The trial coordinator will be able to give you more information.

6. May I get a copy of the protocol document? In some cases, the trial coordinator may be allowed to release the full, detailed protocol document to you. However, the protocol summary and the informed consent document will probably answer most of your questions about the trial's design and intention.

7. May I get a copy of the informed consent document? The U.S. Food and Drug Administration requires that potential participants receive complete information about the study. This process is known as "informed consent" and must be in writing. It may be helpful to see a copy of this document before you decide whether or not to join the trial.

8. Is there a chance I will receive a placebo? Placebos are rarely used in cancer treatment trials, but be sure you understand what possible treatments you may or may not receive for any trial you are thinking of joining.

9. Is the trial randomized? In a randomized clinical trial, participants are assigned, by chance, to separate groups or "arms." Each arm receives a different treatment, and the results are compared. In a randomized trial, you may or may not receive the new treatment.

10. What is the treatment dose and schedule in each arm of the trial? You will want to consider this when you are discussing your various treatment options with your health care team. Does the dose seem reasonable? Is the treatment schedule manageable for you?

11. What costs will I be responsible for? In many cases, the research costs are paid by the group sponsoring the trial. Research costs include the treatments under study and any test performed purely for research purposes. However, you or your insurance plan would be responsible for paying "routine patient care costs." These are the costs of medical care (e.g., doctor visits, hospital stays, x-rays) that you would receive whether or not you were in a clinical trial. Some insurance plans don't cover these costs once you join a trial. Consult your health plan, if you have one.

12. If I have to travel, who will pay for travel and lodging? Some trials may pay for your travel and lodging expenses. Otherwise, you will be responsible for these costs.

13. Will participation in this trial require more time than if I had elected to receive standard care? Will participation require a hospital stay? Understanding how much time is involved may influence your decision and help you make plans.

14. How will participating in the clinical trial affect my everyday life? A cancer diagnosis can be very disrupting to the routine of everyday life. Many patients seek to keep those routines intact as they deal with their diagnosis and treatment. This information will be useful in evaluating any additional help you may need at home.

After Finding a Trial: Step 9

Discuss your options with your doctor: To make a final decision, you will want to know the possible risks and benefits of all the various treatment options open to you. You may decide that joining a trial for which you are eligible is your best option, or you may decide not to join a trial. It is your choice.

After Finding a Trial: Step 10

If you want to join a trial, schedule an appointment: If you decide to participate in a clinical trial for which you are eligible, schedule an appointment with the trial coordinator you spoke to during Step 8.

You might also want your doctor to contact the study's principal investigator to further discuss your medical history and overall current state of your health.

The principal investigator's name should be listed in the protocol summary.

Your doctor might disagree with your decision to participate in a clinical trial. If so, be sure you understand his or her concerns. You also may wish to seek a second opinion about your treatment options at this time. Ultimately, it is up to you to decide what treatment is in your best interest.

Chapter 70

Access to Investigational Drugs

What is an investigational drug?

An investigational drug is one that is under study but does not have permission from the U.S. Food and Drug Administration (FDA) to be legally marketed and sold in the United States.

FDA approval is the final step in the process of drug development. The first step is for the new drug to be tested in the laboratory. If the results are promising, the drug company or sponsor must apply for FDA approval to test the drug in people. This is called an Investigational New Drug (IND) Application. Once the IND is approved, clinical trials can begin. Clinical trials are research studies to determine the safety and measure the effectiveness of the drug in people. Once clinical trials are completed, the sponsor submits the study results in a New Drug Application (NDA) or Biologics License Application (BLA) to the FDA. This application is carefully reviewed and, if the drug is found to be reasonably safe and effective, it is approved.

How do patients get investigational drugs?

By far, the most common way that patients get investigational drugs is by taking part in a clinical trial sponsored under an IND. A patient's doctor may suggest a clinical trial as one treatment option. Or a patient or family member can ask the doctor about clinical trials or new drugs available for cancer treatment.

From "Access to Investigational Drugs," National Cancer Institute (www .cancer.gov), August 8, 2009.

Another way patients and their families can learn about new drugs being tested in clinical trials is through the National Cancer Institute's (NCI) PDQ® database. This database contains information on a large number of ongoing studies. Individuals can search this database at http://www.cancer.gov/clinicaltrials, or they can call the NCI's Cancer Information Service at 800-4-CANCER (800-422-6237). Information specialists can search the database and provide a list of trials for individuals to discuss with their doctor.

Are there other ways to get investigational drugs?

Less common ways that patients can receive investigational drugs include mechanisms such as an expanded access protocol or a special or compassionate exception. The sponsor must agree to provide the drug for this use.

Investigational drugs given under these mechanisms must meet the following criteria:

- There must be substantial clinical evidence that the drug may benefit persons with particular types of cancer.

- The drug must be able to be given safely outside a clinical trial.

- The drug must be in sufficient supply for ongoing and planned clinical trials.

Expanded access: The purpose of an expanded access protocol is to make investigational drugs that have significant activity against specific cancers available to patients before the FDA approval process has been completed. Expanded access protocols allow a larger group of people to be treated with the drug.

The sponsor must apply to the FDA to make the drug available through an expanded access protocol. There must be enough evidence from studies already completed to show that the drug is likely to be effective against a specific type of cancer and that it does not have unreasonable risks. The FDA generally approves expanded access only if there are no other satisfactory treatments available for the disease.

The NCI's Treatment Referral Center (TRC) protocols are one type of expanded access protocol. The NCI establishes a TRC protocol when clinical evidence suggests that an investigational drug should be made more widely available to patients, even though the FDA approval process has not been completed. The TRC protocol is made available at NCI-designated cancer centers and other institutions selected to provide wide geographic availability of the drug to patients.

Special exception/compassionate exemption: Patients who do not meet the eligibility criteria for a clinical trial of an investigational drug may be eligible to receive the drug under a mechanism known as a special exception or a compassionate exemption to the policy of administering investigational drugs only in a clinical trial. The patient's doctor contacts the sponsor of the investigational agent and provides the patient's medical information and treatment history. The sponsor (the drug company or NCI) evaluates the requests on a case-by-case basis. There should be reasonable expectation that the drug will prolong survival or improve quality of life.

In some cases, even patients who qualify for treatment with an investigational drug on a compassionate basis might not be able to obtain the drug if the supply is limited and the demand is high.

Are all investigational drugs available through an expanded access or special exception mechanism?

No. The sponsor decides whether to provide an investigational drug outside a clinical trial. Availability may be limited in part by drug supply, patient demand, or other factors.

What is the NCI's role in providing access to investigational drugs?

The NCI acts as the sponsor for many, but not all, investigational drugs. When acting as sponsor, the NCI provides the investigational drug to the physicians who are participating in clinical trials or TRC protocols. A physician who wishes to treat a patient with the investigational drug as a special exception must request the drug from the NCI. These requests are reviewed on a case-by-case basis.

Who can provide access to investigational drugs being developed by pharmaceutical companies?

In the case of investigational drugs sponsored by a drug company, the drug company in collaboration with the FDA provides access to the drug. The process is similar to that described above.

The patient's physician must submit a request to the drug company and to the FDA. The drug company can provide the name of the appropriate reviewing division at the FDA. (FDA reviewing divisions are prohibited from divulging proprietary information such as whether a sponsor has filed an IND or the status of an IND.)

Are there specific criteria used to determine whether patients can receive an investigational drug outside a clinical trial?

To be considered for treatment with an investigational drug outside a clinical trial, generally patients must meet the following criteria:

- Have undergone standard treatment that has not been successful
- Be ineligible for any ongoing clinical trials of this drug
- Have no acceptable treatment alternatives
- Have a cancer diagnosis for which the investigational drug has demonstrated activity
- Be likely to experience benefits that outweigh the risks involved

What should patients do if they are interested in receiving an investigational drug through a special exception or expanded access mechanism?

Patients interested in gaining access to investigational drugs should talk to their physician about available options. Physicians can make requests for special exceptions by contacting the study sponsor. Physicians will be required to follow strict guidelines, including gaining approval from their Institutional Review Board and obtaining informed consent from the patient. Informed consent is a process that includes a document to be signed by the patient which outlines the known risks and benefits of the treatment, as well as the rights and responsibilities of the patient.

What are the costs involved in receiving an investigational drug?

In general, the drug is provided free of charge. However, there may be other costs associated with the treatment. Before beginning treatment, patients should check with their insurer about coverage of these costs.

What are some of the potential drawbacks to receiving an investigational drug?

It is not known whether an investigational drug is better than standard therapy for treating a disease, and a patient may not receive any benefit. Side effects (both long-term and short-term) from the drug may not be fully understood, especially if the drug is in early phases of testing. Finally, a patient's health insurance company may not pay expenses associated with receiving the investigational drug.

How can patients find out more information about a specific investigational drug?

Patients can find out more about a specific drug by contacting the drug company that is developing the drug. Information may also be available from the NCI's Cancer Information Service at 800-4-CANCER (800-422-6237).

Chapter 71

Cancer Vaccines

What are vaccines?

Vaccines are medicines that boost the immune system's natural ability to protect the body against "foreign invaders" that may cause disease. These invaders are primarily microbes, which can be seen only under a microscope. Microbes include bacteria, viruses, parasites, and fungi.

The immune system is a complex network of organs, tissues, and specialized cells that act collectively to defend the body. When a particular type of microbe invades the body, the immune system recognizes it as foreign, destroys it, and "remembers" it to prevent another infection. Vaccines take advantage of this response.

Traditional vaccines usually contain harmless versions of microbes—killed or weakened microbes, or parts of microbes—that do not cause disease but are able to stimulate an immune response. When the immune system encounters these substances through vaccination, it responds to them, eliminates them from the body, and develops a memory of them. This vaccine-induced memory enables the immune system to act quickly to protect the body if it becomes infected by the same microbe in the future.

The immune system's role in defending against disease-causing microbes has long been recognized. Scientists have also discovered that the

Excerpted from "Cancer Vaccines," National Cancer Institute, March 17, 2009. The complete text of this document, including references, is available online at http://www.cancer.gov/cancertopics/factsheet/Therapy/cancer-vaccines.

immune system can protect the body against threats posed by certain types of damaged, diseased, or abnormal cells, including cancer cells.

How do vaccines stimulate the immune system?

White blood cells, or leukocytes, play the main role in immune responses. These cells carry out the many tasks required to protect the body against disease-causing microbes and abnormal cells.

Some types of leukocytes patrol the body, seeking foreign invaders and diseased, damaged, or dead cells. These white blood cells provide a general—or nonspecific—level of immune protection.

Other types of leukocytes, known as lymphocytes, provide targeted protection against specific threats, whether from a specific microbe or a diseased or abnormal cell. The most important groups of lymphocytes responsible for carrying out immune responses against such threats are B cells and cytotoxic (cell-killing) T cells.

B cells make antibodies, which are large proteins secreted by B cells that bind to, inactivate, and help destroy foreign invaders or abnormal cells. Most preventive vaccines, including those aimed at hepatitis B virus (HBV) and human papillomavirus (HPV), stimulate the production of antibodies that bind to specific, targeted microbes and block their ability to cause infection. Cytotoxic T cells, which are also known as killer T cells, kill infected or abnormal cells by releasing toxic chemicals or by prompting the cells to self-destruct (apoptosis).

Other types of lymphocytes and leukocytes play supporting roles to ensure that B cells and killer T cells do their jobs effectively. Cells that help fine-tune the activities of B cells and killer T cells include helper T cells and dendritic cells, which help activate killer T cells and enable them to recognize specific threats.

Cancer treatment vaccines work by activating B cells and killer T cells and directing them to recognize and act against specific types of cancer. They do this by introducing one or more molecules known as antigens into the body, usually by injection. An antigen is a substance that stimulates a specific immune response. An antigen can be a protein or another type of molecule found on the surface of or inside a cell.

Microbes carry antigens that "tell" the immune system they are foreign—or "non-self"—and, therefore, represent a potential threat that should be destroyed. In contrast, normal cells in the body have antigens that identify them as "self." Self-antigens tell the immune system that normal cells are not a threat and should be ignored.

Cancer cells can carry both types of antigens. They have self-antigens, which they share in common with normal cells, but they may also have antigens that are unique to cancer cells. These cancer-associated antigens mark cancer cells as abnormal, or non-self, and can cause B cells and killer T cells to mount an attack against the cancer.

Cancer cells may also make much larger than normal amounts of certain self-antigens. These overly abundant self-antigens may be viewed by the immune system as being foreign and, therefore, may trigger an immune response against the cancer.

What are cancer vaccines?

Cancer vaccines are medicines that belong to a class of substances known as biological response modifiers. Biological response modifiers work by stimulating or restoring the immune system's ability to fight infections and disease. There are two broad types of cancer vaccines:

- Preventive (or prophylactic) vaccines, which are intended to prevent cancer from developing in healthy people; and

- Treatment (or therapeutic) vaccines, which are intended to treat already existing cancers by strengthening the body's natural defenses against cancer.

Two types of cancer preventive vaccines have been successfully developed and are available in the United States. However, cancer treatment vaccines remain an experimental form of therapy.

How do cancer preventive vaccines work?

Cancer preventive vaccines target infectious agents that cause or contribute to the development of cancer. They are similar to traditional vaccines, which help prevent infectious diseases such as measles or polio by protecting the body against infection. Both cancer preventive vaccines and traditional vaccines are based on antigens that are carried by the infectious agents and that are relatively easy for the immune system to recognize as foreign.

Have any cancer preventive vaccines been approved for use in the United States?

In 2006, the U.S. Food and Drug Administration (FDA) approved the vaccine known as Gardasil®, which protects against infection by two types of HPV—specifically, types 16 and 18—that cause approximately 70% of all cases of cervical cancer worldwide. At least 17 other types of HPV are responsible for the remaining 30% of cervical cancer cases. Gardasil also protects against HPV types 6 and 11, which are responsible for about 90% of all cases of genital warts. However, these two HPV types do not cause cervical cancer.

In 2008, the FDA expanded Gardasil's approval to include its use in the prevention of HPV-associated vulvar and vaginal cancers.

Gardasil, manufactured by Merck & Company, is based on HPV antigens that are proteins. These proteins are used in the laboratory to make four different types of "virus-like particles," or VLPs, which correspond to HPV types 6, 11, 16, and 18. The four types of VLPs are then combined to make the vaccine. Because Gardasil targets four HPV types, it is called a quadrivalent vaccine. In contrast with traditional vaccines, which are often composed of weakened, whole microbes, the VLPs in Gardasil are not infectious. However, they are still able to stimulate the production of antibodies against HPV types 6, 11, 16, and 18.

A second HPV vaccine manufactured by GlaxoSmithKline and known by the name Cervarix® has also been developed. In October 2009, Cervarix was approved by the FDA for use in the United States. In contrast with Gardasil, Cervarix is a bivalent vaccine. It is composed of VLPs made with proteins from HPV types 16 and 18. Therefore, it provides protection only against these two HPV types.

The public health benefits of vaccines against HPV types 16 and 18 may extend beyond reducing the risks of cervical cancer, vaginal cancer, and vulvar cancer. Evidence suggests that chronic infection by one or both of these virus types is also associated with cancers of the anus, penis, and oropharynx.

The FDA has approved one other type of cancer preventive vaccine, which protects against HBV infection. Chronic HBV infection can lead to liver cancer. The first HBV vaccine was approved in 1981, making it the first cancer preventive vaccine to be successfully developed and marketed. Today, most children in the United States are vaccinated against HBV shortly after birth.

Have other microbes been associated with cancer?

Many scientists believe that microbes cause or contribute to between 15% and 25% of all cancers diagnosed worldwide each year, with the percentages being lower in developed countries than in developing countries. The International Agency for Research on Cancer (IARC) has classified several microbes as carcinogenic (causing or contributing to the development of cancer in people), including HPV and HBV. These infectious agents—bacteria, viruses, and parasites—and the cancer types with which they are most strongly associated are listed in Table 71.1.

Table 71.1. Microbes Associated with Cancer

Infectious Agents	Type of Organism	Associated Cancer(s)
hepatitis B virus (HBV)	virus	hepatocellular carcinoma (a type of liver cancer)
hepatitis C virus (HCV)	virus	hepatocellular carcinoma (a type of liver cancer)
human papillomavirus (HPV) types 16 and 18, as well as other HPV types	virus	cervical cancer; vaginal cancer; vulvar cancer; oropharyngeal cancer (cancers of the base of the tongue, tonsils, or upper throat); anal cancer; penile cancer
Epstein-Barr virus	virus	Burkitt lymphoma; non-Hodgkin lymphoma; Hodgkin lymphoma; nasopharyngeal carcinoma (cancer of the upper part of the throat behind the nose)
human T-cell lymphotropic virus 1 (HTLV1)	virus	acute T-cell leukemia
Helicobacter pylori	bacterium	stomach cancer
schistosomes (*Schistosoma hematobium*)	parasite	bladder cancer
liver flukes (*Opisthorchis viverrini*)	parasite	cholangiocarcinoma (a type of liver cancer)

How do cancer treatment vaccines work?

Cancer treatment vaccines are designed to treat cancers that have already occurred. They are intended to delay or stop cancer cell growth; cause tumor shrinkage; prevent cancer from coming back; or eliminate cancer cells that are not killed by other forms of treatment, such as surgery, radiation therapy, or chemotherapy.

Developing effective cancer treatment vaccines requires a detailed understanding of how immune system cells and cancer cells interact. The immune system often does not "see" cancer cells as dangerous or foreign, as it generally does with microbes. Therefore, the immune system does not mount a strong attack against the cancer cells.

There are many reasons the immune system does not easily recognize the threat posed by an already growing cancer. Most important is the fact that cancer cells carry normal self-antigens in addition to any cancer-associated antigens. Furthermore, cancer cells sometimes undergo genetic changes that lead to the loss of cancer-associated antigens. Finally, cancer cells can produce chemical messages that suppress specific anticancer immune responses by killer T cells. As a result, even when the immune system recognizes a growing cancer as a threat, the cancer may still escape a strong attack by the immune system.

Has the FDA approved any cancer treatment vaccines?

The FDA has not approved any type of cancer treatment vaccine. Producing effective treatment vaccines has proved much more difficult and challenging than developing cancer preventive vaccines.

To be effective, cancer treatment vaccines must achieve two goals. First, similar to traditional vaccines and cancer preventive vaccines, cancer treatment vaccines must stimulate specific immune responses and direct them against the correct target. Second, the immune responses stimulated by cancer treatment vaccines must be powerful enough to overcome the barriers that cancer cells use to protect themselves from attack by B cells and killer T cells. Recent advances in understanding how cancer cells escape recognition and attack by the immune system are now giving researchers the knowledge required to design cancer treatment vaccines that can accomplish both goals.

What types of vaccines are being studied in clinical trials?

Vaccines to prevent HPV infection and to treat several types of cancer are being studied in clinical trials.

The list below shows the types of cancer that are being targeted in active cancer prevention or treatment clinical trials using vaccines.

Active clinical trials of cancer treatment vaccines by type of cancer:

- Bladder cancer
- Brain tumors
- Breast cancer
- Cervical cancer
- Kidney cancer
- Melanoma

- Multiple myeloma
- Leukemia
- Lung cancer
- Pancreatic cancer
- Prostate cancer
- Solid tumors

Active clinical trials of cancer preventive vaccines by type of cancer:

- Cervical cancer

How are cancer vaccines made, and what antigens are used?

Scientists make cancer preventive vaccines using antigens from microbes that cause or contribute to the development of cancer. The cancer preventive vaccines currently approved by the FDA are made using antigens from HBV and specific types of HPV. These antigens are proteins that help make up the outer surface of the viruses. Because only part of these microbes is used, the resulting vaccines are not infectious and, therefore, cannot cause disease.

Researchers can also create synthetic versions of antigens in the laboratory for use in vaccines. In doing this, they often modify the chemical structure of the antigens to stimulate immune responses that are stronger than those caused by the original antigens.

Similar to cancer preventive vaccines, cancer treatment vaccines can be made using antigens from cancer cells—either directly or by making modified versions of them. Antigens that have been used thus far include proteins; carbohydrates (sugars); glycoproteins or glycopeptides, which are carbohydrate-protein combinations; and gangliosides, which are carbohydrate-lipid (fat) combinations.

Cancer treatment vaccines can also be made using weakened or killed cancer cells that carry a specific cancer-associated antigen. These cells can be from a patient's own cancer (called an autologous vaccine) or from another person's cancer (called an allogeneic vaccine).

Other types of cancer treatment vaccines can be made using molecules of deoxyribonucleic acid (DNA) or ribonucleic acid (RNA) that contain the genetic instructions for cancer-associated antigens. The DNA or RNA can be injected alone into a patient as a "naked nucleic acid" vaccine, or researchers can insert the DNA or RNA into a harmless virus. After the naked nucleic acid or virus is injected into the body, the DNA or RNA is taken up by cells, which begin to manufacture the tumor-associated antigens. Researchers hope that the cells will make enough of the tumor-associated antigens to stimulate a strong immune response.

Scientists have identified a large number of cancer-associated antigens, several of which are now being used to make experimental cancer treatment vaccines. Some of these antigens are found on or in many or most types of cancer cells. Others are unique to specific cancer types.

Antigens associated with more than one type of cancer include the following:

- **Carcinoembryonic antigen (CEA):** A glycoprotein found in developing fetal tissues and in certain types of cancer, including colorectal cancer, stomach cancer, pancreatic cancer, breast cancer, and non-small cell lung cancer.

- **Cancer/testis antigens, such as NY-ESO-1:** A large family of proteins found in male germ cells (sperm) and a wide variety of cancer types, including melanoma and cancers of the ovary, tongue, pharynx, brain, lung, colon, and breast.

- **Mucin-1 (MUC1):** A glycoprotein found in the outer membrane of mucus-producing epithelial cells (cells that make up the skin and line internal organs) and many types of cancer cells, including breast, prostate, colon, pancreatic, and non-small cell lung cancer cells. Sialyl Tn (STn) is a carbohydrate antigen related to mucin-1 that is being used in some treatment vaccines.

- **Gangliosides, such as GM3 and GD2:** Molecules that are found in the outer membrane of several types of cancer cells, including melanoma, neuroblastoma, small cell lung cancer, and soft tissue sarcomas.

- **p53 protein:** A protein produced by the tumor suppressor gene TP53. Mutation of TP53, which results in a loss of p53 protein function, is the most common abnormality in human cancer. Mutant p53 protein often accumulates in cancer cells, which makes p53 an attractive target for a vaccine.

- **HER2/neu protein (also known as ERBB2):** A protein that is overexpressed—or overproduced—in breast, ovarian, and several other types of cancer. Overexpression of HER2/neu is associated with more aggressive disease and a worse outcome. Targeting HER2/neu with a monoclonal antibody called trastuzumab (Herceptin®) has proven to be an effective treatment for breast cancers that overexpress this protein.

Antigens unique to a specific type of cancer include the following:

- **A mutant form of the epidermal growth factor receptor, called EGFRvIII:** An abnormal protein that contributes to uncontrolled tumor growth and is found in glioblastoma (a type of brain cancer), but not in normal brain tissue.

- **Melanocyte/melanoma differentiation antigens, such as tyrosinase, MART1, and gp100:** Proteins found in mature melanocytes (pigment-producing cells of the skin and eye) and in melanoma cells.

- **Prostate-specific antigen (PSA):** A protein that is often produced in much greater amounts by prostate cancer cells than by normal prostate cells.

- **Idiotype (Id) antibodies:** Antibodies produced by cancerous B cells that serve as antigen markers for diseases such as multiple myeloma and several types of lymphoma. Id antibodies are unique to an individual patient's cancer.

Are other substances used to make cancer treatment vaccines?

Yes. Researchers can use certain immune system cells and their products, as well as antibodies created in the laboratory, to make cancer treatment vaccines. Some examples include the following:

Dendritic cells and costimulatory molecules: Scientists can use a type of white blood cell known as a dendritic cell to make cancer treatment vaccines. Dendritic cells are powerful stimulators of immune responses. They process and present cancer-associated antigens to T cells and B cells, and they produce costimulatory molecules that enhance the cell-killing properties of killer T cells.

To make autologous dendritic-cell vaccines, researchers often harvest dendritic cells from the blood of a cancer patient and grow the cells in the laboratory while "feeding" them cancer-associated antigens. Dendritic cells can be fed antigens directly, or they can be exposed to DNA, RNA, or viruses that contain the genetic instructions for the antigens. After taking up the DNA, RNA, or virus genetic material, the dendritic cells manufacture and process the antigens for display on their cell surface to other immune system cells. Researchers then inject these "antigen-presenting cells" into the patient's bloodstream. In the body, the dendritic cells interact with killer T cells and other immune system cells to generate anticancer immune responses.

Researchers can also create synthetic versions of the costimulatory molecules produced by dendritic cells and add them to other types of treatment vaccines to strengthen killer-T-cell responses. Costimulatory molecules that are frequently used in treatment vaccines include ICAM-1, B7.1, and LFA-3. When used together in a vaccine, these three molecules are designated by the abbreviation TRICOM.

Idiotype (Id) vaccines: Normal B cells and cancerous B cells, such as those produced in multiple myeloma and several types of lymphoma, each make only one type of antibody. In a patient with a B cell cancer, these unique antibodies, also called idiotype (Id) antibodies, can serve as antigen markers for the patient's disease. Id antibodies can also be used to create personalized, autologous vaccines. When injected into a patient in large amounts, Id antibodies may be able to stimulate an immune response that will target cancerous B cells for destruction.

Autologous Id vaccines typically include other substances called adjuvants, which increase the potency of immune responses. Id antibodies can also be used as antigens in making autologous dendritic-cell vaccines.

Anti-idiotype (anti-Id) monoclonal antibody vaccines: Monoclonal antibodies are substances created in the laboratory; each type of monoclonal antibody targets one specific antigen. Anti-Id antibodies have been developed that mimic antigens found on several types of cancer cells. These antibodies can trigger immune responses against cancer cells that bear the antigens that the anti-Id antibodies mimic.

Cancer types for which anti-Id monoclonal antibodies have been developed include melanoma, breast cancer, small cell lung cancer, colorectal cancer, ovarian cancer, peritoneal cancer, and cancer of the fallopian tube.

What are adjuvants, and how are they used in making cancer vaccines?

Antigens are often not enough to make effective cancer treatment vaccines. Researchers often add extra ingredients, known as adjuvants, to treatment vaccines. These substances serve to boost immune responses that have been set in motion by exposure to antigens or other means. Patients undergoing treatment with a cancer vaccine sometimes receive adjuvants separately from the vaccine itself.

Adjuvants used for cancer vaccines come from many different sources. Some microbes, such as the bacterium bacillus Calmette-Guérin (BCG) originally used as a vaccine against tuberculosis, can serve as adjuvants.

Substances produced by bacteria, such as Detox B, are frequently used. Biological products derived from nonmicrobial organisms can also be used as adjuvants. One example is keyhole limpet hemocyanin (KLH), which is a large protein produced by a sea animal. Attaching antigens to KLH has been shown to increase their ability to stimulate immune responses. Even some nonbiological substances, such as the emulsified oil montanide ISA–51, can be used as adjuvants.

Scientists can also use natural or synthetic cytokines as adjuvants. Cytokines are substances that are naturally produced by white blood cells to regulate and fine-tune immune responses. Some cytokines increase the activity of B cells and killer T cells, while other cytokines suppress the activities of these cells. Cytokines frequently used in cancer treatment vaccines or given with them include interleukin 2 (IL2, also known as aldesleukin), interferon alpha (INF–a), and granulocyte-macrophage colony-stimulating factor (GM–CSF, also known as sargramostim).

What side effects have been seen with cancer vaccines?

Vaccines intended to prevent or treat cancer appear to have safety profiles comparable to those of traditional vaccines. However, the side effects of cancer vaccines can vary widely from one vaccine formulation to another and from one person to another.

The most commonly reported side effect of cancer vaccines is inflammation at the site where the vaccine is injected into the body. Reported symptoms include redness, pain, swelling, heightened temperature (the skin surrounding the injection site feels hot to the touch), itchiness, and occasionally a rash.

People sometimes experience flulike symptoms after receiving a cancer vaccine, including fever, chills, weakness, dizziness, nausea or vomiting, muscle ache, fatigue, headache, and occasional breathing difficulties. Blood pressure may also be affected.

Other, more serious health problems have been reported in smaller numbers of people after receiving a cancer vaccine. These problems may or may not have been caused by the vaccine. The reported problems have included asthma, appendicitis, pelvic inflammatory disease, and certain autoimmune diseases, including arthritis and systemic lupus erythematosus.

Vaccines, like any other medication affecting the immune system, can cause adverse effects that may prove life threatening. For example, severe hypersensitivity (allergic) reactions to specific vaccine ingredients have occurred following vaccination. However, such severe reactions are quite rare.

Can cancer treatment vaccines be combined with other types of cancer therapy?

Yes. In many of the clinical trials of cancer treatment vaccines that are now under way, vaccines are being administered with other forms of cancer therapy. Therapies that have been combined with cancer treatment vaccines include surgery, chemotherapy, radiation therapy, and some forms of targeted therapy, including therapies based on boosting immune system responses against cancer with biological response modifiers.

Several studies have suggested that cancer treatment vaccines may be most effective when given in combination with other forms of cancer therapy. In addition, in some clinical trials, cancer treatment vaccines have appeared to increase the effectiveness of other cancer therapies.

Additional evidence suggests that surgical removal of large tumor masses may enhance the effectiveness of cancer treatment vaccines. In patients with extensive disease, the immune system may be overwhelmed by the cancer and effective immune responses cannot be achieved. Surgical removal of the tumor may make it easier for the body to develop an immune response.

Researchers are also designing clinical trials to answer questions such as whether a specific cancer treatment vaccine works best when it is administered before chemotherapy, after chemotherapy, or at the same time as chemotherapy. Answers to such questions may not only provide information about how best to use a specific cancer treatment vaccine but also reveal additional basic principles to guide the future development of combination therapies involving vaccines.

What additional research is under way?

Although researchers have identified many cancer-associated antigens, these molecules vary widely in their capacity to stimulate a strong anticancer immune response. Two major areas of research aimed at developing better cancer treatment vaccines involve the discovery of new cancer-associated antigens that may prove more effective in stimulating immune responses than the already known antigens and the development of new methods to enhance the ability of cancer-associated antigens to stimulate the immune system. Research is also under way to determine how to combine multiple antigens within a single cancer treatment vaccine to produce optimal anticancer immune responses.

Another area of study is how best to combine cancer treatment vaccines with other types of anticancer therapy, whether surgery, chemotherapy, radiation therapy, targeted therapy, or other types of immune system therapy, including adoptive cell transfer. In adoptive cell transfer, which is also known as cellular adoptive immunotherapy, researchers harvest killer T cells that have anticancer activity from a patient's tumor and, in the laboratory, both stimulate their growth to greatly increase their numbers and treat them to enhance their tumor-killing activity. The T cells are then injected into the patient.

Perhaps the most promising avenue of cancer vaccine research is aimed at better understanding the basic biology underlying how immune system cells and cancer cells interact. New technologies are being created as part of this effort. For example, a group of scientists recently developed a new type of imaging technology that allows researchers to observe killer T cells and cancer cells interacting on a one-to-one basis inside the body.

In addition, researchers are trying to identify the mechanisms by which cancer cells evade or suppress anticancer immune responses. A better understanding of how cancer cells manipulate the immune system could lead to the development of new drugs that block those processes and thereby improve the effectiveness of cancer treatment vaccines. For example, research has shown that some cancer cells produce chemical signals that attract white blood cells known as regulatory T cells, or Tregs, to a tumor site. Tregs produce cytokines that can either stimulate or suppress the activity of killer T cells. When Tregs move close to a tumor, they often release cytokines that suppress the activity of nearby killer T cells. The combination of a cancer treatment vaccine with a drug that would block the negative effects of one or more of these suppressive cytokines on killer T cells might improve the vaccine's effectiveness in generating potent killer T cell antitumor responses.

Chapter 72

Gene Therapy for Cancer

What are genes?

Genes are the biological units of heredity. Genes determine obvious traits, such as hair and eye color, as well as more subtle characteristics, such as the ability of the blood to carry oxygen. Complex characteristics, such as physical strength, may be shaped by the interaction of a number of different genes along with environmental influences.

Genes are located on chromosomes inside cells and are made of deoxyribonucleic acid (DNA), which is a type of biological molecule. Humans have between 30,000 and 40,000 genes. Genes carry the instructions that allow cells to produce specific proteins, such as enzymes.

To make proteins, a cell must first copy the information stored in genes into another type of biological molecule called ribonucleic acid (RNA). The cell's protein synthesizing machinery then decodes the information in the RNA to manufacture specific proteins. Only certain genes in a cell are active at any given moment. As cells mature, many genes become permanently inactive. The pattern of active and inactive genes in a cell and the resulting protein composition determine what kind of cell it is and what it can and cannot do. Flaws in genes can result in disease.

From "Gene Therapy for Cancer: Questions and Answers," National Cancer Institute (www.cancer.gov), August 31, 2006.

What is gene therapy?

Advances in understanding and manipulating genes have set the stage for scientists to alter a person's genetic material to fight or prevent disease. Gene therapy is an experimental treatment that involves introducing genetic material (DNA or RNA) into a person's cells to fight disease. Gene therapy is being studied in clinical trials (research studies with people) for many different types of cancer and for other diseases. It is not currently available outside a clinical trial.

How is gene therapy being studied in the treatment of cancer?

Researchers are studying several ways to treat cancer using gene therapy. Some approaches target healthy cells to enhance their ability to fight cancer. Other approaches target cancer cells, to destroy them or prevent their growth. Some gene therapy techniques under study are described below.

In one approach, researchers replace missing or altered genes with healthy genes. Because some missing or altered genes (for example, p53) may cause cancer, substituting "working" copies of these genes may be used to treat cancer.

Researchers are also studying ways to improve a patient's immune response to cancer. In this approach, gene therapy is used to stimulate the body's natural ability to attack cancer cells. In one method under investigation, researchers take a small blood sample from a patient and insert genes that will cause each cell to produce a protein called a T-cell receptor (TCR). The genes are transferred into the patient's white blood cells (called T lymphocytes) and are then given back to the patient. In the body, the white blood cells produce TCRs, which attach to the outer surface of the white blood cells. The TCRs then recognize and attach to certain molecules found on the surface of the tumor cells. Finally, the TCRs activate the white blood cells to attack and kill the tumor cells.

Scientists are investigating the insertion of genes into cancer cells to make them more sensitive to chemotherapy, radiation therapy, or other treatments. In other studies, researchers remove healthy blood-forming stem cells from the body, insert a gene that makes these cells more resistant to the side effects of high doses of anticancer drugs, and then inject the cells back into the patient.

In another approach, researchers introduce "suicide genes" into a patient's cancer cells. A pro-drug (an inactive form of a toxic drug) is then given to the patient. The pro-drug is activated in cancer cells containing these "suicide genes, " which leads to the destruction of those cancer cells.

Other research is focused on the use of gene therapy to prevent cancer cells from developing new blood vessels (angiogenesis).

How are genes transferred into cells so that gene therapy can take place?

In general, a gene cannot be directly inserted into a person's cell. It must be delivered to the cell using a carrier, or "vector." The vectors most commonly used in gene therapy are viruses. Viruses have a unique ability to recognize certain cells and insert genetic material into them.

In some gene therapy clinical trials, cells from the patient's blood or bone marrow are removed and grown in the laboratory. The cells are exposed to the virus that is carrying the desired gene. The virus enters the cells and inserts the desired gene into the cells' DNA. The cells grow in the laboratory and are then returned to the patient by injection into a vein. This type of gene therapy is called ex vivo because the cells are grown outside the body. The gene is transferred into the patient's cells while the cells are outside the patient's body.

In other studies, vectors (often viruses) or liposomes (fatty particles) are used to deliver the desired gene to cells in the patient's body. This form of gene therapy is called in vivo, because the gene is transferred to cells inside the patient's body.

What types of viruses are used in gene therapy, and how can they be used safely?

Many gene therapy clinical trials rely on retroviruses to deliver the desired gene. Other viruses used as vectors include adenoviruses, adeno-associated viruses, lentiviruses, poxviruses, and herpes viruses. These viruses differ in how well they transfer genes to the cells they recognize and are able to infect, and whether they alter the cell's DNA permanently or temporarily. Thus, researchers may use different vectors, depending on the specific characteristics and requirements of the study.

Scientists alter the viruses used in gene therapy to make them safe for humans and to increase their ability to deliver specific genes to a patient's cells. Depending on the type of virus and the goals of the research study, scientists may inactivate certain genes in the viruses to prevent them from reproducing or causing disease. Researchers may also alter the virus so that it better recognizes and enters the target cell.

933

What risks are associated with current gene therapy trials?

Viruses can usually infect more than one type of cell. Thus, when viral vectors are used to carry genes into the body, they might infect healthy cells as well as cancer cells. Another danger is that the new gene might be inserted in the wrong location in the DNA, possibly causing harmful mutations to the DNA or even cancer.

In addition, when viruses or liposomes are used to deliver DNA to cells inside the patient's body, there is a slight chance that this DNA could unintentionally be introduced into the patient's reproductive cells. If this happens, it could produce changes that may be passed on if a patient has children after treatment.

Other concerns include the possibility that transferred genes could be "overexpressed," producing so much of the missing protein as to be harmful; that the viral vector could cause inflammation or an immune reaction; and that the virus could be transmitted from the patient to other individuals or into the environment. Scientists use animal testing and other precautions to identify and avoid these risks before any clinical trials are conducted in humans.

What major problems must scientists overcome before gene therapy becomes a common technique for treating disease?

Scientists need to identify more efficient ways to deliver genes to the body. To treat cancer and other diseases effectively with gene therapy, researchers must develop vectors that can be injected into the patient and specifically focus on the target cells located throughout the body. More work is also needed to ensure that the vectors will successfully insert the desired genes into each of these target cells.

Researchers also need to be able to deliver genes consistently to a precise location in the patient's DNA, and ensure that transplanted genes are precisely controlled by the body's normal physiologic signals.

Although scientists are working hard on these problems, it is impossible to predict when they will have effective solutions.

The first disease approved for treatment with gene therapy was adenosine deaminase (ADA) deficiency. What is this disease and why was it selected?

ADA deficiency is a rare genetic disease. The normal ADA gene produces an enzyme called adenosine deaminase, which is essential to the body's immune system. Patients with ADA deficiency do not have normal ADA genes and do not produce functional ADA enzymes.

ADA-deficient children are born with severe immunodeficiency and are prone to repeated serious infections, which may be life-threatening. Although ADA deficiency can be treated with a drug called PEG-ADA, the drug is extremely costly and must be taken for life by injection into a vein.

ADA deficiency was selected for the first approved human gene therapy trial for several reasons:

- The disease is caused by a defect in a single gene, which increases the likelihood that gene therapy will succeed.

- The gene is regulated in a simple, "always-on" fashion, unlike many genes whose regulation is complex.

- The amount of ADA present does not need to be precisely regulated. Even small amounts of the enzyme are known to be beneficial, while larger amounts are also tolerated well.

How do gene therapy trials receive approval?

A proposed gene therapy trial, or protocol, must be approved by at least two review boards at the scientists' institution. Gene therapy protocols must also be approved by the U.S. Food and Drug Administration (FDA), which regulates all gene therapy products. In addition, trials that are funded by the National Institutes of Health (NIH) must be registered with the NIH Recombinant DNA Advisory Committee (RAC). The NIH, which includes 27 Institutes and Centers, is the federal focal point for biomedical research in the United States.

Why are there so many steps in this process?

Any studies involving humans must be reviewed with great care. Gene therapy in particular is potentially a very powerful technique, is relatively new, and could have profound implications. These factors make it necessary for scientists to take special precautions with gene therapy.

What are some of the social and ethical issues surrounding human gene therapy?

In large measure, the issues are the same as those faced whenever a powerful new technology is developed. Such technologies can accomplish great good, but they can also result in great harm if applied unwisely.

Gene therapy is currently focused on correcting genetic flaws and curing life-threatening disease, and regulations are in place for conducting these types of studies. But in the future, when the techniques of gene therapy have become simpler and more accessible, society will need to deal with more complex questions.

One such question is related to the possibility of genetically altering human eggs or sperm, the reproductive cells that pass genes on to future generations. (Because reproductive cells are also called germ cells, this type of gene therapy is referred to as germ-line therapy.) Another question is related to the potential for enhancing human capabilities—for example, improving memory and intelligence—by genetic intervention. Although both germ-line gene therapy and genetic enhancement have the potential to produce benefits, possible problems with these procedures worry many scientists. Germ-line gene therapy would forever change the genetic makeup of an individual's descendants. Thus, the human gene pool would be permanently affected. Although these changes would presumably be for the better, an error in technology or judgment could have far-reaching consequences. The NIH does not approve germ-line gene therapy in humans.

In the case of genetic enhancement, there is concern that such manipulation could become a luxury available only to the rich and powerful. Some also fear that widespread use of this technology could lead to new definitions of "normal" that would exclude individuals who are, for example, of merely average intelligence. And, justly or not, some people associate all genetic manipulation with past abuses of the concept of "eugenics," or the study of methods of improving genetic qualities through selective breeding.

What is being done to address these social and ethical issues?

Scientists working on the Human Genome Project (HGP), which completed mapping and sequencing all of the genes in humans, recognized that the information gained from this work would have profound implications for individuals, families, and society. The Ethical, Legal, and Social Implications (ELSI) Research Program was established in 1990 as part of the HGP to address these issues. The ELSI Research Program fosters basic and applied research on the ethical, legal, and social implications of genetic and genomic research for individuals, families, and communities. The ELSI Research Program sponsors and manages studies and supports workshops, research consortia, and policy conferences on these topics. More information about the HGP and the ELSI Research Program can be found on the National Human Genome Research Institute (NHGRI) website at http://www.genome.gov on the internet.

Chapter 73

Proton Therapy

How does proton therapy work in relation to other mainstream radiation therapy and chemotherapy?

Proton therapy is the most precise and advanced form of radiation treatment today. It primarily radiates the tumor site, leaving surrounding healthy tissue and organs intact. Conventional x-ray radiation often radiates healthy tissue in its path and surrounding the tumor site. Chemotherapy moves throughout the entire body, unlike radiation and surgery which are considered "site specific" treatments.

What are the side effects from proton therapy?

Minimal to no side effects, compared to conventional forms of radiation. Much more easily tolerated than standard radiation therapy.

What kinds of tumors are best treated by proton therapy?

Tumors that are localized and have not spread to distant areas of the body.

From "Frequently Asked Questions," © 2010 National Association for Proton Therapy (www.proton-therapy.org). Reprinted with permission.

How would I know if proton therapy is the appropriate treatment option for myself or a loved one?

Do your homework. Learn as much as possible about all the treatment options available for your condition. Ask lots of questions and discuss them thoroughly with your doctors.

Can proton therapy be used in conjunction with other forms of cancer treatment?

Yes. Depending on the case, proton therapy may be used in combination with traditional radiation, chemotherapy and/or as a follow-up to surgery.

My doctor never mentioned proton therapy as a cancer treatment option? How long has proton therapy been in use for medical purposes?

Proton therapy was first proposed in 1954, but primarily had been available for very limited use. There was no hospital-based treatment centers in the world until the Proton Treatment Center opened in 1990 at Loma Linda University Medical Center. Most radiation oncologists know about proton therapy, but have not had experience working with the proton technology, making it difficult for them to advise patients on this form of treatment. But the benefits of proton treatment are expanding to other regions of the U.S., including the southwest, midwest, southeast, and mid-Atlantic.

How long does proton therapy take? How soon will I know if the treatment is successful?

Proton therapy can take anywhere from one day to seven weeks depending on the tumor site. The length of treatment time will also decrease over time as heavier doses begin to increase. With most cancer cases, success is determined if the cancer does not re-occur within five years after treatment.

Does proton therapy cost more than conventional forms of cancer treatment? Is it covered by most insurance plans?

Nearly all insurance providers nationwide cover proton therapy as does the U.S. medicare program. Proton therapy costs more than conventional radiation, but generally less than surgery.

Why is proton therapy so limited in its availability?

Proton therapy had been limited to physics research labs until 1990. And, like most new technologies, developing and building a proton center can be an expensive endeavor for most universities and academic medical centers. There are currently only seven operating proton centers in the U.S., with four currently under construction and three in development.

Chapter 74

The Potential of Nanotechnology in Cancer Care

Nanotechnology Basics

A nanometer is a billionth of a meter. It's difficult to imagine anything so small, but think of something only 1/80,000 the width of a human hair. Ten hydrogen atoms could be laid side-by-side in a single nanometer.

Nanotechnology is the creation of useful materials, devices, and systems through the manipulation of matter on this miniscule scale. The emerging field of nanotechnology involves scientists from many different disciplines, including physicists, chemists, engineers, and biologists.

Much of today's nanoscale research is designed to reach a better understanding of how matter behaves on this small scale. The factors that govern larger systems do not necessarily apply at the nanoscale. Because nanomaterials have large surface areas relative to their volumes, phenomena like friction and sticking are more important than they are in larger systems.

There are two basic approaches for creating nanodevices. Scientists refer to these methods as the top-down approach and the bottom-up approach. The top-down approach involves molding or etching materials into smaller components. This approach has traditionally been used in making parts for computers and electronics. The bottom-up approach

From "Understanding Cancer Series: Nanodevices," National Cancer Institute (www.cancer.gov), January 28, 2005. Reviewed by David A. Cooke, MD, FACP, September 2010.

involves assembling structures atom-by-atom or molecule-by-molecule, and it may prove useful in manufacturing devices used in medicine.

Nanodevices in the Body

Other challenges apply specifically to the use of nanostructures within biological systems. Nanostructures can be so small that the body may clear them too rapidly for them to be effective in detection or imaging. Larger nanoparticles may accumulate in vital organs, creating a toxicity problem. Scientists will need to consider these factors as they attempt to create nanodevices the body will accept.

Most animal cells are 10,000 to 20,000 nanometers in diameter. This means that nanoscale devices (less than 100 nanometers) can enter cells and the organelles inside them to interact with DNA and proteins. Tools developed through nanotechnology may be able to detect disease in a very small amount of cells or tissue. They may also be able to enter and monitor cells within a living body.

There are many interesting nanodevices being developed that have a potential to improve cancer detection, diagnosis, and treatment.

Detection of cancer at early stages is a critical step in improving cancer treatment. Currently, detection and diagnosis of cancer usually depend on changes in cells and tissues that are detected by a doctor's physical touch or imaging expertise. Instead, scientists would like to make it possible to detect the earliest molecular changes, long before a physical exam or imaging technology is effective. To do this, they need a new set of tools.

In order to successfully detect cancer at its earliest stages, scientists must be able to detect molecular changes even when they occur only in a small percentage of cells. This means the necessary tools must be extremely sensitive. The potential for nanostructures to enter and analyze single cells suggests they could meet this need.

Nanodevices and Medical Tests

Many nanotechnology tools will make it possible for clinicians to run tests without physically altering the cells or tissue they take from a patient. This is important because the samples clinicians use to screen for cancer are often in limited supply. It is also important because it can capture and preserve cells in their active state. Scientists would like to perform tests without altering cells, so the cells can be used again if further tests are needed.

Miniaturization will allow the tools for many different tests to be situated together on the same small device. Researchers hope that nanotechnology will allow them to run many diagnostic tests simultaneously.

Cantilevers

One nanodevice that can improve cancer detection and diagnosis is the cantilever. These tiny levers, which are anchored at one end, can be engineered to bind to molecules that represent some of the changes associated with cancer. They may bind to altered DNA sequences or proteins that are present in certain types of cancer. When these molecules bind to the cantilevers, surface tension changes, causing the cantilevers to bend. By monitoring the bending of the cantilevers, scientists can tell whether molecules are present. Scientists hope this property will prove effective when cancer-associated molecules are present—even in very low concentrations—making cantilevers a potential tool for detecting cancer in its early stages.

Nanopores

Another interesting nanodevice is the nanopore. Improved methods of reading the genetic code will help researchers detect errors in genes that may contribute to cancer. Scientists believe nanopores, tiny holes that allow DNA to pass through one strand at a time, will make DNA sequencing more efficient. As DNA passes through a nanopore, scientists can monitor the shape and electrical properties of each base, or letter, on the strand. Because these properties are unique for each of the four bases that make up the genetic code, scientists can use the passage of DNA through a nanopore to decipher the encoded information, including errors in the code known to be associated with cancer.

Nanotubes

Another nanodevice that will help identify DNA changes associated with cancer is the nanotube. Nanotubes are carbon rods about half the diameter of a molecule of DNA that not only can detect the presence of altered genes, but they may help researchers pinpoint the exact location of those changes.

To prepare DNA for nanotube analysis, scientists must attach a bulky molecule to regions of the DNA that are associated with cancer. They can design tags that seek out specific mutations in the DNA and bind to them.

Once the mutation has been tagged, researchers use a nanotube tip resembling the needle on a record player to trace the physical shape of

DNA and pinpoint the mutated regions. The nanotube creates a map showing the shape of the DNA molecule, including the tags identifying important mutations. Since the location of mutations can influence the effects they have on a cell, these techniques will be important in predicting disease.

Quantum Dots

Another minuscule molecule that will be used to detect cancer is a quantum dot. Quantum dots are tiny crystals that glow when they are stimulated by ultraviolet light. The wavelength, or color, of the light depends on the size of the crystal. Latex beads filled with these crystals can be designed to bind to specific DNA sequences. By combining different sized quantum dots within a single bead, scientists can create probes that release distinct colors and intensities of light. When the crystals are stimulated by UV light, each bead emits light that serves as a sort of spectral bar code, identifying a particular region of DNA.

To detect cancer, scientists can design quantum dots that bind to sequences of DNA that are associated with the disease. When the quantum dots are stimulated with light, they emit their unique bar codes, or labels, making the critical, cancer-associated DNA sequences visible.

The diversity of quantum dots will allow scientists to create many unique labels, which can identify numerous regions of DNA simultaneously. This will be important in the detection of cancer, which results from the accumulation of many different changes within a cell.

Another advantage of quantum dots is that they can be used in the body, eliminating the need for biopsy.

Improving Cancer Treatment

Nanotechnology may also be useful for developing ways to eradicate cancer cells without harming healthy, neighboring cells. Scientists hope to use nanotechnology to create therapeutic agents that target specific cells and deliver their toxin in a controlled, time-released manner.

Nanoshells

Nanoshells are miniscule beads coated with gold. By manipulating the thickness of the layers making up the nanoshells, scientists can design these beads to absorb specific wavelengths of light. The most useful nanoshells are those that absorb near-infrared light, which can easily penetrate several centimeters of human tissue. The absorption of light by the nanoshells creates an intense heat that is lethal to cells.

Researchers can already link nanoshells to antibodies that recognize cancer cells. Scientists envision letting these nanoshells seek out their cancerous targets, then applying near-infrared light. In laboratory cultures, the heat generated by the light-absorbing nanoshells has successfully killed tumor cells while leaving neighboring cells intact.

Linking Detection, Diagnosis, and Treatment

Researchers aim eventually to create nanodevices that do much more than deliver treatment. The goal is to create a single nanodevice that will do many things: assist in imaging inside the body, recognize precancerous or cancerous cells, release a drug that targets only those cells, and report back on the effectiveness of the treatment.

Dendrimers

Research is being done on a number of nanoparticles created to facilitate drug delivery. One such molecule with potential to link treatment with detection and diagnosis is known as a dendrimer. Dendrimers are man-made molecules about the size of an average protein and have a branching shape. This shape gives them vast amounts of surface area to which scientists can attach therapeutic agents or other biologically active molecules. Researchers aim eventually to create nanodevices that do much more than deliver treatment.

A single dendrimer can carry a molecule that recognizes cancer cells, a therapeutic agent to kill those cells, and a molecule that recognizes the signals of cell death. Researchers hope to manipulate dendrimers to release their contents only in the presence of certain trigger molecules associated with cancer. Following drug release, the dendrimers may also report back whether they are successfully killing their targets.

Nanotechnologies in Patient Care

Nanotechnologies that will aid in cancer care are in various stages of discovery and development. Experts believe that quantum dots, nanopores, and other devices for detection and diagnosis may be available for clinical use in five to 15 years. Therapeutic agents are expected to be available within a similar time frame. Devices that integrate detection and therapy could be used clinically in about 15 or 20 years.

Part Six

Additional Help and Information

Chapter 75

A Glossary of Cancer-Related Terms

ABCD rating: A staging system for prostate cancer that uses ABCD. "A" and "B" refer to cancer that is confined to the prostate. "C" refers to cancer that has grown out of the prostate but has not spread to lymph nodes or other places in the body. "D" refers to cancer that has spread to lymph nodes or to other places in the body. Also called Jewett staging system and Whitmore-Jewett staging system.

abdominal ultrasound: A procedure used to examine the organs in the abdomen. An ultrasound transducer (probe) is pressed firmly against the skin of the abdomen. High-energy sound waves from the transducer bounce off tissues and create echoes. The echoes are sent to a computer, which makes a picture called a sonogram. Also called transabdominal ultrasound.

abdominoperineal resection: Surgery to remove the anus, the rectum, and part of the sigmoid colon through an incision made in the abdomen. The end of the intestine is attached to an opening in the surface of the abdomen and body waste is collected in a disposable bag outside of the body. This opening is called a colostomy. Lymph nodes that contain cancer may also be removed during this operation.

ablation: In medicine, the removal or destruction of a body part or tissue or its function. Ablation may be performed by surgery, hormones, drugs, radiofrequency, heat, or other methods.

Excerpted from "Dictionary of Cancer Terms," National Cancer Institute (www.cancer.gov), undated; accessed December 2010.

abnormal: Not normal. An abnormal lesion or growth may be cancer, premalignant (likely to become cancer), or benign (not cancer).

accelerated radiation therapy: Radiation treatment in which the total dose of radiation is given over a shorter period of time (fewer days) compared to standard radiation therapy.

accelerated-fraction radiation therapy: Radiation treatment in which the total dose of radiation is divided into small doses and the treatments are given more than once a day. The total dose of radiation is also given over a shorter period of time (fewer days) compared to standard radiation therapy.

actinic keratosis: A thick, scaly patch of skin that may become cancer. It usually forms on areas exposed to the sun, such as the face, scalp, back of the hands, or chest. It is most common in people with fair skin. Also called senile keratosis and solar keratosis.

active surveillance: Closely watching a patient's condition but not giving treatment unless there are changes in test results. Active surveillance avoids problems that may be caused by treatments such as radiation or surgery. It is used to find early signs that the condition is getting worse. During active surveillance, patients will be given certain exams and tests done on a regular schedule. It is sometimes used in prostate cancer. It is a type of expectant management.

acute: Symptoms or signs that begin and worsen quickly; not chronic.

adenocarcinoma: Cancer that begins in cells that line certain internal organs and that have gland-like (secretory) properties.

adenoma: A tumor that is not cancer. It starts in gland-like cells of the epithelial tissue (thin layer of tissue that covers organs, glands, and other structures within the body).

adenosarcoma: A tumor that is a mixture of an adenoma (a tumor that starts in the gland-like cells of epithelial tissue) and a sarcoma (a tumor that starts in bone, cartilage, fat, muscle, blood vessels, or other connective or supportive tissue). An example of an adenosarcoma is Wilms tumor.

adjunct therapy: Another treatment used together with the primary treatment. Its purpose is to assist the primary treatment. Also called adjunctive therapy.

adjuvant therapy: Additional cancer treatment given after the primary treatment to lower the risk that the cancer will come back. Adjuvant therapy may include chemotherapy, radiation therapy, hormone therapy, targeted therapy, or biological therapy.

adrenal cancer: Cancer that forms in the tissues of the adrenal glands (two glands located just above the kidneys). The adrenal glands make hormones that control heart rate, blood pressure, and other important body functions. Adrenal cancer that starts in the outside layer of the adrenal gland is called adrenocortical carcinoma. Adrenal cancer that starts in the center of the adrenal gland is called malignant pheochromocytoma.

adrenocortical carcinoma: A rare cancer that forms in the outer layer of tissue of the adrenal gland (a small organ on top of each kidney that makes steroid hormones, adrenaline, and noradrenaline to control heart rate, blood pressure, and other body functions).

advance directive: A legal document that states the treatment or care a person wishes to receive or not receive if he or she becomes unable to make medical decisions (for example, due to being unconscious or in a coma). Some types of advance directives are living wills and do-not-resuscitate (DNR) orders.

advanced cancer: Cancer that has spread to other places in the body and usually cannot be cured or controlled with treatment.

aggressive: In medicine, describes a tumor or disease that forms, grows, or spreads quickly. It may also describe treatment that is more severe or intense than usual.

AIDS-related cancer: Certain cancer types that are more likely to occur in people who are infected with the human immunodeficiency virus (HIV). The most common types are Kaposi sarcoma and non-Hodgkin lymphoma. Other AIDS-related cancers include Hodgkin disease and cancers of the lung, mouth, cervix, and digestive system.

allogenic: Taken from different individuals of the same species.

allograft: The transplant of an organ, tissue, or cells from one individual to another individual of the same species who is not an identical twin.

alopecia: The lack or loss of hair from areas of the body where hair is usually found. Alopecia can be a side effect of some cancer treatments.

alveolar rhabdomyosarcoma: A soft tissue tumor that is most common in older children and teenagers. It begins in embryonic muscle cells (cells that develop into muscles in the body). It can occur at many places in the body, but usually occurs in the trunk, arms, or legs. Also called ARMS.

alveolar soft part sarcoma: A soft tissue tumor that is most common in older children and teenagers. It begins in the soft supporting tissue that connects and surrounds the organs and other tissues. Alveolar soft part sarcoma usually occurs in the legs, but can also occur in the arms, hands, head, or neck. It can cause the growth of new blood vessels that help the tumor grow and spread. Also called ASPS.

anal cancer: Cancer that forms in tissues of the anus. The anus is the opening of the rectum (last part of the large intestine) to the outside of the body.

anaplastic: A term used to describe cancer cells that divide rapidly and have little or no resemblance to normal cells.

androblastoma: A rare type of ovarian tumor in which the tumor cells secrete a male sex hormone. This may cause virilization (the appearance of male physical characteristics in females). Also called arrhenoblastoma and Sertoli-Leydig cell tumor of the ovary.

androgen receptor positive: Describes cells that have a protein that binds to androgens (male hormones). Cancer cells that are androgen receptor positive may need androgens to grow. These cells may stop growing or die when they are treated with substances that block the binding and actions of androgen hormones. Also called AR+.

angiogenesis inhibitor: A substance that may prevent the formation of blood vessels. In anticancer therapy, an angiogenesis inhibitor may prevent the growth of new blood vessels that tumors need to grow.

angiosarcoma: A type of cancer that begins in the cells that line blood vessels or lymph vessels. Cancer that begins in blood vessels is called hemangiosarcoma. Cancer that begins in lymph vessels is called lymphangiosarcoma.

anorexia: An abnormal loss of the appetite for food. Anorexia can be caused by cancer, AIDS, a mental disorder (anorexia nervosa), or other diseases.

antagonist: In medicine, a substance that stops the action or effect of another substance. For example, a drug that blocks the stimulating effect of estrogen on a tumor cell is called an estrogen receptor antagonist.

antiandrogen: A substance that prevents cells from making or using androgens (hormones that play a role in the formation of male sex characteristics). Antiandrogens may stop some cancer cells from growing. Some antiandrogens are used to treat prostate cancer, and others are being studied for this use. An antiandrogen is a type of hormone antagonist.

antiestrogen: A substance that keeps cells from making or using estrogen (a hormone that plays a role in female sex characteristics, the menstrual cycle, and pregnancy). Antiestrogens may stop some cancer cells from growing and are used to prevent and treat breast cancer. They are also being studied in the treatment of other types of cancer. An antiestrogen is a type of hormone antagonist. Also called estrogen blocker.

antihormone therapy: Treatment with drugs, surgery, or radiation in order to block the production or action of a hormone. Antihormone therapy may be used in cancer treatment because certain hormones are able to stimulate the growth of some types of tumors.

antimitotic agent: A type of drug that blocks cell growth by stopping mitosis (cell division). They are used to treat cancer. Also called mitotic inhibitor.

antineoplastic: Blocking the formation of neoplasms (growths that may become cancer).

antiprogestin: A substance that prevents cells from making or using progesterone (a hormone that plays a role in the menstrual cycle and pregnancy). Antiprogestins may stop some cancer cells from growing and they are being studied in the treatment of breast cancer. An antiprogestin is a type of hormone antagonist.

astrocytoma: A tumor that begins in the brain or spinal cord in small, star-shaped cells called astrocytes.

asymptomatic: Having no signs or symptoms of disease.

atypical ductal hyperplasia: A benign (not cancer) condition in which there are more cells than normal in the lining of breast ducts and the cells look abnormal under a microscope. Having atypical ductal hyperplasia increases the risk of breast cancer.

atypical hyperplasia: A benign (not cancer) condition in which cells look abnormal under a microscope and are increased in number.

atypical lobular hyperplasia: A benign (not cancer) condition in which there are more cells than normal in the breast lobules and the cells look abnormal under a microscope. Having atypical lobular hyperplasia increases the risk of breast cancer.

atypical squamous cells of undetermined significance: Abnormal cells from the outer walls of the cervix (the lower, narrow end of the uterus). Abnormal squamous cells (thin, flat cells that look like fish scales) are found in a low number of Pap smears (a procedure used to detect cervical cancer) and may indicate infection with the human papillomavirus (HPV) or another infectious agent. The risk of developing cervical cancer is very low for patients with atypical squamous cells of undetermined significance without HPV infection. Also called ASC-US and ASCUS.

autologous bone marrow transplantation: A procedure in which bone marrow is removed from a person, stored, and then given back to the person after intensive treatment.

autologous stem cell transplantation: A procedure in which blood-forming stem cells (cells from which all blood cells develop) are removed, stored, and later given back to the same person.

axillary: Pertaining to the armpit area, including the lymph nodes that are located there.

axillary dissection: Surgery to remove lymph nodes found in the armpit region. Also called axillary lymph node dissection.

axillary lymph node: A lymph node in the armpit region that drains lymph from the breast and nearby areas.

Barrett esophagus: A condition in which the cells lining the lower part of the esophagus have changed or been replaced with abnormal cells that could lead to cancer of the esophagus. The backing up of stomach contents (reflux) may irritate the esophagus and, over time, cause Barrett esophagus.

basal cell: A small, round cell found in the lower part (or base) of the epidermis, the outer layer of the skin.

basal cell carcinoma: Cancer that begins in the lower part of the epidermis (the outer layer of the skin). It may appear as a small white or flesh-colored bump that grows slowly and may bleed. Basal cell carcinomas are usually found on areas of the body exposed to the sun. Basal cell carcinomas rarely metastasize (spread) to other parts of the body. They are the most common form of skin cancer.

benign: Not cancerous. Benign tumors may grow larger but do not spread to other parts of the body. Also called nonmalignant.

benign breast disease: A common condition marked by benign (not cancer) changes in breast tissue. These changes may include irregular lumps or cysts, breast discomfort, sensitive nipples, and itching. These symptoms may change throughout the menstrual cycle and usually stop after menopause. Also called fibrocystic breast changes, fibrocystic breast disease, and mammary dysplasia.

benign prostatic hyperplasia: A benign (not cancer) condition in which an overgrowth of prostate tissue pushes against the urethra and the bladder, blocking the flow of urine. Also called benign prostatic hypertrophy and BPH.

beta cell neoplasm: An abnormal mass that grows in the beta cells of the pancreas that make insulin. Beta cell neoplasms are usually benign (not cancer). They secrete insulin and are the most common cause of low blood sugar caused by having too much insulin in the body. Also called beta cell tumor of the pancreas, insulinoma, and pancreatic insulin-producing tumor.

bilateral cancer: Cancer that occurs in both of a pair of organs, such as both breasts, ovaries, eyes, lungs, kidneys, or adrenal glands, at the same time.

bile duct cancer: Cancer that forms in a bile duct. A bile duct is a tube that carries bile (fluid made by the liver that helps digest fat) between the liver and gallbladder and the intestine. Bile ducts include the common hepatic, cystic, and common bile ducts. Bile duct cancer may be found inside the liver (intrahepatic) or outside the liver (extrahepatic).

biliary: Having to do with the liver, bile ducts, and/or gallbladder.

biopsy: The removal of cells or tissues for examination by a pathologist. The pathologist may study the tissue under a microscope or perform other tests on the cells or tissue. There are many different types of biopsy procedures. The most common types include: (1) incisional biopsy, in which only a sample of tissue is removed; (2) excisional biopsy, in which an entire lump or suspicious area is removed; and (3) needle biopsy, in which a sample of tissue or fluid is removed with a needle. When a wide needle is used, the procedure is called a core biopsy. When a thin needle is used, the procedure is called a fine-needle aspiration biopsy.

bladder cancer: Cancer that forms in tissues of the bladder (the organ that stores urine). Most bladder cancers are transitional cell carcinomas (cancer that begins in cells that normally make up the inner lining of the bladder). Other types include squamous cell carcinoma (cancer that begins in thin, flat cells) and adenocarcinoma (cancer that begins in cells that make and release mucus and other fluids). The cells that form squamous cell carcinoma and adenocarcinoma develop in the inner lining of the bladder as a result of chronic irritation and inflammation.

bone cancer: Primary bone cancer is cancer that forms in cells of the bone. Some types of primary bone cancer are osteosarcoma, Ewing sarcoma, malignant fibrous histiocytoma, and chondrosarcoma. Secondary bone cancer is cancer that spreads to the bone from another part of the body (such as the prostate, breast, or lung).

bone marrow aspiration: A procedure in which a small sample of bone marrow is removed, usually from the hip bone, breastbone, or thigh bone. A small area of skin and the surface of the bone underneath are numbed with an anesthetic. Then, a special wide needle is pushed into the bone. A sample of liquid bone marrow is removed with a syringe attached to the needle. The bone marrow is sent to a laboratory to be looked at under a microscope. This procedure may be done at the same time as a bone marrow biopsy.

bone marrow biopsy: A procedure in which a small sample of bone with bone marrow inside it is removed, usually from the hip bone. A small area of skin and the surface of the bone underneath are numbed with an anesthetic. Then, a special, wide needle is pushed into the bone and rotated to remove a sample of bone with the bone marrow inside it. The sample is sent to a laboratory to be looked at under a microscope. This procedure may be done at the same time as a bone marrow aspiration.

bone marrow cancer: Cancer that forms in the blood-forming stem cells of the bone marrow (soft sponge-like tissue in the center of most bones). Bone marrow cancer includes leukemias and multiple myeloma.

bone marrow transplantation: A procedure to replace bone marrow that has been destroyed by treatment with high doses of anticancer drugs or radiation. Transplantation may be autologous (an individual's own marrow saved before treatment), allogeneic (marrow donated by someone else), or syngeneic (marrow donated by an identical twin).

brachytherapy: A type of radiation therapy in which radioactive material sealed in needles, seeds, wires, or catheters is placed directly into or near a tumor. Also called implant radiation therapy, internal radiation therapy, and radiation brachytherapy.

brain metastasis: Cancer that has spread from the original (primary) tumor to the brain.

brain stem glioma: A tumor located in the part of the brain that connects to the spinal cord (the brain stem). It may grow rapidly or slowly, depending on the grade of the tumor.

brain tumor: The growth of abnormal cells in the tissues of the brain. Brain tumors can be benign (not cancer) or malignant (cancer).

BRCA1: A gene on chromosome 17 that normally helps to suppress cell growth. A person who inherits certain mutations (changes) in a BRCA1 gene has a higher risk of getting breast, ovarian, prostate, and other types of cancer.

BRCA2: A gene on chromosome 13 that normally helps to suppress cell growth. A person who inherits certain mutations (changes) in a BRCA2 gene has a higher risk of getting breast, ovarian, prostate, and other types of cancer.

breakthrough pain: Intense increases in pain that occur with rapid onset even when pain-control medication is being used. Breakthrough pain can occur spontaneously or in relation to a specific activity.

breast cancer: Cancer that forms in tissues of the breast, usually the ducts (tubes that carry milk to the nipple) and lobules (glands that make milk). It occurs in both men and women, although male breast cancer is rare.

breast carcinoma in situ: There are two types of breast carcinoma in situ: ductal carcinoma in situ (DCIS) and lobular carcinoma in situ (LCIS). DCIS is a noninvasive condition in which abnormal cells are found in the lining of a breast duct (a tube that carries milk to the nipple). The abnormal cells have not spread outside the duct to other tissues in the breast. In some cases, DCIS may become invasive cancer and spread to other tissues, although it is not known how to predict which lesions will become invasive cancer. LCIS is a condition in which abnormal cells are found in the lobules (small sections of tissue involved with making milk) of the breast. This condition seldom becomes invasive cancer; however, having LCIS in one breast increases the risk of developing breast cancer in either breast. Also called stage 0 breast carcinoma in situ.

breast reconstruction: Surgery to rebuild the shape of the breast after a mastectomy.

breast self-exam: An exam by a woman of her breasts to check for lumps or other changes.

breast-conserving surgery: An operation to remove the breast cancer but not the breast itself. Types of breast-conserving surgery include lumpectomy (removal of the lump), quadrantectomy (removal of one quarter, or quadrant, of the breast), and segmental mastectomy (removal of the cancer as well as some of the breast tissue around the tumor and the lining over the chest muscles below the tumor). Also called breast-sparing surgery.

bronchial adenoma: Cancer that forms in tissues of the bronchi (large air passages in the lungs including those that lead to the lungs from the windpipe).

bronchial brush biopsy: A procedure in which cells are taken from the inside of the airways that lead to the lungs. A bronchoscope (a thin, tube-like instrument with a light and a lens for viewing) is inserted through the nose or mouth into the lungs. A small brush is then used to remove cells from the airways. These cells are then looked at under a microscope. A bronchial brush biopsy is used to find cancer and changes in cells that may lead to cancer. It is also used to help diagnose other lung conditions. Also called bronchial brushing.

bronchogenic carcinoma: Cancer that begins in the tissue that lines or covers the airways of the lungs, including small cell and non-small cell lung cancer.

bronchoscopy: A procedure that uses a bronchoscope to examine the inside of the trachea, bronchi (air passages that lead to the lungs), and lungs. A bronchoscope is a thin, tube-like instrument with a light and a lens for viewing. It may also have a tool to remove tissue to be checked under a microscope for signs of disease. The bronchoscope is inserted through the nose or mouth. Bronchoscopy may be used to detect cancer or to perform some treatment procedures.

bronchus: A large airway that leads from the trachea (windpipe) to a lung. The plural of bronchus is bronchi.

CA 19-9: A substance released into the bloodstream by both cancer cells and normal cells. Too much CA 19-9 in the blood can be a sign of pancreatic cancer or other types of cancer or conditions. The amount of CA 19-9 in the blood can be used to help keep track of how well cancer treatments are working or if cancer has come back. It is a type of tumor marker.

CA-125: A substance that may be found in high amounts in the blood of patients with certain types of cancer, including ovarian cancer. CA-125 levels may also help monitor how well cancer treatments are working or if cancer has come back. Also called cancer antigen 125.

cachexia: Loss of body weight and muscle mass, and weakness that may occur in patients with cancer, AIDS, or other chronic diseases.

calcification: Deposits of calcium in the tissues. Calcification in the breast can be seen on a mammogram, but cannot be detected by touch. There are two types of breast calcification, macrocalcification and microcalcification. Macrocalcifications are large deposits and are usually not related to cancer. Microcalcifications are specks of calcium that may be found in an area of rapidly dividing cells. Many microcalcifications clustered together may be a sign of cancer.

cancer: A term for diseases in which abnormal cells divide without control and can invade nearby tissues. Cancer cells can also spread to other parts of the body through the blood and lymph systems. There are several main types of cancer. Carcinoma is a cancer that begins in the skin or in tissues that line or cover internal organs. Sarcoma is a cancer that begins in bone, cartilage, fat, muscle, blood vessels, or other connective or supportive tissue. Leukemia is a cancer that starts in blood-forming tissue such as the bone marrow, and causes large numbers of abnormal blood cells to be produced and enter the blood. Lymphoma and multiple myeloma are cancers that begin in the cells of the immune system. Central nervous system cancers are cancers that begin in the tissues of the brain and spinal cord. Also called malignancy.

cancer of unknown primary origin: A case in which cancer cells are found in the body, but the place where the cells first started growing (the origin or primary site) cannot be determined. Also called carcinoma of unknown primary and CUP.

carcinoembryonic antigen: A substance that is sometimes found in an increased amount in the blood of people who have certain cancers, other diseases, or who smoke. It is used as a tumor marker for colorectal cancer. Also called CEA.

carcinogen: Any substance that causes cancer.

carcinoid: A slow-growing type of tumor usually found in the gastrointestinal system (most often in the appendix), and sometimes in the lungs or other sites. Carcinoid tumors may spread to the liver or other sites in the body, and they may secrete substances such as serotonin or prostaglandins, causing carcinoid syndrome.

carcinoma: Cancer that begins in the skin or in tissues that line or cover internal organs.

carcinoma in situ: A group of abnormal cells that remain in the place where they first formed. They have not spread. These abnormal cells may become cancer and spread into nearby normal tissue. Also called stage 0 disease.

carcinosarcoma: A malignant tumor that is a mixture of carcinoma (cancer of epithelial tissue, which is skin and tissue that lines or covers the internal organs) and sarcoma (cancer of connective tissue, such as bone, cartilage, and fat).

carcinosis: A condition in which cancer is spread widely throughout the body, or, in some cases, to a relatively large region of the body. Also called carcinomatosis.

central nervous system primitive neuroectodermal tumor: A type of cancer that arises from a particular type of cell within the brain or spinal cord. Also called CNS PNET.

cervical cancer: Cancer that forms in tissues of the cervix (the organ connecting the uterus and vagina). It is usually a slow-growing cancer that may not have symptoms but can be found with regular Pap tests (a procedure in which cells are scraped from the cervix and looked at under a microscope). Cervical cancer is almost always caused by human papillomavirus (HPV) infection.

cervical intraepithelial neoplasia: Growth of abnormal cells on the surface of the cervix. Numbers from one to three may be used to describe how abnormal the cells are and how much of the cervical tissue is involved.

cervicectomy: Surgery to remove the cervix (the end of the uterus that forms a canal between the uterus and the vagina).The upper part of the vagina and certain pelvic lymph nodes may also be removed. Also called trachelectomy.

chemoimmunotherapy: Chemotherapy combined with immunotherapy. Chemotherapy uses different drugs to kill or slow the growth of cancer cells; immunotherapy uses treatments to stimulate or restore the ability of the immune system to fight cancer.

chemoprevention: The use of drugs, vitamins, or other agents to try to reduce the risk of, or delay the development or recurrence of, cancer.

chemotherapy: Treatment with drugs that kill cancer cells.

cholangiocarcinoma: A rare type of cancer that develops in cells that line the bile ducts in the liver. Cancer that forms where the right and left ducts meet is called Klatskin tumor.

cholangiosarcoma: A tumor of the connective tissues of the bile ducts.

chondrosarcoma: A type of cancer that forms in bone cartilage. It usually starts in the pelvis (between the hip bones), the shoulder, the ribs, or at the ends of the long bones of the arms and legs. A rare type of chondrosarcoma called extraskeletal chondrosarcoma does not form in bone cartilage. Instead, it forms in the soft tissues of the upper part of the arms and legs. Chondrosarcoma can occur at any age but is more common in people older than 40 years. It is a type of bone cancer.

chordoma: A type of bone cancer that usually starts in the lower spinal column or at the base of the skull.

chorioblastoma: A malignant, fast-growing tumor that develops from trophoblastic cells (cells that help an embryo attach to the uterus and help form the placenta). Almost all chorioblastomas form in the uterus after fertilization of an egg by a sperm, but a small number form in a testis or an ovary. Chorioblastomas spread through the blood to other organs, especially the lungs. They are a type of gestational trophoblastic disease. Also called choriocarcinoma, chorioepithelioma, and chorionic carcinoma.

chronic: A disease or condition that persists or progresses over a long period of time.

Clark levels: A system for describing how deep skin cancer has spread into the skin. Levels I-V describe the layers of skin involved.

clear cell carcinoma: A rare type of tumor, usually of the female genital tract, in which the insides of the cells look clear when viewed under a microscope. Also called clear cell adenocarcinoma and mesonephroma.

clear cell sarcoma of soft tissue: A soft tissue tumor that begins in a tendon (tough, fibrous, cord-like tissue that connects muscle to bone or to another structure). Clear cell sarcoma of soft tissue has certain markers that are also found on malignant melanoma (a type of skin cancer). It usually occurs in the leg or arm. Also called malignant melanoma of soft parts.

clear cell sarcoma of the kidney: A rare type of kidney cancer, in which the inside of the cells look clear when viewed under a microscope. Clear cell sarcoma can spread from the kidney to other organs, most commonly the bone, but also including the lungs, brain, and soft tissues of the body.

clinical stage: The stage of cancer (amount or spread of cancer in the body) that is based on tests that are done before surgery. These include physical exams, imaging tests, laboratory tests (such as blood tests), and biopsies.

colon cancer: Cancer that forms in the tissues of the colon (the longest part of the large intestine). Most colon cancers are adenocarcinomas (cancers that begin in cells that make and release mucus and other fluids).

colon polyp: An abnormal growth of tissue in the lining of the bowel. Polyps are a risk factor for colon cancer.

colonoscopy: Examination of the inside of the colon using a colonoscope, inserted into the rectum. A colonoscope is a thin, tube-like instrument with a light and a lens for viewing. It may also have a tool to remove tissue to be checked under a microscope for signs of disease.

colorectal cancer: Cancer that develops in the colon (the longest part of the large intestine) and/or the rectum (the last several inches of the large intestine before the anus).

colostomy: An opening into the colon from the outside of the body. A colostomy provides a new path for waste material to leave the body after part of the colon has been removed.

colposcopy: Examination of the vagina and cervix using a lighted magnifying instrument called a colposcope.

comfort care: Care given to improve the quality of life of patients who have a serious or life-threatening disease. The goal of comfort care is to prevent or treat as early as possible the symptoms of a disease, side effects caused by treatment of a disease, and psychological, social, and spiritual problems related to a disease or its treatment. Also called palliative care, supportive care, and symptom management.

compassionate use trial: A way to provide an investigational therapy to a patient who is not eligible to receive that therapy in a clinical trial, but who has a serious or life-threatening illness for which other treatments are not available. Compassionate use trials allow patients to receive promising but not yet fully studied or approved cancer therapies when no other treatment option exists. Also called expanded access trial.

complete remission: The disappearance of all signs of cancer in response to treatment. This does not always mean the cancer has been cured. Also called complete response.

computerized axial tomography scan: A series of detailed pictures of areas inside the body taken from different angles. The pictures are created by a computer linked to an x-ray machine. Also called CAT scan, computed tomography scan, computerized tomography, and CT scan.

condyloma: A raised growth on the surface of the genitals caused by human papillomavirus (HPV) infection. The HPV in condyloma is very contagious and can be spread by skin-to-skin contact, usually during oral, anal, or genital sex with an infected partner. Also called genital wart.

cone biopsy: Surgery to remove a cone-shaped piece of tissue from the cervix and cervical canal. Cone biopsy may be used to diagnose or treat a cervical condition. Also called conization.

core biopsy: The removal of a tissue sample with a wide needle for examination under a microscope. Also called core needle biopsy.

corpus: The body of the uterus.

cryosurgery: A procedure in which tissue is frozen to destroy abnormal cells. Liquid nitrogen or liquid carbon dioxide is used to freeze the tissue. Also called cryoablation and cryosurgical ablation.

cyst: A sac or capsule in the body. It may be filled with fluid or other material.

cystectomy: Surgery to remove all or part of the bladder (the organ that holds urine) or to remove a cyst (a sac or capsule in the body).

D&C: A procedure to remove tissue from the cervical canal or the inner lining of the uterus. The cervix is dilated (made larger) and a curette (spoon-shaped instrument) is inserted into the uterus to remove tissue. Also called dilatation and curettage and dilation and curettage.

de novo: In cancer, the first occurrence of cancer in the body.

desmoid tumor: A tumor of the tissue that surrounds muscles, usually in the abdomen. A desmoid tumor rarely metastasizes (spreads to other parts of the body). It may be called aggressive fibromatosis when the tumor is outside of the abdomen.

diethylstilbestrol: A synthetic form of the hormone estrogen that was prescribed to pregnant women between about 1940 and 1971 because it was thought to prevent miscarriages. Diethylstilbestrol may increase the risk of uterine, ovarian, or breast cancer in women who took it. It also has been linked to an increased risk of clear cell carcinoma of the vagina or cervix in daughters exposed to diethylstilbestrol before birth. Also called DES.

digital mammography: The use of a computer, rather than x-ray film, to create a picture of the breast.

digital rectal examination: An examination in which a doctor inserts a lubricated, gloved finger into the rectum to feel for abnormalities. Also called DRE.

disease-free survival: The length of time after treatment for a specific disease during which a patient survives with no sign of the disease. Disease-free survival may be used in a clinical study or trial to help measure how well a new treatment works.

ductal carcinoma in situ: A noninvasive condition in which abnormal cells are found in the lining of a breast duct. The abnormal cells have not spread outside the duct to other tissues in the breast. In some cases, ductal carcinoma in situ may become invasive cancer and spread to other tissues, although it is not known at this time how to predict which lesions will become invasive. Also called DCIS and intraductal carcinoma.

ductal lavage: A method used to collect cells from milk ducts in the breast. A hair-size catheter (tube) is inserted into the nipple, and a small amount of salt water is released into the duct. The water picks up breast cells, and is removed. The cells are checked under a microscope. Ductal lavage may be used in addition to clinical breast examination and mammography to detect breast cancer.

Dukes classification: A staging system used to describe the extent of colorectal cancer. Stages range from A (early stage) to D (advanced stage).

dysplasia: Cells that look abnormal under a microscope but are not cancer.

dysplastic nevus: A type of nevus (mole) that looks different from a common mole. A dysplastic nevus is often larger with borders that are not easy to see. Its color is usually uneven and can range from pink to dark brown. Parts of the mole may be raised above the skin surface. A dysplastic nevus may develop into malignant melanoma (a type of skin cancer).

early-stage cancer: A term used to describe cancer that is early in its growth, and may not have spread to other parts of the body. What is called early stage may differ between cancer types.

edema: Swelling caused by excess fluid in body tissues.

embryonal tumor: A mass of rapidly growing cells that begins in embryonic (fetal) tissue. Embryonal tumors may be benign or malignant, and include neuroblastomas and Wilms tumors. Also called embryoma.

enchondroma: A benign (not cancer) growth of cartilage in bones or in other areas where cartilage is not normally found.

endocrine cancer: Cancer that occurs in endocrine tissue, the tissue in the body that secretes hormones.

endocrine therapy: Treatment that adds, blocks, or removes hormones. For certain conditions (such as diabetes or menopause), hormones are given to adjust low hormone levels. To slow or stop the growth of certain cancers (such as prostate and breast cancer), synthetic hormones or other drugs may be given to block the body's natural hormones. Sometimes surgery is needed to remove the gland that makes a certain hormone. Also called hormonal therapy, hormone therapy, and hormone treatment.

endometrial biopsy: A procedure in which a sample of tissue is taken from the endometrium (inner lining of the uterus) for examination under a microscope. A thin tube is inserted through the cervix into the uterus, and gentle scraping and suction are used to remove the sample.

endometrial cancer: Cancer that forms in the tissue lining the uterus (the small, hollow, pear-shaped organ in a woman's pelvis in which a fetus develops). Most endometrial cancers are adenocarcinomas (cancers that begin in cells that make and release mucus and other fluids).

endometrial hyperplasia: An abnormal overgrowth of the endometrium (the layer of cells that lines the uterus). There are four types of endometrial hyperplasia: simple endometrial hyperplasia, complex endometrial hyperplasia, simple endometrial hyperplasia with atypia, and complex endometrial hyperplasia with atypia. These differ in terms of how abnormal the cells are and how likely it is that the condition will become cancer.

endoscopy: A procedure that uses an endoscope to examine the inside of the body. An endoscope is a thin, tube-like instrument with a light and a lens for viewing. It may also have a tool to remove tissue to be checked under a microscope for signs of disease.

enucleation: In medicine, the removal of an organ or tumor in such a way that it comes out clean and whole, like a nut from its shell.

ependymoma: A type of brain tumor that begins in cells lining the spinal cord central canal (fluid-filled space down the center) or the ventricles (fluid-filled spaces of the brain). Ependymomas may also form in the choroid plexus (tissue in the ventricles that makes cerebrospinal fluid). Also called ependymal tumor.

epithelial carcinoma: Cancer that begins in the cells that line an organ.

esophageal cancer: Cancer that forms in tissues lining the esophagus (the muscular tube through which food passes from the throat to the stomach). Two types of esophageal cancer are squamous cell carcinoma (cancer that begins in flat cells lining the esophagus) and adenocarcinoma (cancer that begins in cells that make and release mucus and other fluids).

esophageal speech: Speech produced by trapping air in the esophagus and forcing it out again. It is used after removal of a person's larynx (voice box).

estrogen blocker: A substance that keeps cells from making or using estrogen (a hormone that plays a role in female sex characteristics, the menstrual cycle, and pregnancy). Estrogen blockers may stop some cancer cells from growing and are used to prevent and treat breast cancer. They are also being studied in the treatment of other types of cancer. An estrogen blocker is a type of hormone antagonist. Also called antiestrogen.

estrogen receptor: A protein found inside the cells of the female reproductive tissue, some other types of tissue, and some cancer cells. The hormone estrogen will bind to the receptors inside the cells and may cause the cells to grow. Also called ER.

estrogen receptor negative: Describes cells that do not have a protein to which the hormone estrogen will bind. Cancer cells that are estrogen receptor negative do not need estrogen to grow, and usually do not stop growing when treated with hormones that block estrogen from binding. Also called ER-.

estrogen receptor positive: Describes cells that have a receptor protein that binds the hormone estrogen. Cancer cells that are estrogen receptor positive may need estrogen to grow, and may stop growing or die when treated with substances that block the binding and actions of estrogen. Also called ER+.

Ewing sarcoma family of tumors: A group of cancers that includes Ewing tumor of bone (ETB or Ewing sarcoma of bone), extraosseous Ewing (EOE) tumors, primitive neuroectodermal tumors (PNET or peripheral neuroepithelioma), and Askin tumors (PNET of the chest wall). These tumors all come from the same type of stem cell. Also called EFTs.

excisional biopsy: A surgical procedure in which an entire lump or suspicious area is removed for diagnosis. The tissue is then examined under a microscope.

exocrine cancer: A disease in which malignant (cancer) cells are found in the tissues of the pancreas. Also called pancreatic cancer.

extracranial germ cell tumor: A rare cancer that forms in germ cells in the testicle or ovary, or in germ cells that have traveled to areas of the body other than the brain (such as the chest, abdomen, or tailbone). Germ cells are reproductive cells that develop into sperm in males and eggs in females.

extrahepatic bile duct cancer: A rare cancer that forms in the part of the bile duct that is outside the liver. The bile duct is the tube that collects bile from the liver and joins a duct from the gallbladder to form the common bile duct, which carries bile into the small intestine when food is being digested.

extrapleural pneumonectomy: Surgery to remove a diseased lung, part of the pericardium (membrane covering the heart), part of the diaphragm (muscle between the lungs and the abdomen), and part of the parietal pleura (membrane lining the chest). This type of surgery is used most often to treat malignant mesothelioma.

eye cancer: Cancer that forms in tissues of and around the eye. Some of the cancers that may affect the eye include melanoma (a rare cancer that begins in cells that make the pigment melanin in the eye), carcinoma (cancer that begins in tissues that cover structures in the eye), lymphoma (cancer that begins in immune system cells), and retinoblastoma (cancer that begins in the retina and usually occurs in children younger than five years).

false-negative test result: A test result that indicates that a person does not have a specific disease or condition when the person actually does have the disease or condition.

false-positive test result: A test result that indicates that a person has a specific disease or condition when the person actually does not have the disease or condition.

familial atypical multiple mole melanoma syndrome: An inherited condition marked by the following: (1) one or more first- or second-degree relatives (parent, sibling, child, grandparent, grandchild, aunt, or uncle) with malignant melanoma; (2) many moles, some of which are atypical (asymmetrical, raised, and/or different shades of tan, brown, black, or red) and often of different sizes; and (3) moles that have specific features when examined under a microscope. FAMMM syndrome increases the risk of melanoma and may increase the risk of pancreatic cancer. Also called FAMMM syndrome.

familial cancer: Cancer that occurs in families more often than would be expected by chance. These cancers often occur at an early age, and may indicate the presence of a gene mutation that increases the risk of cancer. They may also be a sign of shared environmental or lifestyle factors.

familial dysplastic nevi: A condition that runs in certain families in which at least two members have dysplastic nevi (atypical moles) and have a tendency to develop melanoma.

familial polyposis: An inherited condition in which numerous polyps (growths that protrude from mucous membranes) form on the inside walls of the colon and rectum. It increases the risk of colorectal cancer. Also called familial adenomatous polyposis.

family medical history: A record of the relationships among family members along with their medical histories. This includes current and past illnesses. A family medical history may show a pattern of certain diseases in a family.

fibrocystic breast disease: A common condition marked by benign (not cancer) changes in breast tissue. These changes may include irregular lumps or cysts, breast discomfort, sensitive nipples, and itching. These symptoms may change throughout the menstrual cycle and usually stop after menopause. Also called benign breast disease, fibrocystic breast changes, and mammary dysplasia.

fibroid: A benign smooth-muscle tumor, usually in the uterus or gastrointestinal tract. Also called leiomyoma.

fine-needle aspiration biopsy: The removal of tissue or fluid with a thin needle for examination under a microscope. Also called FNA biopsy.

first-degree relative: The parents, brothers, sisters, or children of an individual.

five-year survival rate: The percentage of people in a study or treatment group who are alive five years after they were diagnosed with or treated for a disease, such as cancer. The disease may or may not have come back.

gallbladder cancer: Cancer that forms in tissues of the gallbladder. The gallbladder is a pear-shaped organ below the liver that collects and stores bile (a fluid made by the liver to digest fat). Gallbladder cancer begins in the innermost layer of tissue and spreads through the outer layers as it grows.

gallium scan: A procedure to detect areas of the body where cells are dividing rapidly. It is used to locate cancer cells or areas of inflammation. A very small amount of radioactive gallium is injected into a vein and travels through the bloodstream. The gallium is taken up by rapidly dividing cells in the bones, tissues, and organs and is detected by a scanner.

Gamma Knife therapy: A treatment using gamma rays, a type of high-energy radiation that can be tightly focused on small tumors or other lesions in the head or neck, so very little normal tissue receives radiation. The gamma rays are aimed at the tumor from many different angles at once, and deliver a large dose of radiation exactly to the tumor in one treatment session. This procedure is a type of stereotactic radiosurgery. Gamma Knife therapy is not a knife and is not surgery. Gamma Knife is a registered trademark of Elekta Instruments, Inc.

gastric cancer: Cancer that forms in tissues lining the stomach. Also called stomach cancer.

gastrinoma: A tumor that causes overproduction of gastric acid. It usually begins in the duodenum (first part of the small intestine that connects to the stomach) or the islet cells of the pancreas. Rarely, it may also begin in other organs, including the stomach, liver, jejunum (the middle part of the small intestine), biliary tract (organs and ducts that make and store bile), mesentery, or heart. It is a type of neuroendocrine tumor, and it may metastasize (spread) to the liver and the lymph nodes.

gastrointestinal carcinoid tumor: An indolent (slow-growing) cancer that forms in cells that make hormones in the lining of the gastrointestinal tract (the stomach and intestines). It usually occurs in the appendix (a small fingerlike pouch of the large intestine), small intestine, or rectum. Having gastrointestinal carcinoid tumor increases the risk of forming other cancers of the digestive system.

gastrointestinal stromal tumor: A type of tumor that usually begins in cells in the wall of the gastrointestinal tract. It can be benign or malignant. Also called GIST.

gene therapy: Treatment that alters a gene. In studies of gene therapy for cancer, researchers are trying to improve the body's natural ability to fight the disease or to make the cancer cells more sensitive to other kinds of therapy.

germ cell tumor: A type of tumor that begins in the cells that give rise to sperm or eggs. Germ cell tumors can occur almost anywhere in the body and can be either benign or malignant.

gestational trophoblastic tumor: Any of a group of tumors that develops from trophoblastic cells (cells that help an embryo attach to the uterus and help form the placenta) after fertilization of an egg by a sperm. The two main types of gestational trophoblastic tumors are hydatidiform mole and choriocarcinoma.

glioblastoma: A fast-growing type of central nervous system tumor that forms from glial (supportive) tissue of the brain and spinal cord and has cells that look very different from normal cells. Glioblastoma usually occurs in adults and affects the brain more often than the spinal cord. Also called GBM, glioblastoma multiforme, and grade IV astrocytoma.

grading: A system for classifying cancer cells in terms of how abnormal they appear when examined under a microscope. The objective of a grading system is to provide information about the probable growth rate of the tumor and its tendency to spread. The systems used to grade tumors vary with each type of cancer. Grading plays a role in treatment decisions.

granulocytic sarcoma: A malignant, green-colored tumor of myeloid cells (a type of immature white blood cell). This tumor is usually associated with myelogenous leukemia. Also called chloroma.

granulosa cell tumor: A type of slow-growing, malignant tumor that usually affects the ovary.

gynecologic cancer: Cancer of the female reproductive tract, including the cervix, endometrium, fallopian tubes, ovaries, uterus, and vagina.

gynecologic oncologist: A doctor who specializes in treating cancers of the female reproductive organs.

hairy cell leukemia: A rare type of leukemia in which abnormal B-lymphocytes (a type of white blood cell) are present in the bone marrow, spleen, and peripheral blood. When viewed under a microscope, these cells appear to be covered with tiny hair-like projections.

Halsted radical mastectomy: Surgery for breast cancer in which the breast, chest muscles, and all of the lymph nodes under the arm are removed. For many years, this was the breast cancer operation used most often, but it is used rarely now. Doctors consider radical mastectomy only when the tumor has spread to the chest muscles. Also called radical mastectomy.

hamartoma: A benign (not cancer) growth made up of an abnormal mixture of cells and tissues normally found in the area of the body where the growth occurs.

Helicobacter pylori: A type of bacterium that causes inflammation and ulcers in the stomach or small intestine. People with *H. pylori* infections may be more likely to develop cancer in the stomach, including MALT (mucosa-associated lymphoid tissue) lymphoma.

hemangiosarcoma: A type of cancer that begins in the cells that line blood vessels.

hematologic cancer: A cancer of the blood or bone marrow, such as leukemia or lymphoma.

hepatoblastoma: A type of liver tumor that occurs in infants and children.

hepatocellular carcinoma: A type of adenocarcinoma and the most common type of liver tumor.

HER1: The protein found on the surface of some cells and to which epidermal growth factor binds, causing the cells to divide. It is found at abnormally high levels on the surface of many types of cancer cells, so these cells may divide excessively in the presence of epidermal growth factor. Also called EGFR, epidermal growth factor receptor, and ErbB1.

HER2/neu: A protein involved in normal cell growth. It is found on some types of cancer cells, including breast and ovarian. Cancer cells removed from the body may be tested for the presence of HER2/neu to help decide the best type of treatment. HER2/neu is a type of receptor tyrosine kinase. Also called c-erbB-2, human EGF receptor 2, and human epidermal growth factor receptor 2.

hereditary nonpolyposis colon cancer: An inherited disorder in which affected individuals have a higher-than-normal chance of developing colorectal cancer and certain other types of cancer, often before the age of 50. Also called HNPCC and Lynch syndrome.

high-dose chemotherapy: An intensive drug treatment to kill cancer cells, but that also destroys the bone marrow and can cause other severe side effects. High-dose chemotherapy is usually followed by bone marrow or stem cell transplantation to rebuild the bone marrow.

high-dose radiation: An amount of radiation that is greater than that given in typical radiation therapy. High-dose radiation is precisely directed at the tumor to avoid damaging healthy tissue, and may kill more cancer cells in fewer treatments.

high-dose-rate remote brachytherapy: A type of internal radiation treatment in which the radioactive source is removed between treatments. Also called high-dose-rate remote radiation therapy and remote brachytherapy.

high-energy photon therapy: A type of radiation therapy that uses high-energy photons (units of light energy). High-energy photons penetrate deeply into tissues to reach tumors while giving less radiation to superficial tissues such as the skin.

high-intensity focused ultrasound therapy: A procedure in which high-energy sound waves are aimed directly at an area of abnormal cells or tissue in the body. The waves create heat that kills the cells. High-intensity focused ultrasound therapy is being studied in the treatment of prostate cancer and some other types of cancer and other diseases.

high-risk cancer: Cancer that is likely to recur (come back), or spread.

Hodgkin lymphoma: A cancer of the immune system that is marked by the presence of a type of cell called the Reed-Sternberg cell. The two major types of Hodgkin lymphoma are classical Hodgkin lymphoma and nodular lymphocyte-predominant Hodgkin lymphoma. Symptoms include the painless enlargement of lymph nodes, spleen, or other immune tissue. Other symptoms include fever, weight loss, fatigue, or night sweats. Also called Hodgkin disease.

hormone: One of many chemicals made by glands in the body. Hormones circulate in the bloodstream and control the actions of certain cells or organs. Some hormones can also be made in the laboratory.

hormone receptor: A cell protein that binds a specific hormone. The hormone receptor may be on the surface of the cell or inside the cell. Many changes take place in a cell after a hormone binds to its receptor.

hormone receptor test: A test to measure the amount of certain proteins, called hormone receptors, in cancer tissue. Hormones can attach to these proteins. A high level of hormone receptors may mean that hormones help the cancer grow.

hospice: A program that provides special care for people who are near the end of life and for their families, either at home, in freestanding facilities, or within hospitals.

hydatidiform mole: A slow-growing tumor that develops from trophoblastic cells (cells that help an embryo attach to the uterus and help form the placenta) after fertilization of an egg by a sperm. A hydatidiform mole contains many cysts (sacs of fluid). It is usually benign (not cancer) but it may spread to nearby tissues (invasive mole). It may also become a malignant tumor called choriocarcinoma. Hydatidiform mole is the most common type of gestational trophoblastic tumor. Also called molar pregnancy.

hyperfractionated radiation therapy: Radiation treatment in which the total dose of radiation is divided into small doses and treatments are given more than once a day. Also called hyperfractionation and superfractionated radiation therapy.

hypofractionated radiation therapy: Radiation treatment in which the total dose of radiation is divided into large doses and treatments are given less than once a day. Also called hypofractionation.

hypopharyngeal cancer: Cancer that forms in tissues of the hypopharynx (the bottom part of the throat). The most common type is squamous cell carcinoma (cancer that begins in flat cells lining the hypopharynx).

hysterectomy: Surgery to remove the uterus and, sometimes, the cervix. When the uterus and the cervix are removed, it is called a total hysterectomy. When only the uterus is removed, it is called a partial hysterectomy.

idiopathic: Describes a disease of unknown cause.

imaging: In medicine, a process that makes pictures of areas inside the body. Imaging uses methods such as x-rays (high-energy radiation), ultrasound (high-energy sound waves), and radio waves.

immunosuppression: Suppression of the body's immune system and its ability to fight infections and other diseases. Immunosuppression may be deliberately induced with drugs, as in preparation for bone marrow or other organ transplantation, to prevent rejection of the donor tissue. It may also result from certain diseases such as AIDS or lymphoma or from anticancer drugs.

immunotherapy: Treatment to boost or restore the ability of the immune system to fight cancer, infections, and other diseases. Also used to lessen certain side effects that may be caused by some cancer treatments. Agents used in immunotherapy include monoclonal antibodies, growth factors, and vaccines. These agents may also have a direct antitumor effect. Also called biological response modifier therapy, biological therapy, biotherapy, and BRM therapy.

in situ: In its original place. For example, in carcinoma in situ, abnormal cells are found only in the place where they first formed. They have not spread.

in vitro: In the laboratory (outside the body). The opposite of in vivo (in the body).

in vivo: In the body. The opposite of in vitro (outside the body or in the laboratory).

incisional biopsy: A surgical procedure in which a portion of a lump or suspicious area is removed for diagnosis. The tissue is then examined under a microscope to check for signs of disease.

indolent: A type of cancer that grows slowly.

infiltrating cancer: Cancer that has spread beyond the layer of tissue in which it developed and is growing into surrounding, healthy tissues. Also called invasive cancer.

inflammatory breast cancer: A type of breast cancer in which the breast looks red and swollen and feels warm. The skin of the breast may also show the pitted appearance called peau d'orange (like the skin of an orange). The redness and warmth occur because the cancer cells block the lymph vessels in the skin.

informed consent: A process in which a person is given important facts about a medical procedure or treatment, a clinical trial, or genetic testing before deciding whether or not to participate. It also includes informing the patient when there is new information that may affect his or her decision to continue. Informed consent includes information about the possible risks, benefits, and limits of the procedure, treatment, trial, or genetic testing.

insulinoma: An abnormal mass that grows in the beta cells of the pancreas that make insulin. Insulinomas are usually benign (not cancer). They secrete insulin and are the most common cause of low blood sugar caused by having too much insulin in the body. Also called beta cell neoplasm, beta cell tumor of the pancreas, and pancreatic insulin-producing tumor.

interferon: A biological response modifier (a substance that can improve the body's natural response to infections and other diseases). Interferons interfere with the division of cancer cells and can slow tumor growth. There are several types of interferons, including interferon-alpha, -beta, and -gamma. The body normally produces these substances. They are also made in the laboratory to treat cancer and other diseases.

interleukin: One of a group of related proteins made by leukocytes (white blood cells) and other cells in the body. Interleukins regulate immune responses. Interleukins made in the laboratory are used as biological response modifiers to boost the immune system in cancer therapy. Also called IL.

interstitial radiation therapy: A type of internal radiation therapy in which radioactive material sealed in needles, seeds, wires, or catheters is placed directly into a tumor or body tissue.

intraductal carcinoma: A noninvasive condition in which abnormal cells are found in the lining of a breast duct. The abnormal cells have not spread outside the duct to other tissues in the breast. In some cases, intraductal carcinoma may become invasive cancer and spread to other tissues, although it is not known at this time how to predict which lesions will become invasive. Also called DCIS and ductal carcinoma in situ.

intraductal papilloma: A benign (not cancer), wart-like growth in a milk duct of the breast. It is usually found close to the nipple and may cause a discharge from the nipple. It may also cause pain and a lump in the breast that can be felt. It usually affects women aged 35–55 years. Having a single papilloma does not increase the risk of breast cancer. When there are multiple intraductal papillomas, they are usually found farther from the nipple. There may not be a nipple discharge and the papillomas may not be felt. Having multiple intraductal papillomas may increase the risk of breast cancer. Also called intraductal breast papilloma.

intraocular melanoma: A rare cancer of melanocytes (cells that produce the pigment melanin) found in the eye. Also called ocular melanoma.

invasive cancer: Cancer that has spread beyond the layer of tissue in which it developed and is growing into surrounding, healthy tissues. Also called infiltrating cancer.

inverted papilloma: A type of tumor in which surface epithelial cells grow downward into the underlying supportive tissue. It may occur in the nose and/or sinuses or in the urinary tract (bladder, renal pelvis, ureter, urethra). When it occurs in the nose or sinuses, it may cause symptoms similar to those caused by sinusitis, such as nasal congestion. When it occurs in the urinary tract, it may cause blood in the urine.

investigational: In clinical trials, refers to a drug (including a new drug, dose, combination, or route of administration) or procedure that has undergone basic laboratory testing and received approval from the U.S. Food and Drug Administration (FDA) to be tested in human subjects. A drug or procedure may be approved by the FDA for use in one disease or condition, but be considered investigational in other diseases or conditions. Also called experimental.

islet cell carcinoma: A rare cancer that forms in the islets of Langerhans cells (a type of cell found in the pancreas). Also called pancreatic endocrine cancer.

islet cell tumor: A mass of abnormal cells that forms in the endocrine (hormone-producing) tissues of the pancreas. Islet cell tumors may be benign (not cancer) or malignant (cancer).

jaundice: A condition in which the skin and the whites of the eyes become yellow, urine darkens, and the color of stool becomes lighter than normal. Jaundice occurs when the liver is not working properly or when a bile duct is blocked.

Jewett staging system: A staging system for prostate cancer that uses ABCD. "A" and "B" refer to cancer that is confined to the prostate. "C" refers to cancer that has grown out of the prostate but has not spread to lymph nodes or other places in the body. "D" refers to cancer that has spread to lymph nodes or to other places in the body. Also called ABCD rating and Whitmore-Jewett staging system.

Kaposi sarcoma: A type of cancer characterized by the abnormal growth of blood vessels that develop into skin lesions or occur internally.

kidney cancer: Cancer that forms in tissues of the kidneys. Kidney cancer includes renal cell carcinoma (cancer that forms in the lining of very small tubes in the kidney that filter the blood and remove waste products) and renal pelvis carcinoma (cancer that forms in the center of the kidney where urine collects). It also includes Wilms tumor, which is a type of kidney cancer that usually develops in children under the age of five.

Klatskin tumor: Cancer that develops in cells that line the bile ducts in the liver, where the right and left ducts meet. It is a type of cholangiocarcinoma.

Klinefelter syndrome: A genetic disorder in males caused by having one or more extra X chromosomes. Males with this disorder may have larger than normal breasts, a lack of facial and body hair, a rounded body type, and small testicles. They may learn to speak much later than other children and may have difficulty learning to read and write. Klinefelter syndrome increases the risk of developing extragonadal germ cell tumors and breast cancer.

Krukenberg tumor: A tumor in the ovary caused by the spread of stomach cancer.

laparoscopic surgery: Surgery done with the aid of a laparoscope. A laparoscope is a thin, tube-like instrument with a light and a lens for viewing. It may also have a tool to remove tissue to be checked under a microscope for signs of disease. Also called laparoscopic-assisted resection.

large cell carcinoma: Lung cancer in which the cells are large and look abnormal when viewed under a microscope.

large intestine: The long, tube-like organ that is connected to the small intestine at one end and the anus at the other. The large intestine has four parts: cecum, colon, rectum, and anal canal. Partly digested food moves through the cecum into the colon, where water and some nutrients and electrolytes are removed. The remaining material, solid waste called stool, moves through the colon, is stored in the rectum, and leaves the body through the anal canal and anus.

laryngeal cancer: Cancer that forms in tissues of the larynx (area of the throat that contains the vocal cords and is used for breathing, swallowing, and talking). Most laryngeal cancers are squamous cell carcinomas (cancer that begins in flat cells lining the larynx).

laryngectomee: A person whose larynx (voice box) has been removed.

laryngectomy: An operation to remove all or part of the larynx (voice box).

laser therapy: Treatment that uses intense, narrow beams of light to cut and destroy tissue, such as cancer tissue. Laser therapy may also be used to reduce lymphedema (swelling caused by a buildup of lymph fluid in tissue) after breast cancer surgery.

late effects: Side effects of cancer treatment that appear months or years after treatment has ended. Late effects include physical and mental problems and second cancers.

late-stage cancer: A term used to describe cancer that is far along in its growth, and has spread to the lymph nodes or other places in the body.

leptomeningeal carcinoma: A serious problem that may occur in cancer in which cancer cells spread from the original (primary) tumor to the meninges (thin layers of tissue that cover and protect the brain and spinal cord). It can happen in many types of cancer, but is the most common in melanoma, breast, lung, and gastrointestinal cancer. The cancer may cause the meninges to be inflamed. Also called carcinomatous meningitis, leptomeningeal metastasis, meningeal carcinomatosis, meningeal metastasis, and neoplastic meningitis.

leukemia: Cancer that starts in blood-forming tissue such as the bone marrow and causes large numbers of blood cells to be produced and enter the bloodstream.

leukopenia: A condition in which there is a lower-than-normal number of leukocytes (white blood cells) in the blood.

leukoplakia: An abnormal patch of white tissue that forms on mucous membranes in the mouth and other areas of the body. It may become cancer. Tobacco (smoking and chewing) and alcohol may increase the risk of leukoplakia in the mouth.

light therapy: The treatment of disease with certain types of light. Light therapy can use lasers, LED, fluorescent lamps, and ultraviolet or infrared radiation. Also called phototherapy.

liver cancer: Primary liver cancer is cancer that forms in the tissues of the liver. Secondary liver cancer is cancer that spreads to the liver from another part of the body.

liver function test: A blood test to measure the blood levels of certain substances released by the liver. A high or low level of certain substances can be a sign of liver disease.

liver metastasis: Cancer that has spread from the original (primary) tumor to the liver.

living will: A type of legal advance directive in which a person describes specific treatment guidelines that are to be followed by health care providers if he or she becomes terminally ill and cannot communicate. A living will usually has instructions about whether to use aggressive medical treatment to keep a person alive (such as CPR, artificial nutrition, use of a respirator).

lobe: A portion of an organ, such as the liver, lung, breast, thyroid, or brain.

lobectomy: Surgery to remove a whole lobe (section) of an organ (such as the lungs, liver, brain, or thyroid gland).

lobular carcinoma in situ: A condition in which abnormal cells are found in the lobules of the breast. Lobular carcinoma in situ seldom becomes invasive cancer; however, having it in one breast increases the risk of developing breast cancer in either breast. Also called LCIS.

lobule: A small lobe or a subdivision of a lobe.

local anesthesia: A temporary loss of feeling in one small area of the body caused by special drugs or other substances called anesthetics. The patient stays awake but has no feeling in the area of the body treated with the anesthetic.

local cancer: An invasive malignant cancer confined entirely to the organ where the cancer began.

local therapy: Treatment that affects cells in the tumor and the area close to it.

localized: Restricted to the site of origin, without evidence of spread.

locally advanced cancer: Cancer that has spread from where it started to nearby tissue or lymph nodes.

locally recurrent cancer: Cancer that has recurred (come back) at or near the same place as the original (primary) tumor, usually after a period of time during which the cancer could not be detected.

loop electrosurgical excision procedure: A technique that uses electric current passed through a thin wire loop to remove abnormal tissue. Also called LEEP and loop excision.

low grade: A term used to describe cells that look nearly normal under a microscope. These cells are less likely to grow and spread more quickly than cells in high-grade cancer or in growths that may become cancer.

lower GI series: X-rays of the colon and rectum that are taken after a person is given a barium enema.

lumbar puncture: A procedure in which a thin needle called a spinal needle is put into the lower part of the spinal column to collect cerebrospinal fluid or to give drugs. Also called spinal tap.

lumpectomy: Surgery to remove abnormal tissue or cancer from the breast and a small amount of normal tissue around it. It is a type of breast-sparing surgery.

lung biopsy: The removal of a small piece of lung tissue to be checked by a pathologist for cancer or other diseases. The tissue may be removed using a bronchoscope (a thin, lighted, tube-like instrument that is inserted through the trachea and into the lung). It may also be removed using a fine needle inserted through the chest wall, by surgery guided by a video camera inserted through the chest wall, or by an open biopsy. In an open biopsy, a doctor makes an incision between the ribs, removes a sample of lung tissue, and closes the wound with stitches.

lung cancer: Cancer that forms in tissues of the lung, usually in the cells lining air passages. The two main types are small cell lung cancer and non-small cell lung cancer. These types are diagnosed based on how the cells look under a microscope.

lung function test: A test used to measure how well the lungs work. It measures how much air the lungs can hold and how quickly air is moved into and out of the lungs. It also measures how much oxygen is used and how much carbon dioxide is given off during breathing. A lung function test can be used to diagnose a lung disease and to see how well treatment for the disease is working. Also called PFT and pulmonary function test.

lung metastasis: Cancer that has spread from the original (primary) tumor to the lung.

lymph node: A rounded mass of lymphatic tissue that is surrounded by a capsule of connective tissue. Lymph nodes filter lymph (lymphatic fluid), and they store lymphocytes (white blood cells). They are located along lymphatic vessels. Also called lymph gland.

lymph node dissection: A surgical procedure in which the lymph nodes are removed and a sample of tissue is checked under a microscope for signs of cancer. For a regional lymph node dissection, some of the lymph nodes in the tumor area are removed; for a radical lymph node dissection, most or all of the lymph nodes in the tumor area are removed. Also called lymphadenectomy.

lymphatic system: The tissues and organs that produce, store, and carry white blood cells that fight infections and other diseases. This system includes the bone marrow, spleen, thymus, lymph nodes, and lymphatic vessels (a network of thin tubes that carry lymph and white blood cells). Lymphatic vessels branch, like blood vessels, into all the tissues of the body.

lymphedema: A condition in which extra lymph fluid builds up in tissues and causes swelling. It may occur in an arm or leg if lymph vessels are blocked, damaged, or removed by surgery.

lymphoma: Cancer that begins in cells of the immune system. There are two basic categories of lymphomas. One kind is Hodgkin lymphoma, which is marked by the presence of a type of cell called the Reed-Sternberg cell. The other category is non-Hodgkin lymphomas, which includes a large, diverse group of cancers of immune system cells. Non-Hodgkin lymphomas can be further divided into cancers that have an indolent (slow-growing) course and those that have an aggressive (fast-growing) course. These subtypes behave and respond to treatment differently. Both Hodgkin and non-Hodgkin lymphomas can occur in children and adults, and prognosis and treatment depend on the stage and the type of cancer.

macrocalcification: A small deposit of calcium in the breast that cannot be felt but can be seen on a mammogram. It is usually caused by aging, an old injury, or inflamed tissue and is usually not related to cancer.

magnetic resonance imaging: A procedure in which radio waves and a powerful magnet linked to a computer are used to create detailed pictures of areas inside the body. These pictures can show the difference between normal and diseased tissue. Magnetic resonance imaging makes better images of organs and soft tissue than other scanning techniques, such as computed tomography (CT) or x-ray. Magnetic resonance imaging is especially useful for imaging the brain, the spine, the soft tissue of joints, and the inside of bones. Also called MRI, NMRI, and nuclear magnetic resonance imaging.

maintenance therapy: Treatment that is given to help keep cancer from coming back after it has disappeared following the initial therapy. It may include treatment with drugs, vaccines, or antibodies that kill cancer cells, and it may be given for a long time.

malignancy: A term for diseases in which abnormal cells divide without control and can invade nearby tissues. Malignant cells can also spread to other parts of the body through the blood and lymph systems. There are several main types of malignancy. Carcinoma is a malignancy that begins in the skin or in tissues that line or cover internal organs. Sarcoma is a malignancy that begins in bone, cartilage, fat, muscle, blood vessels, or other connective or supportive tissue. Leukemia is a malignancy that starts in blood-forming tissue such as the bone marrow, and causes large numbers of abnormal blood cells to be produced and enter the blood. Lymphoma and multiple myeloma are malignancies that begin in the cells of the immune system. Central nervous system cancers are malignancies that begin in the tissues of the brain and spinal cord. Also called cancer.

mammary dysplasia: A common condition marked by benign (not cancer) changes in breast tissue. These changes may include irregular lumps or cysts, breast discomfort, sensitive nipples, and itching. These symptoms may change throughout the menstrual cycle and usually stop after menopause. Also called benign breast disease, fibrocystic breast changes, and fibrocystic breast disease.

mammography: The use of film or a computer to create a picture of the breast.

margin: The edge or border of the tissue removed in cancer surgery. The margin is described as negative or clean when the pathologist finds no cancer cells at the edge of the tissue, suggesting that all of the cancer has been removed. The margin is described as positive or involved when the pathologist finds cancer cells at the edge of the tissue, suggesting that all of the cancer has not been removed.

mass: In medicine, a lump in the body. It may be caused by the abnormal growth of cells, a cyst, hormonal changes, or an immune reaction. A mass may be benign (not cancer) or malignant (cancer).

mastectomy: Surgery to remove the breast (or as much of the breast tissue as possible).

medullary thyroid cancer: Cancer that develops in C cells of the thyroid. The C cells make a hormone (calcitonin) that helps maintain a healthy level of calcium in the blood.

medulloblastoma: A malignant brain tumor that begins in the lower part of the brain and that can spread to the spine or to other parts of the body. Medulloblastomas are a type of primitive neuroectodermal tumor (PNET).

melanoma: A form of cancer that begins in melanocytes (cells that make the pigment melanin). It may begin in a mole (skin melanoma), but can also begin in other pigmented tissues, such as in the eye or in the intestines.

meningioma: A type of slow-growing tumor that forms in the meninges (thin layers of tissue that cover and protect the brain and spinal cord). Meningiomas usually occur in adults.

Merkel cell carcinoma: A rare type of cancer that forms on or just beneath the skin, usually in parts of the body that have been exposed to the sun. It is most common in older people and in people with weakened immune systems. Also called Merkel cell cancer, neuroendocrine carcinoma of the skin, and trabecular cancer.

mesothelioma: A benign (not cancer) or malignant (cancer) tumor affecting the lining of the chest or abdomen. Exposure to asbestos particles in the air increases the risk of developing malignant mesothelioma.

metaplastic carcinoma: A general term used to describe cancer that begins in cells that have changed into another cell type (for example, a squamous cell of the esophagus changing to resemble a cell of the stomach). In some cases, metaplastic changes alone may mean there is an increased chance of cancer developing at the site.

metastasis: The spread of cancer from one part of the body to another. A tumor formed by cells that have spread is called a "metastatic tumor" or a "metastasis." The metastatic tumor contains cells that are like those in the original (primary) tumor. The plural form of metastasis is metastases (meh-TAS-tuh-SEEZ).

microcalcification: A tiny deposit of calcium in the breast that cannot be felt but can be detected on a mammogram. A cluster of these very small specks of calcium may indicate that cancer is present.

micrometastasis: Small numbers of cancer cells that have spread from the primary tumor to other parts of the body and are too few to be picked up in a screening or diagnostic test.

microstaging: A technique used to help determine the stage (extent) of melanoma and certain squamous cell cancers. A sample of skin that contains tumor tissue is examined under a microscope to find out how thick the tumor is and/or how deeply the tumor has grown into the skin or connective tissues.

microwave thermotherapy: A type of treatment in which body tissue is exposed to high temperatures to damage and kill cancer cells or to make cancer cells more sensitive to the effects of radiation and certain anticancer drugs. Also called microwave therapy.

Mohs surgery: A surgical procedure used to treat skin cancer. Individual layers of cancer tissue are removed and examined under a microscope one at a time until all cancer tissue has been removed.

mole: A benign (not cancer) growth on the skin that is formed by a cluster of melanocytes (cells that make a substance called melanin, which gives color to skin and eyes). A mole is usually dark and may be raised from the skin. Also called nevus.

molecularly targeted therapy: In cancer treatment, substances that kill cancer cells by targeting key molecules involved in cancer cell growth.

monoclonal antibody: A type of protein made in the laboratory that can bind to substances in the body, including tumor cells. There are many kinds of monoclonal antibodies. Each monoclonal antibody is made to find one substance. Monoclonal antibodies are being used to treat some types of cancer and are being studied in the treatment of other types. They can be used alone or to carry drugs, toxins, or radio-active materials directly to a tumor.

multicentric breast cancer: Breast cancer in which there is more than one tumor, all of which have formed separately from one another. The tumors are likely to be in different quadrants (sections) of the breast. Multicentric breast cancers are rare.

multifocal breast cancer: Breast cancer in which there is more than one tumor, all of which have arisen from one original tumor. The tumors are likely to be in the same quadrant (section) of the breast.

multiple endocrine neoplasia syndrome: An inherited condition that may result in the development of cancers of the endocrine system. There are several types of multiple endocrine neoplasia syndrome, and patients with each type may develop different types of cancer. The altered genes that cause each type can be detected with a blood test. Also called MEN syndrome.

multiple myeloma: A type of cancer that begins in plasma cells (white blood cells that produce antibodies). Also called Kahler disease, my-elomatosis, and plasma cell myeloma.

mutation: Any change in the DNA of a cell. Mutations may be caused by mistakes during cell division, or they may be caused by exposure to DNA-damaging agents in the environment. Mutations can be harm-ful, beneficial, or have no effect. If they occur in cells that make eggs or sperm, they can be inherited; if mutations occur in other types of cells, they are not inherited. Certain mutations may lead to cancer or other diseases.

myeloablative chemotherapy: High-dose chemotherapy that kills cells in the bone marrow, including cancer cells. It lowers the number of normal blood-forming cells in the bone marrow, and can cause severe side effects. Myeloablative chemotherapy is usually followed by a bone marrow or stem cell transplant to rebuild the bone marrow.

myelodysplastic syndromes: A group of diseases in which the bone marrow does not make enough healthy blood cells. Also called preleukemia and smoldering leukemia.

myelogenous: Having to do with, produced by, or resembling the bone marrow. Sometimes used as a synonym for myeloid; for example, acute myeloid leukemia and acute myelogenous leukemia are the same disease.

myeloid: Having to do with or resembling the bone marrow. May also refer to certain types of hematopoietic (blood-forming) cells found in the bone marrow. Sometimes used as a synonym for myelogenous.

myeloma: Cancer that arises in plasma cells, a type of white blood cell.

myelomatosis: A type of cancer that begins in plasma cells (white blood cells that produce antibodies). Also called Kahler disease, multiple myeloma, and plasma cell myeloma.

myeloproliferative disorder: A group of slow growing blood cancers, including chronic myelogenous leukemia, in which large numbers of abnormal red blood cells, white blood cells, or platelets grow and spread in the bone marrow and the peripheral blood.

nasopharyngeal cancer: Cancer that forms in tissues of the nasopharynx (upper part of the throat behind the nose). Most nasopharyngeal cancers are squamous cell carcinomas (cancer that begins in flat cells lining the nasopharynx).

neck dissection: Surgery to remove lymph nodes and other tissues in the neck.

necrosis: Refers to the death of living tissues.

needle biopsy: The removal of tissue or fluid with a needle for examination under a microscope. When a wide needle is used, the procedure is called a core biopsy. When a thin needle is used, the procedure is called a fine-needle aspiration biopsy.

negative axillary lymph node: A lymph node in the armpit that is free of cancer.

neoadjuvant therapy: Treatment given as a first step to shrink a tumor before the main treatment, which is usually surgery, is given. Examples of neoadjuvant therapy include chemotherapy, radiation therapy, and hormone therapy. It is a type of induction therapy.

neoplasm: An abnormal mass of tissue that results when cells divide more than they should or do not die when they should. Neoplasms may be benign (not cancer), or malignant (cancer). Also called tumor.

neuroblastoma: Cancer that arises in immature nerve cells and affects mostly infants and children.

neuroectodermal tumor: A tumor of the central or peripheral nervous system.

neuroendocrine tumor: A tumor that forms from cells that release hormones in response to a signal from the nervous system. Some examples of neuroendocrine tumors are carcinoid tumors, islet cell tumors, medullary thyroid carcinomas, pheochromocytomas, and neuroendocrine carcinomas of the skin (Merkel cell cancer). These tumors may secrete higher-than-normal amounts of hormones, which can cause many different symptoms.

neurofibroma: A benign tumor that develops from the cells and tissues that cover nerves.

neuroma: A tumor that arises in nerve cells.

neuropathy: A nerve problem that causes pain, numbness, tingling, swelling, or muscle weakness in different parts of the body. It usually begins in the hands or feet and gets worse over time. Neuropathy may be caused by physical injury, infection, toxic substances, disease (such as cancer, diabetes, kidney failure, or malnutrition), or drugs, including anticancer drugs.

nevus: A benign (not cancer) growth on the skin that is formed by a cluster of melanocytes (cells that make a substance called melanin, which gives color to skin and eyes). A nevus is usually dark and may be raised from the skin. Also called mole.

node-negative: Cancer that has not spread to the lymph nodes.

node-positive: Cancer that has spread to the lymph nodes.

nodule: A growth or lump that may be malignant (cancer) or benign (not cancer).

non-Hodgkin lymphoma: Any of a large group of cancers of lymphocytes (white blood cells). Non-Hodgkin lymphomas can occur at any age and are often marked by lymph nodes that are larger than normal, fever, and weight loss. There are many different types of non-Hodgkin lymphoma. These types can be divided into aggressive (fast-growing) and indolent (slow-growing) types, and they can be formed from either B-cells or T-cells. B-cell non-Hodgkin lymphomas include Burkitt lymphoma, chronic lymphocytic leukemia/small lymphocytic lymphoma (CLL/SLL), diffuse large B-cell lymphoma, follicular lymphoma, immunoblastic large cell lymphoma, precursor B-lymphoblastic lymphoma, and mantle cell lymphoma. T-cell non-Hodgkin lymphomas include mycosis fungoides, anaplastic large cell lymphoma, and precursor T-lymphoblastic lymphoma. Lymphomas that occur after bone marrow or stem cell transplantation are usually B-cell non-Hodgkin lymphomas. Prognosis and treatment depend on the stage and type of disease. Also called NHL.

non-small cell lung cancer: A group of lung cancers that are named for the kinds of cells found in the cancer and how the cells look under a microscope. The three main types of non-small cell lung cancer are squamous cell carcinoma, large cell carcinoma, and adenocarcinoma. Non-small cell lung cancer is the most common kind of lung cancer.

nonfunctioning tumor: A tumor that is found in endocrine tissue but does not make extra hormones. Nonfunctioning tumors usually do not cause symptoms until they grow large or spread to other parts of the body. Also called endocrine-inactive tumor.

noninvasive: In medicine, it describes a procedure that does not require inserting an instrument through the skin or into a body opening. In cancer, it describes disease that has not spread outside the tissue in which it began.

nonmalignant: Not cancerous. Nonmalignant tumors may grow larger but do not spread to other parts of the body. Also called benign.

nonmelanoma skin cancer: Skin cancer that forms in the lower part of the epidermis (the outer layer of the skin) or in squamous cells, but not in melanocytes (skin cells that make pigment).

nonmetastatic: Cancer that has not spread from the primary site (place where it started) to other places in the body.

nonseminoma: A group of testicular cancers that begin in the germ cells (cells that give rise to sperm). Nonseminomas are identified by the type of cell in which they begin and include embryonal carcinoma, teratoma, choriocarcinoma, and yolk sac carcinoma.

nuclear medicine scan: A method of diagnostic imaging that uses very small amounts of radioactive material. The patient is injected with a liquid that contains the radioactive substance, which collects in the part of the body to be imaged. Sophisticated instruments detect the radioactive substance in the body and process that information into an image. Also called nuclear scan.

occult primary tumor: Cancer in which the site of the primary (original) tumor cannot be found. Most metastases from occult primary tumors are found in the head and neck.

occult stage non-small cell lung cancer: Cancer cells are found in sputum (mucus coughed up from the lungs), but no tumor can be found in the lung by imaging tests or bronchoscopy, or the tumor is too small to be checked.

ocular melanoma: A rare cancer of melanocytes (cells that produce the pigment melanin) found in the eye. Also called intraocular melanoma.

oncogene: A gene that is a mutated (changed) form of a gene involved in normal cell growth. Oncogenes may cause the growth of cancer cells. Mutations in genes that become oncogenes can be inherited or caused by being exposed to substances in the environment that cause cancer.

oncologist: A doctor who specializes in treating cancer. Some oncologists specialize in a particular type of cancer treatment. For example, a radiation oncologist specializes in treating cancer with radiation.

open biopsy: A procedure in which a surgical incision (cut) is made through the skin to expose and remove tissues. The biopsy tissue is examined under a microscope by a pathologist. An open biopsy may be done in the doctor's office or in the hospital, and may use local anesthesia or general anesthesia. A lumpectomy to remove a breast tumor is a type of open biopsy.

open resection: Surgery to remove part or all of an organ or a tumor and nearby lymph nodes. The incision is large enough to let the surgeon see into the body.

oral cancer: Cancer that forms in tissues of the oral cavity (the mouth) or the oropharynx (the part of the throat at the back of the mouth).

oral cavity cancer: Cancer that forms in tissues of the oral cavity (the mouth). The tissues of the oral cavity include the lips, the lining inside the cheeks and lips, the front two thirds of the tongue, the upper and lower gums, the floor of the mouth under the tongue, the bony roof of the mouth, and the small area behind the wisdom teeth.

oropharyngeal cancer: Cancer that forms in tissues of the oropharynx (the part of the throat at the back of the mouth, including the soft palate, the base of the tongue, and the tonsils). Most oropharyngeal cancers are squamous cell carcinomas (cancer that begins in flat cells lining the oropharynx).

osteosarcoma: A cancer of the bone that usually affects the large bones of the arm or leg. It occurs most commonly in young people and affects more males than females. Also called osteogenic sarcoma.

ovarian cancer: Cancer that forms in tissues of the ovary (one of a pair of female reproductive glands in which the ova, or eggs, are formed). Most ovarian cancers are either ovarian epithelial carcinomas (cancer that begins in the cells on the surface of the ovary) or malignant germ cell tumors (cancer that begins in egg cells).

ovarian germ cell tumor: An abnormal mass of tissue that forms in germ (egg) cells in the ovary (female reproductive gland in which the eggs are formed). These tumors usually occur in teenage girls or young women, usually affect just one ovary, and can be benign (not cancer) or malignant (cancer). The most common ovarian germ cell tumor is called dysgerminoma.

ovarian low malignant potential tumor: A condition in which cells that may become cancer form in the thin layer of tissue that covers an ovary (female reproductive gland in which eggs are made). In this condition, tumor cells rarely spread outside of the ovary. Also called ovarian borderline malignant tumor.

p53 gene: A tumor suppressor gene that normally inhibits the growth of tumors. This gene is altered in many types of cancer.

Paget disease of the nipple: A form of breast cancer in which the tumor grows from ducts beneath the nipple onto the surface of the nipple. Symptoms commonly include itching and burning and an eczema-like condition around the nipple, sometimes accompanied by oozing or bleeding.

palliative care: Care given to improve the quality of life of patients who have a serious or life-threatening disease. The goal of palliative care is to prevent or treat as early as possible the symptoms of a disease, side effects caused by treatment of a disease, and psychological, social, and spiritual problems related to a disease or its treatment. Also called comfort care, supportive care, and symptom management.

palliative therapy: Treatment given to relieve the symptoms and reduce the suffering caused by cancer and other life-threatening diseases. Palliative cancer therapies are given together with other cancer treatments, from the time of diagnosis, through treatment, survivorship, recurrent or advanced disease, and at the end of life.

palpable disease: A term used to describe cancer that can be felt by touch, usually present in lymph nodes, skin, or other organs of the body such as the liver or colon.

pancreatic cancer: A disease in which malignant (cancer) cells are found in the tissues of the pancreas. Also called exocrine cancer.

pancreatic endocrine cancer: A rare cancer that forms in the islets of Langerhans cells (a type of cell found in the pancreas). Also called islet cell carcinoma.

pancreatic insulin-producing tumor: An abnormal mass that grows in the beta cells of the pancreas that make insulin. Pancreatic insulin-producing tumors are usually benign (not cancer). They secrete insulin and are the most common cause of low blood sugar caused by having too much insulin in the body. Also called beta cell neoplasm, beta cell tumor of the pancreas, and insulinoma.

Pap smear: A procedure in which cells are scraped from the cervix for examination under a microscope. It is used to detect cancer and changes that may lead to cancer. A Pap smear can also show conditions, such as infection or inflammation, that are not cancer. Also called Pap test and Papanicolaou test.

papillary serous carcinoma: An aggressive cancer that usually affects the uterus/endometrium, peritoneum, or ovary.

papillary tumor: A tumor shaped like a small mushroom, with its stem attached to the epithelial layer (inner lining) of an organ.

paraganglioma: A rare, usually benign tumor that develops from cells of the paraganglia. Paraganglia are a collection of cells that came from embryonic nervous tissue, and are found near the adrenal glands and some blood vessels and nerves. Paragangliomas that develop in the adrenal gland are called pheochromocytomas. Those that develop outside of the adrenal glands near blood vessels or nerves are called glomus tumors or chemodectomas.

paranasal sinus and nasal cavity cancer: Cancer that forms in tissues of the paranasal sinuses (small hollow spaces in the bones around the nose) or nasal cavity (the inside of the nose). The most common type of paranasal sinus and nasal cavity cancer is squamous cell carcinoma (cancer that begins in flat cells lining these tissues and cavities).

parathyroid cancer: A rare cancer that forms in tissues of one or more of the parathyroid glands (four pea-sized glands in the neck that make parathyroid hormone, which helps the body store and use calcium).

parotid gland cancer: Cancer that forms in a parotid gland, the largest of the salivary glands, which make saliva and release it into the mouth. There are two parotid glands, one in front of and just below each ear. Most salivary gland tumors begin in parotid glands.

partial-breast irradiation: A type of radiation therapy given only to the part of the breast that has cancer in it. Partial-breast irradiation gives a higher dose over a shorter time than is given in standard whole-breast radiation therapy. Partial-breast irradiation may be given using internal or external sources of radiation. Also called accelerated partial-breast irradiation.

pathological stage: The stage of cancer (amount or spread of cancer in the body) that is based on how different from normal the cells in samples of tissue look under a microscope.

pathologist: A doctor who identifies diseases by studying cells and tissues under a microscope.

pathology report: The description of cells and tissues made by a pathologist based on microscopic evidence, and sometimes used to make a diagnosis of a disease.

pelvic lymphadenectomy: Surgery to remove lymph nodes in the pelvis for examination under a microscope to see if they contain cancer.

penile cancer: A rare cancer that forms in the penis (an external male reproductive organ). Most penile cancers are squamous cell carcinomas (cancer that begins in flat cells lining the penis).

periampullary cancer: A cancer that forms near the ampulla of Vater (an enlargement of the ducts from the liver and pancreas where they join and enter the small intestine).

peripheral primitive neuroectodermal tumor: A type of cancer that forms in bone or soft tissue. Also called Ewing sarcoma and pPNET.

peritoneal cancer: Cancer of the tissue that lines the abdominal wall and covers organs in the abdomen.

Peutz-Jeghers syndrome: A genetic disorder in which polyps form in the intestine and dark spots appear on the mouth and fingers. Having PJS increases the risk of developing gastrointestinal and many other types of cancer. Also called PJS.

pharyngeal cancer: Cancer that forms in tissues of the pharynx (the hollow tube inside the neck that starts behind the nose and ends at the top of the windpipe and esophagus). Pharyngeal cancer includes cancer of the nasopharynx (the upper part of the throat behind the nose), the oropharynx (the middle part of the pharynx), and the hypopharynx (the bottom part of the pharynx). Cancer of the larynx (voice box) may also be included as a type of pharyngeal cancer. Most pharyngeal cancers are squamous cell carcinomas (cancer that begins in thin, flat cells that look like fish scales). Also called throat cancer.

phase I trial: The first step in testing a new treatment in humans. These studies test the best way to give a new treatment (for example, by mouth, intravenous infusion, or injection) and the best dose. The dose is usually increased a little at a time in order to find the highest dose that does not cause harmful side effects. Because little is known about the possible risks and benefits of the treatments being tested, phase I trials usually include only a small number of patients who have not been helped by other treatments.

phase I/II trial: A trial to study the safety, dosage levels, and response to a new treatment.

phase II trial: A study to test whether a new treatment has an anticancer effect (for example, whether it shrinks a tumor or improves blood test results) and whether it works against a certain type of cancer.

phase II/III trial: A trial to study response to a new treatment and the effectiveness of the treatment compared with the standard treatment regimen.

phase III trial: A study to compare the results of people taking a new treatment with the results of people taking the standard treatment (for example, which group has better survival rates or fewer side effects). In most cases, studies move into phase III only after a treatment seems to work in phases I and II. Phase III trials may include hundreds of people.

phase IV trial: After a treatment has been approved and is being marketed, it is studied in a phase IV trial to evaluate side effects that were not apparent in the phase III trial. Thousands of people are involved in a phase IV trial. Also called post-marketing surveillance trials.

pheochromocytoma: Tumor that forms in the center of the adrenal gland (gland located above the kidney) that causes it to make too much adrenaline. Pheochromocytomas are usually benign (not cancer) but can cause high blood pressure, pounding headaches, heart palpitations, flushing of the face, nausea, and vomiting.

photon beam radiation therapy: A type of radiation therapy that uses x-rays or gamma rays that come from a special machine called a linear accelerator (linac). The radiation dose is delivered at the surface of the body and goes into the tumor and through the body. Photon beam radiation therapy is different from proton beam therapy.

phototherapy: The treatment of disease with certain types of light. Phototherapy can use lasers, LED, fluorescent lamps, and ultraviolet or infrared radiation. Also called light therapy.

pineal region tumor: A type of brain tumor that occurs in or around the pineal gland, a tiny organ near the center of the brain.

pineoblastoma: A fast growing type of brain tumor that occurs in or around the pineal gland, a tiny organ near the center of the brain.

pineocytoma: A slow growing type of brain tumor that occurs in or around the pineal gland, a tiny organ near the center of the brain.

pituitary tumor: A tumor that forms in the pituitary gland. The pituitary is a pea-sized organ in the center of the brain above the back of the nose. It makes hormones that affect other glands and many body functions, especially growth. Most pituitary tumors are benign (not cancer).

placebo: An inactive substance or treatment that looks the same as, and is given the same way as, an active drug or treatment being tested. The effects of the active drug or treatment are compared to the effects of the placebo.

plaque radiotherapy: A type of radiation therapy used to treat eye tumors. A thin piece of metal (usually gold) with radioactive seeds placed on one side is sewn onto the outside wall of the eye with the seeds aimed at the tumor. It is removed at the end of treatment, which usually lasts for several days

plasma cell tumor: A tumor that begins in plasma cells (white blood cells that produce antibodies). Multiple myeloma, monoclonal gammopathy of undetermined significance (MGUS), and plasmacytoma are types of plasma cell tumors.

plasmacytoma: A type of cancer that begins in plasma cells (white blood cells that produce antibodies). A plasmacytoma may turn into multiple myeloma.

polycystic ovary syndrome: A condition marked by infertility, enlarged ovaries, menstrual problems, high levels of male hormones, excess hair on the face and body, acne, and obesity. Women with polycystic ovary syndrome have an increased risk of diabetes, high blood pressure, heart disease, and endometrial cancer. Also called PCOS.

polyp: A growth that protrudes from a mucous membrane.

port-a-cath: An implanted device through which blood may be withdrawn and drugs may be infused without repeated needle sticks. Also called port.

positive axillary lymph node: A lymph node in the area of the armpit (axilla) to which cancer has spread. This spread is determined by surgically removing some of the lymph nodes and examining them under a microscope to see whether cancer cells are present.

positron emission tomography scan: A procedure in which a small amount of radioactive glucose (sugar) is injected into a vein, and a scanner is used to make detailed, computerized pictures of areas inside the body where the glucose is used. Because cancer cells often use more glucose than normal cells, the pictures can be used to find cancer cells in the body. Also called PET scan.

postremission therapy: Treatment that is given after cancer has disappeared following the initial therapy. Postremission therapy is used to kill any cancer cells that may be left in the body. It may include radiation therapy, a stem cell transplant, or treatment with drugs that kill cancer cells. Also called consolidation therapy and intensification therapy.

predictive factor: A condition or finding that can be used to help predict whether a person's cancer will respond to a specific treatment. Predictive factor may also describe something that increases a person's risk of developing a condition or disease.

preleukemia: A group of diseases in which the bone marrow does not make enough healthy blood cells. Also called myelodysplastic syndromes and smoldering leukemia.

premalignant: A term used to describe a condition that may (or is likely to) become cancer. Also called precancerous.

primary CNS lymphoma: Cancer that forms in the lymph tissue of the brain, spinal cord, meninges (outer covering of the brain), or eye (called ocular lymphoma). Also called PCNSL and primary central nervous system lymphoma.

primary therapy: Initial treatment used to reduce a cancer. Primary therapy is followed by other treatments, such as chemotherapy, radiation therapy, and hormone therapy to get rid of cancer that remains. Also called first-line therapy, induction therapy, and primary treatment.

primary tumor: The original tumor.

primitive neuroectodermal tumor: One of a group of cancers that develop from the same type of early cells, and share certain biochemical and genetic features. Some primitive neuroectodermal tumors develop in the brain and central nervous system (CNS-PNET), and others develop in sites outside of the brain such as the limbs, pelvis, and chest wall (peripheral PNET). Also called PNET.

progesterone receptor positive: Describes cells that have a protein to which the hormone progesterone will bind. Cancer cells that are PR+ need progesterone to grow and will usually stop growing when treated with hormones that block progesterone from binding. Also called PR+.

progesterone receptor negative: Describes cells that do not have a protein to which the hormone progesterone will bind. Cancer cells that are PR- do not need progesterone to grow, and usually do not stop growing when treated with hormones that block progesterone from binding. Also called PR-.

prognostic factor: A situation or condition, or a characteristic of a patient, that can be used to estimate the chance of recovery from a disease or the chance of the disease recurring (coming back).

programmed cell death: A type of cell death in which a series of molecular steps in a cell leads to its death. This is the body's normal way of getting rid of unneeded or abnormal cells. The process of programmed cell death may be blocked in cancer cells. Also called apoptosis.

prostate-specific antigen: A protein made by the prostate gland and found in the blood. Prostate-specific antigen blood levels may be higher than normal in men who have prostate cancer, benign prostatic hyperplasia (BPH), or infection or inflammation of the prostate gland. Also called PSA.

proton beam radiation therapy: A type of radiation therapy that uses streams of protons (tiny particles with a positive charge) that come from a special machine. This type of radiation kills tumor cells but does not damage nearby tissues. It is used to treat cancers in the head and neck and in organs such as the brain, eye, lung, spine, and prostate. Proton beam radiation is different from x-ray radiation.

pulmonary sulcus tumor: A type of lung cancer that begins in the upper part of a lung and spreads to nearby tissues such as the ribs and vertebrae. Most pulmonary sulcus tumors are non-small cell cancers. Also called Pancoast tumor.

punch biopsy: Removal of a small disk-shaped sample of tissue using a sharp, hollow device. The tissue is then examined under a microscope.

radiation enteritis: Inflammation of the small intestine caused by radiation therapy to the abdomen, pelvis, or rectum. Symptoms include nausea, vomiting, abdominal pain and cramping, frequent bowel movements, watery or bloody diarrhea, fatty stools, and weight loss. Some of these symptoms may continue for a long time.

radiation therapy: The use of high-energy radiation from x-rays, gamma rays, neutrons, protons, and other sources to kill cancer cells and shrink tumors. Radiation may come from a machine outside the body (external-beam radiation therapy), or it may come from radioactive material placed in the body near cancer cells (internal radiation therapy). Systemic radiation therapy uses a radioactive substance, such as a radiolabeled monoclonal antibody, that travels in the blood to tissues throughout the body. Also called irradiation and radiotherapy.

radical local excision: Surgery to remove a tumor and a large amount of normal tissue surrounding it. Nearby lymph nodes may also be removed.

radical lymph node dissection: A surgical procedure to remove most or all of the lymph nodes that drain lymph from the area around a tumor. The lymph nodes are then examined under a microscope to see if cancer cells have spread to them.

radioactive iodine: A radioactive form of iodine, often used for imaging tests or to treat an overactive thyroid, thyroid cancer, and certain other cancers. For imaging tests, the patient takes a small dose of radioactive iodine that collects in thyroid cells and certain kinds of tumors and can be detected by a scanner. To treat thyroid cancer, the patient takes a large dose of radioactive iodine, which kills thyroid cells. Radioactive iodine is also used in internal radiation therapy for prostate cancer, intraocular (eye) melanoma, and carcinoid tumors. Radioactive iodine is given by mouth as a liquid or in capsules, by infusion, or sealed in seeds, which are placed in or near the tumor to kill cancer cells.

radiofrequency ablation: A procedure that uses radio waves to heat and destroy abnormal cells. The radio waves travel through electrodes (small devices that carry electricity). Radiofrequency ablation may be used to treat cancer and other conditions.

radiosurgery: A type of external radiation therapy that uses special equipment to position the patient and precisely give a single large dose of radiation to a tumor. It is used to treat brain tumors and other brain disorders that cannot be treated by regular surgery. It is also being studied in the treatment of other types of cancer. Also called radiation surgery, stereotactic radiosurgery, and stereotaxic radiosurgery.

randomized clinical trial: A study in which the participants are assigned by chance to separate groups that compare different treatments; neither the researchers nor the participants can choose which group. Using chance to assign people to groups means that the groups will be similar and that the treatments they receive can be compared objectively. At the time of the trial, it is not known which treatment is best. It is the patient's choice to be in a randomized trial.

recurrent cancer: Cancer that has recurred (come back), usually after a period of time during which the cancer could not be detected. The cancer may come back to the same place as the original (primary) tumor or to another place in the body. Also called recurrence.

Reed-Sternberg cell: A type of cell that appears in people with Hodgkin disease. The number of these cells increases as the disease advances.

refractory cancer: Cancer that does not respond to treatment. The cancer may be resistant at the beginning of treatment or it may become resistant during treatment. Also called resistant cancer.

regional lymph node dissection: A surgical procedure to remove some of the lymph nodes that drain lymph from the area around a tumor. The lymph nodes are then examined under a microscope to see if cancer cells have spread to them.

remission: A decrease in or disappearance of signs and symptoms of cancer. In partial remission, some, but not all, signs and symptoms of cancer have disappeared. In complete remission, all signs and symptoms of cancer have disappeared, although cancer still may be in the body.

remote brachytherapy: A type of internal radiation treatment in which the radioactive source is removed between treatments. Also called high-dose-rate remote brachytherapy and high-dose-rate remote radiation therapy.

renal cell carcinoma: The most common type of kidney cancer. It begins in the lining of the renal tubules in the kidney. The renal tubules filter the blood and produce urine. Also called hypernephroma, renal cell adenocarcinoma, and renal cell cancer.

resectable: Able to be removed by surgery.

resection: Surgery to remove tissue or part or all of an organ.

retinoblastoma: Cancer that forms in the tissues of the retina (the light-sensitive layers of nerve tissue at the back of the eye). Retinoblastoma usually occurs in children younger than five years. It may be hereditary or nonhereditary (sporadic).

rhabdoid tumor: A malignant tumor of either the central nervous system (CNS) or the kidney. Malignant rhabdoid tumors of the CNS often have an abnormality of chromosome 22. These tumors usually occur in children younger than two years.

rhabdomyosarcoma: Cancer that forms in the soft tissues in a type of muscle called striated muscle. Rhabdomyosarcoma can occur anywhere in the body.

risk factor: Something that increases the chance of developing a disease. Some examples of risk factors for cancer are age, a family history of certain cancers, use of tobacco products, being exposed to radiation or certain chemicals, infection with certain viruses or bacteria, and certain genetic changes.

salivary gland cancer: A rare cancer that forms in tissues of a salivary gland (gland in the mouth that makes saliva). Most salivary gland cancers occur in older people.

salpingo-oophorectomy: Surgical removal of the fallopian tubes and ovaries.

salvage therapy: Treatment that is given after the cancer has not responded to other treatments.

sarcoma: A cancer of the bone, cartilage, fat, muscle, blood vessels, or other connective or supportive tissue.

sarcomatoid carcinoma: A type of cancer that begins in the skin or in tissues that line or cover internal organs and that contains long spindle-shaped cells. Also called spindle cell cancer.

satellite tumor: A type of skin cancer on or under the skin that has spread from the primary tumor through the lymph system and is not more than two centimeters away from the original tumor.

schwannoma: A tumor of the peripheral nervous system that arises in the nerve sheath (protective covering). It is almost always benign, but rare malignant schwannomas have been reported.

second primary cancer: Refers to a new primary cancer in a person with a history of cancer.

second-line therapy: Treatment that is given when initial treatment (first-line therapy) doesn't work, or stops working.

secondary cancer: A term that is used to describe either a new primary cancer or cancer that has spread from the place in which it started to other parts of the body.

segmental resection: Surgery to remove part of an organ or gland. It may also be used to remove a tumor and normal tissue around it. In lung cancer surgery, segmental resection refers to removing a section of a lobe of the lung. Also called segmentectomy.

seminoma: A type of cancer of the testicles. Seminomas may spread to the lung, bone, liver, or brain.

sentinel lymph node biopsy: Removal and examination of the sentinel node(s) (the first lymph node(s) to which cancer cells are likely to spread from a primary tumor). To identify the sentinel lymph node(s), the surgeon injects a radioactive substance, blue dye, or both near the tumor. The surgeon then uses a probe to find the sentinel lymph node(s) containing the radioactive substance or looks for the lymph node(s) stained with dye. The surgeon then removes the sentinel node(s) to check for the presence of cancer cells.

Sertoli-Leydig cell tumor of the ovary: A rare type of ovarian tumor in which the tumor cells secrete a male sex hormone. This may cause virilization (the appearance of male physical characteristics in females). Also called androblastoma and arrhenoblastoma.

sex cord tumor: A rare type of cancer that forms in the tissues that support the ovaries or testes. These tumors may release sex hormones. Sex cord tumors include granulosa cell, Sertoli cell, and Leydig cell tumors. Also called sex cord-gonadal stromal tumor and sex cord-stromal tumor.

Sézary syndrome: A cancer that affects the skin. It is a form of cutaneous T-cell lymphoma.

shave biopsy: A procedure in which a skin abnormality and a thin layer of surrounding skin are removed with a small blade for examination under a microscope. Stitches are not needed with this procedure.

Shwachman-Diamond syndrome: A rare, inherited disorder in which the pancreas and bone marrow do not work the way they should. Symptoms include problems digesting food, a low number of neutrophils (a type of white blood cell), bone problems, and being short. Infants with the disorder get bacterial infections and are at an increased risk of aplastic anemia, myelodysplastic syndrome, and leukemia. Also called SDS and Shwachman syndrome.

sigmoidoscopy: Examination of the lower colon using a sigmoidoscope, inserted into the rectum. A sigmoidoscope is a thin, tube-like instrument with a light and a lens for viewing. It may also have a tool to remove tissue to be checked under a microscope for signs of disease. Also called proctosigmoidoscopy.

signet ring cell carcinoma: A highly malignant type of cancer typically found in glandular cells that line the digestive organs. The cells resemble signet rings when examined under a microscope.

single-photon emission computed tomography: A special type of computed tomography (CT) scan in which a small amount of a radioactive drug is injected into a vein and a scanner is used to make detailed images of areas inside the body where the radioactive material is taken up by the cells. Single-photon emission computed tomography can give information about blood flow to tissues and chemical reactions (metabolism) in the body. Also called SPECT.

skin cancer: Cancer that forms in the tissues of the skin. There are several types of skin cancer. Skin cancer that forms in melanocytes (skin cells that make pigment) is called melanoma. Skin cancer that forms in the lower part of the epidermis (the outer layer of the skin) is called basal cell carcinoma. Skin cancer that forms in squamous cells (flat cells that form the surface of the skin) is called squamous cell carcinoma. Skin cancer that forms in neuroendocrine cells (cells that release hormones in response to signals from the nervous system) is called neuroendocrine carcinoma of the skin. Most skin cancers form in older people on parts of the body exposed to the sun or in people who have weakened immune systems.

sleeve resection: Surgery to remove a lung tumor in a lobe of the lung and a part of the main bronchus (airway). The ends of the bronchus are rejoined and any remaining lobes are reattached to the bronchus. This surgery is done to save part of the lung. Also called sleeve lobectomy.

small cell lung cancer: An aggressive (fast-growing) cancer that forms in tissues of the lung and can spread to other parts of the body. The cancer cells look small and oval-shaped when looked at under a microscope.

small intestine cancer: A rare cancer that forms in tissues of the small intestine (the part of the digestive tract between the stomach and the large intestine). The most common type is adenocarcinoma (cancer that begins in cells that make and release mucus and other fluids). Other types of small intestine cancer include sarcoma (cancer that begins in connective or supportive tissue), carcinoid tumor (a slow-growing type of cancer), gastrointestinal stromal tumor (a type of soft tissue sarcoma), and lymphoma (cancer that begins in immune system cells).

smoldering leukemia: A group of diseases in which the bone marrow does not make enough healthy blood cells. Also called myelodysplastic syndromes and preleukemia.

smoldering myeloma: A very slow-growing type of myeloma in which abnormal plasma cells (a type of white blood cell) make too much of a single type of monoclonal antibody (a protein). This protein builds up in the blood or is passed in the urine. Patients with smoldering myeloma usually have no symptoms, but need to be checked often for signs of progression to fully developed multiple myeloma.

soft tissue sarcoma: A cancer that begins in the muscle, fat, fibrous tissue, blood vessels, or other supporting tissue of the body.

solid tumor: An abnormal mass of tissue that usually does not contain cysts or liquid areas. Solid tumors may be benign (not cancer), or malignant (cancer). Different types of solid tumors are named for the type of cells that form them. Examples of solid tumors are sarcomas, carcinomas, and lymphomas. Leukemias (cancers of the blood) generally do not form solid tumors.

spindle cell cancer: A type of cancer that begins in the skin or in tissues that line or cover internal organs and that contains long spindle-shaped cells. Also called sarcomatoid carcinoma.

spine cancer: Cancer that begins in the spinal column (backbone) or spinal cord. The spinal column is made up of linked bones, called vertebrae. The spinal cord is a column of nerve tissue that runs from the base of the skull down the back. It is surrounded by three protective membranes, and is enclosed within the vertebrae. Many different types of cancer may form in the bones, tissues, fluid, or nerves of the spine.

spiral CT scan: A detailed picture of areas inside the body. The pictures are created by a computer linked to an x-ray machine that scans the body in a spiral path. Also called helical computed tomography.

sputum cytology: Examination under a microscope of cells found in sputum (mucus and other matter brought up from the lungs by coughing). The test checks for abnormal cells, such as lung cancer cells.

squamous cell carcinoma: Cancer that begins in squamous cells, which are thin, flat cells that look like fish scales. Squamous cells are found in the tissue that forms the surface of the skin, the lining of the hollow organs of the body, and the passages of the respiratory and digestive tracts. Also called epidermoid carcinoma.

stage: The extent of a cancer in the body. Staging is usually based on the size of the tumor, whether lymph nodes contain cancer, and whether the cancer has spread from the original site to other parts of the body.

stage 0 disease: A group of abnormal cells that remain in the place where they first formed. They have not spread. These abnormal cells may become cancer and spread into nearby normal tissue. Also called carcinoma in situ.

staging: Performing exams and tests to learn the extent of the cancer within the body, especially whether the disease has spread from the original site to other parts of the body. It is important to know the stage of the disease in order to plan the best treatment.

standard therapy: In medicine, treatment that experts agree is appropriate, accepted, and widely used. Health care providers are obligated to provide patients with standard therapy. Also called best practice, standard medical care, and standard of care.

Stanford V regimen: An abbreviation for a chemotherapy combination that is used to treat Hodgkin lymphoma and is being studied in the treatment of other types of cancer. It includes the drugs mechlorethamine, doxorubicin hydrochloride, vinblastine sulfate, vincristine sulfate, bleomycin sulfate, etoposide phosphate, and prednisone and was developed at Stanford University.

statistically significant: Describes a mathematical measure of difference between groups. The difference is said to be statistically significant if it is greater than what might be expected to happen by chance alone.

stem cell transplant: A method of replacing immature blood-forming cells in the bone marrow that have been destroyed by drugs, radiation, or disease. Stem cells are injected into the patient and make healthy blood cells. A stem cell transplant may be autologous (using a patient's own stem cells that were saved before treatment), allogeneic (using stem cells donated by someone who is not an identical twin), or syngeneic (using stem cells donated by an identical twin).

stereotactic biopsy: A biopsy procedure that uses a computer and a three-dimensional scanning device to find a tumor site and guide the removal of tissue for examination under a microscope.

stereotactic radiation therapy: A type of external radiation therapy that uses special equipment to position the patient and precisely deliver radiation to a tumor. The total dose of radiation is divided into several smaller doses given over several days. Stereotactic radiation therapy is used to treat brain tumors and other brain disorders. It is also being studied in the treatment of other types of cancer, such as lung cancer. Also called stereotactic external-beam radiation therapy and stereotaxic radiation therapy.

stoma: A surgically created opening from an area inside the body to the outside.

stomach cancer: Cancer that forms in tissues lining the stomach. Also called gastric cancer.

stromal tumor: A tumor that arises in the supporting connective tissue of an organ.

subcutaneous port: A tube surgically placed into a blood vessel and attached to a disk placed under the skin. It is used for the administration of intravenous fluids and drugs; it can also be used to obtain blood samples.

superior vena cava syndrome: A condition in which a tumor presses against the superior vena cava (the large vein that carries blood from the head, neck, arms, and chest to the heart). This pressure blocks blood flow to the heart and may cause coughing, difficulty in breathing, and swelling of the face, neck, and upper arms.

supportive care: Care given to improve the quality of life of patients who have a serious or life-threatening disease. The goal of supportive care is to prevent or treat as early as possible the symptoms of a disease, side effects caused by treatment of a disease, and psychological, social, and spiritual problems related to a disease or its treatment. Also called comfort care, palliative care, and symptom management.

survivorship: In cancer, survivorship covers the physical, psychosocial, and economic issues of cancer, from diagnosis until the end of life. It focuses on the health and life of a person with cancer beyond the diagnosis and treatment phases. Survivorship includes issues related to the ability to get health care and follow-up treatment, late effects of treatment, second cancers, and quality of life. Family members, friends, and caregivers are also part of the survivorship experience.

synovial sarcoma: A malignant tumor that develops in the synovial membrane of the joints.

systemic chemotherapy: Treatment with anticancer drugs that travel through the blood to cells all over the body.

systemic radiation therapy: A type of radiation therapy in which a radioactive substance, such as radioactive iodine or a radioactively labeled monoclonal antibody, is swallowed or injected into the body and travels through the blood, locating and killing tumor cells.

targeted therapy: A type of treatment that uses drugs or other substances, such as monoclonal antibodies, to identify and attack specific cancer cells. Targeted therapy may have fewer side effects than other types of cancer treatments.

teratocarcinoma: A type of germ cell cancer that usually forms in the testes (testicles).

teratoma: A type of germ cell tumor that may contain several different types of tissue, such as hair, muscle, and bone. Teratomas occur most often in the ovaries in women, the testicles in men, and the tailbone in children. Not all teratomas are malignant.

terminal disease: Disease that cannot be cured and will cause death.

testicular cancer: Cancer that forms in tissues of the testis (one of two egg-shaped glands inside the scrotum that make sperm and male hormones). Testicular cancer usually occurs in young or middle-aged men. Two main types of testicular cancer are seminomas (cancers that grow slowly and are sensitive to radiation therapy) and nonseminomas (different cell types that grow more quickly than seminomas).

thermal ablation: A procedure using heat to remove tissue or a part of the body, or destroy its function. For example, to remove the lining of the uterus, a catheter is inserted through the cervix into the uterus, a balloon at the end of the catheter is inflated, and fluid inside the balloon is heated to destroy the lining of the uterus.

third-line therapy: Treatment that is given when both initial treatment (first-line therapy) and subsequent treatment (second-line therapy) don't work, or stop working.

thymic carcinoma: A rare type of thymus gland cancer. It usually spreads, has a high risk of recurrence, and has a poor survival rate. Thymic carcinoma is divided into subtypes, depending on the types of cells in which the cancer began. Also called type C thymoma.

thymoma: A tumor of the thymus, an organ that is part of the lymphatic system and is located in the chest, behind the breastbone.

thyroid cancer: Cancer that forms in the thyroid gland (an organ at the base of the throat that makes hormones that help control heart rate, blood pressure, body temperature, and weight). Four main types of thyroid cancer are papillary, follicular, medullary, and anaplastic thyroid cancer. The four types are based on how the cancer cells look under a microscope.

TNM staging system: A system developed by the American Joint Committee on Cancer (AJCC) that uses TNM to describe the extent of cancer in a patient's body. T describes the size of the tumor and whether it has invaded nearby tissue. N describes whether cancer has spread to nearby lymph nodes, and M describes whether cancer has metastasized (spread to distant parts of the body). The TNM staging system is used to describe most types of cancer. Also called AJCC staging system.

tongue cancer: Cancer that begins in the tongue. When the cancer begins in the front two-thirds of the tongue, it is considered to be a type of oral cavity cancer; when the cancer begins in the back third of the tongue, it is considered to be a type of oropharyngeal or throat cancer.

topical chemotherapy: Treatment with anticancer drugs in a lotion or cream applied to the skin.

total-body irradiation: Radiation therapy to the entire body. It is usually followed by bone marrow or peripheral stem cell transplantation.

transitional cell cancer: Cancer that forms in transitional cells in the lining of the bladder, ureter, or renal pelvis (the part of the kidney that collects, holds, and drains urine). Transitional cells are cells that can change shape and stretch without breaking apart.

transperineal biopsy: A procedure in which a sample of tissue is removed from the prostate for examination under a microscope. The sample is removed with a thin needle that is inserted through the skin between the scrotum and rectum and into the prostate.

transplantation: A surgical procedure in which tissue or an organ is transferred from one area of a person's body to another area, or from one person (the donor) to another person (the recipient).

transrectal biopsy: A procedure in which a sample of tissue is removed from the prostate using a thin needle that is inserted through the rectum and into the prostate. Transrectal ultrasound (TRUS) is usually used to guide the needle. The sample is examined under a microscope to see if it contains cancer.

transurethral biopsy: A procedure in which a sample of tissue is removed from the prostate for examination under a microscope. A thin, lighted tube is inserted through the urethra into the prostate, and a small piece of tissue is removed with a cutting loop.

transurethral needle ablation: A procedure that is used to treat benign prostatic hypertrophy (BPH). A small probe that gives off low-level radiofrequency energy is inserted through the urethra into the prostate. The energy from the probe heats and destroys the abnormal prostate tissue without damaging the urethra. Also called transurethral radiofrequency ablation and TUNA.

transurethral resection of the prostate: Surgery to remove tissue from the prostate using an instrument inserted through the urethra. Also called TURP.

transvaginal ultrasound: A procedure used to examine the vagina, uterus, fallopian tubes, ovaries, and bladder. An instrument is inserted into the vagina that causes sound waves to bounce off organs inside the pelvis. These sound waves create echoes that are sent to a computer, which creates a picture called a sonogram. Also called transvaginal sonography and TVS.

triple-negative breast cancer: Describes breast cancer cells that do not have estrogen receptors, progesterone receptors, or large amounts of HER2/neu protein. Also called ER-negative PR-negative HER2/neu-negative and ER-PR-HER2/neu-.

tumor: An abnormal mass of tissue that results when cells divide more than they should or do not die when they should. Tumors may be benign (not cancer), or malignant (cancer). Also called neoplasm.

tumor debulking: Surgical removal of as much of a tumor as possible. Tumor debulking may increase the chance that chemotherapy or radiation therapy will kill all the tumor cells. It may also be done to relieve symptoms or help the patient live longer.

tumor marker: A substance that may be found in tumor tissue or released from a tumor into the blood or other body fluids. A high level of a tumor marker may mean that a certain type of cancer is in the body. Examples of tumor markers include CA 125 (in ovarian cancer), CA 15-3 (in breast cancer), CEA (in ovarian, lung, breast, pancreas, and gastrointestinal tract cancers), and PSA (in prostate cancer).

tumor necrosis factor: A protein made by white blood cells in response to an antigen (substance that causes the immune system to make a specific immune response) or infection. Tumor necrosis factor can also be made in the laboratory. It may boost a person's immune response, and also may cause necrosis (cell death) of some types of tumor cells. Tumor necrosis factor is being studied in the treatment of some types of cancer. It is a type of cytokine. Also called TNF.

ultrasound: A procedure in which high-energy sound waves are bounced off internal tissues or organs and make echoes. The echo patterns are shown on the screen of an ultrasound machine, forming a picture of body tissues called a sonogram.

ultrasound-guided biopsy: A biopsy procedure that uses an ultrasound imaging device to find an abnormal area of tissue and guide its removal for examination under a microscope.

ultraviolet radiation: Invisible rays that are part of the energy that comes from the sun. Ultraviolet radiation that reaches the Earth's surface is made up of two types of rays, called UVA and UVB. Ultraviolet radiation also comes from sun lamps and tanning beds. It can cause skin damage, premature aging, melanoma, and other types of skin cancer. It can also cause problems with the eyes and the immune system. Skin specialists recommend that people use sunscreens that protect the skin from both kinds of ultraviolet radiation. In medicine, ultraviolet radiation also comes from special lamps or a laser and is used to treat certain skin conditions such as psoriasis, vitiligo, and skin tumors of cutaneous T-cell lymphoma. Also called UV radiation.

unresectable: Unable to be removed with surgery.

unsealed internal radiation therapy: Radiation therapy given by injecting a radioactive substance into the bloodstream or a body cavity, or by swallowing it. This substance is not sealed in a container.

upper GI series: A series of x-ray pictures of the esophagus, stomach, and duodenum (the first part of the small intestine). The x-ray pictures are taken after the patient drinks a liquid containing barium sulfate (a form of the silver-white metallic element barium). The barium sulfate coats and outlines the inner walls of the upper gastrointestinal tract so that they can be seen on the x-ray pictures. Also called upper gastrointestinal series.

upstaging: In cancer, changing the stage used to describe a patient's cancer from a lower stage (less extensive) to a higher stage (more extensive). Upstaging is based on the results of additional staging tests. It is important to know the stage of the disease in order to plan the best treatment.

urethral cancer: A rare cancer that forms in tissues of the urethra (the tube through which urine empties the bladder and leaves the body). Types of urethral cancer include transitional cell carcinoma (cancer that begins in cells that can change shape and stretch without breaking apart), squamous cell carcinoma (cancer that begins in flat cells lining the urethra), and adenocarcinoma (cancer that begins in cells that make and release mucus and other fluids).

uterine cancer: Cancer that forms in tissues of the uterus (the small, hollow, pear-shaped organ in a woman's pelvis in which a fetus develops). Two types of uterine cancer are endometrial cancer (cancer that begins in cells lining the uterus) and uterine sarcoma (a rare cancer that begins in muscle or other tissues in the uterus).

uterine sarcoma: A rare type of uterine cancer that forms in muscle or other tissues of the uterus (the small, hollow, pear-shaped organ in a woman's pelvis in which a fetus develops). It usually occurs after menopause. The two main types are leiomyosarcoma (cancer that begins in smooth muscle cells) and endometrial stromal sarcoma (cancer that begins in connective tissue cells).

vacuum-assisted biopsy: A procedure in which a small sample of tissue is removed from the breast. An imaging device is used to guide a hollow probe connected to a vacuum device. The probe is inserted through a tiny cut made in numbed skin on the breast. The tissue sample is removed using gentle vacuum suction and a small rotating knife within the probe. Then the tissue sample is studied under a microscope to check for signs of disease. This procedure causes very little scarring and no stitches are needed. Also called VACB and vacuum-assisted core biopsy.

vaginal cancer: Cancer that forms in the tissues of the vagina (birth canal). The vagina leads from the cervix (the opening of the uterus) to the outside of the body. The most common type of vaginal cancer is squamous cell carcinoma, which starts in the thin, flat cells lining the vagina. Another type of vaginal cancer is adenocarcinoma, cancer that begins in glandular cells in the lining of the vagina.

video-assisted resection: Surgery that is aided by the use of a video camera that projects and enlarges the image on a television screen. Also called video-assisted surgery.

villous adenoma: A type of polyp that grows in the colon and other places in the gastrointestinal tract and sometimes in other parts of the body. These adenomas may become malignant (cancer).

viral therapy: Treatment using a virus that has been changed in the laboratory to find and destroy cancer cells without harming healthy cells. It is a type of targeted therapy. Also called oncolytic virotherapy, oncolytic virus therapy, and virotherapy.

virtual colonoscopy: A method to examine the inside of the colon by taking a series of x-rays. A computer is used to make two-dimensional (2-D) and three-dimensional (3-D) pictures of the colon from these x-rays. The pictures can be saved, changed to give better viewing angles, and reviewed after the procedure, even years later. Also called computed tomographic colonography, computed tomography colonography, CT colonography, and CTC.

vulvar cancer: Cancer of the vulva (the external female genital organs, including the clitoris, vaginal lips, and the opening to the vagina).

WAGR syndrome: A rare, genetic disorder that is present at birth and has two or more of the following symptoms: Wilms tumor (a type of kidney cancer); little or no iris (the colored part of the eye); defects in the sexual organs and urinary tract (the organs that make urine and pass it from the body); and below average mental ability. This syndrome occurs when part of chromosome 11 is missing. Also called Wilms tumor-aniridia-genitourinary anomalies-mental retardation syndrome.

Waldenström macroglobulinemia: An indolent (slow-growing) type of non-Hodgkin lymphoma marked by abnormal levels of IgM antibodies in the blood and an enlarged liver, spleen, or lymph nodes. Also called lymphoplasmacytic lymphoma.

watchful waiting: Closely watching a patient's condition but not giving treatment unless symptoms appear or change. Watchful waiting is used in conditions that progress slowly, are hard to diagnose, or may get better without treatment. It is also used when the risks of treatment are greater than the possible benefits. During watchful waiting, patients may be given certain tests and exams. Watchful waiting is sometimes used in prostate cancer. It is a type of expectant management.

wedge resection: Surgery to remove a triangle-shaped slice of tissue. It may be used to remove a tumor and a small amount of normal tissue around it.

Whipple procedure: A type of surgery used to treat pancreatic cancer. The head of the pancreas, the duodenum, a portion of the stomach, and other nearby tissues are removed.

whole-brain radiation therapy: A type of external radiation therapy used to treat patients who have cancer in the brain. It is often used to treat patients whose cancer has spread to the brain, or who have more than one tumor or tumors that cannot be removed by surgery. Radiation is given to the whole brain over a period of many weeks.

wide local excision: Surgery to cut out the cancer and some healthy tissue around it.

Wilms tumor: A disease in which malignant (cancer) cells are found in the kidney, and may spread to the lungs, liver, or nearby lymph nodes. Wilms tumor usually occurs in children younger than five years old.

wound: A break in the skin or other body tissues caused by injury or surgical incision (cut).

x-ray: A type of high-energy radiation. In low doses, x-rays are used to diagnose diseases by making pictures of the inside of the body. In high doses, x-rays are used to treat cancer.

x-ray therapy: A type of radiation therapy that uses high-energy radiation from x-rays to kill cancer cells and shrink tumors.

yttrium: A metal of the rare earth group of elements. A radioactive form of yttrium may be attached to a monoclonal antibody or other molecule that can locate and bind to cancer cells and be used to diagnose or treat some types of cancer.

Chapter 76

National Organizations Offering Cancer-Related Services

General Cancer Information and Cancer Survivorship

American Academy of Family Physicians
11400 Tomahawk Creek Parkway
Leawood, KS 66211-2672
Toll-Free: 800-274-2237
Phone: 913-906-6000
Website: http://www.aafp.org
E-mail: fp@aafp.org

American Cancer Fund
3401 Quebec St. Suite 3200
Denver, CO 80207
Toll-Free: 800-321-1557
Website: http://www.amc.org
E-mail: contactus@amc.org

American Cancer Society
250 Williams Street NW, Suite 600
Atlanta, GA 30303-1002
Toll-Free: 800-227-2345
Phone: 404-320-3333
Website: http://www.cancer.org

American Childhood Cancer Organization
P.O. Box 498
Kensington, MD 20895
Toll-Free: 800-366-2223
Phone: 301-962-3520
Website: http://www
.americanchildhoodcancer.org
E-mail: staff@
americanchildhoodcancer.org

Information in this chapter was compiled from "National Organizations That Offer Cancer-Related Services," National Cancer Institute (www.cancer.gov), 2010, and other sources deemed reliable. Inclusion does not constitute endorsement and there is no implication associated with omission. All contact information was updated and verified in October 2010.

American Institute for Cancer Research
1759 R Street, NW
Washington, DC 20009
Toll-Free: 800-843-8114
Phone: 202-328-7744
Website:
http://www.aicr.org
E-mail: aicrweb@aicr.org

Bloch Cancer Foundation, Inc.
One H&R Block Way
Kansas City, MO 64105
Toll-Free: 800-433-0464
Phone: 816-854-5050
Website:
http://www.blochcancer.org
E-mail:
hotline@hrblock.com

Canadian Cancer Society
565 W. 10th Ave.
Vancouver, BC V5Z 4J4
Tel: 604-872-4400
Website:
www.bc.cancer.ca
E-mail:
inquiries@bc.cancer.ca

Cancer Hope Network
2 North Road
Suite A
Chester, NJ 07930
Toll-Free: 800-552-4366
Phone: 908-879-4039
Website: http://www
.cancerhopenetwork.org
E-mail: info@
cancerhopenetwork.org

Cancer Project
5100 Wisconsin Avenue
Suite 400
Washington, DC 20016
Phone: 202-244-5038
Website: http://www.
CancerProject.org
E-mail: info@CancerProject.org

Cancer Research and Prevention Foundation
1600 Duke Street, Suite 500
Alexandria, VA 22314
Toll-Free: 800-227-2732
Phone: 703-836-4412
Website:
http://www.preventcancer.org
E-mail: info@preventcancer.org

Cancer Support Community
1050 17th St., NW
Suite 500
Washington, DC 20036
Toll-Free: 888-793-9355
Phone: 202-659-9709
Website: http://www
.cancersupportcommunity.org
E-mail: help@
cancersupportcommunity.org

CancerCare
275 Seventh Avenue
22nd Floor
New York, NY 10001
Toll-Free: 800-813-4673
Website:
http://www.cancercare.org
E-mail: info@cancercare.org

CancerEducation.com
Website: http://www
.cancereducation.com

CancerWise
Website:
http://www.cancerwise.org

Cleveland Clinic
9500 Euclid Avenue NA31
Cleveland, OH 44195
Toll-Free: 800-223-2273
Phone: 216-444-2200
TTY: 216-444-0261
Website: http://www
.clevelandclinic.org
E-mail: healthl@ccf.org

Cure Search for Children's Cancer
4600 East West Highway
Suite 600
Bethesda, MD 20814
Toll-Free: 800-458-6223
Website:
http://www.curesearch.org
E-mail: info@curesearch.org

Facing Our Risk of Cancer Empowered (FORCE)
16057 Tampa Palms Blvd. W
PMB #373
Tampa, FL 33647
Toll-Free: 866-824-7475
Website: www.facingourrisk.org
E-mail: info@facingourrisk.org

Intercultural Cancer Council
Baylor College of Medicine
1720 Dryden Rd.
Suite #1025
Houston, TX 77030
Phone: 713-798-4614
Website: http://iccnetwork.org
E-mail: info@iccnetwork.org

International Union Against Cancer
62 Route de Frontenex
1205 Geneva
Switzerland
Phone: + 41 22 809 18 11
Website:
http://www.uicc.org

Lance Armstrong Foundation
2201 E. Sixth St.
Austin, TX 78702
Toll-Free:
866-673-7205 (English)
866-927-7205 (Spanish)
Phone: 512-236-8820
Website:
http://www.livestrong.org

Macmillan Cancer Support
89 Albert Embankment
London, SE1 7UQ
United Kingdom
Phone:
011-44-020-7840-7840
Website:
http://www.macmillan.org.uk

Mayo Foundation for Medical Education and Research
200 First Street SW
Rochester, MN 55905
Website:
http://www.mayoclinic.com
E-mail:
comments@mayoclinic.com

M. D. Anderson Cancer Center
1515 Holcombe Blvd.
Houston, TX 77030
Toll-Free: 800-392-1611
Phone: 713-792-6161
Website:
http://www.mdanderson.org

Memorial Sloan-Kettering Cancer Center
1275 York Avenue
New York, NY 10065
Toll-Free: 800-525-2225
Phone: 212-639-2000
Website: www.mskcc.org

National Association for Proton Therapy
1301 Highland Drive
Silver Spring, MD 20910
Phone: 301-587-6100
Website:
http://www.proton-therapy.org

National Cancer Institute (NCI)
Public Inquiries Office
Suite 300
6116 Executive Boulevard
MSC8322
Bethesda, MD 20892-8322
Toll-Free: 800-4-CANCER
(800-422-6237)
TTY: 800-332-8615
Website:
http://www.cancer.gov

National Children's Cancer Society
One South Memorial Drive
Suite 800
St. Louis, MO 63102
Toll-Free: 800-532-6459
Phone: 314-241-1600
Website:
http://www.children-cancer.org

National Coalition for Cancer Survivorship
1010 Wayne Avenue
Suite 770
Silver Spring, MD 20910
Toll-Free: 888-650-9127
Phone: 301-650-9127
Website:
http://www.canceradvocacy.org
E-mail: info@canceradvocacy.org

National Women's Health Information Center
8270 Willow Oaks
Corporate Drive
Fairfax, VA 22031
Toll-Free: 800-994-9662
TTY: 888-220-5446
Website: http://www.4woman.gov

OncoLink
Abramson Cancer Center of the
University of Pennsylvania
3400 Spruce Street, 2 Donner
Philadelphia, PA 19104-4283
Website:
http://www.oncolink.com

Oncologychannel.com
Healthcommunities, Inc.
Website:
http://www.oncologychannel.com

Teens Living with Cancer

1000 Elmood Avenue, Suite 300
Rochester, NY 14620
Phone: 585-563-6221
Website: http://www
.teenslivingwithcancer.org
E-mail: info@
teenslivingwithcancer.org

Vital Options International

4419 Coldwater Canyon Avenue
Suite I
Studio City, CA 91604
Toll-Free: 800-477-7666
Phone: 818-508-5657
Website:
http://www.vitaloptions.org
E-mail: info@vitaloptions.org

Information about Specific Cancers

To make it easier to find information about cancer in specific sites, the organizations listed in this section are alphabetized by key word.

Bladder Cancer Advocacy
Network
4813 St. Elmo Avenue
Bethesda, MD 20814
Toll-Free: 888-901-2226
Phone: 301-215-9099
Website: http://www.bcan.org

National **Bladder** Foundation
Website:
http://www.bladder.org

American Association of
Neurological Surgeons
[**Brain Tumor**]
Website: http://www
.neurosurgerytoday.org

American **Brain Tumor**
Association
2720 River Road
Des Plaines, IL 60018
Toll-Free: 800-886-2282
Phone: 847-827-9910
Website:
http://www.abta.org
E-mail: info@abta.org

National **Brain Tumor** Society
East Coast Office
124 Watertown Street
Suite 2D
Watertown, MA 02472
Toll-Free: 800-770-8287
Phone: 617-924-9997
Website: http://www.tbts.org
E-mail: info@tbts.org
West Coast Office
22 Battery Street, Suite 612
San Francisco, CA 94111-5520
Toll-Free: 800-934-2873
Phone: 415-834-9970
Website:
http://www.braintumor.org
E-mail: nbtf@braintumor.org

Children's **Brain
Tumor** Foundation
274 Madison Avenue, Suite 1004
New York, NY 10016
Toll-Free: 866-228-4673
Phone: 212-448-9494
Website: http://www.cbtf.org
E-mail: info@cbtf.org

American **Breast Cancer**
Foundation
1220 B East Joppa Road, Suite 332
Baltimore, MD 21286
Toll-Free: 877-539-2543
(Enrollment Hotline)
Phone: 877-323-ICAN (4226)
Website: www.abcf.org
E-mail: contact@abcf.org

BreastCancer.org
Website: www.breastcancer.org

Breast Cancer Action
55 New Montgomery, Suite 323
San Francisco, CA 94105
Toll-Free: 877-278-6722
Phone: 415-243-9301
Website: http://www.bcaction.org
E-mail: info@bcaction.org

Breast Cancer
Network of Strength
135 S. LaSalle Street
Suite 2000
Chicago, IL 60603
Toll-Free: 800-221-2141 (English
only); 800-986-9505 (Spanish)
Phone: 312-986-8338
Website: http://www
.networkofstrength.org

Imaginis **[Breast Cancer]**
Website: www.imaginis.com
E-mail: learnmore@imaginis.com

Komen **Breast Cancer**
Foundation
5005 LBJ Freeway, Suite 250
Dallas, TX 75244
Toll-Free: 800-462-9273
Phone: 972-855-1600
Website: http://ww5.komen.org
E-mail: helpline@komen.org

Kushner **Breast Cancer**
Advisory Center
P.O. Box 757
Malaga, CA 90274
Website: www.rkbcac.org

Living Beyond **Breast Cancer**
354 West Lancaster Avenue
Suite 224
Haverford, PA 19041
Toll-Free: 888-753-5222
Phone: 484-708-1550;
610-645-4567
Website: http://www.lbbc.org
E-mail: mail@lbbc.org

National **Breast
Cancer** Coalition
1101 17th Street, NW
Suite 1300
Washington, DC 20036
Toll-Free: 800-622-2838
Phone: 202-296-7477
Website:
http://www.stopbreastcancer.org
E-mail:
info@stopbreastcancer.org

Young Survival Coalition
[Breast Cancer]
61 Broadway, Suite 2235
New York, NY 10006
Toll-Free: 877-972-1011
Phone: 646-257-3000
Website:
http://www.youngsurvival.org
E-mail: info@youngsurvival.org

Carcinoid Cancer Foundation
333 Mamaroneck Avenue, #492
White Plains, NY 10605
Phone: 888-722-3132
Website: http://www.carcinoid.org

Caring for **Carcinoid**
Foundation
198 Tremont St.
Box 456
Boston, MA 02116
Phone: 617-848-3977
Website: http://www
.caringforcarcinoid.org

Alliance for **Cervical**
Cancer Prevention
Website:
http://www.alliance-cxca.org
E-mail: accp@path.org

National **Cervical Cancer**
Coalition
6520 Platt Avenue, #693
West Hills, CA 91307
Toll-Free: 800-685-5531
Phone: 818-992-4242
Website:
http://www.nccc-online.org
E-mail: info@nccc-online.org

National HPV and **Cervical**
Cancer Prevention
Resource Center
P.O. Box 13827
Research Triangle Park,
NC 27709
Website:
http://www.ashastd.org/hpvccrc

Cholangiocarcinoma
Foundation
5526 West 13400 South, #510
Salt Lake City, UT 84096
Phone: 801-999-0455
Website: http://www
.cholangiocarcinoma.org
E-mail: info@
cholangiocarcinoma.org

Colon Cancer Alliance
1200 G Street, NW
Suite 800
Washington, DC 20005
Toll-Free: 877-422-2030
Phone: 202-434-8980
Website:
http://www.ccalliance.org
E-mail: info@ccalliance.org

American Gastroenterological
Association [**Colorectal**
Cancer]
4930 Del Ray Avenue
Bethesda, MD 20814
Phone: 301-654-2055
Website:
http://www.gastro.org
E-mail: member@gstro.org

C3: **Colorectal**
Cancer Coalition
1414 Prince Street
Suite 204
Washington DC 20008
Alexandria, VA 22314
Toll-Free: 877-427-2111
Phone: 703-548-1225
Website: http://www
.fightcolorectalcancer.org
E-mail: info@
fightcolorectalcancer.org

Bascom Palmer
Eye Institute
University of Miami
School of Medicine
900 Northwest 17th Street
Miami, FL 33136
Toll-Free: 800-329-7000
Phone: 305-326-6000
Website:
http://www.eyecancermd.org

Eye Cancer Network
115 East 61st St.
New York City, NY 10021
Phone: 212-832-8170
Website: http://www.eyecancer.com

Gynecologic Cancer
Foundation/Women's Cancer
Network
230 W. Monroe, Suite 2528
Chicago, IL 60606
Phone: 312-578-1439
Website: http://www.wcn.org
E-mail: info@thegcf.org

International **Gynecologic Cancer** Society
P.O. Box 6387
Louisville, KY 40206
Phone: 502-891-4575
Website: http://www.igcs.org
E-mail: adminoffice@igcs.org

American Academy of
Otolaryngology-**Head and Neck** Surgery
1650 Diagonal Rd.
Alexandria, VA, 22314
Phone: 703-836-4444
Website: www.entnet.org
E-mail: webmaster@entnet.org

National Institute of Dental
and Craniofacial Research
[**Head and Neck Cancer**]
One NOHIC Way
Bethesda, MD 20892-3500
National Oral Health
Information Clearinghouse:
301-402-7364
Website:
http://www.nidcr.nih.gov
E-mail: nidcrinfo@mail.nih.gov

American Association of
Kidney Patients
3505 E. Frontage Rd.
Suite 315
Tampa, FL 33607
Phone: 800-749-2257
Website: http://www.aakp.org
E-mail: info@aakp.org

Kidney Cancer Association
Post Office Box 96503
Washington, DC 20090
Toll-Free: 800-850-9132
Phone: 847-332-1051
Website:
http://www.kidneycancer.org
E-mail:
kidney.cancer@hotmail.com

National Institute of
Diabetes and Digestive and
Kidney Diseases
National Institutes of Health
Building 31
Room 9A06
31 Center Drive, MSC 2560
Bethesda, MD 20892-2560
Toll-Free: 800-891-5390
(Information Clearinghouse)
Website:
http://www.niddk.nih.gov
E-mail: dkwebmaster@extra
.niddk.nih.gov

National **Kidney** Foundation
30 East 33rd Street
New York, NY 10016
Toll-Free: 800-622-9010
Phone: 212-889-2210
Website: http://www.kidney.org

Leukemia and
Lymphoma Society
1311 Mamaroneck Avenue
Suite 310
White Plains, NY 10605-5221
Toll-Free: 800-955-4572
Phone: 914-949-5213
Website: http://www
.leukemia-lymphoma.org
E-mail: infocenter@
leukemia-lymphoma.org

American **Liver** Foundation
75 Maiden Lane, Suite 603
New York, NY 10038
Toll-Free: 800-GO-Liver
(465-4837)
Phone: 212-668-1000
Website:
http://www.liverfoundation.org

LiverTumor.org
Website:
http://www.livertumor.org

American **Lung** Association
1301 Pennsylvania Ave., NW
Suite 800
Washington, DC 20004
Toll-Free: 800-LUNGUSA
(586-4872)
Website: http://www.lungusa.org

Lung Cancer Alliance
888 16th Street, NW
Suite 150
Washington, DC 20006
Toll-Free: 800-298-2436
Phone: 202-463-2080
Website: http://www
.lungcanceralliance.org
E-mail:
info@lungcanceralliance.org

LungCancer.org
Website: http://www.lungcancer.org

Lymphoma Foundation
of America
1100 North Main Street
Ann Arbor, MI 48104
Toll-Free Patient Hotline:
800-385-1060
Patient Hotline: 734-222-1133
Website:
http://www.lymphomahelp.org
E-mail: LFA@lymphomahelp.org

Lymphoma Research
Foundation
115 Broadway, Suite 1301
New York, NY 10006
Toll-Free: 800-500-9976
Phone 212-349-2910
Website:
http://www.lymphoma.org
E-mail for general information:
LRF@lymphoma.org
E-mail for patient services:
helpline@lymphoma.org

Melanoma International
Foundation
250 Mapleflower Road
Glenmoore, PA 19343
Toll-Free: 866-463-6663
Phone: 610-942-3432
Website:
http://www.safefromthesun.org

Melanoma Education
Foundation
P.O. Box 2023
Peabody, MA 01960
Phone: 978-535-3080
Website: http://www.skincheck.org
E-mail: mef@skincheck.org

Asbestos Disease Awareness
Organization [**Mesothelioma**]
Website: http://www
.asbestosdiseaseawareness.org

Mesothelioma Applied
Research Foundation
1317 King St.
Alexandria, VA 22314
Toll-Free: 877-363-6376
Phone: 805-563-8400
Website:
http://www.curemeso.org
E-mail: info@curemeso.org

Mesothelioma Information
and Resource Group
Coady Law Firm
205 Portland Street
Boston, MA 02114
Website: http://www.mirg.org

Multiple Myeloma
Research Foundation
383 Main Ave.
5th floor
Norwalk, CT 06851
Phone: 203-229-0464
Website:
http://www.themmrf.org
E-mail: info@themmrf.org

International **Myeloma**
Foundation (IMF)
12650 Riverside Drive
Suite 206
North Hollywood, CA
91607-3421
Toll-Free: 800-452-2873
Phone: 818-487-7455
E-mail: TheIMF@myeloma.org
Website:
http://www.myeloma.org

Oral Cancer Foundation
3419 Via Lido
#205
Newport Beach, CA 92663
Phone: 949-646-8000
Website: http://www
.oralcancerfoundation.org
E-mail: info@
oralcancerfoundation.org

Support for People with **Oral**
and Head and Neck Cancer
P.O. Box 53
Locust Valley, NY 11560
Toll-Free: 800-377-0928
Website: http://www.spohnc.org
E-mail: info@spohnc.org

Osteosarcoma Online
Website: http://iucc.iu.edu/
osteosarcoma

National **Ovarian Cancer**
Association
101-145 Front Street East
Toronto, Ontario M5A 1E3
Canada
Phone: 416-962-2700
Website:
http://www.ovariancanada.org
E-mail: noca@ovariancanada.org

National **Ovarian Cancer**
Coalition
2501 Oak Lawn Avenue
Suite 435
Dallas, TX 75219
Toll-Free: 888-682-7426
Phone: 214-273-4200
Website: http://www.ovarian.org
E-mail: nocc@ovarian.org

Ovarian Cancer
National Alliance
910 17th Street, NW
Suite 1190
Washington, DC 20006
Website:
http://www.ovariancancer.org
E-mail: ocna@ovariancancer.org

Ovarian Cancer
Research Fund, Inc.
14 Pennsylvania Plaza
Suite 1400
New York, NY 10122
Toll-Free: 800-873-9569
Phone: 212-268-1002
Website: http://www.ocrf.org
E-mail: info@ocrf.org

Lustgarten Foundation for
Pancreatic Cancer Research
1111 Stewart Avenue
Bethpage, NY 11714
Toll-Free: 866-789-1000
Phone: 516-803-2304
Website: http://www
.lustgartenfoundation.org

Pancreatic Cancer Action
Network (PanCAN)
2141 Rosecrans Avenue
Suite 7000
El Segundo, CA 90245
Toll-Free: 877-272-6226
Phone: 310-725-0025
Website:
http://www.pancan.org
E-mail:
information@pancan.org

Hormone Foundation
[Pituitary Tumor]
8401 Connecticut Ave., Suite 900
Chevy Chase, MD 20815-5817
Phone: 800-HORMONE
(467-6663)
Website: http://www.hormone.org
E-mail:
hormone@endo-society.org

Pituitary Network Association
Website: http://www.pituitary.org

American **Prostate** Society
Toll-Free: 800-308-1106
Website: http://www.ameripros.org

Canadian **Prostate Cancer**
145 Front St. E., Suite 306
Toronto, Ontario M5A 1E3
Canada
Toll-Free: 888-255-0333
Website: http://www.cpcn.org

Prostate Cancer Foundation
1250 Fourth Street
Santa Monica, CA 90401
Toll-Free: 800-757-2873
Phone: 310-570-4700
Website: http://www
.prostatecancerfoundation.org
E-mail: info@pcf.org

Prostate Cancer
Foundation of Australia
P.O. Box 1332
Lane Cove, NSW 1595
Australia
Phone: 011 61 2 9438 7000
Website:
http://www.prostate.org.au
E-mail:
enquiries@prostate.org.au

Prostate Cancer
Research Institute
5777 W. Century Blvd.
Suite 800
Los Angeles, CA 90045
Toll-Free Helpline:
 800-641-PCRI (7274)
Phone: 310-743-2116
Website:
http://www.prostate-cancer.org
E-mail: info@pcri.org

Us Too International, Inc.
[Prostate Cancer]
5003 Fairview Avenue
Downers Grove, IL 60515
Toll-Free: 800-808-7866
Phone: 630-795-1002
Website:
http://www.ustoo.org
E-mail: ustoo@ustoo.org

ZERO: The Project To End
Prostate Cancer
10 G St. NE
Suite 601
Washington, DC 20002
Toll-Free: 888-245-9455
Phone: 202-463-9455
Website:
http://www.zerocancer.org
E-mail: info@zerocancer.org

Sarcoma Alliance
775 East Blithedale
#334
Mill Valley, CA 94941
Phone: 415-381-7236
Website:
http://www.sarcomaalliance.org
E-mail:
info@sarcomaalliance.org

American Academy of
Dermatology [**Skin Cancer**]
P.O. Box 4014
Schaumburg, IL 60173
Toll-Free: 888-462-3376;
866-503-7546
Phone: 847-330-0230
Website: http://www.aad.org

National Institute of
Arthritis and Musculoskeletal
and **Skin** Diseases
1 AMS Circle
Bethesda, MD 20892-3675
Toll-Free: 877-226-4267
Phone: 301-495-4484
TTY: 301-565-2966
Website: http://www.niams.nih.gov
E-mail: niamsinfo@mail.nih.gov

New Zealand Dermatological
Society, Inc. [**Skin Cancer**]
Website: http://dermnetnz.org

Skin Cancer Foundation
149 Madison, Suite 901
New York, NY 10016
Toll-Free: 800-754-6490
Phone: 212-725-5176
Website:
http://www.skincancer.org
E-mail: info@skincancer.org

Testicular Cancer
Resource Center
Website: http://tcrc.acor.org

American **Thyroid** Association
6066 Leesburg Pike, Suite 550
Falls Church, VA 22041
Phone: 703-998-8890
Website: http://www.thyroid.org
E-mail: admin@thyroid.org

Thyroid Cancer Survivors'
Association, Inc.
P.O. Box 1545
New York, NY 10159-1545
Toll-Free: 877-588-7904
Website: http://www.thyca.org
E-mail: thyca@thyca.org

American **Urological**
Association Foundation
1000 Corporate Boulevard,
Suite 410
Linthicum, MD 21090
Hotline: 800-828-7866
Toll-Free: 866-746-4282
Phone: 410-689-3700
Website: http://www.
UrologyHealth.org

International **Waldenström's
Macroglobulinemia**
Foundation
3932 D Swift Road
Sarasota, FL 34231
Phone: 941-927-4963
Website: http://www.iwmf.com
E-mail: info@iwmf.com

Selected Resources for End-of-Life Issues

*American Academy of
Hospice and Palliative
Medicine*
4700 W. Lake Ave.
Glenview IL 60025
Phone: 847-375-4712
Website:
http://www.aahpm.org
E-mail: info@aahpm.org

*American Chronic Pain
Association*
P.O. Box 850
Rocklin, CA 95677
Toll-Free: 800-533-3231
Website:
http://www.theacpa.org

*American Hospice
Foundation*
2120 L Street, NW
Suite 200
Washington, DC 20037
Phone: 202-223-0204
Website:
http://www.americanhospice.org
E-mail:
ahf@americanhospice.org

American Pain Foundation
201 N. Charles St.
Suite 710
Baltimore, MD 21201-4111
Toll-Free: 888-615-7246
(message line)
Website:
http://www.painfoundation.org
E-mail:
info@painfoundation.org

American Pain Society
4700 W. Lake Ave.
Glenview IL 60025
Phone: 847-375-4715
Website:
http://www.ampainsoc.org
E-mail: info@ampainsoc.org

Children's Hospice International
1101 King Street
Suite 360
Alexandria, VA 22314
Phone: 703-684-0330
Website:
http://www.chionline.org
E-mail: info@chionline.org

Family Caregiver Alliance
180 Montgomery St.
Suite 900
San Francisco, CA 94104
Toll-Free: 800-445-8106
Phone: 415-434-3388
Website: http://caregiver.org
E-mail: info@caregiver.org

Hospice Education Institute
Three Unity Square
P.O. Box 98
Machiasport, ME 04655-0098
Toll-Free: 800-331-1620
Phone: 207-255-8800
Website:
http://www.hospiceworld.org
E-mail:
info@hospiceworld.org

Hospice Foundation of America
1710 Rhode Island Ave., NW
Suite 400
Washington, DC 20036
Toll-Free: 800-854-3402
Website: http://www
.hospicefoundation.org
E-mail:
info@hospicefoundation.org

Hospice Net
401 Bowling Avenue
Suite 51
Nashville, TN 37205-5124
Website:
http://www.hospicenet.org
E-mail: info@hospicenet.org

Hospice Patients Alliance
Website:
http://www.hospicepatients.org

National Association for Home Care
Hospice Association of America
228 Seventh Street, SE
Washington, DC 20003
Phone: 202-547-7424
Website: http://www.nahc.org

National Family Caregivers
10400 Connecticut Ave.
Suite 500
Kensington, MD 20895-3944
Toll-Free: 800-896-3650
Phone: 301-942-6430
Website: http://www
.thefamilycaregiver.org
E-mail:
info@thefamilycaregiver.org

*National Hospice
and Palliative Care
Organization*
1731 King St. Suite 100
Alexandria, VA 22314
Helpline: 800-658-8898
Phone: 703-837-1500
Website: http://www.nhpco.org
E-mail: info@nhpco.org

*National Institute
on Aging (NIA)*
Bldg. 31, Room 5C27
31 Center Dr., MSC 2292
Bethesda, MD 20892
Toll-Free: 800-222-2225
Toll-Free TTY: 800-222-4225
Website: http://www.nia.nih.gov

*Visiting Nurse
Associations of America*
900 19th St., NW
Suite 200
Washington, DC 20006
Phone: 202-384-1420
Website:
http://www.vnaa.org
E-mail: vnaa@vnaa.org

Chapter 77

How to Find Resources in Your Own Community If You Have Cancer

If you have cancer or are undergoing cancer treatment, there are places in your community to turn to for help. There are many local organizations throughout the country that offer a variety of practical and support services to people with cancer. However, people often don't know about these services or are unable to find them. National cancer organizations can assist you in finding these resources, and there are a number of things you can do for yourself.

Whether you are looking for a support group, counseling, advice, financial assistance, transportation to and from treatment, or information about cancer, most neighborhood organizations, local health care providers, or area hospitals are a good place to start. Often, the hardest part of looking for help is knowing the right questions to ask.

The Kind of Help You Can Get

Until now, you probably never thought about the many issues and difficulties that arise with a diagnosis of cancer. There are support services to help you deal with almost any type of problem that might occur. The first step in finding the help you need is knowing what types of services are available. The following information describes some of these services and the next section explains how to find them.

Excepted from "How to Find Resources in Your Own Community If You Have Cancer," National Cancer Institute (www.cancer.gov), August 5, 2005; accessed October 5, 2010.

Information on Cancer

Most national cancer organizations provide a range of information services, including materials on different types of cancer, treatments, and treatment-related issues.

Counseling

While some people are reluctant to seek counseling, studies show that having someone to talk to reduces stress and helps people both mentally and physically. Counseling can also provide emotional support to cancer patients and help them better understand their illness. Different types of counseling include individual, group, family, self-help (sometimes called peer counseling), bereavement, patient-to-patient, and sexuality.

Medical Treatment Decisions

Often, people with cancer need to make complicated medical decisions. Many organizations provide hospital and physician referrals for second opinions and information on clinical trials (research studies with people), which may expand treatment options.

Prevention and Early Detection

While cancer prevention may never be 100 percent effective, many things (such as quitting smoking and eating healthy foods) can greatly reduce a person's risk for developing cancer. Prevention services usually focus on smoking cessation and nutrition. Early detection services, which are designed to detect cancer when a person has no symptoms of disease, can include referrals for screening mammograms, Pap tests, or prostate exams.

Home Health Care

Home health care assists patients who no longer need to stay in a hospital or nursing home, but still require professional medical help. Skilled nursing care, physical therapy, social work services, and nutrition counseling are all available at home.

Hospice Care

Hospice is care focused on the special needs of terminally ill cancer patients. Sometimes called palliative care, it centers around providing comfort, controlling physical symptoms, and giving emotional support to patients who can no longer benefit from curative treatment. Hospice programs provide services in various settings, including the patient's home, hospice centers, hospitals, or skilled nursing facilities. Your doctor or social worker can provide a referral for these services.

Rehabilitation

Rehabilitation services help people adjust to the effects of cancer and its treatment. Physical rehabilitation focuses on recovery from the physical effects of surgery or the side effects associated with chemotherapy. Occupational or vocational therapy helps people readjust to everyday routines, get back to work, or find employment.

Advocacy

Advocacy is a general term that refers to promoting or protecting the rights and interests of a certain group, such as cancer patients. Advocacy groups may offer services to assist with legal, ethical, medical, employment, legislative, or insurance issues, among others. For instance, if you feel your insurance company has not handled your claim fairly, you may want to advocate for a review of its decision.

Financial

Having cancer can be a tremendous financial burden to cancer patients and their families. There are programs sponsored by the Government and nonprofit organizations to help cancer patients with problems related to medical billing, insurance coverage, and reimbursement issues. There are also sources for financial assistance, and ways to get help collecting entitlements from Medicaid, Medicare, and the Social Security Administration.

Housing/Lodging

Some organizations provide lodging for the family of a patient undergoing treatment, especially if it is a child who is ill and the parents are required to accompany the child to treatment.

Children's Services

A number of organizations provide services for children with cancer, including summer camps, make-a-wish programs, and help for parents seeking child-care.

How to Find These Services

Often, the services that people with cancer are looking for are right in their own neighborhood or city. The following is a list of places where you can begin your search for help.

The hospital, clinic, or medical center where you see your doctor, received your diagnosis, or where you undergo treatment should be able to give you information. Your doctor or nurse may be able to tell you about your specific medical condition, pain management, rehabilitation services, home nursing, or hospice care.

Most hospitals also have a social work, home care, or discharge planning department. This department may be able to help you find a support group, a nonprofit agency that helps people who have cancer, or the government agencies that oversee Social Security, Medicare, and Medicaid. While you are undergoing treatment, be sure to ask the hospital about transportation, practical assistance, or even temporary child care. Talk to a hospital financial counselor in the business office about developing a monthly payment plan if you need help with hospital expenses.

The public library is an excellent source of information, as are patient libraries at many cancer centers. A librarian can help you find books and articles through a literature search.

A local church, synagogue, YMCA or YWCA, or fraternal order may provide financial assistance, or may have volunteers who can help with transportation and home care. Catholic Charities or the American Red Cross may also operate local offices. Some of these organizations may provide home care.

Local or county government agencies may offer low-cost transportation (sometimes called para-transit) to individuals unable to use public transportation. Most states also have an Area Agency on Aging that offers low-cost services to people over 60. Your hospital or community social worker can direct you to government agencies for entitlements, including Social Security, state disability, Medicaid, income maintenance, and food stamps. (Keep in mind that most applications to entitlement programs take some time to process.) The federal government also runs the Hill-Burton program (800-638-0742), which funds certain medical facilities and hospitals to provide cancer patients with free or low-cost care if they are in financial need.

Getting the Most from a Service: What to Ask

No matter what type of help you are looking for, the only way to find resources to fit your needs is to ask the right questions. When you are calling an organization for information, it is important to think about what questions you are going to ask before you call. Many people find it helpful to write out their questions in advance, and to take notes during the call. Another good tip is to ask the name of the person with whom you are speaking in case you have follow-up questions. Below are some of the questions you may want to consider if you are calling or visiting a new agency and want to learn about how they can help:

- How do I apply [for this service]?

- Are there eligibility requirements? What are they?

- Is there an application process? How long will it take? What information will I need to complete the application process?

- Will I need anything else to get the service?

- Do you have any other suggestions or ideas about where I can find help?

The most important thing to remember is that you will rarely receive help unless you ask for it. In fact, asking can be the hardest part of getting help. Don't be afraid or ashamed to ask for assistance. Cancer is a very difficult disease, but there are people and services that can ease your burdens and help you focus on your treatment and recovery.

Chapter 78

Beware of Online Cancer Fraud

While health fraud is a cruel form of greed, fraud involving cancer treatments can be particularly heartless—especially because fraudulent information can travel around the Web in an instant.

"Anyone who suffers from cancer, or knows someone who does, understands the fear and desperation that can set in," says Gary Coody, R.Ph., the National Health Fraud Coordinator and a Consumer Safety Officer with the Food and Drug Administration's (FDA) Office of Regulatory Affairs. "There can be a great temptation to jump at anything that appears to offer a chance for a cure."

Medicinal products and devices intended to treat cancer must gain FDA approval before they are marketed. The agency's review process helps ensure that these products are safe and effective.

Nevertheless, it's always possible to find someone or some company hawking bogus cancer "treatments." Such "treatments" come in many forms, including pills, tonics, and creams. "They're frequently offered as natural treatments and 'dietary supplements,'" says Coody. Many of these fraudulent cancer products even appear completely harmless, but may cause indirect harm by delaying or interfering with proven, beneficial treatments.

"Advertisements and other promotional materials touting bogus cancer 'cures' have probably been around as long as the printing press," says Coody. "However, the Internet has compounded the problem by providing the peddlers of these often dangerous products a whole new outlet."

From "Beware of Online Cancer Fraud," U.S. Food and Drug Administration (www.fda.gov), September 18, 2008.

Unproven 'Remedies,' False Promises

Coody cites black salves as one of the fake cancer "remedies" that indeed have proven to be harmful. "Although it is illegal to market these salves as a cancer treatment, they are readily available online," he says.

The salves are sold with false promises that they will cure cancer by "drawing out" the disease from beneath the skin. "However, there is no scientific evidence that black salves are effective," says Janet Woodcock, Director of FDA's Center for Drug Evaluation and Research (CDER). "Even worse, black salves can cause direct harm to the patient."

The corrosive, oily salves "essentially burn off layers of the skin and surrounding normal tissue," says Woodcock. "This is not a simple, painless process. There are documented cases of these salves destroying large parts of people's skin and underlying tissue, leaving terrible scars."

Another unproven "remedy" that has been hawked for decades is an herbal regimen known as the Hoxsey Cancer Treatment. "FDA has taken regulatory and enforcement action against this discredited course of therapy beginning in the 1950s," says Coody.

"There is no scientific evidence that it has any value to treat cancer," he adds. "Yet consumers can go online right now and find all sorts of false claims that Hoxsey treatment is effective against the disease."

Red Flags

Coody says that firms engaged in cancer treatment or prevention fraud often use exaggerated and bogus claims to promote these products. He adds that consumers should recognize the following phrases as red flags:

- "Treats all forms of cancer"

- "Skin cancers disappear"

- "Shrinks malignant tumors"

- "Non-toxic"

- "Doesn't make you sick"

- "Avoid painful surgery, radiotherapy, chemotherapy, or other conventional treatments"

- "Treat non-melanoma skin cancers easily and safely"

"Unproven claims are also found in unverified testimonials, re-search results, or even in product and website names," says Coody. He offers important points that consumers seeking cancer treatments should keep in mind:

- Always consult with your health care professional before start-ing a new treatment or adding one to existing therapies. "Some products may interact with your medicines or keep them from working the way they are supposed to," says Coody.

- Understand the difference between fraudulent drug products and what FDA calls "investigational drugs." Investigational drugs undergo clinical testing to determine if they are safe and effective for their intended uses. Fraudulent products, on the other hand, are unapproved and typically have never been clini-cally tested or reviewed by FDA for safety and effectiveness. Marketing them is a violation of federal law.

"There are legal ways for patients to access investigational drugs," says Coody. "The most common way is by taking part in clinical trials. But patients can also receive investigational drugs outside of clinical trials in some cases."

Agencies Take Action

FDA and the U.S. Federal Trade Commission (FTC), in collaboration with other North American government agencies, have announced a new initiative to prevent these deceptive products from reaching con-sumers. Coody says that as part of the joint campaign, FDA and FTC have sent approximately 135 warning letters and two advisory letters to firms that market these products online.

The initiative originated not only from consumer complaints, he says, but also from a Web surf for fraudulent cancer products by FDA and members of the Mexico-United States-Canada Health fraud work-ing group (MUCH).

Signs of Health Fraud

All consumers seeking information about any health product or medical treatment should be familiar with the following signs of health fraud:

- Statements that the product is a quick and effective cure-all or a diagnostic tool for a wide variety of ailments.

- Suggestions that a product can treat or cure serious or incurable diseases.

- Claims such as "scientific breakthrough," "miraculous cure," "secret ingredient," and "ancient remedy."

- Impressive-sounding terms, such as "hunger stimulation point" and "thermogenesis" for a weight loss product.

- Claims that the product is safe because it is "natural."

- Undocumented case histories or personal testimonials by consumers or doctors claiming amazing results.

- Claims of limited availability and advance payment requirements.

- Promises of no-risk, money-back guarantees.

- Promises of an "easy" fix for problems like excess weight, hair loss, or impotency.

Index

Index

H

V

Health Reference Series
Complete Catalog
List price $93 per volume. School and library price $84 per volume.

Adolescent Health Sourcebook, 3rd Edition

Basic Consumer Health Information about Adolescent Growth and Development, Puberty, Sexuality, Reproductive Health, and Physical, Emotional, Social, and Mental Health Concerns of Teens and Their Parents, Including Facts about Nutrition, Physical Activity, Weight Management, Acne, Allergies, Cancer, Diabetes, Growth Disorders, Juvenile Arthritis, Infections, Substance Abuse, and More

Along with Information about Adolescent Safety Concerns, Youth Violence, a Glossary of Related Terms, and a Directory of Resources

Edited by Amy L. Sutton. 600 pages. 2010. 978-0-7808-1140-9.

Adult Health Concerns Sourcebook

Basic Consumer Health Information about Medical and Mental Concerns of Adults, Including Facts about Choosing Healthcare Providers, Navigating Insurance Options, Maintaining Wellness, Preventing Cancer, Heart Disease, Stroke, Diabetes, and Osteoporosis, and Understanding Aging-Related Health Concerns, Including Menopause, Cognitive Changes, and Changes in the Coronary and Vascular Systems

Along with Tips on Caring for Aging Parents and Dealing with Health-Related Work and Travel Issues, a Glossary, and a Directory of Resources for Additional Help and Information

Edited by Sandra J. Judd. 648 pages. 2008. 978-0-7808-0999-4.

"Provides a thorough list of topics that are important to adult health and for caregivers."
—*CHOICE, Nov '08*

"Written in easy-to-understand language... the content is well-organized and is intended to aid adults in making health care-related decisions."
—*AORN Journal, Dec '08*

AIDS Sourcebook, 4th Edition

Basic Consumer Health Information about Human Immunodeficiency Virus (HIV) and Acquired Immunodeficiency Syndrome (AIDS), Featuring Updated Statistics and Facts about Risks, Prevention, Screening, Diagnosis, Treatments, Side Effects, and Complications, and Including a Section about the Impact of HIV/AIDS on the Health of Women, Children, and Adolescents

Along with Tips on Managing Life with AIDS, Reports on Current Research Initiatives and Clinical Trials, a Glossary of Related Terms, and Resource Directories for Further Help and Information

Edited by Ivy L. Alexander. 680 pages. 2008. 978-0-7808-0997-0.

SEE ALSO *Contagious Diseases Sourcebook, 2nd Edition*

Alcoholism Sourcebook, 3rd Edition

Basic Consumer Health Information about Alcohol Use, Abuse, and Dependence, Featuring Facts about the Physical, Mental, and Social Health Effects of Alcohol Addiction, Including Alcoholic Liver Disease, Pancreatic Disease, Cardiovascular Disease, Neurological Disorders, and the Effects of Drinking during Pregnancy

Along with Information about Alcohol Treatment, Medications, and Recovery Programs, in Addition to Tips for Reducing the Prevalence of Underage Drinking, Statistics about Alcohol Use, a Glossary of Related Terms, and Directories of Resources for More Help and Information

Edited by Joyce Brennfleck Shannon. 600 pages. 2010. 978-0-7808-1141-6.

SEE ALSO *Drug Abuse Sourcebook, 3rd Edition*

Allergies Sourcebook, 3rd Edition

Basic Consumer Health Information about Allergic Disorders, Such as Anaphylaxis, Hives,

Eczema, Rhinitis, Sinusitis, and Conjunctivitis, and Their Triggers, Including Pollen, Mold, Dust Mites, Animal Dander, Insects, Chemicals, Food, Food Additives, and Medications

Along with Advice about the Diagnosis and Treatment of Allergy Symptoms, a Glossary of Related Terms, a Directory of Resources for Help and Information, and Suggestions for Additional Reading

Edited by Amy L. Sutton. 588 pages. 2007. 978-0-7808-0950-5.

SEE ALSO Asthma Sourcebook, 2nd Edition

Alzheimer Disease Sourcebook, 4th Edition

Basic Consumer Health Information about Alzheimer Disease, Other Dementias, and Related Disorders, Including Multi-Infarct Dementia, Dementia with Lewy Bodies, Frontotemporal Dementia (Pick Disease), Wernicke-Korsakoff Syndrome (Alcohol-Related Dementia), AIDS Dementia Complex, Huntington Disease, Creutzfeldt-Jacob Disease, and Delirium

Along with Information about Coping with Memory Loss and Forgetfulness, Maintaining Skills, and Long-Term Planning for People with Dementia, and Suggestions Addressing Common Caregiver Concerns, Updated Information about Current Research Efforts, a Glossary of Related Terms, and Directories of Sources for Additional Help and Information

Edited by Karen Bellenir. 603 pages. 2008. 978-0-7808-1001-3.

"An invaluable resource for persons who have received a diagnosis, for caregivers, and for family members dealing with this insidious disease. It is recommended for public, community college, and ready-reference sections in academic libraries."
—American Reference Books Annual, 2009

SEE ALSO Brain Disorders Sourcebook, 3rd Edition

Arthritis Sourcebook, 3rd Edition

Basic Consumer Health Information about the Risk Factors, Symptoms, Diagnosis, and Treatment of Osteoarthritis, Rheumatoid Arthritis, Juvenile Arthritis, Gout, Infectious Arthritis, and Autoimmune Disorders Associated with Arthritis

Along with Facts about Medications, Surgeries, and Self-Care Techniques to Manage Pain and Disability, Tips on Living with Arthritis, a Glossary of Related Terms, and Resources for Additional Help and Information

Edited by Amy L. Sutton. 600 pages. 2010. 978-0-7808-1077-8.

Asthma Sourcebook, 2nd Edition

Basic Consumer Health Information about the Causes, Symptoms, Diagnosis, and Treatment of Asthma in Infants, Children, Teenagers, and Adults, Including Facts about Different Types of Asthma, Common Co-Occurring Conditions, Asthma Management Plans, Triggers, Medications, and Medication Delivery Devices

Along with Asthma Statistics, Research Updates, a Glossary, a Directory of Asthma-Related Resources, and More

Edited by Karen Bellenir. 581 pages. 2006. 978-0-7808-0866-9.

SEE ALSO Lung Disorders Sourcebook; Respiratory Disorders Sourcebook, 2nd Edition

Attention Deficit Disorder Sourcebook

Basic Consumer Health Information about Attention Deficit/Hyperactivity Disorder in Children and Adults, Including Facts about Causes, Symptoms, Diagnostic Criteria, and Treatment Options Such as Medications, Behavior Therapy, Coaching, and Homeopathy

Along with Reports on Current Research Initiatives, Legal Issues, and Government Regulations, and Featuring a Glossary of Related Terms, Internet Resources, and a List of Additional Reading Material

Edited by Dawn D. Matthews. 447 pages. 2002. 978-0-7808-0624-5.

"Recommended reference source."
—Booklist, Jan '03

SEE ALSO Learning Disabilities Sourcebook, 3rd Edition

Autism and Pervasive Developmental Disorders Sourcebook

Basic Consumer Health Information about Autism Spectrum and Pervasive Developmental Disorders, Such as Classical Autism, Asperger Syndrome, Rett Syndrome, and Childhood Disintegrative Disorder, Including Information about Related Genetic Disorders and Medical Problems and Facts about Causes, Screening Methods, Diagnostic Criteria, Treatments and Interventions, and Family and Education Issues

Along with a Glossary of Related Terms, Tips for Evaluating the Validity of Health Claims, and a Directory of Resources for Additional Help and Information

Edited by Sandra J. Judd. 603 pages. 2007. 978-0-7808-0953-6.

"This book provides a current overview of disorders on the autism spectrum and information about various therapies, educational resources, and help for families with practical issues such as workplace adjustments, living arrangements, and estate planning. It is a useful resource for public and consumer health libraries."
—*American Reference Books Annual, 2009*

SEE ALSO *Learning Disabilities Sourcebook, 3rd Edition*

Back and Neck Disorders Sourcebook, 2nd Edition

Basic Consumer Health Information about Spinal Pain, Spinal Cord Injuries, and Related Disorders, Such as Degenerative Disk Disease, Osteoarthritis, Scoliosis, Sciatica, Spina Bifida, and Spinal Stenosis, and Featuring Facts about Maintaining Spinal Health, Self-Care, Pain Management, Rehabilitative Care, Chiropractic Care, Spinal Surgeries, and Complementary Therapies

Along with Suggestions for Preventing Back and Neck Pain, a Glossary of Related Terms, and a Directory of Resources

Edited by Amy L. Sutton. 607 pages. 2004. 978-0-7808-0738-9.

"Recommended... An easy to use, comprehensive medical reference book."
—*E-Streams, Sep '05*

"For anyone who has back or neck problems, this book is ideal. Its easy-to-understand language and variety of topics makes this sourcebook a worthwhile read. The price... is reasonable for the amount of information contained in the book"
—*Occupational Therapy in Health Care, 2007*

Blood & Circulatory Disorders Sourcebook, 3rd Edition

Basic Consumer Health Information about Blood and Circulatory System Disorders, Such as Anemia, Leukemia, Lymphoma, Rh Disease, Hemophilia, Thrombophilia, Other Bleeding and Clotting Deficiencies, and Artery, Vascular, and Venous Diseases, Including Facts about Blood Types, Blood Donation, Bone Marrow and Stem Cell Transplants, Tests and Medications, and Tips for Maintaining Circulatory Health

Along with a Glossary of Related Terms and a List of Resources for Additional Help and Information

Edited by Sandra J. Judd. 600 pages. 2010. 978-0-7808-1081-5.

SEE ALSO *Leukemia Sourcebook*

Brain Disorders Sourcebook, 3rd Edition

Basic Consumer Health Information about Acquired and Traumatic Brain Injuries, Brain Tumors, Cerebral Palsy and Other Genetic and Congenital Brain Disorders, Infections of the Brain, Epilepsy, and Degenerative Neurological Disorders Such as Dementia, Huntington Disease, and Amyotrophic Lateral Sclerosis (ALS)

Along with Information on Brain Structure and Function, Treatment and Rehabilitation Options, a Glossary of Terms Related to Brain Disorders, and a Directory of Resources for More Information

Edited by Joyce Brennfleck Shannon. 600 pages. 2010. 978-0-7808-1083-9.

SEE ALSO *Alzheimer Disease Sourcebook, 4th Edition*

Breast Cancer Sourcebook, 3rd Edition

Basic Consumer Health Information about Breast Health and Breast Cancer, Including Facts about Environmental, Genetic, and Other Risk Factors, Prevention Efforts, Screening and Diagnostic Methods, Surgical Treatment Options and Other Care Choices, Complementary and Alternative Therapies, and Post-Treatment Concerns

Along with Statistical Data, News about Research Advances, a Glossary of Related Terms, and Directories of Resources for Additional Information and Support

Edited by Karen Bellenir. 606 pages. 2009. 978-0-7808-1030-3.

"A very useful reference for people wanting to learn more about breast cancer and how to negotiate their care or the care of a loved one. The third edition is necessary as information/treatment options continue to evolve."
— *Doody's Review Service, 2009*

SEE ALSO *Cancer Sourcebook for Women, 3rd Edition, Women's Health Concerns Sourcebook, 3rd Edition*

Breastfeeding Sourcebook

Basic Consumer Health Information about the Benefits of Breastmilk, Preparing to Breastfeed, Breastfeeding as a Baby Grows, Nutrition, and More, Including Information on Special Situations and Concerns Such as Mastitis, Illness, Medications, Allergies, Multiple Births, Prematurity, Special Needs, and Adoption

Along with a Glossary and Resources for Additional Help and Information

Edited by Jenni Lynn Colson. 367 pages. 2002. 978-0-7808-0332-9.

SEE ALSO *Pregnancy and Birth Sourcebook, 3rd Edition*

Burns Sourcebook

Basic Consumer Health Information about Various Types of Burns and Scalds, Including Flame, Heat, Cold, Electrical, Chemical, and Sun Burns

Along with Information on Short-Term and Long-Term Treatments, Tissue Reconstruction, Plastic Surgery, Prevention Suggestions, and First Aid

Edited by Allan R. Cook. 604 pages. 1999. 978-0-7808-0204-9.

"This is an exceptional addition to the series and is highly recommended for all consumer health collections, hospital libraries, and academic medical centers."
— *E-Streams, Mar '00*

"This key reference guide is an invaluable addition to all health care and public libraries in confronting this ongoing health issue."
— *American Reference Books Annual, 2000*

SEE ALSO *Dermatological Disorders Sourcebook, 2nd Edition*

Cancer Sourcebook, 5th Edition

Basic Consumer Health Information about Major Forms and Stages of Cancer, Featuring Facts about Head and Neck Cancers, Lung Cancers, Gastrointestinal Cancers, Genitourinary Cancers, Lymphomas, Blood Cell Cancers, Endocrine Cancers, Skin Cancers, Bone Cancers, Metastatic Cancers, and More

Along with Facts about Cancer Treatments, Cancer Risks and Prevention, a Glossary of Related Terms, Statistical Data, and a Directory of Resources for Additional Information

Edited by Karen Bellenir. 1105 pages. 2007. 978-0-7808-0947-5.

"The 5th, updated edition of Cancer Sourcebook should be in every public and health lending library collection... An unparalleled discussion essential for any health collections considering an all-in-one basic general reference."
— *California Bookwatch, Aug '07*

SEE ALSO *Breast Cancer Sourcebook, 3rd Edition, Cancer Survivorship Sourcebook, Leukemia Sourcebook*

Cancer Sourcebook for Women, 4th Edition

Basic Consumer Health Information about Gynecologic Cancers and Other Cancers of Special Concern to Women, Including Cancers of the Breast, Cervix, Colon, Lung, Ovaries, Thyroid, and Uterus

Along with Facts about Benign Conditions of the Female Reproductive System, Cancer Risk

Factors, Diagnostic and Treatment Procedures, Side Effects of Cancer and Cancer Treatments, Women's Issues in Cancer Survivorship, a Glossary of Related Terms, and a Directory of Resources for Additional Help and Information

Edited by Karen Bellenir. 600 pages. 2010. 978-0-7808-1139-3.

SEE ALSO Breast Cancer Sourcebook, 3rd Edition, Women's Health Concerns Sourcebook, 3rd Edition

---

Cancer Survivorship Sourcebook

Basic Consumer Health Information about the Physical, Educational, Emotional, Social, and Financial Needs of Cancer Patients from Diagnosis, through Cancer Treatment, and Beyond, Including Facts about Researching Specific Types of Cancer and Learning about Clinical Trials and Treatment Options, and Featuring Tips for Coping with the Side Effects of Cancer Treatments and Adjusting to Life after Cancer Treatment Concludes

Along with Suggestions for Caregivers, Friends, and Family Members of Cancer Patients, a Glossary of Cancer Care Terms, and Directories of Related Resources

Edited by Karen Bellenir. 633 pages. 2007. 978-0-7808-0985-7.

"Well organized and comprehensive in coverage, the book speaks to issues encountered both during and after cancer treatment. Recommended for consumer health and public libraries."
—*Library Journal, Aug 1 '07*

"Cancer Survivorship Sourcebook will be useful to anyone who has a friend or loved one with a cancer diagnosis."
—*American Reference Books Annual, 2008*

SEE ALSO *Cancer Sourcebook, 5th Edition, Disease Management Sourcebook*

Cardiovascular Disorders Sourcebook, 4th Edition

Basic Consumer Health Information about Heart and Blood Vessel Diseases and Disorders, Such as Angina, Heart Attack, Heart Failure, Cardiomyopathy, Arrhythmias, Valve Disease, Atherosclerosis, Aneurysms, and

Congenital Heart Defects, Including Information about Cardiovascular Disease in Women, Men, Children, Adolescents, and Minorities

Along with Facts about Diagnosing, Managing, and Preventing Cardiovascular Disease, a Glossary of Related Medical Terms, and a Directory of Resources for Additional Information

Edited by Amy L. Sutton. 600 pages. 2010. 978-0-7808-1080-8.

Caregiving Sourcebook

Basic Consumer Health Information for Caregivers, Including a Profile of Caregivers, Caregiving Responsibilities and Concerns, Tips for Specific Conditions, Care Environments, and the Effects of Caregiving

Along with Facts about Legal Issues, Financial Information, and Future Planning, a Glossary, and a Listing of Additional Resources

Edited by Joyce Brennfleck Shannon. 583 pages. 2001. 978-0-7808-0331-2.

"Essential for most collections."
—*Library Journal, Apr 1 '02*

"An ideal addition to the reference collection of any public library. Health sciences information professionals may also want to acquire the Caregiving Sourcebook for their hospital or academic library for use as a ready reference tool by health care workers interested in aging and caregiving."
—*E-Streams, Jan '02*

Child Abuse Sourcebook, 2nd Edition

Basic Consumer Health Information about the Physical, Sexual, and Emotional Abuse of Children, Neglect, Münchhausen Syndrome by Proxy (MSBP), and Shaken Baby Syndrome, and Featuring Facts about Withholding Medical Care, Corporal Punishment, Child Maltreatment in Youth Sports, and Parental Substance Abuse

Along with Information about Child Protective Services, Foster Care, Adoption, Parenting Challenges, Abuse Prevention Programs, and Intervention, Treatment, and Recovery Guidelines, a Glossary of Related Terms, and Resources for Additional Help and Information

Edited by Joyce Brennfleck Shannon. 600 pages. 2009. 978-0-7808-1037-2.

SEE ALSO Domestic Violence Sourcebook, 3rd Edition

Childhood Diseases and Disorders Sourcebook, 2nd Edition

Basic Consumer Health Information about the Physical, Mental, and Developmental Health of Pre-Adolescent Children, Including Facts about Infectious Diseases, Asthma, Allergies, Diabetes, and Other Acute and Chronic Conditions Affecting the Gastrointestinal Tract, Ears, Nose, Throat, Liver, Kidneys, Heart, Blood, Brain, Muscles, Bones, and Skin

Along with Reports on Recommended Childhood Vaccinations, Wellness Guidelines, a Glossary of Related Medical Terms, and a List of Resources for Parents

Edited by Sandra J. Judd. 694 pages. 2009. 978-0-7808-1031-0.

"The strength of this source is the wide range of information given about childhood health issues... It is most appropriate for public libraries and academic libraries that field medical questions."
—American Reference Books Annual, 2009

SEE ALSO Healthy Children Sourcebook

Colds, Flu and Other Common Ailments Sourcebook

Basic Consumer Health Information about Common Ailments and Injuries, Including Colds, Coughs, the Flu, Sinus Problems, Headaches, Fever, Nausea and Vomiting, Menstrual Cramps, Diarrhea, Constipation, Hemorrhoids, Back Pain, Dandruff, Dry and Itchy Skin, Cuts, Scrapes, Sprains, Bruises, and More

Along with Information about Prevention, Self-Care, Choosing a Doctor, Over-the-Counter Medications, Folk Remedies, and Alternative Therapies, and Including a Glossary of Important Terms and a Directory of Resources for Further Help and Information

Edited by Chad T. Kimball. 622 pages. 2001. 978-0-7808-0435-7.

"A good starting point for research on common illnesses. It will be a useful addition to public and consumer health library collections."
—American Reference Books Annual, 2002

"Will prove valuable to any library seeking to maintain a current, comprehensive reference collection of health resources... Excellent reference."
—The Bookwatch, Aug '01

SEE ALSO Contagious Diseases Sourcebook, 2nd Edition

Communication Disorders Sourcebook

Basic Information about Deafness and Hearing Loss, Speech and Language Disorders, Voice Disorders, Balance and Vestibular Disorders, and Disorders of Smell, Taste, and Touch

Edited by Linda M. Ross. 533 pages. 1996. 978-0-7808-0077-9.

"This is skillfully edited and is a welcome resource for the layperson. It should be found in every public and medical library."
—Booklist Health Sciences Supplement, Oct '97

Complementary & Alternative Medicine Sourcebook, 4th Edition

Basic Consumer Health Information about Ayurveda, Acupuncture, Aromatherapy, Chiropractic Care, Diet-Based Therapies, Guided Imagery, Herbal and Vitamin Supplements, Homeopathy, Hypnosis, Massage, Meditation, Naturopathy, Pilates, Reflexology, Reiki, Shiatsu, Tai Chi, Traditional Chinese Medicine, Yoga, and Other Complementary and Alternative Medical Therapies

Along with Statistics, Tips for Selecting a Practitioner, Treatments for Specific Health Conditions, a Glossary of Related Terms, and a Directory of Resources for Additional Help and Information

Edited by Amy L. Sutton. 600 pages. 2010. 978-0-7808-1082-2.

Congenital Disorders Sourcebook, 2nd Edition

Basic Consumer Health Information about Nonhereditary Birth Defects and Disorders

Related to Prematurity, Gestational Injuries, Congenital Infections, and Birth Complications, Including Heart Defects, Hydrocephalus, Spina Bifida, Cleft Lip and Palate, Cerebral Palsy, and More

Along with Facts about the Prevention of Birth Defects, Fetal Surgery and Other Treatment Options, Research Initiatives, a Glossary of Related Terms, and Resources for Additional Information and Support

Edited by Sandra J. Judd. 619 pages. 2007. 978-0-7808-0945-1.

"Congenital Disorders Sourcebook provides an excellent, non-technical overview of many aspects of pregnancy with the focus on congenital disorders."

—American Reference Books Annual, 2008

"An excellent readable reference aimed at the lay public for difficult to understand medical problems. An excellent starting point for the interested parent or family member who may then be motivated to seek more information."

—Doody's Review Service, 2007

SEE ALSO Pregnancy and Birth Sourcebook, 3rd Edition

Contagious Diseases Sourcebook, 2nd Edition

Basic Consumer Health Information about Diseases Spread from Person to Person through Direct Physical Contact, Airborne Transmissions, Sexual Contact, or Contact with Blood or Other Body Fluids, Including Pneumococcal, Staphylococcal, and Streptococcal Diseases, Colds, Influenza, Lice, Measles, Mumps, Tuberculosis, and Others

Along with Facts about Self-Care and Over-the-Counter Medications, Antibiotics and Drug Resistance, Disease Prevention, Vaccines, and Bioterrorism, a Glossary, and a Directory of Resources for More Information

Edited by Joyce Brennfleck Shannon. 600 pages. 2010. 978-0-7808-1075-4.

SEE ALSO AIDS Sourcebook, 4th Edition, Hepatitis Sourcebook

Cosmetic and Reconstructive Surgery Sourcebook, 2nd Edition

Basic Consumer Information about Plastic Surgery and Non-Surgical Appearance-Enhancing Procedures, Including Facts about Botulinum Toxin, Collagen Replacement, Dermabrasion, Chemical Peels, Eyelid Surgery, Nose Reshaping, Lip Augmentation, Liposuction, Breast Enlargement and Reduction, Tummy Tucking, and Other Skin, Hair, Facial, and Body Shaping Procedures

Along with Information about Reconstructive Procedures for Congenital Disorders, Disfiguring Diseases, Burns, and Traumatic Injuries, a Glossary of Related Terms, and a Directory of Additional Resources

Edited by Karen Bellenir. 483 pages. 2007. 978-0-7808-0951-2.

"A comprehensive source for people considering cosmetic surgery... also recommended for medical students who will perform these procedures later in their careers; and public librarians and academic medical librarians who may assist patrons interested in this information."

—Medical Reference Services Quarterly, Fall '08

"A practical guide for health care consumers and health care workers... This easy-to-read reference guide would be useful for novice and veteran health care consumers, surgical technology students, nursing students, and perioperative nurses new to plastic and reconstructive surgery. It also may be helpful for medical-surgical nurses as a guide for patient teaching in their practices."

—AORN Journal, Aug '08

SEE ALSO Surgery Sourcebook, 2nd Edition

Death and Dying Sourcebook, 2nd Edition

Basic Consumer Health Information about End-of-Life Care and Related Perspectives and Ethical Issues, Including End-of-Life Symptoms and Treatments, Pain Management, Quality-of-Life Concerns, the Use of Life Support, Patients' Rights and Privacy Issues, Advance Directives, Physician-Assisted Suicide, Caregiving, Organ and Tissue Donation, Autopsies, Funeral Arrangements, and Grief

Along with Statistical Data, Information about the Leading Causes of Death, a Glossary, and Directories of Support Groups and Other Resources

Edited by Joyce Brennfleck Shannon. 626 pages. 2006. 978-0-7808-0871-3.

Dental Care and Oral Health Sourcebook, 3rd Edition

Basic Consumer Health Information about Dental Care and Oral Health Throughout the Lifespan, Including Facts about Cavities, Bad Breath, Cold and Canker Sores, Dry Mouth, Toothaches, Gum Disease, Malocclusion, Temporomandibular Joint and Muscle Disorders, Oral Cancers, and Dental Emergencies

Along with Information about Mouth Hygiene, Crowns, Bridges, Implants, and Fillings, Surgical, Orthodontic, and Cosmetic Dental Procedures, Pain Management, Health Conditions that Impact Oral Care, a Glossary of Related Terms, and a Directory of Additional Resources

Edited by Amy L. Sutton. 619 pages. 2008. 978-0-7808-1032-7.

"Could serve as turning point in the battle to educate consumers in issues concerning oral health. Tightly written in terms the average person can understand, yet comprehensive in scope and authoritative in tone, it is another excellent sourcebook in the Health Reference Series... Should be in the reference department of all public libraries, and in academic libraries that have a public constituency."
—American Reference Books Annual, 2009

Depression Sourcebook, 2nd Edition

Basic Consumer Health Information about Unipolar Depression, Bipolar Disorder, Dysthymia, Seasonal Affective Disorder, Postpartum Depression, and Other Depressive Disorders, Including Facts about Populations at Special Risk, Coexisting Medical Conditions, Symptoms, Treatment Options, and Suicide Prevention

Along with Statistical Data, a Glossary of Related Terms, and a Directory of Resources for Additional Help and Information

Edited by Sandra J. Judd. 646 pages. 2008. 978-0-7808-1003-7.

"Recommended for public libraries."
—American Reference Books Annual, 2009

SEE ALSO Mental Health Disorders Sourcebook, 4th Edition

Dermatological Disorders Sourcebook, 2nd Edition

Basic Consumer Health Information about Conditions and Disorders Affecting the Skin, Hair, and Nails, Such as Acne, Rosacea, Rashes, Dermatitis, Pigmentation Disorders, Birthmarks, Skin Cancer, Skin Injuries, Psoriasis, Scleroderma, and Hair Loss, Including Facts about Medications and Treatments for Dermatological Disorders and Tips for Maintaining Healthy Skin, Hair, and Nails

Along with Information about How Aging Affects the Skin, a Glossary of Related Terms, and a Directory of Resources for Additional Help and Information

Edited by Amy L. Sutton. 617 pages. 2006. 978-0-7808-0795-2.

"Well organized... presents a plethora of information in a manner that is appropriate in style and readability for the intended audience."
—Physical Therapy, Nov '06

"Helpfully brings together... sources in one convenient place, saving the user hours of research time."
—American Reference Books Annual, 2006

SEE ALSO Burns Sourcebook

Diabetes Sourcebook, 4th Edition

Basic Consumer Health Information about Type 1 and Type 2 Diabetes Mellitus, Gestational Diabetes, Monogenic Forms of Diabetes, and Insulin Resistance, with Guidelines for Lifestyle Modifications and the Medical Management of Diabetes, Including Facts about Insulin, Insulin Delivery Devices, Oral Diabetes Medications, Self-Monitoring of Blood Glucose, Meal Planning, Physical Activity Recommendations, Foot Care, and Treatment Options for People with Kidney Failure

Along with a Section about Diabetes Complications and Co-Occurring Conditions, a Glossary of Related Terms, and Directories of Resources for Additional Help and Information

Edited by Karen Bellenir. 627 pages. 2008. 978-0-7808-1005-1.

"Completely and comprehensively covering almost everything a student or physician would need to know... well worth the investment."
—*Internet Bookwatch, Dec '08*

SEE ALSO *Endocrine and Metabolic Disorders Sourcebook, 2nd Edition*

Diet and Nutrition Sourcebook, 3rd Edition

Basic Consumer Health Information about Dietary Guidelines and the Food Guidance System, Recommended Daily Nutrient Intakes, Serving Proportions, Weight Control, Vitamins and Supplements, Nutrition Issues for Different Life Stages and Lifestyles, and the Needs of People with Specific Medical Concerns, Including Cancer, Celiac Disease, Diabetes, Eating Disorders, Food Allergies, and Cardiovascular Disease

Along with Facts about Federal Nutrition Support Programs, a Glossary of Nutrition and Dietary Terms, and Directories of Additional Resources for More Information about Nutrition

Edited by Joyce Brennfleck Shannon. 605 pages. 2006. 978-0-7808-0800-3.

"A valuable resource tool for any individual."
—*Journal of Dental Hygiene, Apr '07*

"From different recommended eating habits to reduce disease and common ailments to nutrition advice for those with specific conditions, Diet and Nutrition Sourcebook is especially important because so much is changing in this area, and so rapidly."
—*California Bookwatch, Jun '06*

SEE ALSO *Eating Disorders Sourcebook, 2nd Edition, Vegetarian Sourcebook*

Digestive Diseases and Disorders Sourcebook

Basic Consumer Health Information about Diseases and Disorders that Impact the Upper and Lower Digestive System, Including Celiac

Disease, Constipation, Crohn's Disease, Cyclic Vomiting Syndrome, Diarrhea, Diverticulosis and Diverticulitis, Gallstones, Heartburn, Hemorrhoids, Hernias, Indigestion (Dyspepsia), Irritable Bowel Syndrome, Lactose Intolerance, Ulcers, and More

Along with Information about Medications and Other Treatments, Tips for Maintaining a Healthy Digestive Tract, a Glossary, and Directory of Digestive Diseases Organizations

Edited by Karen Bellenir. 323 pages. 2000. 978-0-7808-0327-5.

"An excellent addition to all public or patient-research libraries."
—*American Reference Books Annual, 2001*

"Recommended reference source."
—*Booklist, May '00*

SEE ALSO *Gastrointestinal Diseases and Disorders Sourcebook, 2nd Edition*

Disabilities Sourcebook

Basic Consumer Health Information about Physical and Psychiatric Disabilities, Including Descriptions of Major Causes of Disability, Assistive and Adaptive Aids, Workplace Issues, and Accessibility Concerns

Along with Information about the Americans with Disabilities Act, a Glossary, and Resources for Additional Help and Information

Edited by Dawn D. Matthews. 602 pages. 2000. 978-0-7808-0389-3.

"A must for libraries with a consumer health section."
—*American Reference Books Annual, 2002*

"A much needed addition to the Omnigraphics Health Reference Series. A current reference work to provide people with disabilities, their families, caregivers or those who work with them, a broad range of information in one volume, has not been available until now... It is recommended for all public and academic library reference collections."
—*E-Streams, May '01*

"An excellent source book in easy-to-read format covering many current topics; highly recommended for all libraries."
—*CHOICE, Jan '01*

Disease Management Sourcebook

Basic Consumer Health Information about Coping with Chronic and Serious Illnesses, Navigating the Health Care System, Communicating with Health Care Providers, Assessing Health Care Quality, and Making Informed Health Care Decisions, Including Facts about Second Opinions, Hospitalization, Surgery, and Medications

Along with a Section about Children with Chronic Conditions, Information about Legal, Financial, and Insurance Issues, a Glossary of Related Terms, and Directories of Additional Resources

Edited by Joyce Brennfleck Shannon. 621 pages. 2008. 978-0-7808-1002-0.

"Consumers need to know how to manage their health care the same way they manage anything else in their lives. The text is very readable and is written for the layperson and consumer. The cost is not prohibitive. This book should be in all collections of health care libraries and public libraries."
— American Reference Books Annual, 2009

"The information is very current, and the selection of font and layout make the book easy to read. A hardback that will stand up to much usage, this is an excellent resource for consumers... Recommended. General readers."
—CHOICE, Nov '08

"Intended for lay readers, this resource clarifies the many confusing and overwhelming details associated with chronic disease care. Meticulous and clearly explained, the book even includes diagrams intended to ease comprehension of over-the-counter medication labels. An essential guide to navigating the health-care rapids."
—Library Journal, Aug '08

Domestic Violence Sourcebook, 3rd Edition

Basic Consumer Health Information about Warning Signs, Risk Factors, and Health Consequences of Intimate Partner Violence, Sexual Violence and Rape, Stalking, Human Trafficking, Child Maltreatment, Teen Dating Violence, and Elder Abuse

Along with Facts about Victims and Perpetrators, Strategies for Violence Prevention, and Emergency Interventions, Safety Plans, and Financial and Legal Tips for Victims, a Glossary of Related Terms, and Directories of Resources for Additional Information and Support

Edited by Joyce Brennfleck Shannon. 634 pages. 2009. 978-0-7808-1038-9.

"A recommended pick for any library interested in consumer health and social issues... A 'must' for any serious health collection."
—California Bookwatch, Jul '09

SEE ALSO Child Abuse Sourcebook, 2nd Edition

Drug Abuse Sourcebook, 3rd Edition

Basic Consumer Health Information about the Abuse of Cocaine, Club Drugs, Hallucinogens, Heroin, Inhalants, Marijuana, and Other Illicit Substances, Prescription Medications, and Over-the-Counter Medicines

Along with Facts about Addiction and Related Health Effects, Drug Abuse Treatment and Recovery, Drug Testing, Prevention Programs, Glossaries of Drug-Related Terms, and Directories of Resources for More Information

Edited by Joyce Brennfleck Shannon. 600 pages. 2010. 978-0-7808-1079-2.

SEE ALSO Alcoholism Sourcebook, 3rd Edition

Ear, Nose, and Throat Disorders Sourcebook, 2nd Edition

Basic Consumer Health Information about Disorders of the Ears, Hearing Loss, Vestibular Disorders, Nasal and Sinus Problems, Throat and Vocal Cord Disorders, and Otolaryngologic Cancers, Including Facts about Ear Infections and Injuries, Genetic and Congenital Deafness, Sensorineural Hearing Disorders, Tinnitus, Vertigo, Ménière Disease, Rhinitis, Sinusitis, Snoring, Sore Throats, Hoarseness, and More

Along with Reports on Current Research Initiatives, a Glossary of Related Medical Terms, and a Directory of Sources for Further Help and Information

Edited by Sandra J. Judd. 631 pages. 2007. 978-0-7808-0872-0.

"A resource book for the general public that provides comprehensive coverage of basic up-to-date medical information about the causes, symptoms, diagnosis, and treatment of diseases and disorders that affect the ears, nose, sinuses, throat, and voice... The majority of information is presented in question and answer format, much like questions a patient might ask of a health care provider. An extensive index facilitates the reader's ability to easily access information on any specific topic."
—*Journal of Dental Hygiene*, Oct '07

"A handy compilation of information on common and some not so common ailments of the ears, nose, and throat."
—*Doody's Review Service*, 2007

▨

Eating Disorders Sourcebook, 2nd Edition

Basic Consumer Health Information about Anorexia Nervosa, Bulimia, Binge Eating, Compulsive Exercise, Female Athlete Triad, and Other Eating Disorders, Including Facts about Body Image and Other Cultural and Age-Related Risk Factors, Prevention Efforts, Adverse Health Effects, Treatment Options, and the Recovery Process

Along with Guidelines for Healthy Weight Control, a Glossary, and Directories of Additional Resources

Edited by Joyce Brennfleck Shannon. 557 pages. 2007. 978-0-7808-0948-2.

"Recommended for the reference collection of large public libraries."
—*American Reference Books Annual*, 2008

"A basic health reference any health or general library needs."
—*Internet Bookwatch*, Jun '07

SEE ALSO *Diet and Nutrition Sourcebook, 3rd Edition, Mental Health Disorders Sourcebook, 4th Edition*

▨

Emergency Medical Services Sourcebook

Basic Consumer Health Information about Preventing, Preparing for, and Managing Emergency Situations, When and Who to Call for Help, What to Expect in the Emergency Room, the Emergency Medical Team,

Patient Issues, and Current Topics in Emergency Medicine

Along with Statistical Data, a Glossary, and Sources of Additional Help and Information

Edited by Jenni Lynn Colson. 472 pages. 2002. 978-0-7808-0420-3.

"Handy and convenient for home, public, school, and college libraries. Recommended."
—*CHOICE*, Apr '03

"This reference can provide the consumer with answers to most questions about emergency care in the United States, or it will direct them to a resource where the answer can be found."
—*American Reference Books Annual*, 2003

SEE ALSO *Injury and Trauma Sourcebook*

▨

Endocrine and Metabolic Disorders Sourcebook, 2nd Edition

Basic Consumer Health Information about Hormonal and Metabolic Disorders that Affect the Body's Growth, Development, and Functioning, Including Disorders of the Pancreas, Ovaries and Testes, and Pituitary, Thyroid, Parathyroid, and Adrenal Glands, with Facts about Growth Disorders, Addison Disease, Cushing Syndrome, Conn Syndrome, Diabetic Disorders, Multiple Endocrine Neoplasia, Inborn Errors of Metabolism, and More

Along with Information about Endocrine Functioning, Diagnostic and Screening Tests, a Glossary of Related Terms, and Directories of Additional Resources

Edited by Joyce Brennfleck Shannon. 597 pages. 2007. 978-0-7808-0952-9.

SEE ALSO *Diabetes Sourcebook, 4th Edition*

▨

Environmental Health Sourcebook, 3rd Edition

Basic Consumer Health Information about the Environment and Its Effects on Human Health, Including Facts about Air, Water, and Soil Contamination, Hazardous Chemicals, Foodborne Hazards and Illnesses, Household Hazards Such as Radon, Mold, and Carbon Monoxide, Consumer Hazards from Toxic Products and Imported Goods, and Disorders

Linked to Environmental Causes, Including Chemical Sensitivity, Cancer, Allergies, and Asthma

Along with Information about the Impact of Environmental Hazards on Specific Populations, a Glossary of Related Terms, and Resources for Additional Help and Information.

Edited by Laura Larsen. 600 pages. 2010. 978-0-7808-1078-5

Ethnic Diseases Sourcebook

Basic Consumer Health Information for Ethnic and Racial Minority Groups in the United States, Including General Health Indicators and Behaviors, Ethnic Diseases, Genetic Testing, the Impact of Chronic Diseases, Women's Health, Mental Health Issues, and Preventive Health Care Services

Along with a Glossary and a Listing of Additional Resources

Edited by Joyce Brennfleck Shannon. 648 pages. 2001. 978-0-7808-0336-7.

"Not many books have been written on this topic to date, and the Ethnic Diseases Sourcebook is a strong addition to the list. It will be an important introductory resource for health consumers, students, health care personnel, and social scientists. It is recommended for public, academic, and large hospital libraries."

— American Reference Books Annual, 2002

"Will prove valuable to any library seeking to maintain a current, comprehensive reference collection of health resources... An excellent source of health information about genetic disorders which affect particular ethnic and racial minorities in the U.S."

—The Bookwatch, Aug '01

Eye Care Sourcebook, 3rd Edition

Basic Consumer Health Information about Eye Care and Eye Disorders, Including Facts about the Diagnosis, Prevention, and Treatment of Refractive Disorders, Cataracts, Glaucoma, Macular Degeneration, and Problems Affecting the Cornea, Retina, and Lacrimal Glands

Along with Advice about Preventing Eye Injuries and Tips for Living with Low Vision or Blindness, a Glossary of Related Terms, and Directories of Resources for More Help and Information

Edited by Amy L. Sutton. 646 pages. 2008. 978-0-7808-1000-6.

"A solid reference tool for eye care and a valuable addition to a collection."

—American Reference Books Annual, 2009

Family Planning Sourcebook

Basic Consumer Health Information about Planning for Pregnancy and Contraception, Including Traditional Methods, Barrier Methods, Hormonal Methods, Permanent Methods, Future Methods, Emergency Contraception, and Birth Control Choices for Women at Each Stage of Life

Along with Statistics, a Glossary, and Sources of Additional Information

Edited by Amy Marcaccio Keyzer. 503 pages. 2001. 978-0-7808-0379-4.

"Recommended for public, health, and undergraduate libraries as part of the circulating collection."

—E-Streams, Mar '02

"Will prove valuable to any library seeking to maintain a current, comprehensive reference collection of health resources... Excellent reference."

—The Bookwatch, Aug '01

SEE ALSO Pregnancy and Birth Sourcebook, 3rd Edition

Fitness and Exercise Sourcebook, 3rd Edition

Basic Consumer Health Information about the Physical and Mental Benefits of Fitness, Including Cardiorespiratory Endurance, Muscular Strength, Muscular Endurance, and Flexibility, with Facts about Sports Nutrition and Exercise-Related Injuries and Tips about Physical Activity and Exercises for People of All Ages and for People with Health Concerns

Along with Advice on Selecting and Using Exercise Equipment, Maintaining Exercise Motivation, a Glossary of Related Terms, and a Directory of Resources for More Help and Information

Edited by Amy L. Sutton. 635 pages. 2007. 978-0-7808-0946-8.

"Updates the consumer information on the physical and mental benefits of physical activity throughout the lifespan offered in earlier editions... Recommended. All readers; all levels."
—*CHOICE, Oct '07*

"An exceptionally well-rounded coverage perfect for any concerned about developing and understanding a fitness program."
—*California Bookwatch, Jun '07*

SEE ALSO *Sports Injuries Sourcebook, 3rd Edition*

Food Safety Sourcebook
Basic Consumer Health Information about the Safe Handling of Meat, Poultry, Seafood, Eggs, Fruit Juices, and Other Food Items, and Facts about Pesticides, Drinking Water, Food Safety Overseas, and the Onset, Duration, and Symptoms of Foodborne Illnesses, Including Types of Pathogenic Bacteria, Parasitic Protozoa, Worms, Viruses, and Natural Toxins

Along with the Role of the Consumer, the Food Handler, and the Government in Food Safety, a Glossary, and Resources for Additional Help and Information

Edited by Dawn D. Matthews. 327 pages. 1999. 978-0-7808-0326-8.

"Recommended reference source."
—*Booklist, May '00*

"This book takes the complex issues of food safety and foodborne pathogens and presents them in an easily understood manner. [It does] an excellent job of covering a large and often confusing topic."
— *American Reference Books Annual, 2000*

Forensic Medicine Sourcebook
Basic Consumer Information for the Layperson about Forensic Medicine, Including Crime Scene Investigation, Evidence Collection and Analysis, Expert Testimony, Computer-Aided Criminal Identification, Digital Imaging in the Courtroom, DNA Profiling, Accident Reconstruction, Autopsies, Ballistics, Drugs and Explosives Detection, Latent Fingerprints,

Product Tampering, and Questioned Document Examination

Along with Statistical Data, a Glossary of Forensics Terminology, and Listings of Sources for Further Help and Information

Edited by Annemarie S. Muth. 574 pages. 1999. 978-0-7808-0232-2.

"Given the expected widespread interest in its content and its easy to read style, this book is recommended for most public and all college and university libraries."
—*E-Streams, Feb '01*

"A wealth of information, useful statistics, references are up-to-date and extremely complete. This wonderful collection of data will help students who are interested in a career in any type of forensic field. It is a great resource for attorneys who need information about types of expert witnesses needed in a particular case. It also offers useful information for fiction and nonfiction writers whose work involves a crime. A fascinating compilation. All levels."
—*CHOICE, Jan '00*

"There are several items that make this book attractive to consumers who are seeking certain forensic data... This is a useful current source for those seeking general forensic medical answers."
—*American Reference Books Annual, 2000*

Gastrointestinal Diseases and Disorders Sourcebook, 2nd Edition
Basic Consumer Health Information about the Upper and Lower Gastrointestinal (GI) Tract, Including the Esophagus, Stomach, Intestines, Rectum, Liver, and Pancreas, with Facts about Gastroesophageal Reflux Disease, Gastritis, Hernias, Ulcers, Celiac Disease, Diverticulitis, Irritable Bowel Syndrome, Hemorrhoids, Gastrointestinal Cancers, and Other Diseases and Disorders Related to the Digestive Process

Along with Information about Commonly Used Diagnostic and Surgical Procedures, Statistics, Reports on Current Research Initiatives and Clinical Trials, a Glossary, and Resources for Additional Help and Information

Edited by Sandra J. Judd. 654 pages. 2006. 978-0-7808-0798-3.

"The text is designed for the general reader seeking information on prevention, disease warning signs, diagnostic and therapeutic questions... It is an excellent resource for the general reader to conveniently locate credible, coordinated and indexed information... The sourcebook will prove very helpful for patients, caregivers and should be available in every physician waiting room."
—*Doody's Review Service, 2006*

SEE ALSO *Diet and Nutrition Sourcebook, 3rd Edition, Digestive Diseases and Disorders Sourcebook*

Genetic Disorders Sourcebook, 4th Edition

Basic Consumer Health Information about Hereditary Diseases and Disorders, Including Facts about the Human Genome, Genetic Inheritance Patterns, Disorders Associated with Specific Genes, Such as Sickle Cell Disease, Hemophilia, and Cystic Fibrosis, Chromosome Disorders, Such as Down Syndrome, Fragile X Syndrome, and Turner Syndrome, and Complex Diseases and Disorders Resulting from the Interaction of Environmental and Genetic Factors, Such as Allergies, Cancer, and Obesity

Along with Facts about Genetic Testing, Suggestions for Parents of Children with Special Needs, Reports on Current Research Initiatives, a Glossary of Genetic Terminology, and Resources for Additional Help and Information

Edited by Sandra J. Judd. 600 pages. 2010. 978-0-7808-1076-1.

Head Trauma Sourcebook

Basic Information for the Layperson about Open-Head and Closed-Head Injuries, Treatment Advances, Recovery, and Rehabilitation

Along with Reports on Current Research Initiatives

Edited by Karen Bellenir. 414 pages. 1997. 978-0-7808-0208-7.

Headache Sourcebook

Basic Consumer Health Information about Migraine, Tension, Cluster, Rebound and Other Types of Headaches, with Facts about

the Cause and Prevention of Headaches, the Effects of Stress and the Environment, Headaches during Pregnancy and Menopause, and Childhood Headaches

Along with a Glossary and Other Resources for Additional Help and Information

Edited by Dawn D. Matthews. 342 pages. 2002. 978-0-7808-0337-4.

"Highly recommended for academic and medical reference collections."
—*Library Bookwatch, Sep '02*

SEE ALSO *Pain Sourcebook, 3rd Edition*

Healthy Aging Sourcebook

Basic Consumer Health Information about Maintaining Health through the Aging Process, Including Advice on Nutrition, Exercise, and Sleep, Help in Making Decisions about Midlife Issues and Retirement, and Guidance Concerning Practical and Informed Choices in Health Consumerism

Along with Data Concerning the Theories of Aging, Different Experiences in Aging by Minority Groups, and Facts about Aging Now and Aging in the Future; and Featuring a Glossary, a Guide to Consumer Help, Additional Suggested Reading, and Practical Resource Directory

Edited by Jenifer Swanson. 537 pages. 1999. 978-0-7808-0390-9.

"Recommended reference source."
—*Booklist, Feb '00*

SEE ALSO *Adult Health Sourcebook, Physical and Mental Issues in Aging Sourcebook*

Healthy Children Sourcebook

Basic Consumer Health Information about the Physical and Mental Development of Children between the Ages of 3 and 12, Including Routine Health Care, Preventative Health Services, Safety and First Aid, Healthy Sleep, Dental Care, Nutrition, and Fitness, and Featuring Parenting Tips on Such Topics as Bedwetting, Choosing Day Care, Monitoring TV and Other Media, and Establishing a Foundation for Substance Abuse Prevention

Along with a Glossary of Commonly Used Pediatric Terms and Resources for Additional Help and Information.

Edited by Chad T. Kimball. 624 pages. 2003. 978-0-7808-0247-6.

"Should be required reading for parents and teachers."
—E-Streams, Jun '04

"It is hard to imagine that any other single resource exists that would provide such a comprehensive guide of timely information on health promotion and disease prevention for children aged 3 to 12."
—American Reference Books Annual, 2004

"This easy-to-read volume is a tremendous resource."
—AORN Journal, May '05

SEE ALSO Childhood Diseases and Disorders Sourcebook, 2nd Edition

Healthy Heart Sourcebook for Women

Basic Consumer Health Information about Cardiac Issues Specific to Women, Including Facts about Major Risk Factors and Prevention, Treatment and Control Strategies, and Important Dietary Issues

Along with a Special Section Regarding the Pros and Cons of Hormone Replacement Therapy and Its Impact on Heart Health, and Additional Help, Including Recipes, a Glossary, and a Directory of Resources

Edited by Dawn D. Matthews. 321 pages. 2000. 978-0-7808-0329-9.

"A good reference source and recommended for all public, academic, medical, and hospital libraries."
—Medical Reference Services Quarterly, Summer '01

"Contains very important information about coronary artery disease that all women should know. The information is current and presented in an easy-to-read format. The book will make a good addition to any library."
—American Medical Writers Association Journal, Summer '00

SEE ALSO Cardiovascular Diseases and Disorders Sourcebook, 4th Edition, Women's Health Concerns Sourcebook, 3rd Edition

Hepatitis Sourcebook

Basic Consumer Health Information about Hepatitis A, Hepatitis B, Hepatitis C, and Other Forms of Hepatitis, Including Autoimmune Hepatitis, Alcoholic Hepatitis, Nonalcoholic Steatohepatitis, and Toxic Hepatitis, with Facts about Risk Factors, Screening Methods, Diagnostic Tests, and Treatment Options

Along with Information on Liver Health, Tips for People Living with Chronic Hepatitis, Reports on Current Research Initiatives, a Glossary of Terms Related to Hepatitis, and a Directory of Sources for Further Help and Information

Edited by Sandra J. Judd. 570 pages. 2006. 978-0-7808-0749-5.

"The breadth of information found in this one book would not be readily found in another source. Highly recommended."
—American Reference Books Annual, 2006

SEE ALSO Contagious Diseases Sourcebook, 2nd Edition

Household Safety Sourcebook

Basic Consumer Health Information about Household Safety, Including Information about Poisons, Chemicals, Fire, and Water Hazards in the Home

Along with Advice about the Safe Use of Home Maintenance Equipment, Choosing Toys and Nursery Furniture, Holiday and Recreation Safety, a Glossary, and Resources for Further Help and Information

Edited by Dawn D. Matthews. 587 pages. 2002. 978-0-7808-0338-1.

"As a sourcebook on household safety this book meets its mark. It is encyclopedic in scope and covers a wide range of safety issues that are commonly seen in the home."
—E-Streams, Jul '02

Hypertension Sourcebook

Basic Consumer Health Information about the Causes, Diagnosis, and Treatment of High Blood Pressure, with Facts about Consequences, Complications, and Co-Occurring Disorders, Such as Coronary Heart Disease, Diabetes, Stroke, Kidney Disease, and Hypertensive Retinopathy, and Issues in Blood Pressure

Control, Including Dietary Choices, Stress Management, and Medications

Along with Reports on Current Research Initiatives and Clinical Trials, a Glossary, and Resources for Additional Help and Information

Edited by Dawn D. Matthews and Karen Bellenir. 588 pages. 2004. 978-0-7808-0674-0.

"Academic, public, and medical libraries will want to add the Hypertension Sourcebook to their collections."
—E-Streams, Aug '05

"The strength of this source is the wide range of information given about hypertension."
—American Reference Books Annual, 2005

SEE ALSO Stroke Sourcebook, 2nd Edition

Immune System Disorders Sourcebook, 2nd Edition

Basic Consumer Health Information about Disorders of the Immune System, Including Immune System Function and Response, Diagnosis of Immune Disorders, Information about Inherited Immune Disease, Acquired Immune Disease, and Autoimmune Diseases, Including Primary Immune Deficiency, Acquired Immunodeficiency Syndrome (AIDS), Lupus, Multiple Sclerosis, Type 1 Diabetes, Rheumatoid Arthritis, and Graves' Disease

Along with Treatments, Tips for Coping with Immune Disorders, a Glossary, and a Directory of Additional Resources

Edited by Joyce Brennfleck Shannon. 643 pages. 2005. 978-0-7808-0748-8.

"Highly recommended for academic and public libraries."
—American Reference Books Annual, 2006

"The updated second edition is a 'must' for any consumer health library seeking a solid resource covering the treatments, symptoms, and options for immune disorder sufferers... An excellent guide."
—MBR Bookwatch, Jan '06

SEE ALSO AIDS Sourcebook, 4th Edition, Arthritis Sourcebook, 3rd Edition

Infant and Toddler Health Sourcebook

Basic Consumer Health Information about the Physical and Mental Development of Newborns, Infants, and Toddlers, Including Neonatal Concerns, Nutrition Recommendations, Immunization Schedules, Common Pediatric Disorders, Assessments and Milestones, Safety Tips, and Advice for Parents and Other Caregivers

Along with a Glossary of Terms and Resource Listings for Additional Help

Edited by Jenifer Swanson. 570 pages. 2000. 978-0-7808-0246-9.

"As a reference for the general public, this would be useful in any library."
—E-Streams, May '01

"Recommended reference source."
—Booklist, Feb '01

Infectious Diseases Sourcebook

Basic Consumer Health Information about Non-Contagious Bacterial, Viral, Prion, Fungal, and Parasitic Diseases Spread by Food and Water, Insects and Animals, or Environmental Contact, Including Botulism, E. Coli, Encephalitis, Legionnaires' Disease, Lyme Disease, Malaria, Plague, Rabies, Salmonella, Tetanus, and Others, and Facts about Newly Emerging Diseases, Such as Hantavirus, Mad Cow Disease, Monkeypox, and West Nile Virus

Along with Information about Preventing Disease Transmission, the Threat of Bioterrorism, and Current Research Initiatives, with a Glossary and Directory of Resources for More Information

Edited by Karen Bellenir. 610 pages. 2004. 978-0-7808-0675-7.

"This reference continues the excellent tradition of the Health Reference Series in consolidating a wealth of information on a selected topic into a format that is easy to use and accessible to the general public."
—American Reference Books Annual, 2005

"Recommended for public and academic libraries."
—E-Streams, Jan '05

SEE ALSO Environmental Health Sourcebook, 3rd Edition

Injury and Trauma Sourcebook

Basic Consumer Health Information about the Impact of Injury, the Diagnosis and Treatment of Common and Traumatic Injuries, Emergency Care, and Specific Injuries Related to Home, Community, Workplace, Transportation, and Recreation

Along with Guidelines for Injury Prevention, a Glossary, and a Directory of Additional Resources

Edited by Joyce Brennfleck Shannon. 675 pages. 2002. 978-0-7808-0421-0.

"Practitioners should be aware of guides such as this in order to facilitate their use by patients and their families."
— *Doody's Health Sciences Book Review Journal, Sep-Oct '02*

"Recommended reference source."
— *Booklist, Sep '02*

"Highly recommended for academic and medical reference collections."
— *Library Bookwatch, Sep '02*

SEE ALSO *Emergency Medical Services Sourcebook, Sports Injuries Sourcebook, 3rd Edition*

Learning Disabilities Sourcebook, 3rd Edition

Basic Consumer Health Information about Dyslexia, Auditory and Visual Processing Disorders, Communication Disorders, Dyscalculia, Dysgraphia, and Other Conditions That Impede Learning, Including Attention Deficit/Hyperactivity Disorder, Autism Spectrum Disorders, Hearing and Visual Impairments, Chromosome-Based Disorders, and Brain Injury

Along with Facts about Brain Function, Assessment, Therapy and Remediation, Accommodations, Assistive Technology, Legal Protections, and Tips about Family Life, School Transitions, and Employment Strategies, a Glossary of Related Terms, and Directories of Additional Resources

Edited by Joyce Brennfleck Shannon. 613 pages. 2009. 978-0-7808-1039-6.

"Intended to be a starting point for people who need to know about learning disabilities. Each chapter on a specific disability includes readable, well-organized descriptions... The book is well indexed and a glossary is included. Chapters on organizations and helpful websites will aid the reader who needs more information."
— *American Reference Books Annual, 2009*

"This book provides the necessary information to better understand learning disabilities and work with children who have them... It would be difficult to find another book that so comprehensively explains learning disabilities without becoming incomprehensible to the average parent who needs this information."
— *Doody's Review Service, 2009*

SEE ALSO *Attention Deficit Disorder Sourcebook, Autism and Pervasive Developmental Disorders Sourcebook*

Leukemia Sourcebook

Basic Consumer Health Information about Adult and Childhood Leukemias, Including Acute Lymphocytic Leukemia (ALL), Chronic Lymphocytic Leukemia (CLL), Acute Myelogenous Leukemia (AML), Chronic Myelogenous Leukemia (CML), and Hairy Cell Leukemia, and Treatments Such as Chemotherapy, Radiation Therapy, Peripheral Blood Stem Cell and Marrow Transplantation, and Immunotherapy

Along with Tips for Life During and After Treatment, a Glossary, and Directories of Additional Resources

Edited by Joyce Brennfleck Shannon. 564 pages. 2003. 978-0-7808-0627-6.

"Unlike other medical books for the layperson... the language does not talk down to the reader... This volume is highly recommended for all libraries."
— *American Reference Books Annual, 2004*

"A fine title which ranges from diagnosis to alternative treatments, staging, and tips for life during and after diagnosis."
— *The Bookwatch, Dec '03*

SEE ALSO *Blood & Circulatory Disorders Sourcebook, 3rd Edition, Cancer Sourcebook, 5th Edition*

Liver Disorders Sourcebook

Basic Consumer Health Information about the Liver and How It Works; Liver Diseases, Including Cancer, Cirrhosis, Hepatitis, and

Toxic and Drug Related Diseases; Tips for Maintaining a Healthy Liver; Laboratory Tests, Radiology Tests, and Facts about Liver Transplantation

Along with a Section on Support Groups, a Glossary, and Resource Listings

Edited by Joyce Brennfleck Shannon. 580 pages. 2000. 978-0-7808-0383-1.

"This title is recommended for health sciences and public libraries with consumer health collections."
—E-Streams, Oct '00

"Recommended reference source."
—Booklist, Jun '00

SEE ALSO Gastrointestinal Diseases and Disorders Sourcebook, 2nd Edition, Hepatitis Sourcebook

Lung Disorders Sourcebook

Basic Consumer Health Information about Emphysema, Pneumonia, Tuberculosis, Asthma, Cystic Fibrosis, and Other Lung Disorders, Including Facts about Diagnostic Procedures, Treatment Strategies, Disease Prevention Efforts, and Such Risk Factors as Smoking, Air Pollution, and Exposure to Asbestos, Radon, and Other Agents

Along with a Glossary and Resources for Additional Help and Information

Edited by Dawn D. Matthews. 657 pages. 2002. 978-0-7808-0339-8.

"Highly recommended for academic and medical reference collections."
—Library Bookwatch, Sep '02

SEE ALSO Asthma Sourcebook, 2nd Edition, Respiratory Disorders Sourcebook, 2nd Edition

Medical Tests Sourcebook, 3rd Edition

Basic Consumer Health Information about X-Rays, Blood Tests, Stool and Urine Tests, Biopsies, Mammography, Endoscopic Procedures, Ultrasound Exams, Computed Tomography, Magnetic Resonance Imaging (MRI), Nuclear Medicine, Genetic Testing, Home-Use Tests, and More

Along with Facts about Preventive Care and Screening Test Guidelines, Screening and

Assessment Tests Associated with Such Specific Concerns as Cancer, Heart Disease, Allergies, Diabetes, Thyroid Disfunction, and Infertility, a Glossary of Related Terms, and a Directory of Resources for Additional Help and Information

Edited by Karen Bellenir. 627 pages. 2008. 978-0-7808-1040-2

"This volume has a wide scope that makes it useful... Can be a valuable reference guide."
—American Reference Books Annual, 2009

"Would be a valuable contribution to any consumer health or public library."
—Doody's Book Review Service, 2009

Men's Health Concerns Sourcebook, 3rd Edition

Basic Consumer Health Information about Wellness in Men and Gender-Related Differences in Health, With Facts about Heart Disease, Cancer, Traumatic Injury, and Other Leading Causes of Death in Men, Reproductive Concerns, Sexual Dysfunction, Disorders of the Prostate, Penis, and Testes, Sex-Linked Genetic Disorders, and Other Medical and Mental Concerns of Men

Along with Statistical Data, a Glossary of Related Terms, and a Directory of Resources for Additional Information

Edited by Sandra J. Judd. 632 pages. 2009. 978-0-7808-1033-4.

"A good addition to any reference shelf in academic, consumer health, or hospital libraries."
—ARBAOnline, Oct '09

SEE ALSO Prostate and Urological Disorders Sourcebook

Mental Health Disorders Sourcebook, 4th Edition

Basic Consumer Health Information about the Causes and Symptoms of Mental Health Problems, Including Depression, Bipolar Disorder, Anxiety Disorders, Posttraumatic Stress Disorder, Obsessive-Compulsive Disorder, Eating Disorders, Addictions, and Personality and Psychotic Disorders

Along with Information about Medications and Treatments, Mental Health Concerns in

Children, Adolescents, and Adults, Tips on Living with Mental Health Disorders, a Glossary of Related Terms, and a Directory of Resources for Additional Help and Information

Edited by Amy L. Sutton. 680 pages. 2009. 978-0-7808-1041-9.

"Mental health concerns are presented in everyday language and intended for patients and their families as well as the general public... This resource is comprehensive and up to date... The easy-to-understand writing style helps to facilitate assimilation of needed facts and specifics on often challenging topics."
—ARBAOnline, Oct '09

"No health collection should be without this resource, which will reach into many a general lending library as well."
—Internet Bookwatch, Oct '09

SEE ALSO Depression Sourcebook, 2nd Edition, Stress-Related Disorders Sourcebook, 2nd Edition

Mental Retardation Sourcebook

Basic Consumer Health Information about Mental Retardation and Its Causes, Including Down Syndrome, Fetal Alcohol Syndrome, Fragile X Syndrome, Genetic Conditions, Injury, and Environmental Sources

Along with Preventive Strategies, Parenting Issues, Educational Implications, Health Care Needs, Employment and Economic Matters, Legal Issues, a Glossary, and a Resource Listing for Additional Help and Information

Edited by Joyce Brennfleck Shannon. 627 pages. 2000. 978-0-7808-0377-0.

"Public libraries will find the book useful for reference and as a beginning research point for students, parents, and caregivers."
—American Reference Books Annual, 2001

"The strength of this work is that it compiles many basic fact sheets and addresses for further information in one volume. It is intended and suitable for the general public."
—E-Streams, Nov '00

"An invaluable overview."
—Reviewer's Bookwatch, Jul '00

Movement Disorders Sourcebook, 2nd Edition

Basic Consumer Health Information about the Symptoms and Causes of Movement Disorders, Including Parkinson Disease, Amyotrophic Lateral Sclerosis, Cerebral Palsy, Muscular Dystrophy, Multiple Sclerosis, Myasthenia, Myoclonus, Spina Bifida, Dystonia, Essential Tremor, Choreatic Disorders, Huntington Disease, Tourette Syndrome, and Other Disorders That Cause Slowed, Absent, or Excessive Movements

Along with Information about Surgical and Nonsurgical Interventions, Physical Therapies, Strategies for Independent Living, a Glossary of Related Terms, and a Directory of Resources for Additional Help and Information

Edited by Amy L. Sutton. 618 pages. 2009. 978-0-7808-1034-1.

"The second updated edition of Movement Disorders Sourcebook is a winner, providing the latest research and health findings on all kinds of movement disorders in children and adults... a top pick for any health or general lending library's health reference collection."
—California Bookwatch, Aug '09

SEE ALSO Muscular Dystrophy Sourcebook

Multiple Sclerosis Sourcebook

Basic Consumer Health Information about Multiple Sclerosis (MS) and Its Effects on Mobility, Vision, Bladder Function, Speech, Swallowing, and Cognition, Including Facts about Risk Factors, Causes, Diagnostic Procedures, Pain Management, Drug Treatments, and Physical and Occupational Therapies

Along with Guidelines for Nutrition and Exercise, Tips on Choosing Assistive Equipment, Information about Disability, Work, Financial, and Legal Issues, a Glossary of Related Terms, and a Directory of Additional Resources

Edited by Joyce Brennfleck Shannon. 553 pages. 2007. 978-0-7808-0998-7.

Muscular Dystrophy Sourcebook

Basic Consumer Health Information about Congenital, Childhood-Onset, and Adult-Onset

Forms of Muscular Dystrophy, Such as Duchenne, Becker, Emery-Dreifuss, Distal, Limb-Girdle, Facioscapulohumeral (FSHD), Myotonic, and Ophthalmoplegic Muscular Dystrophies, Including Facts about Diagnostic Tests, Medical and Physical Therapies, Management of Co-Occurring Conditions, and Parenting Guidelines

Along with Practical Tips for Home Care, a Glossary, and Directories of Additional Resources

Edited by Joyce Brennfleck Shannon. 552 pages. 2004. 978-0-7808-0676-4.

"This book is highly recommended for public and academic libraries as well as health care offices that support the information needs of patients and their families."
—E-Streams, Apr '05

"Excellent reference."
—The Bookwatch, Jan '05

SEE ALSO Movement Disorders Sourcebook, 2nd Edition

Obesity Sourcebook

Basic Consumer Health Information about Diseases and Other Problems Associated with Obesity, and Including Facts about Risk Factors, Prevention Issues, and Management Approaches

Along with Statistical and Demographic Data, Information about Special Populations, Research Updates, a Glossary, and Source Listings for Further Help and Information

Edited by Wilma Caldwell and Chad T. Kimball. 360 pages. 2001. 978-0-7808-0333-6.

"The book synthesizes the reliable medical literature on obesity into one easy-to-read and useful resource for the general public."
—American Reference Books Annual, 2002

"Well suited for the health reference collection of a public library or an academic health science library that serves the general population."
—E-Streams, Sep '01

Osteoporosis Sourcebook

Basic Consumer Health Information about Primary and Secondary Osteoporosis and Juvenile Osteoporosis and Related Conditions, Including Fibrous Dysplasia, Gaucher Disease, Hyperthyroidism, Hypophosphatasia,

Myeloma, Osteopetrosis, Osteogenesis Imperfecta, and Paget's Disease

Along with Information about Risk Factors, Treatments, Traditional and Non-Traditional Pain Management, a Glossary of Related Terms, and a Directory of Resources

Edited by Allan R. Cook. 568 pages. 2001. 978-0-7808-0239-1.

"This resource is recommended as a great reference source for public, health, and academic libraries, and is another triumph for the editors of Omnigraphics."
—American Reference Books Annual, 2002

"Will prove valuable to any library seeking to maintain a current, comprehensive reference collection of health resources... From prevention to treatment and associated conditions, this provides an excellent survey."
—The Bookwatch, Aug '01

SEE ALSO Healthy Aging Sourcebook, Women's Health Concerns Sourcebook, 3rd Edition

Pain Sourcebook, 3rd Edition

Basic Consumer Health Information about Acute and Chronic Pain, Including Nerve Pain, Bone Pain, Muscle Pain, Cancer Pain, and Disorders Characterized by Pain, Such as Arthritis, Temporomandibular Muscle and Joint (TMJ) Disorder, Carpal Tunnel Syndrome, Headaches, Heartburn, Sciatica, and Shingles, and Facts about Diagnostic Tests and Treatment Options for Pain, Including Over-the-Counter and Prescription Drugs, Physical Rehabilitation, Injection and Infusion Therapies, Implantable Technologies, and Complementary Medicine

Along with Tips for Living with Pain, a Glossary of Related Terms, and a Directory of Additional Resources

Edited by Joyce Brennfleck Shannon. 644 pages. 2008. 978-0-7808-1006-8.

"Excellent for ready-reference users and can be used for beginning students in health fields... appropriate for the consumer health collection in both public and academic libraries."
—American Reference Books Annual, 2009

SEE ALSO Arthritis Sourcebook, 3rd Edition; Back and Neck Sourcebook, 2nd Edition;

Headache Sourcebook; Sports Injuries Sourcebook, 3rd Edition

SEE ALSO Healthy Aging Sourcebook

Pediatric Cancer Sourcebook

Basic Consumer Health Information about Leukemias, Brain Tumors, Sarcomas, Lymphomas, and Other Cancers in Infants, Children, and Adolescents, Including Descriptions of Cancers, Treatments, and Coping Strategies

Along with Suggestions for Parents, Caregivers, and Concerned Relatives, a Glossary of Cancer Terms, and Resource Listings

Edited by Edward J. Prucha. 575 pages. 1999. 978-0-7808-0245-2.

"An excellent source of information. Recommended for public, hospital, and health science libraries with consumer health collections."
—E-Streams, Jun '00

"A valuable addition to all libraries specializing in health services and many public libraries."
—American Reference Books Annual, 2000

SEE ALSO Childhood Diseases and Disorders Sourcebook, 2nd Edition, Healthy Children Sourcebook

Physical and Mental Issues in Aging Sourcebook

Basic Consumer Health Information on Physical and Mental Disorders Associated with the Aging Process, Including Concerns about Cardiovascular Disease, Pulmonary Disease, Oral Health, Digestive Disorders, Musculoskeletal and Skin Disorders, Metabolic Changes, Sexual and Reproductive Issues, and Changes in Vision, Hearing, and Other Senses

Along with Data about Longevity and Causes of Death, Information on Acute and Chronic Pain, Descriptions of Mental Concerns, a Glossary of Terms, and Resource Listings for Additional Help

Edited by Jenifer Swanson. 660 pages. 1999. 978-0-7808-0233-9.

"This is a treasure of health information for the layperson."
—CHOICE Health Sciences Supplement, May '00

Podiatry Sourcebook, 2nd Edition

Basic Consumer Health Information about Disorders, Diseases, and Deformities that Affect the Foot and Ankle, Including Sprains, Corns, Calluses, Bunions, Plantar Warts, Plantar Fasciitis, Neuromas, Clubfoot, Flat Feet, Achilles Tendonitis, and Much More

Along with Information about Selecting a Foot Care Specialist, Foot Fitness, Shoes and Socks, Diagnostic Tests and Corrective Procedures, Financial Assistance for Corrective Devices, a Glossary of Related Terms, and a Directory of Resources for Additional Help and Information

Edited by Ivy L. Alexander. 516 pages. 2007. 978-0-7808-0944-4.

"An excellent resource... Although there have been various types of 'foot books' published in the past, none are as comprehensive as this one. 5 Stars (out of 5)!"
—Doody's Review Service, 2007

"Perfect for both health libraries and general-interest lending collections."
—Internet Bookwatch, Jul '07

Pregnancy and Birth Sourcebook, 3rd Edition

Basic Consumer Health Information about Pregnancy and Fetal Development, Including Facts about Fertility and Conception, Physical and Emotional Changes during Pregnancy, Prenatal Care and Diagnostic Tests, High-Risk Pregnancies and Complications, Labor, Delivery, and the Postpartum Period

Along with Tips on Maintaining Health and Wellness during Pregnancy and Caring for Newborn Infants, a Glossary of Related Terms, and Directories of Resources for Additional Help and Information

Edited by Amy L. Sutton. 645 pages. 2009. 978-0-7808-1074-7.

SEE ALSO Breastfeeding Sourcebook, Congenital Disorders Sourcebook, 2nd Edition, Family Planning Sourcebook, Women's Health Concerns Sourcebook, 3rd Edition

Prostate and Urological Disorders Sourcebook

Basic Consumer Health Information about Urogenital and Sexual Disorders in Men, Including Prostate and Other Andrological Cancers, Prostatitis, Benign Prostatic Hyperplasia, Testicular and Penile Trauma, Cryptorchidism, Peyronie Disease, Erectile Dysfunction, and Male Factor Infertility, and Facts about Commonly Used Tests and Procedures, Such as Prostatectomy, Vasectomy, Vasectomy Reversal, Penile Implants, and Semen Analysis

Along with a Glossary of Andrological Terms and a Directory of Resources for Additional Information

Edited by Karen Bellenir. 604 pages. 2006. 978-0-7808-0797-6.

"Certain to be a popular pick among library reference holdings... No prior knowledge is assumed for any of the conditions or terms herein, making it a most accessible general-interest reference."
—California Bookwatch, Apr '06

SEE ALSO *Men's Health Concerns Sourcebook, 3rd Edition, Urinary Tract and Kidney Diseases and Disorders Sourcebook, 2nd Edition*

Prostate Cancer Sourcebook

Basic Consumer Health Information about Prostate Cancer, Including Information about the Associated Risk Factors, Detection, Diagnosis, and Treatment of Prostate Cancer

Along with Information on Non-Malignant Prostate Conditions, and Featuring a Section Listing Support and Treatment Centers and a Glossary of Related Terms

Edited by Dawn D. Matthews. 340 pages. 2001. 978-0-7808-0324-4.

"Recommended reference source."
—Booklist, Jan '02

"A valuable resource for health care consumers seeking information on the subject... All text is written in a clear, easy-to-understand language that avoids technical jargon. Any library that collects consumer health resources would strengthen their collection with the addition of the Prostate Cancer Sourcebook."
—American Reference Books Annual, 2002

SEE ALSO *Cancer Sourcebook, 5th Edition, Men's Health Concerns Sourcebook, 3rd Edition*

Rehabilitation Sourcebook

Basic Consumer Health Information about Rehabilitation for People Recovering from Heart Surgery, Spinal Cord Injury, Stroke, Orthopedic Impairments, Amputation, Pulmonary Impairments, Traumatic Injury, and More, Including Physical Therapy, Occupational Therapy, Speech/Language Therapy, Massage Therapy, Dance Therapy, Art Therapy, and Recreational Therapy

Along with Information on Assistive and Adaptive Devices, a Glossary, and Resources for Additional Help and Information

Edited by Dawn D. Matthews. 519 pages. 2000. 978-0-7808-0236-0.

"This is an excellent resource for public library reference and health collections."
—American Reference Books Annual, 2001

"Recommended reference source."
—Booklist, May '00

Respiratory Disorders Sourcebook, 2nd Edition

Basic Consumer Health Information about Infectious, Inflammatory, and Chronic Conditions Affecting the Lungs and Respiratory System, Including Pneumonia, Bronchitis, Influenza, Tuberculosis, Sarcoidosis, Asthma, Cystic Fibrosis, Chronic Obstructive Pulmonary Disease, Lung Abscesses, Pulmonary Embolism, Occupational Lung Diseases, and Other Bacterial, Viral, and Fungal Infections

Along with Facts about the Structure and Function of the Lungs and Airways, Methods of Diagnosing Respiratory Disorders, and Treatment and Rehabilitation Options, a Glossary of Related Terms, and a Directory of Resources for Additional Help and Information

Edited by Sandra L. Judd. 638 pages. 2008. 978-0-7808-1007-5.

"An excellent book for patients, their families, or for those who are just curious about respiratory disease. Public libraries and physician offices would find this a valuable resource as well. 4 Stars! (out of 5)"
—Doody's Review Service, 2009

"A great addition for public and school libraries because it provides concise health information... readers can start with this reference source and get satisfactory answers before proceeding to other medical reference tools for

more in depth information... A good guide for health education on lung disorders."
—*American Reference Books Annual, 2009*

SEE ALSO Asthma Sourcebook, 2nd Edition, Lung Disorders Sourcebook

Sexually Transmitted Diseases Sourcebook, 4th Edition

Basic Consumer Health Information about Chlamydial Infections, Gonorrhea, Hepatitis, Herpes, HIV/AIDS, Human Papillomavirus, Pubic Lice, Scabies, Syphilis, Trichomoniasis, Vaginal Infections, and Other Sexually Transmitted Diseases, Including Facts about Risk Factors, Symptoms, Diagnosis, Treatment, and the Prevention of Sexually Transmitted Infections

Along with Updates on Current Research Initiatives, a Glossary of Related Terms, and Resources for Additional Help and Information

Edited by Laura Larsen. 623 pages. 2009. 978-0-7808-1073-0.

"**Extremely beneficial... The question-and-answer format along with the index and table of contents make this well-organized resource extremely easy to reference, read, and comprehend... an invaluable medical reference source for lay readers, and a highly appropriate addition for public library collections, health clinics, and any library with a consumer health collection"**
—*ARBAOnline, Oct '09*

SEE ALSO AIDS Sourcebook, 4th Edition, Contagious Diseases Sourcebook, 2nd Edition, Men's Health Concerns Sourcebook, 3rd Edition, Women's Health Concerns Sourcebook, 3rd Edition

Sleep Disorders Sourcebook, 3rd Edition

Basic Consumer Health Information about Sleep Disorders, Including Insomnia, Sleep Apnea and Snoring, Jet Lag and Other Circadian Rhythm Disorders, Narcolepsy, and Parasomnias, Such as Sleep Walking and Sleep Talking, and Featuring Facts about Other Health Problems that Affect Sleep, Why Sleep Is Necessary, How Much Sleep Is Needed, the Physical and Mental Effects of Sleep Deprivation, and Pediatric Sleep Issues

Along with Tips for Diagnosing and Treating Sleep Disorders, a Glossary of Related Terms, and a List of Resources for Additional Help and Information

Edited by Sandra J. Judd. 600 pages. 2010. 978-0-7808-1084-6.

Smoking Concerns Sourcebook

Basic Consumer Health Information about Nicotine Addiction and Smoking Cessation, Featuring Facts about the Health Effects of Tobacco Use, Including Lung and Other Cancers, Heart Disease, Stroke, and Respiratory Disorders, Such as Emphysema and Chronic Bronchitis

Along with Information about Smoking Prevention Programs, Suggestions for Achieving and Maintaining a Smoke-Free Lifestyle, Statistics about Tobacco Use, Reports on Current Research Initiatives, a Glossary of Related Terms, and Directories of Resources for Additional Help and Information

Edited by Karen Bellenir. 595 pages. 2004. 978-0-7808-0323-7.

"**Provides everything needed for the student or general reader seeking practical details on the effects of tobacco use."**
—*The Bookwatch, Mar '05*

"**Public libraries and consumer health care libraries will find this work useful."**
—*American Reference Books Annual, 2005*

SEE ALSO Respiratory Disorders Sourcebook, 2nd Edition

Sports Injuries Sourcebook, 3rd Edition

Basic Consumer Health Information about Sprains and Strains, Fractures, Growth Plate Injuries, Overtraining Injuries, and Injuries to the Head, Face, Shoulders, Elbows, Hands, Spinal Column, Knees, Ankles, and Feet, and with Facts about Heat-Related Illness, Steroids and Sport Supplements, Protective Equipment, Diagnostic Procedures, Treatment Options, and Rehabilitation

Along with a Glossary of Related Terms and a Directory of Resources for Additional Help and Information

Edited by Sandra J. Judd. 623 pages. 2007. 978-0-7808-0949-9.

SEE ALSO *Fitness and Exercise Sourcebook, 3rd Edition, Podiatry Sourcebook, 2nd Edition*

Stress-Related Disorders Sourcebook, 2nd Edition

Basic Consumer Health Information about Stress and Stress-Related Disorders, Including Types of Stress, Sources of Acute and Chronic Stress, the Impact of Stress on the Body's Systems, and Mental and Emotional Health Problems Associated with Stress, Such as Depression, Anxiety Disorders, Substance Abuse, Posttraumatic Stress Disorder, and Suicide

Along with Advice about Getting Help for Stress-Related Disorders, Information about Stress Management Techniques, a Glossary of Stress-Related Terms, and a Directory of Resources for Additional Help and Information

Edited by Amy L. Sutton. 608 pages. 2007. 978-0-7808-0996-3.

"Accessible to the lay reader. Highly recommended for medical and psychiatric collections."
—*Library Journal, Mar '08*

"Well-written for a general readership, the 2ⁿᵈ Edition of Stress-Related Disorders Sourcebook is a useful addition to the health reference literature."
—*American Reference Books Annual, 2008*

SEE ALSO *Mental Health Disorders Sourcebook, 4th Edition*

Stroke Sourcebook, 2nd Edition

Basic Consumer Health Information about Stroke, Including Ischemic, Hemorrhagic, and Mini Strokes, as Well as Risk Factors, Prevention Guidelines, Diagnostic Tests, Medications and Surgical Treatments, and Complications of Stroke

Along with Rehabilitation Techniques and Innovations, Tips on Staying Healthy and Maintaining Independence after Stroke, a Glossary of Related Terms, and a Directory of Resources for Stroke Survivors and Their Families

Edited by Amy L. Sutton. 626 pages. 2008. 978-0-7808-1035-8.

"An encyclopedic handbook on stroke that is written in a language the layperson can understand... This is one of the most helpful, readable books on stroke. This volume is highly recommended and should be in every medical, hospital and public library; in addition, every family practitioner should have a copy in his or her office."
—*American Reference Books Annual, 2009*

SEE ALSO *Brain Disorders Sourcebook, 3rd Edition, Hypertension Sourcebook*

Surgery Sourcebook, 2nd Edition

Basic Consumer Health Information about Common Inpatient and Outpatient Surgeries, Including Critical Care and Trauma, Gastrointestinal, Gynecologic and Obstetric, Cardiac and Vascular, Neurologic, Ophthalmologic, Orthopedic, Reconstructive and Cosmetic, and Other Major and Minor Surgeries

Along with Information about Anesthesia and Pain Relief Options, Risks and Complications, Postoperative Recovery Concerns, and Innovative Surgical Techniques and Tools, a Glossary of Related Terms, and a Directory of Additional Resources

Edited by Amy L. Sutton. 645 pages. 2008. 978-0-7808-1004-4.

"Large public libraries and medical libraries would benefit from this material in their reference collections."
—*American Reference Books Annual, 2009*

SEE ALSO *Cosmetic and Reconstructive Surgery Sourcebook, 2nd Edition*

Thyroid Disorders Sourcebook

Basic Consumer Health Information about Disorders of the Thyroid and Parathyroid Glands, Including Hypothyroidism, Hyperthyroidism, Graves Disease, Hashimoto Thyroiditis, Thyroid Cancer, and Parathyroid Disorders, Featuring Facts about Symptoms, Risk Factors, Tests, and Treatments

Along with Information about the Effects of Thyroid Imbalance on Other Body Systems, Environmental Factors That Affect the Thyroid Gland, a Glossary, and a Directory of Additional Resources

Edited by Joyce Brennfleck Shannon. 573 pages. 2005. 978-0-7808-0745-7.

"Recommended for consumer health collections."
—American Reference Books Annual, 2006

"Highly recommended pick for Basic Consumer health reference holdings at all levels."
—The Bookwatch, Aug '05

SEE ALSO Endocrine and Metabolic Disorders Sourcebook, 2nd Edition

Transplantation Sourcebook
Basic Consumer Health Information about Organ and Tissue Transplantation, Including Physical and Financial Preparations, Procedures and Issues Relating to Specific Solid Organ and Tissue Transplants, Rehabilitation, Pediatric Transplant Information, the Future of Transplantation, and Organ and Tissue Donation

Along with a Glossary and Listings of Additional Resources

Edited by Joyce Brennfleck Shannon. 610 pages. 2002. 978-0-7808-0322-0.

"Recommended for libraries with an interest in offering consumer health information."
—E-Streams, Jul '02

"This is a unique and valuable resource for patients facing transplantation and their families."
—Doody's Review Service, Jun '02

Traveler's Health Sourcebook
Basic Consumer Health Information for Travelers, Including Physical and Medical Preparations, Transportation Health and Safety, Essential Information about Food and Water, Sun Exposure, Insect and Snake Bites, Camping and Wilderness Medicine, and Travel with Physical or Medical Disabilities

Along with International Travel Tips, Vaccination Recommendations, Geographical Health Issues, Disease Risks, a Glossary, and a Listing of Additional Resources

Edited by Joyce Brennfleck Shannon. 619 pages. 2000. 978-0-7808-0384-8.

"Recommended reference source."
—Booklist, Feb '01

"This book is recommended for any public library, any travel collection, and especially any collection for the physically disabled."
—American Reference Books Annual, 2001

SEE ALSO Worldwide Health Sourcebook

Urinary Tract and Kidney Diseases and Disorders Sourcebook, 2nd Edition
Basic Consumer Health Information about the Urinary System, Including the Bladder, Urethra, Ureters, and Kidneys, with Facts about Urinary Tract Infections, Incontinence, Congenital Disorders, Kidney Stones, Cancers of the Urinary Tract and Kidneys, Kidney Failure, Dialysis, and Kidney Transplantation

Along with Statistical and Demographic Information, Reports on Current Research in Kidney and Urologic Health, a Summary of Commonly Used Diagnostic Tests, a Glossary of Related Terms, and a Directory of Resources for Additional Help and Information

Edited by Ivy L. Alexander. 621 pages. 2005. 978-0-7808-0750-1.

"A good choice for a consumer health information library or for a medical library needing information to refer to their patients."
—American Reference Books Annual, 2006

SEE ALSO Prostate and Urological Disorders Sourcebook

Vegetarian Sourcebook
Basic Consumer Health Information about Vegetarian Diets, Lifestyle, and Philosophy, Including Definitions of Vegetarianism and Veganism, Tips about Adopting Vegetarianism, Creating a Vegetarian Pantry, and Meeting Nutritional Needs of Vegetarians, with Facts Regarding Vegetarianism's Effect on Pregnant and Lactating Women, Children, Athletes, and Senior Citizens

Along with a Glossary of Commonly Used Vegetarian Terms and Resources for Additional Help and Information

Edited by Chad T. Kimball. 337 pages. 2002. 978-0-7808-0439-5.

"Organizes into one concise volume the answers to the most common questions concerning vegetarian diets and lifestyles. This title is

1115

recommended for public and secondary school libraries."

—E-Streams, Apr '03

"Invaluable reference for public and school library collections alike."
—Library Bookwatch, Apr '03

"The articles in this volume are easy to read and come from authoritative sources. The book does not necessarily support the vegetarian diet but instead provides the pros and cons of this important decision... Recommended for public libraries and consumer health libraries."
—American Reference Books Annual, 2003

SEE ALSO Diet and Nutrition Sourcebook, 3rd Edition

Women's Health Concerns Sourcebook, 3rd Edition

Basic Consumer Health Information about Issues and Trends in Women's Health and Health Conditions of Special Concern to Women, Including Endometriosis, Uterine Fibroids, Menstrual Irregularities, Menopause, Sexual Dysfunction, Infertility, Cancer in Women, and Other Such Chronic Disorders as Lupus, Fibromyalgia, and Thyroid Disease

Along with Statistical Data, Tips for Maintaining Wellness, a Glossary, and a Directory of Resources for Further Help and Information

Edited by Sandra J. Judd. 679 pages. 2009. 978-0-7808-1036-5.

"This useful resource provides information about a wide range of topics that will help women understand their bodies, prevent or treat disease, and maintain health... A detailed index helps readers locate information. This is a useful addition to public and consumer health library collections"
—ARBAOnline, Jun '09

SEE ALSO Breast Cancer Sourcebook, 3rd Edition, Cancer Sourcebook for Women, 4th Edition, Healthy Heart Sourcebook for Women

Workplace Health and Safety Sourcebook

Basic Consumer Health Information about Workplace Health and Safety, Including the Effect of Workplace Hazards on the Lungs, Skin, Heart, Ears, Eyes, Brain, Reproductive Organs, Musculoskeletal System, and Other Organs and Body Parts

Along with Information about Occupational Cancer, Personal Protective Equipment, Toxic and Hazardous Chemicals, Child Labor, Stress, and Workplace Violence

Edited by Chad T. Kimball. 610 pages. 2000. 978-0-7808-0231-5.

"As a reference for the general public, this would be useful in any library."
—E-Streams, Jun '01

"Provides helpful information for primary care physicians and other caregivers interested in occupational medicine... General readers; professionals."
—CHOICE, May '01

Worldwide Health Sourcebook

Basic Information about Global Health Issues, Including Malnutrition, Reproductive Health, Disease Dispersion and Prevention, Emerging Diseases, Risky Health Behaviors, and the Leading Causes of Death

Along with Global Health Concerns for Children, Women, and the Elderly, Mental Health Issues, Research and Technology Advancements, and Economic, Environmental, and Political Health Implications, a Glossary, and a Resource Listing for Additional Help and Information

Edited by Joyce Brennfleck Shannon. 597 pages. 2001. 978-0-7808-0330-5.

"Named an Outstanding Academic Title."
—CHOICE, Jan '02

"Yet another handy but also unique compilation in the extensive Health Reference Series, this is a useful work because many of the international publications reprinted or excerpted are not readily available. Highly recommended."
—CHOICE, Nov '01

SEE ALSO Traveler's Health Sourcebook

Teen Health Series
Complete Catalog
List price $69 per volume. School and library price $62 per volume.

Abuse and Violence Information for Teens
Health Tips about the Causes and Consequences of Abusive and Violent Behavior
Including Facts about the Types of Abuse and Violence, the Warning Signs of Abusive and Violent Behavior, Health Concerns of Victims, and Getting Help and Staying Safe

Edited by Sandra Augustyn Lawton. 411 pages. 2008. 978-0-7808-1008-2.

"A useful resource for schools and organizations providing services to teens and may also be a starting point in research projects."
—*Reference and Research Book News, Aug '08*

"Violence is a serious problem for teens... This resource gives teens the information they need to face potential threats and get help—either for themselves or for their friends."
—*American Reference Books Annual, 2009*

Accident and Safety Information for Teens
Health Tips about Medical Emergencies, Traumatic Injuries, and Disaster Preparedness
Including Facts about Motor Vehicle Accidents, Burns, Poisoning, Firearms, Natural Disasters, National Security Threats, and More

Edited by Karen Bellenir. 420 pages. 2008. 978-0-7808-1046-4.

"Aimed at teenage audiences, this guide provides practical information for handling a comprehensive list of emergencies, from sport injuries and auto accidents to alcohol poisoning and natural disasters."
—*Library Journal, Apr 1, '09*

"Useful in the young adult collections of public libraries as well as high school libraries."
—*American Reference Books Annual, 2009*

SEE ALSO *Sports Injuries Information for Teens, 2nd Edition*

Alcohol Information for Teens, 2nd Edition
Health Tips about Alcohol and Alcoholism
Including Facts about Alcohol's Effects on the Body, Brain, and Behavior, the Consequences of Underage Drinking, Alcohol Abuse Prevention and Treatment, and Coping with Alcoholic Parents

Edited by Lisa Bakewell. 410 pages. 2009. 978-0-7808-1043-3.

"This handbook, written for a teenage audience, provides information on the causes, effects, and preventive measures related to alcohol abuse among teens... The chapters are quick to make a connection to their teenage reading audience. The prose is straightforward and the book lends itself to spot reading. It should be useful both for practical information and for research, and it is suitable for public and school libraries."
—*ARBAOnline, Jun '09*

SEE ALSO *Drug Information for Teens, 2nd Edition*

Allergy Information for Teens
Health Tips about Allergic Reactions Such as Anaphylaxis, Respiratory Problems, and Rashes
Including Facts about Identifying and Managing Allergies to Food, Pollen, Mold, Animals, Chemicals, Drugs, and Other Substances

Edited by Karen Bellenir. 410 pages. 2006. 978-0-7808-0799-0.

"This is a comprehensive, readable text on the subject of allergic diseases in teenagers. 5 Stars (out of 5)!"
—*Doody's Review Service, Jun '06*

"This authoritative and useful self-help title is a solid addition to YA collections, whether for personal interest or reports."
—*School Library Journal, Jul '06*

Asthma Information for Teens, 2nd Ed.
Health Tips about Managing Asthma and Related Concerns

Including Facts about Asthma Causes, Triggers and Symptoms, Diagnosis, and Treatment

Edited by Kim Wohlenhaus. 400 pages. 2010. 978-0-7808-1086-0.

Body Information for Teens
Health Tips about Maintaining Well-Being for a Lifetime
Including Facts about the Development and Functioning of the Body's Systems, Organs, and Structures and the Health Impact of Lifestyle Choices

Edited by Sandra Augustyn Lawton. 458 pages. 2007. 978-0-7808-0443-2.

Cancer Information for Teens, 2nd Edition
Health Tips about Cancer Awareness, Symptoms, Prevention, Diagnosis, and Treatment
Including Facts about Common Cancers Affecting Teens, Causes, Detection, Coping Strategies, Clinical Trials, Nutrition and Exercise, Cancer in Friends or Family, and More

Edited by Karen Bellenir and Lisa Bakewell. 445 pages. 2010. 978-0-7808-1085-3.

Complementary and Alternative Medicine Information for Teens
Health Tips about Non-Traditional and Non-Western Medical Practices
Including Information about Acupuncture, Chiropractic Medicine, Dietary and Herbal Supplements, Hypnosis, Massage Therapy, Prayer and Spirituality, Reflexology, Yoga, and More

Edited by Sandra Augustyn Lawton. 407 pages. 2007. 978-0-7808-0966-6.

"This volume covers CAM specifically for teenagers but of general use also. It should be a welcome addition to both public and academic libraries."
—American Reference Books Annual, 2008

"This volume provides a solid foundation for further investigation of the subject, making it useful for both public and high school libraries."
—VOYA: Voice of Youth Advocates, Jun '07

Diabetes Information for Teens
Health Tips about Managing Diabetes and Preventing Related Complications
Including Information about Insulin, Glucose Control, Healthy Eating, Physical Activity, and Learning to Live with Diabetes

Edited by Sandra Augustyn Lawton. 410 pages. 2006. 978-0-7808-0811-9.

"A comprehensive instructional guide for teens... some of the material may also be directed towards parents or teachers. 5 stars (out of 5)!"
—Doody's Review Service, 2006

"Students dealing with their own diabetes or that of a friend or family member or those writing reports on the topic will find this a valuable resource."
—School Library Journal, Aug '06

"This text is directed to the teen population and would be an excellent library resource for a health class or for the teacher as a reference for class preparation. It can, however, serve a much wider audience. The clinical educator on diabetes may find it valuable to educate the newly diagnosed client regardless of age. It also would be an excellent reference and education tool for a preventive medicine seminar on diabetes."
—Physical Therapy, Mar '07

Diet Information for Teens, 2nd Edition
Health Tips about Diet and Nutrition
Including Facts about Dietary Guidelines, Food Groups, Nutrients, Healthy Meals, Snacks, Weight Control, Medical Concerns Related to Diet, and More

Edited by Karen Bellenir. 432 pages. 2006. 978-0-7808-0820-1.

"A very quick and pleasant read in spite of the fact that it is very detailed in the information it gives... A book for anyone concerned about diet and nutrition."
—American Reference Books Annual, 2007

SEE ALSO *Eating Disorders Information for Teens, 2nd Edition*

Drug Information for Teens, 2nd Edition

Health Tips about the Physical and Mental Effects of Substance Abuse

Including Information about Marijuana, Inhalants, Club Drugs, Stimulants, Hallucinogens, Opiates, Prescription and Over-the-Counter Drugs, Herbal Products, Tobacco, Alcohol, and More

Edited by Sandra Augustyn Lawton. 468 pages. 2006. 978-0-7808-0862-1.

"As with earlier installments in Omnigraphics' Teen Health Series, Drug Information for Teens is designed specifically to meet the needs and interests of middle and high school students... Strongly recommended for both academic and public libraries."
—American Reference Books Annual, 2007

"Solid thoughtful advice is given about how to handle peer pressure, drug-related health concerns, and treatment strategies."
—School Library Journal, Dec '06

SEE ALSO Alcohol Information for Teens, 2nd Edition, Tobacco Information for Teens, 2nd Edition

Eating Disorders Information for Teens, 2nd Edition

Health Tips about Anorexia, Bulimia, Binge Eating, And Other Eating Disorders

Including Information about Risk Factors, Diagnosis and Treatment, Prevention, Related Health Concerns, and Other Issues

Edited by Sandra Augustyn Lawton. 377 pages. 2009. 978-0-7808-1044-0.

"This handy reference offers basic information and addresses specific disorders, consequences, prevention, diagnosis and treatment, healthy eating, and more. It is written in a conversational style that is easy to understand... Will provide plenty of facts for reports as well as browsing potential for students with an interest in the topic.
—School Library Journal, Jun '09

"Written in a straightforward style that will appeal to its teenage audience. The author does not play down the danger of living with an eating disorder and urges those struggling with this problem to seek professional help.

This work, as well as others in this series, will be a welcome addition to high school and undergraduate libraries."
—American Reference Books Annual, 2009

SEE ALSO Diet Information for Teens, 2nd Edition

Fitness Information for Teens, 2nd Edition

Health Tips about Exercise, Physical Well-Being, and Health Maintenance

Including Facts about Conditioning, Stretching, Strength Training, Body Shape and Body Image, Sports Nutrition, and Specific Activities for Athletes and Non-Athletes

Edited by Lisa Bakewell. 432 pages. 2009. 978-0-7808-1045-7.

"This no-nonsense guide packs a great deal into its pages... This is a helpful reference for basic diet and exercise information for health reports or personal use."
—School Library Journal, April 2009

"An excellent source for general information on why teens should be active, making time to exercise, the equipment people might need, various types of activities to try, how to maintain health and wellness, and how to avoid barriers to becoming healthier... This would still be an excellent addition to a public library ready-reference collection or a high school health library collection."
—American Reference Books Annual, 2009

"This easy to read, well-written, up-to-date overview of fitness for teenagers provides excellent wellness and exercise tips, information, and directions... It is a useful tool for them to obtain a base knowledge in fitness topics and different sports."
—Doody's Review Service, 2009

SEE ALSO Diet Information for Teens, 2nd Edition, Sports Injuries Information for Teens, 2nd Edition

Learning Disabilities Information for Teens

Health Tips about Academic Skills Disorders and Other Disabilities That Affect Learning

Including Information about Common Signs of Learning Disabilities, School Issues, Learning to Live with a Learning Disability, and Other Related Issues

Edited by Sandra Augustyn Lawton. 400 pages. 2006. 978-0-7808-0796-9.

"This book provides a wealth of information for any reader interested in the signs, causes, and consequences of learning disabilities, as well as related legal rights and educational interventions... Public and academic libraries should want this title for both students and general readers."
—*American Reference Books Annual, 2006*

Mental Health Information for Teens, 3rd Edition
Health Tips about Mental Wellness and Mental Illness
Including Facts about Mental and Emotional Health, Depression and Other Mood Disorders, Anxiety Disorders, Behavior Disorders, Self-Injury, Psychosis, Schizophrenia, and More

Edited by Karen Bellenir. 400 pages. 2010. 978-0-7808-1087-7.

SEE ALSO *Stress Information for Teens, Suicide Information for Teens, 2nd Edition*

Pregnancy Information for Teens
Health Tips about Teen Pregnancy and Teen Parenting
Including Facts about Prenatal Care, Pregnancy Complications, Labor and Delivery, Postpartum Care, Pregnancy-Related Lifestyle Concerns, and More

Edited by Sandra Augustyn Lawton. 434 pages. 2007. 978-0-7808-0984-0.

Sexual Health Information for Teens, 2nd Edition
Health Tips about Sexual Development, Reproduction, Contraception, and Sexually Transmitted Infections
Including Facts about Puberty, Sexuality, Birth Control, Chlamydia, Gonorrhea, Herpes, Human Papillomavirus, Syphilis, and More

Edited by Sandra Augustyn Lawton. 430 pages. 2008. 978-0-7808-1010-5.

"This offering represents the most up-to-date information available on an array of topics including abstinence-only sexual education and pregnancy-prevention methods... The range of coverage—from puberty and anatomy to sexually transmitted diseases—is thorough and extensive. Each chapter includes a bibliographic citation, and the three back sections containing additional resources, further reading, and the index are all first-rate... This volume will be well used by students in need of the facts, whether for educational or personal reasons."
—*School Library Journal, Nov '08*

"Presents information related to the emotional, physical, and biological development of both males and females that occurs during puberty. It also strives to address some of the issues and questions that may arise... The text is easy to read and understand for young readers, with satisfactory definitions within the text to explain new terms."
—*American Reference Books Annual, 2009*

Skin Health Information for Teens, 2nd Edition
Health Tips about Dermatological Concerns and Skin Cancer Risks
Including Facts about Acne, Warts, Hives, and Other Conditions and Lifestyle Choices, Such as Tanning, Tattooing, and Piercing, That Affect the Skin, Nails, Scalp, and Hair

Edited by Edited by Kim Wohlenhaus. 418 pages. 2009. 978-0-7808-1042-6.

"The material in this work will be easily understood by teenagers and young adults. The publisher has liberally used bulleted lists and sidebars to keep the reader's attention... A useful addition to school and public library collections."
—*ARBAOnline, Oct '09*

Sleep Information for Teens
Health Tips about Adolescent Sleep Requirements, Sleep Disorders, and the Effects of Sleep Deprivation
Including Facts about Why People Need Sleep, Sleep Patterns, Circadian Rhythms, Dreaming, Insomnia, Sleep Apnea, Narcolepsy, and More

Edited by Karen Bellenir. 355 pages. 2008. 978-0-7808-1009-9.

"Clear, concise, and very readable and would be a good source of sleep information for anyone—not just teenagers. This work is highly recommended for medical libraries, public school libraries, and public libraries."
—*American Reference Books Annual, 2009*

SEE ALSO Body Information for Teens

Sports Injuries Information for Teens, 2nd Edition
Health Tips about Acute, Traumatic, and Chronic Injuries in Adolescent Athletes
Including Facts about Sprains, Fractures, and Overuse Injuries, Treatment, Rehabilitation, Sport-Specific Safety Guidelines, Fitness Suggestions, and More

Edited by Karen Bellenir. 429 pages. 2008. 978-0-7808-1011-2.

"An engaging selection of informative articles about the prevention and treatment of sports injuries... The value of this book is that the articles have been vetted and are often augmented with inserts of useful facts, definitions of technical terms, and quick tips. Sensitive topics like injuries to genitalia are discussed openly and responsibly. This revised edition contains updated articles and defines sport more broadly than the first edition."
—*School Library Journal, Nov '08*

"This work will be useful in the young adult collections of public libraries as well as high school libraries... A useful resource for student research."
—*American Reference Books Annual, 2009*

SEE ALSO Accident and Safety Information for Teens

Stress Information for Teens
Health Tips about the Mental and Physical Consequences of Stress
Including Information about the Different Kinds of Stress, Symptoms of Stress, Frequent Causes of Stress, Stress Management Techniques, and More

Edited by Sandra Augustyn Lawton. 392 pages. 2008. 978-0-7808-1012-9.

"Understanding what stress is, what causes it, how the body and the mind are impacted by it, and what teens can do are the general categories addressed here... The chapters are brief but informative, and the list of community-help organizations is exhaustive. Report writers will find information quickly and easily, as will those who have personal concerns. The print is clear and the format is readable, making this an accessible resource for struggling readers and researchers."
—*School Library Journal, Dec '08*

"The articles selected will specifically appeal to young adults and are designed to answer their most common questions."
— *American Reference Books Annual, 2009*

SEE ALSO Mental Health Information for Teens, 3rd Edition

Suicide Information for Teens, 2nd Edition
Health Tips about Suicide Causes and Prevention
Including Facts about Depression, Risk Factors, Getting Help, Survivor Support, and More

Edited by Kim Wohlenhaus. 400 pages. 2010. 978-0-7808-1088-4.

SEE ALSO Mental Health Information for Teens, 3rd Edition

Tobacco Information for Teens, 2nd Edition
Health Tips about the Hazards of Using Cigarettes, Smokeless Tobacco, and Other Nicotine Products
Including Facts about Nicotine Addiction, Nicotine Delivery Systems, Secondhand Smoke, Health Consequences of Tobacco Use, Related Cancers, Smoking Cessation, and Tobacco Use Statistics

Edited by Karen Bellenir. 400 pages. 2010. 978-0-7808-1153-9.

SEE ALSO Drug Information for Teens, 2nd Edition

Health Reference Series